AMERICAN PSYCHIATRIC PRESS

REVIEW
OF
PSYCHIATRY

VOLUME

13

AMERICAN PSYCHIATRIC PRESS

REVIEW
OF
PSYCHIATRY

VOLUME

13

EDITED BY

JOHN M. OLDHAM, M.D., and
MICHELLE B. RIBA, M.D.

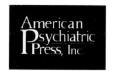

Washington, DC
London, England

Note: The authors have worked to ensure that all information in this book concerning drug dosages, schedules, and routes of administration is accurate as of the time of publication and consistent with standards set by the U.S. Food and Drug Administration and the general medical community. As medical research and practice advance, however, therapeutic standards may change. For this reason and because human and mechanical errors sometimes occur, we recommend that readers follow the advice of a physician who is directly involved in their care or the care of a member of their family.

Copyright © 1994 American Psychiatric Press, Inc.
97 96 95 94   4 3 2 1
ALL RIGHTS RESERVED
Manufactured in the United States of America on acid-free paper

American Psychiatric Press, Inc.
1400 K Street, N.W.
Washington, DC   20005

American Psychiatric Press Review of Psychiatry, Volume 13
ISSN 1041-5882
ISBN 0-88048-440-3

The correct citation for this book is *American Psychiatric Press Review of Psychiatry,* Volume 13. Edited by Oldham JM, Riba MB. Washington, DC, American Psychiatric Press, 1994.

**AMERICAN PSYCHIATRIC PRESS REVIEW OF PSYCHIATRY,
VOLUME 8** (1989)

*Allan Tasman, M.D., Robert E. Hales, M.D., and Allen J. Frances, M.D.,
Editors*

Borderline Personality Disorder
John G. Gunderson, M.D., Section Editor

Child Psychiatry
Jerry M. Wiener, M.D., Section Editor

Alcoholism
Roger E. Meyer, M.D., Section Editor

Psychiatry and the Law
Paul S. Appelbaum, M.D., Section Editor

Difficult Situations in Clinical Practice
William S. Sledge, M.D., Section Editor

**AMERICAN PSYCHIATRIC PRESS REVIEW OF PSYCHIATRY,
VOLUME 9** (1990)

*Allan Tasman, M.D., Stephen M. Goldfinger, M.D.,
and Charles A. Kaufmann, M.D., Editors*

Treatment of Refractory Mood Disorders
Robert M. Post, M.D., Section Editor

Recent Advances in Geriatric Psychiatry
Charles A. Shamoian, M.D., Ph.D., Section Editor

Contributions of Self Psychology to Psychotherapy
Jerald Kay, M.D., Section Editor

Consultation-Liaison Psychiatry
Robert E. Hales, M.D., and Troy L. Thompson, M.D., Section Editors

AIDS and HIV Infections
*Stephen M. Goldfinger, M.D., and Carolyn B. Robinowitz, M.D.,
Section Editors*

AMERICAN PSYCHIATRIC PRESS REVIEW OF PSYCHIATRY, VOLUME 10 (1991)

Allan Tasman, M.D., and Stephen M. Goldfinger, M.D., Editors

Schizophrenia
Daniel R. Weinberger, M.D., Section Editor

Dissociative Disorders
David Spiegel, M.D., Section Editor

Sexual Abuse of Children and Adolescents
Elissa P. Benedek, M.D., Section Editor

Neuroscience
Joseph T. Coyle, M.D., Section Editor

New Perspectives on Human Development
Leah J. Dickstein, M.D., Section Editor

AMERICAN PSYCHIATRIC PRESS REVIEW OF PSYCHIATRY, VOLUME 11 (1992)

Allan Tasman, M.D., and Michelle B. Riba, M.D., Editors

Severe Personality Disorders
Thomas A. Widiger, Ph.D., and John G. Gunderson, M.D., Section Editors

Brain, Behavior, and the Immune System
Marvin Stein, M.D., and Andrew H. Miller, M.D., Section Editors

Anxiety Disorders
Jack M. Gorman, M.D., and Laszlo A. Papp, M.D., Section Editors

Concurrent Diagnoses
Joel Yager, M.D., Section Editor

Hospital Psychiatry
Richard L. Munich, M.D., and Glen O. Gabbard, M.D., Section Editors

**AMERICAN PSYCHIATRIC PRESS REVIEW OF PSYCHIATRY,
VOLUME 12** (1993)

*John M. Oldham, M.D., Michelle B. Riba, M.D.,
and Allan Tasman, M.D., Editors*

Changing Perspectives on Homosexuality
Terry S. Stein, M.D., Section Editor

Posttraumatic Stress Disorder
Robert S. Pynoos, M.D., M.P.H., Section Editor

Brain Imaging
Nancy C. Andreasen, M.D., Ph.D., Section Editor

Combined Treatments
Bernard D. Beitman, M.D., Section Editor

The Neuropsychiatry of Memory
Stuart C. Yudofsky, M.D., and Robert E. Hales, M.D., Section Editors

**AMERICAN PSYCHIATRIC PRESS REVIEW OF PSYCHIATRY,
VOLUME 14** (1995)

John M. Oldham, M.D., and Michelle B. Riba, M.D., Editors

Substance Abuse
Herbert Kleber, M.D., Section Editor

Psychiatric Disorders in Women and Women's Health Care
Myrna Weissman, Ph.D., and Michelle B. Riba, M.D., Section Editors

Psychiatric Genetics
Elliott Gershon, M.D., Section Editor

Cross-Cultural Psychiatry
Pedro Ruiz, M.D., Section Editor

Sexual Disorders
Judith Becker, Ph.D., and Taylor Segraves, M.D., Section Editors

Contents

Section

III
Ethics

Section

IV

**Psychotherapy With Children
and Adolescents**

Contributors

Kenneth Z. Altshuler, M.D.
Stanton Sharp Professor and Chairman, Department of Psychiatry, University of Texas Southwestern Medical School, Dallas, Texas

Thomas A. Ban, M.D.
Professor, Department of Psychiatry, Vanderbilt University, Nashville, Tennessee

R. Joffree Barrnett, M.D.
Adjunct Faculty, Department of Psychiatry, Division of Child and Adolescent Psychiatry, Dartmouth College Medical School, Lebanon, New Hampshire

Kathleen L. Benson, Ph.D.
Research Associate, Psychiatry Service, Department of Veterans Affairs Medical Center; and Department of Psychiatry and Behavioral Sciences, Stanford University School of Medicine, Palo Alto, California

Efrain Bleiberg, M.D.
Vice President and Director, Child and Adolescent Services, The Menninger Clinic, Topeka, Kansas

Donald L. Bliwise, Ph.D.
Associate Professor of Neurology, Sleep Disorders Center, Emory University Medical School, Atlanta, Georgia

Alan S. Brown, M.D.
Assistant Professor of Clinical Psychiatry and Postdoctoral Fellow, Columbia University College of Physicians and Surgeons, New York, New York

Daniel J. Buysse, M.D.
Assistant Professor of Psychiatry, Sleep and Chronobiology Center, Western Psychiatric Institute and Clinic, University of Pittsburgh School of Medicine, Pittsburgh, Pennsylvania

Irene Chatoor, M.D.
Associate Professor of Psychiatry and Behavioral Sciences and of Pediatrics, George Washington University School of Medicine, Washington, DC

Patricia A. Coble, R.N.
Assistant Professor of Psychiatry, Department of Psychiatry, Western Psychiatric Institute and Clinic, University of Pittsburgh Medical Center, Pittsburgh, Pennsylvania

Donald J. Cohen, M.D.
Irving B. Harris Professor of Child Psychiatry, Psychology, and Pediatrics, Yale University Child Study Center, New Haven, Connecticut

Jeremy Coplan, M.D.
Assistant Professor of Clinical Psychiatry, Columbia University, New York, New York

Ronald E. Dahl, M.D.
Associate Professor of Psychiatry and Pediatrics, Department of Psychiatry, Western Psychiatric Institute and Clinic, University of Pittsburgh Medical Center, Pittsburgh, Pennsylvania

Donna Elliott Frick, M.D.
Private practice in psychiatry, Chapel Hill; and Associate Professor of Psychiatry, University of North Carolina, Chapel Hill, North Carolina

Glen O. Gabbard, M.D.
Vice President for Adult Services, The Menninger Clinic; and Clinical Professor of Psychiatry, University of Kansas School of Medicine, Topeka, Kansas

Donna E. Giles, Ph.D.
Associate Professor of Psychiatry, Department of Psychiatry, Western Psychiatric Institute and Clinic, University of Pittsburgh Medical Center, Pittsburgh, Pennsylvania

Judith H. Gold, M.D., F.R.C.P.C.
Private practice in psychiatry, Halifax, Nova Scotia, Canada

Jack M. Gorman, M.D.
Professor of Clinical Psychiatry, Columbia University; and Chief, Department of Clinical Psychobiology, New York State Psychiatric Institute, New York, New York

Arthur H. Green, M.D.
Clinical Professor of Psychiatry, Columbia University; and Clinical Director of the Family Center and Therapeutic Nursery, The Presbyterian Hospital, New York, New York

Dorothy E. Grice, M.D.
Postdoctoral Fellow, Yale University Child Study Center, New Haven, Connecticut

Katherine A. Halmi, M.D.
Professor of Psychiatry and Director, Eating Disorders Program, New York Hospital—Cornell Medical Center, Westchester Division, White Plains, New York

Denise M. Heebink, M.D.
Instructor of Psychiatry and Chief, Inpatient Eating Disorders Unit, New York Hospital—Cornell Medical Center, Westchester Division, White Plains, New York

Joanne Intrator, M.D.
Assistant Professor of Psychiatry, Mt. Sinai School of Medicine; and Assistant Chief of Psychiatry, Bronx Veteran's Affairs Medical Center, New York, New York

Jay E. Kantor, Ph.D.
Adjunct Associate Professor of Psychiatry (Medical Humanities), New York University School of Medicine, Bellevue Hospital 19 West, New York, New York

Clarice J. Kestenbaum, M.D.
Clinical Professor of Psychiatry, Columbia University College of Physicians and Surgeons, New York, New York

Robert A. King, M.D.
Assistant Professor of Child Psychiatry, Yale University Child Study Center, New Haven, Connecticut

David J. Kupfer, M.D.
Professor and Chairman, Department of Psychiatry, University of Pittsburgh School of Medicine, Pittsburgh, Pennsylvania

Jeremy A. Lazarus, M.D.
Assistant Clinical Professor of Psychiatry, University of Colorado Health Sciences Center, Denver, Colorado

James F. Leckman, M.D.
Neison Harris Professor of Child Psychiatry and Pediatrics, Yale University Child Study Center, New Haven, Connecticut

Heinz E. Lehmann, M.D.
Professor Emeritus, Department of Psychiatry, McGill University, Montreal, Quebec, Canada

Gregory B. Leong, M.D.
Assistant Professor of Psychiatry, School of Medicine, University of California, Los Angeles; and Staff Psychiatrist, West Los Angeles Veterans Affairs Medical Center, Los Angeles, California

Owen Lewis, M.D.
Associate Clinical Professor of Psychiatry, Columbia University College of Physicians and Surgeons, New York, New York

Jeffrey A. Lieberman, M.D.
Director of Research, Hillside Hospital, Long Island Jewish Medical Center; and Professor of Psychiatry, Albert Einstein College of Medicine, Glen Oaks, New York

John S. McIntyre, M.D.
Chair, Department of Psychiatry, St. Mary's Hospital, and Clinical Professor of Psychiatry, University of Rochester, Rochester, New York

Timothy H. Monk, Ph.D.
Associate Professor of Psychiatry, Sleep and Chronobiology Center, Western Psychiatric Institute and Clinic, University of Pittsburgh School of Medicine, Pittsburgh, Pennsylvania

Kalpana I. Nathan, M.D.
Research Fellow, Department of Psychiatry, Stanford University Hospital, Stanford, California

Eric A. Nofzinger, M.D.
Assistant Professor of Psychiatry, Sleep and Chronobiology Center, Western Psychiatric Institute and Clinic, University of Pittsburgh School of Medicine, Pittsburgh, Pennsylvania

John M. Oldham, M.D.
Director, New York State Psychiatric Institute; and Professor and Associate Chairman, Department of Psychiatry, Columbia University College of Physicians and Surgeons, New York, New York

Laszlo A. Papp, M.D.
Assistant Professor of Clinical Psychiatry, Columbia University;
Associate Director, Department of Clinical Psychobiology, New York
State Psychiatric Institute; and Director, Anxiety Disorders Program,
Hillside Hospital, New York, New York

Ann M. Rasmusson, M.D.
Fellow in Psychiatry, Department of Psychiatry, Yale University,
New Haven, Connecticut

Charles F. Reynolds III, M.D.
Professor of Psychiatry and Neurology, University of Pittsburgh
School of Medicine, Pittsburgh, Pennsylvania

Michelle B. Riba, M.D.
Assistant Clinical Professor of Psychiatry and Director, Ambulatory
Consultation-Liaison Psychiatry, University of Michigan Medical
Center; and Department of Family Practice, Oakwood Hospital,
Dearborn, Michigan

Timothy A. Roehrs, Ph.D.
Director of Research, Sleep Disorders and Research Center, Henry
Ford Hospital, Detroit, Michigan

John Romano, M.D.
Distinguished University Professor of Psychiatry Emeritus,
University of Rochester, Rochester, New York

Leon Rosenthal, M.D.
Staff Scientist, Sleep Disorders and Research Center, Henry Ford
Hospital, Detroit, Michigan

Thomas Roth, Ph.D.
Chief, Division of Sleep Disorders Medicine, Sleep Disorders and
Research Center, Henry Ford Hospital, Detroit, Michigan

Alan F. Schatzberg, M.D.
Chairman and Professor, Department of Psychiatry, Stanford
University Hospital, Stanford, California

Marc A. Schuckit, M.D.
Professor of Psychiatry, Veterans Affairs Medical Center and
University of California, San Diego

Steven S. Sharfstein, M.D.
Medical Director and CEO, The Sheppard and Enoch Pratt Hospital;
and Clinical Professor of Psychiatry, University of Maryland Medical
School, Baltimore, Maryland

Larry J. Siever, M.D.
Professor of Psychiatry and Director, Outpatient Psychiatry Division,
Bronx Veteran's Affairs Medical Center and Mt. Sinai School of
Medicine, New York, New York

J. Arturo Silva, M.D.
Associate Professor of Psychiatry, University of Texas Health Science
Center at San Antonio; and Staff Psychiatrist, Audie L. Murphy
Memorial Veterans Hospital, San Antonio, Texas

Bonnie J. Steinberg, M.D.
Clinical Fellow, Bronx Veteran's Affairs Medical Center and Mt. Sinai
School of Medicine, New York, New York

John A. Talbott, M.D.
Professor and Chairman, Department of Psychiatry, University of
Maryland School of Medicine; and Director, Institute of Psychiatry
and Human Behavior, University of Maryland Medical Center,
Baltimore, Maryland

Robert L. Trestman, Ph.D., M.D.
Assistant Professor of Psychiatry, Bronx Veteran's Affairs Medical
Center and Mt. Sinai School of Medicine, New York, New York

Michael J. Vergare, M.D.
Associate Chairman, Department of Psychiatry, Albert Einstein
Medical Center, Philadelphia, Pennsylvania

Robert Weinstock, M.D.
Associate Clinical Professor of Psychiatry, School of Medicine,
University of California, Los Angeles; Director, Forensic Psychiatry
Fellowship Program, University of California, Los Angeles; and Staff
Psychiatrist, West Los Angeles Veterans Affairs Medical Center,
Los Angeles, California

Robert M. Wettstein, M.D.
Codirector, Law and Psychiatry Program, Western Psychiatric
Institute and Clinic, University of Pittsburgh School of Medicine,
Pittsburgh, Pennsylvania

Vincent P. Zarcone, Jr., M.D.
Professor, Psychiatry Service, Department of Veterans Affairs
Medical Center; and Department of Psychiatry and Behavioral
Sciences, Stanford University School of Medicine,
Palo Alto, California

Foreword to Volume 13

John M. Oldham, M.D, and Michelle B. Riba, M.D.

In this sesquicentennial year of the American Psychiatric Association (APA), it seemed fitting to plan Volume 13 of the *Review of Psychiatry* with the year's presidential theme in mind: "Our Heritage, Our Future." The profession of psychiatry has a rich and fascinating history, from its origins in colonial Philadelphia to the present day. In the early days of American psychiatry, treatment was primitive and limited, and influential leaders in the field focused on the importance of humane psychosocial settings in which to care for mentally ill people. As a new millennium approaches, the field of psychiatry has changed dramatically in a changing world, and advances in knowledge about the etiology and treatment of mental illness have grown exponentially. We have become appropriately preoccupied with neurotransmitters, molecules, and genes, made possible by enormous advances in research. As these technologies are being developed, however, new treatments such as genetic engineering appear on the horizon that have staggering implications, and major new challenges are at our doorstep to consider the economics and ethics of the new technology. These are exciting times for psychiatry, and the future promises even more as we expand our attention to include more and better treatment as well as prevention of mental illness. Throughout these 150 years, one of the most important constants has been the patient, whose need for help—not just for new medications developed from new findings in molecular biology, but also for new psychosocial interventions—remains a foremost concern.

To address the scope of developments from the origins of American psychiatry to the frontiers of future neuroscience in a single volume is an impossible task indeed. We have attempted to select a few samples that will, we hope, be representative of the field. The volume begins, appropriately, with a section on American psychiatry's beginnings—a look at some aspects of the history of psychiatry in the United States. This section is edited by Michael Vergare, M.D., who chaired the Sesquicentennial Committee for the APA, and John S. McIntyre, M.D., President of the APA during this, its sesquicentennial year. Among the contributors to this section include two "senior statesmen" of psychiatry, John Romano and Heinz Lehmann, who give us a wonderful personal perspective on education and research, spanning the many decades of their own rich and productive careers.

The second section of the volume brings us forward to an area of rapid progress in current biological psychiatry—the developing understanding of biological markers as ways of identifying populations at risk, a window toward better methods of prevention. Section Editors Jack M. Gorman, M.D., and Laszlo A. Papp, M.D., have put together a set of outstanding contributors to present the newest information available in this important area.

The third section of Volume 13, after moving from history to the cutting edge of the present and the future, takes us into a timeless realm that has been equally important for the field throughout its entire history—that is, the ethics of psychiatry. Jeremy A. Lazarus, M.D., immediate past Chair of the Ethics Committee of the APA, serves as editor of this section. Ethical issues relating to research, confidentiality concerns, forensics, boundary violations and sexual misconduct, and, important in these recent times, economics and managed care are reviewed in depth.

One of the most important forms of treatment, with its own lengthy history, is psychotherapy, and the fourth section takes a look at the current status of psychotherapy with children and adolescents, edited by Clarice J. Kestenbaum, M.D., and Owen Lewis, M.D. In this section, several major categories of psychopathology have been selected, and psychotherapeutic approaches with each have been reviewed. The section includes a chapter on current psychotherapy research and a chapter on psychotherapeutic interventions for children and adolescents who have been victims of abuse.

The final section brings us back to a subject that has been long identified as having healing and restorative powers—that is, sleep. New developments have accumulated rapidly in our understanding of not just the architecture of normal sleep, but of the broad importance and impact of sleep disorders. Charles F. Reynolds III, M.D., and David J. Kupfer, M.D., coedit this section, bringing us the very latest about developmental and familial aspects of sleep; patterns of disturbed sleep in depression, psychotic disorders, and the dementias; normal sleep patterns; and the impact of shift work and international travel on sleep.

As always, this project would not have been possible without the good work of all of the section editors and authors, but most particularly without the terrific administrative coordination and editorial assistance of Helen ("Sam") McGowan. Claire Reinburg, Pam Harley, and Lindsay Edmunds, along with many others, have also provided enormously helpful guidance and assistance from American Psychiatric Press, Inc.

I

History of Psychiatry in America

Section I

History of Psychiatry in America

Foreword

Michael J. Vergare, M.D., and John S. McIntyre, M.D.,
Section Editors

On the occasion of the celebration of the sesquicentennial of the American Psychiatric Association, it is fitting that a section of the *Review of Psychiatry* series is devoted to the history of American psychiatry over these 150 years—in particular, over the last 50 years. Although some previous volumes of the *Review of Psychiatry* have incorporated summations of the history related to the topics addressed, none has taken history itself as a major focus.

Clearly, during the last 50 years tremendous upheavals and changes have taken place in our field. These changes built on a long history of psychiatrists seeking new ways to understand the workings of the mind and to utilize this knowledge to help those with mental illness. Benjamin Rush, M.D., who is considered the father of American psychiatry, began this mission to put to use the best thinking of his time to help his patients. At the same time, he applied himself as a teacher and researcher.

Today's psychiatrists continue in the tradition of Rush. As reflected in this and prior reviews, our field is rich with new refinements in our understanding of mental illness. That has been especially true during the last 50 years. Authors of chapters in this section try to capture aspects of this history as it has unfolded since colonial times.

Chapter 1 focuses on the evolution of psychiatric education in America. John Romano, M.D., begins with the first physician to be appointed a professor of psychiatry, Samuel Mitchel Smith. From there we move to the influence of Adolf Meyer, the impact of the Flexner report, and the formalization of the educator role throughout medicine during the twentieth century. This chapter is rich in firsthand accounts of critical moments in psychiatric education that have led to medical school and residency training in our field as we know it today.

In Chapter 2, Heinz E. Lehmann, M.D., and Thomas A. Ban, M.D., trace the evolution of research in psychiatry in America by first going back to its European roots. Starting with the work of Pinel, Reil, Griesinger, and Heinroth, they then explore how Rush and his followers developed their own theories about mental illness and its treatment. Drs. Lehman and Ban divide their review into separate sections that focus on therapy, nosology, pathology, and epidemiology. Each of these areas is covered up to the present.

In Chapter 3, Kenneth Z. Altshuler, M.D., narrows the historical focus to the last 50 years as he takes on the daunting task of reviewing the evolution of our thinking concerning psychotherapy. He starts with psychoanalysis in the post–World War II era, noting the tremendous influence it had because it resonated with "the notion of man's limitless reach and . . . the idea that the mind has the power to liberate itself." He moves from psychoanalysis to review the beginnings of change, focusing on briefer treatments such as behavior therapy, transactional analysis, and other psychotherapies of the 1960s and 1970s. He brings us up to the present with a discussion of the consolidation of theories, the integration of psychopharmacology with psychotherapy, the newer cognitive theories, and the proliferation of therapists in many disciplines. He closes with a view of the future and the impact of insurance reform.

Chapter 4 focuses on women and psychiatry over the last five decades. In this review, Judith H. Gold, M.D., F.R.C.P.C., first discusses how thinking has changed during this time concerning gender differences and mental illness. She describes the attention given to gender-specific disorders and the resulting controversies that coincided with the rise of feminism in the 1970s. The revisions in thinking during the latter half of this century concerning theories of psychodynamics and underlying female development are also examined. DSM-IV is previewed, with an emphasis on the common pitfalls associated with gender-related diagnosis. She concludes with a discussion of the changing perceptions in the 1990s of women's social roles and notes that women still make up the majority of psychiatric patients. She suggests that the increase in the number of women psychiatrists might influence future directions for research and treatment.

The section closes with Chapter 5, in which John A. Talbott, M.D., reviews changes in the treatment of patients with chronic mental illness during the last 50 years. He first provides a brief review of the evolution of institutions from 1492 to 1854, followed by the devolution that occurred from the late nineteenth century. He sets the stage for the changes that exploded after World War II and the pharmacological revolution. From the early days of deinstitutionalization to the community mental health center movement, along with the expansion of psychiatry in general hospitals and the attempts to fix the system in the late 1970s and early 1980s, he traces the decline in the role of large institutions as providers of care. New services are described, with their emphasis on community-based care, "consumer" empowerment, and the integration of rehabilitation into the care of mentally ill patients. He concludes with a look at current experiments in mental health services, the impact of "new economics," and how we might do better by "picking up the pieces of our previous policies . . . before moving on to new services."

Chapter 1

Evolution of Psychiatric Education in the United States, 1849–1993

John Romano, M.D.

Although I found no separate section or chapter devoted to psychiatric education in the centennial volume *One Hundred Years of American Psychiatry* (American Psychiatric Association 1944), I did find throughout the text reference to several aspects of psychiatric education: undergraduate, graduate, and military. However, in the centennial anniversary issue of the *American Journal of Psychiatry*, Franklin G. Ebaugh, with the considerable acknowledged assistance of Cotter Hirschberg, wrote a very detailed account of the history of psychiatric education in the United States from 1844 to 1944 (Ebaugh 1944). Particular attention should be directed to the thorough bibliography that accompanied that article. In it, Pliny Earle was cited as giving the first course of lectures on mental disease in 1853.

Later, we found that Samuel Mitchel Smith was the first professor of psychiatry appointed to the faculty of any United States medical school (Rond 1958). Smith had received two medical degrees—one in 1839 from the University of Cincinnati and the second in 1840 from the University of Pennsylvania. Smith's appointment was made at Willoughby University, soon to be renamed the Starling Medical College and eventually Ohio State University College of Medicine at Columbus. Smith was chairman of the departments of psychiatry, jurisprudence, materia medica, and therapeutics, and later became dean.

Until the 1870s, even occasional lectures on nervous and mental diseases, not to speak of systemic courses, were rarities in our medical colleges. This appalling lack of psychiatric instruction was formally recognized in 1871, when the Association of Medical Superintendents of American Institutions for the Insane, at its annual meeting, adopted a series of resolutions vigorously recommending the need for lectures and clinical experiences for medical students. This recommendation was repeated at the end of the nineteenth century and continued to be made in the twentieth century.

Insufficient tribute has been paid to Adolf Meyer, who more than any other person persisted in pointing out deficiencies and the urgent need to develop a systematic curriculum in psychiatry in the medical

---

schools. Recently, a tribute was paid to Adolf Meyer for his establishment of educational objectives in the early days of the New York State Psychiatric Institute (Kolb and Roizin 1992).

In 1909, the Council on Medical Education of the American Medical Colleges set a minimum standard of 20 hours of instruction in psychiatry in medical schools. Largely through Adolf Meyer's efforts, surveys were done by Graves (1914), Noble (1933), and Ebaugh and Rymer (1942). The first two surveys were followed by conferences supported by the National Committee for Mental Hygiene. The first was held in 1933 to consider the formation of the American Board of Psychiatry and Neurology; the second in 1934 to discuss the curriculum for psychiatric teaching; the third in 1935 to discuss psychiatry and pediatrics; and the fourth in 1936 to discuss the methods of teaching psychiatry. The Commonwealth Fund supported one conference that took place during World War II (February 1945).

The two Ithaca conferences were held in the summers of 1951 and 1952. The significance of these conferences is well known. Whatever success followed the Ithaca conferences depended in great part on what had preceded them, but there was one difference that distinguished these conferences from previous ventures. The Ithaca conferences and the recommendations that ensued from them were generously nourished by federal funds available for the development of both undergraduate and graduate teaching programs (American Psychiatric Association 1952, 1953).

In 1962, the World Health Organization submitted an additional report on the teaching of psychiatry, and at the Psychiatry and Medical Education Conference in 1967 the increase in behavioral sciences during the first 2 years of medical school, the increase in elective curriculum hours, and the increase in interdepartmental teaching were identified as significant trends (American Psychiatric Association 1969). The increase in behavioral sciences during the first 2 years of medical school was due to several factors, including an increase in the number of courses being offered, an increase in the number of students enrolled in these courses, and the participation by the departments of preventive medicine, pediatrics, and medicine, as well as psychiatry. Although the amount of instruction in psychiatry and behavioral science has been increasing for over 70 years, the greatest increase occurred at the end of World War II. Most of us acknowledge that the single most important determinant of change in the departments of psychiatry in the United States since the end of World War II was the enactment of the National Mental Health Act (passed by the 79th Congress in 1946), which made possible the allocations of funds for education and research.

Other determinants that brought about changes in the teaching of psychiatry to medical students included the establishment of psychiatric services in general hospitals. In the almost five decades that have elapsed since the enactment of the National Mental Health Act, the remarkable growth in the number, size, and diversity of funds provided to the academic departments has been influenced by additional factors. Political factors include the provision of government health insurance for elderly and poor people and the community mental health movement. Biological factors include the introduction of rauwolfia and the phenothiazines in the early 1950s. Psychosocial factors include the notion of the open hospital, the therapeutic community, and deinstitutionalization.

We are apt to look on psychiatry as being quite young, younger than our sister clinical disciplines, particularly medicine and surgery. However, even in my salad days as a medical student in the early 1930s, 20 years after the publication of Abraham Flexner's influential report to the Carnegie Foundation for the Advancement of Teaching, only a few medical schools could boast a full-time faculty in any of the clinical disciplines. Psychiatry may not have been much younger, but surely we were poorer and less prestigious. As a result, we had less to begin with and more to gain from whatever support we could receive.

After World War II, although national health insurance was defeated, the government under Harry S. Truman once again began providing aid for hospital construction through the Hill-Burton Program. This program made possible matching funds for the building of psychiatric services in general hospitals. Over 90% of psychiatric units in university teaching hospitals and in community general hospitals were established after 1948. But more important was the generous and unprecedented support given for medical research and education through the National Institutes of Health and the National Science Foundation. I have a most vivid memory of the excitement and promise of the first meeting of the Council of the National Institute of Mental Health on August 15, 1946, held in the American Red Cross Building in Washington, D.C., presided over by that resolute person, Thomas Parran, probably the most distinguished surgeon general of the century. Quite appropriately, the meeting was covered for *PM* newspaper by Albert Deutsch, later to become the muckraker of his day through the publication of his camera-documented survey of the shocking conditions in our state mental hospitals entitled *The Shame of the States* (Deutsch 1948). This action of the federal government indicated a basic change in its prior posture of peripheral support to that of more direct support of medicine. Over the next two decades, the federal government's primary commitment was to the support of research, to professional education, and to the provision of facilities.

But what of our origins? At the turn of the century, opportunities for the education of the career psychiatrist, much less that of the medical student, were more by happenstance than by design. In the latter part of the nineteenth century, the real mental hospitals were built throughout the world. Reform had separated the criminals from the insane patients, and hospitals were used for treatment rather than for detention.

With these changes came hospitals for acutely insane patients, hospitals for chronically insane patients, asylums for criminally insane patients, institutions for feeble-minded patients, and colonies for epileptic patients. In addition to the public institutions for poor people and the institutions that served soldiers and veterans, there were several well-appointed retreats, homes, and sanitariums for the rich. In our country, there were built the great private mental hospitals like McLean, Bloomingdale, Pennsylvania, Pratt, and others.

In the first decade of this century, a number of psychopathic hospitals were established, usually associated with university medical centers. Modeled after the Psychiatrische Klinik of the German universities, these were small, compact hospitals of 60–100 beds, built in Ann Arbor, Michigan; Boston, Massachusetts; Iowa City, Iowa; Denver, Colorado; Galveston, Texas; and later in New York City. Fully equipped for diagnostic study and with adequate treatment facilities to handle a considerable number of acutely ill patients needing brief hospital stays, they also made possible the beginning of outpatient treatment (Peterson 1911). These hospitals, together with the psychiatric wards built in the large city hospitals (Bellevue, Philadelphia, Cincinnati), began to replace and supplement the famous nineteenth-century large public mental hospitals and several of the private hospitals as theaters for the systematic education of career psychiatrists and for laboratory and clinical investigative work, but with little attention to the education of the medical student.

Other events that may have played some part in the eventual establishment of the departments of psychiatry were the mental hygiene movement, born in the first decade of this century, which reflected much of our characteristic American evangelical optimism and pragmatism, and the child guidance movement, nourished in great part by the Commonwealth Fund and undoubtedly influenced greatly by John Dewey. This was to be the century of the child. Both of these movements contributed support by conducting surveys, establishing clinics, and providing opportunities for clinical instruction to psychiatrists, psychologists, and social workers.

World War I, particularly through the influence of Thomas P. Salmon, led to increasing concern about mental health and mental illness. In the decade before World War II, there was a considerable surge of therapeutic enthusiasm following the introduction of the somatic therapies—insulin, metrazol, dauerschlaf, electroconvulsive therapy (ECT), and lobotomy. These ventures supported the basic idea of a physical cause for madness, particularly for the enigma of schizophrenia. One must remember that two great mental scourges of this century, neurosyphilis and pellagra, were reduced—if not eliminated—by biochemical means. With the exception of the remarkable benefits obtained from the use of ECT with depressed patients, the methods of physical treatment did not fulfill their promise, eventually were used less and less, and finally were abandoned by most practitioners. As a result of this disillusionment, the pendulum quite predictably swung again from physical causality toward reconsidering schizophrenia as a psychosocial disorder. After World War II, there was a great increase and interest in all aspects of psychotherapy, with many psychiatrists seeking further training in psychoanalytic techniques. Consequently, a number of psychoanalysts attempted to extend their psychotherapeutic efforts toward the psychotic patient.

So far as I can determine, the first statistical record of hospitals approved for advanced internships or residencies was published in 1927 ("Hospitals Approved for Advanced Internships or Residencies" 1927). Two hundred seventy hospitals, with a bed capacity of 155,962, had been approved for 1,699 residencies in the special fields. The report continued: "It is interesting to note that the largest number of residencies at present, 360 in number, is found in neuropsychiatry, owing to the fact, probably, that more of these hospitals have been investigated for residencies, as the type of patients cared for prevents their obtaining interns." Neuropsychiatry had 80 hospital programs that offered opportunities for 360 residencies. Surgery provided the next largest number of residencies (249), followed by 200 residencies in internal medicine, 157 in tuberculosis, 133 in pediatrics, and 105 in obstetrics and gynecology. Of the 80 hospital programs that offered residencies in neuropsychiatry, 50 were hospitals with more than 1,000 beds. Of those 50, 40 were large federal and state mental hospitals that provided 242 of the 360 residency opportunities, or two-thirds of the total.

Unknown are how many residencies were filled, how many were devoted primarily to neurology and to mental retardation, the length of the assignment (probably no more than 1 year), and the design of the curriculum, if such existed. The only residencies that were associated with university medical centers were those at Stanford (1 resident), Colorado Psychopathic Hospital (3 residents), Johns Hopkins (6 residents), Boston Psychopathic Hospital (8 residents), Michigan (1 resident), Minnesota (1 resident), Barnes Hospital, St. Louis (1 resident), Cincinnati (1 resident), and Wisconsin (1 resident)—a total of 23, or 6% of the total of 360 neuropsychiatry residencies. Residencies offered for the year 1973–1974 for the same number of universities were 418 in general psychiatry and 83 in child psychiatry, about 22 times the number offered in 1927.

As is evident, before World War II the situation facing the candidate for special training in psychiatry was not very promising. There was no regular curriculum, and periods of study and experience were usually

1 or 2 years. A limited number of fellowship opportunities were offered by both the Rockefeller Foundation and the Commonwealth Fund. A few recipients used their fellowships to obtain psychoanalytic training abroad; others studied neurology at Queen's Square in London; but most of the recipients took resident training in the available psychopathic hospitals, such as I undertook in Colorado in the middle 1930s. Many of the psychiatrists at that time sought neurological training in the United States as well as abroad, in addition to training in clinical psychiatry. A small handful pursued psychoanalytic study. The number of programs was limited, as was the number of residencies offered.

And what has happened since? Fifteen years ago I noted that there were 300 approved programs, with about 4,800 residents in training. Of the 300 programs, about 10% were in child psychiatry, 60% were in general psychiatry, and 30% were in combined general and child psychiatry programs. About one-third of the programs were conducted under the administrative sponsorship of a medical school. The most recent data obtained from the Residency Review Committee for Psychiatry and from the Office of Education of the American Psychiatric Association, together with data from the *Journal of the American Medical Association* ("Graduate Medical Education in the Changing Environment of Medicine" 1992), indicated that there was a total of 322 programs—200 adult programs and 122 child programs—with a total of 6,095 residents. The article stated that fewer than 20% of the programs are freestanding (i.e., not associated with a university).

I was told that the biggest change in psychiatric education in recent years was a change in the special requirements; this change was introduced by the Residency Review Committee for Psychiatry in 1987 (J. H. Scully, M.D., Director, Office of Education, American Psychiatric Association, personal communication). Requirements in the curricular patterns became quite specific. Not only are required clinical rotations and didactic topics outlined in a very specific manner, but residents have to maintain a record of specific cases treated that is reviewed to assess progress. Although it is said that the biopsychosocial model has become the official conceptual model, I do not believe that this model represents a wide departure from the past. Over the years, few programs were narrowly defined according to biological or psychological extremes, and most programs were pluralistic in their espousal of psychosocial, as well as genetic and biological, determinants. This pluralism existed long before the somewhat hackneyed use of the biopsychosocial concept.

The site visits of programs have become more like accreditation visits from the Joint Commission on Accreditation of Healthcare Organizations rather than like the older visits from the Residency Review Committee, which I remember as quite perfunctory. I assume that one of the reasons for the structured rigidity in the special requirements is to ensure the maintenance of minimal standards, particularly in those programs not affiliated with a university. Nevertheless, I still have some mixed feelings about the structured special requirements. In the past, I was concerned about the increasing intrusion of accrediting bodies into the functions and responsibilities of the university medical centers. It is my understanding that the various graduate boards were established over the years by practitioners of specific disciplines to ensure minimal standards of conduct. The university, on the other hand, is, or should be, concerned principally with the imaginative acquisition of knowledge, as Alfred North Whitehead put it—in other words, to be constantly critical of existing knowledge, to pursue new knowledge, and to try to do things better than they had been done before.

In 1967, at the Detroit meeting of the Association of Professors and Chairmen of Departments of Psychiatry in U.S. Medical Schools, I challenged a recent action of the Residency Review Committee that insisted that we teach a certain subject in a certain way. I acknowledged the right of the Residency Review Committee to set standards, but I believed the university should have the right to determine how best to achieve them. In other words, I found this action of the Residency Review Committee to be intrusive on the freedom of the university to accomplish its tasks.

Shortly after that, I wrote a serious critique of actions taken by the American Board of Psychiatry and Neurology that led to the elimination of the traditional internship as a prerequisite to training in psychiatry (Romano 1970). I pointed out that the elimination of the internship requirement would seriously undermine the future psychiatrist's unique contributions to his or her own field, as well as to other areas of medical practice. It was evident that the implications of such a change had not been fully discussed, and clarification was needed as to how the desirable features of the internship were to be incorporated into psychiatric residency training programs. I warned that blind acceptance of the trend toward earlier specialization in medical education would lead to neglect of the major issue, the provision of quality education for future psychiatrists. The internship requirement was reinstated in 1977.

The move toward subspecialization in the field of psychiatry continues. In 1953, subspecialization with certification in the field of administrative psychiatry was established. Although this subspecialty still exists, certification is done under the auspices of the American Psychiatric Association rather than the Residency Review Committee of the American Board of Psychiatry and Neurology. With that exception, after many years of no subspecialty other than child and adolescent psychiatry, four new subspecialties requiring an additional year of training are in various stages of approval. Geriatric psychiatry has been approved by the American Board of Medical Specialty and the American Board of Psychiatry and Neurology, and examinations have been given. I understand that these boards also have accredited the subspecialty of clinical neurophysiology, an area of study especially directed toward neurologists but also open to psychiatrists. The subspecialty of addiction was accredited in 1993 by the same boards, and the subspecialty of forensic psychiatry is to be accredited in 1994. The subspecialty of consultation-liaison psychiatry has not been reviewed, but it is thought that this review will take place in the near future. The Accreditation Council on Graduate Medical Education has yet to accredit fellowship training programs because of the moratorium imposed by it in 1992 on all new specialties.

The subspecialty movement has been viewed critically by many because of concerns about fragmenting the field. Restricting the practices of those who do not have certificates of subspecialization could result in a situation where these subspecialties are not taught to general psychiatry residents. It has been stated that both pediatrics and internal medicine faced this problem earlier, and although the advent of subspecialization in these disciplines led to some fragmentation, the overall strengthening of these fields has been impressive (Shore 1993).

I have not been impressed with the evidence supporting the movement toward subspecialization. I do not believe that existing scholarship and skills attributed to the subspecialties in psychiatry warrant such separation. The fact that medicine and pediatrics have divided their fields into 15 or 16 divisions is not a necessary or logical argument for insisting that psychiatry do the same. In my view, the move toward subspecialization in our field has not only led to the weakening of the generalist but to increasing divisiveness within the profession and to selfish, self-serving, mercenary objectives. The movement also presents a major training problem in that it reduces the number of persons with overall generalist capacities.

Fortunately, the education of medical students is less structured than the education of residents. In the preclinical period, there may be a variety of courses, including those relating to human development, psychopathology, interviewing techniques, and behavioral neuroscience. In our school, medical students have elective opportunities in the following areas: inpatient, outpatient, day treatment program, and psychosomatic research. The number of hours in the curriculum varies as well. Some schools have only 10–20 hours of behavioral science, whereas others have hundreds of hours. Clerkship length in the third year is more uniform. The median length of a psychiatry clerkship is 6 weeks. The shortest clerkship is 4 weeks, and the longest is 8 weeks. The average duration of psychiatry rotations is about 6.2 weeks. Most clerkships are hospital based, with consultation-liaison rotations. Some clerkships have an outpatient rotation.

Recruitment has again become a problem. Match results over the past several years have been disappointing because of continual decline, but the census of residents has remained high because of international medical graduates and people choosing psychiatry several years after graduating from medical school, although data supporting the latter statement are questionable. Sidney Weissman, who is immediate past president of Directors of Psychiatry Residency Training, reported on the results of a conference held May 28–29, 1992, on the recruitment of U.S. medical school graduates into psychiatry (Weissman 1992). He indicated that the number of students entering psychiatry peaked at 745 in 1988, and since then, there has been a considerable decline in the number of candidates. The recommendations of the conference were quite detailed, including attempts to enhance high school and college students' awareness of psychiatry. The principal recommendations concerned reinforcement and strengthening of educational programs for undergraduate medical students.

More recently, a note in *Psychiatric News* stated that, on average, U.S. medical centers had 41.5% of their psychiatric residency positions filled by new graduates from U.S. medical schools (Cody 1993). International medical graduates, osteopathic graduates, and U.S. graduates from earlier years, however, bring the percentage of positions filled to 63.4%. Since peaking in 1988 at 745 students, recruitment of U.S. medical school graduates had declined by over one-third to 477. Intended action to decrease medical costs may reduce the number of psychiatrists. Even though psychiatry is a field with acknowledged shortages, the present movement to increase the number of general practitioners may further reduce the number of psychiatrists.

Concern about recruitment of American graduates of medical schools to the field of psychiatry is not new, nor are the possible reasons for the decline. In 1980, I commented on this matter in some detail (Romano 1980). A portion of this 1980 article is included below.[1]

> Departments of psychiatry are particularly concerned with the decline in the number of medical students who choose psychiatric careers. In 1970–1971, approximately 12% of the American medical graduates went into psychiatry. This figure dropped to 8% by 1974–1975 and to 4% by 1979. Further evidence has been obtained through an as-yet unpublished nationwide study of fourth-year medical students conducted by the American Association for Cancer Education (Bakemeier and Black 1979). Students were asked to designate in terms of their own future professional development the most attractive and the least attractive of each of the clinical specialties. Psychiatry was the least attractive of the

---

[1] Adapted from Romano J: "On the Teaching of Psychiatry to Medical Students: Does It Have to Get Worse Before It Gets Better?" *Psychosomatic Medicine* 42 (suppl):103–111, 1980. Used with permission. Copyright 1980 American Psychosomatic Society.

major clinical divisions, including family practice. Only oncology and surgical pathology had lower ratings.

Many ask, Why is this happening? Obviously, it is a complex matter, but the following factors may contribute to the change. A principal reason offered is the attraction of students to family medicine programs. It is claimed that family medicine programs are attracting many bright, thoughtful, psychologically perceptive, and socially conscious young men and women who, 10 or more years ago, would have chosen careers in psychiatry. From my limited experience with the family medicine program at the University of Rochester and with several other programs I visited, I, too, have been impressed with the high caliber of the residents. However, I am not sure that this is the principal factor because recent studies show that dropouts from the family medicine program and, for that matter, graduates of it rarely change their careers to psychiatry.

I believe that family medicine—which has as its central concerns entry, coordination, and longitudinal responsibility—is a separate universe from that of psychiatry. At the moment, I believe that family medicine is in great part illusory and that it sounds better than it really is, because I have seen no evidence of its being anything but a health delivery service to members of a family as individuals. If family medicine is to become more than a service function (i.e., an academic discipline), it will need to create its intellectual raison d'etre—most likely the study of the family in sickness and in health. With the exception of one study, I am not aware of any basic curiosity about, much less systematic inquiry into, the nature of the family or those events that transpire among members of the family that may promote health or lead to disability (Medalie and Goldbourt 1976).

A second factor that is thought to explain the decline of interest in psychiatry is the preference of medical school admission committees for students with interest and competence in the physical and biological sciences. I am sure that policies in this matter vary from school to school, and I am not sure that students with interest and competence in the physical and biological sciences are less interested in or sensitive to psychological matters.

A third factor is the downgrading of the teaching of psychiatry to medical students. As I go about the country, I have found very few chairpersons or senior professorial staff working intimately with medical students. Part-time faculties appeared to be harassed in their hurried visits to their patients. Much of the teaching has been relegated to residents and to junior staff without adequate models for them to emulate and with questionable reward systems. Another point is the reduced opportunity the student has for clinical scholarship. In the past, the fourth year of medical school provided advanced clinical clerkships in all the major clinical disciplines, but with the change to an elective year, most students were deprived of the opportunity for sustained responsible clinical assignments.

The fourth factor in many schools is thought to be the lack of prestige of the psychiatric faculty among their peers and their negligible influence on the governance of the medical school as a whole. Further, few models of psychiatrists engaged in research (basic or applied) are available for the students to emulate. At best, the student may meet, at random, the occasional research assistant, who is often seen in a swirl of computer printouts.

The fifth factor is confusion, worse confounded, resulting from the elimination of the freestanding internship, the obvious second-rate quality of the current colonialized internship provisions, and the sheer absurdity of assuming that the parent department of psychiatry could ensure proper surveillance.

A sixth factor is financial. I am informed that psychiatrists are close to the bottom, if not at the bottom, of the medical professional income market and that they make less money now than pediatricians do. We must remember that medical students—most of them married, with and without children—finish medical school with considerable burdens of indebtedness approximating $20,000–$25,000. Is it not likely that they may look to careers with assured high incomes?[2]

A seventh factor may stem from our medical students and residents, who look about them in the urban areas with which they are familiar and find those areas to be saturated with practicing psychiatrists. In my lifetime, there has been an increase from 2 psychiatrists per 100,000 to over 12 per 100,000.[3] It is claimed that there are more psychiatrists than pediatricians and obstetricians in the nation. In 1934, when I began my resident training at Yale University, the total membership of the American Psychiatric Association was 1,064. Today it is over 25,000.[4] A relevant question is how many additional psychiatrists we need per year. Is it a matter of distribution rather than of numbers, as it is in the rest of medicine?

Eighth is the fundamental concern of the psychiatrist with the definition of his or her professional role. Who am I, and what am I to do that is different from what others do? This difference is clearly perceived by both students and residents on the inpatient psychiatric floors. When students come to these floors, unlike the other clinical services, they find that most of the staff are not in uniform. Students find that staff wear open shirts, loose gypsy blouses, hip-hugging jeans, wooden shoes, and Indian beads and have an abundance of hair. There are nurses, nursing assistants, nurse practitioners, nurse clinicians, assistant clinicians, psychiatric technicians, social workers, social work assistants, mental health aides, program coordinators, psychology students, primary therapists, occupational therapists, recreational therapists, physical therapists, family and group therapists, mental health information service clerks, junior psychiatric faculty, and senior psychiatric faculty (not many of these). Staff members may work full-time (fewer of these), part-time (often in a hurry), sometimes, one time, and regrettably, most of them never on time.

---

[2] In 1993, the indebtedness was at least three times what it was in 1980.

[3] Currently, it is 16 per 100,000.

[4] Currently, it is almost 40,000.

From time to time, from out of the medical mist emerges a silent white-coated person with a stethoscope who conducts a physical examination of the patient, records such on the ever-burgeoning chart, and leaves almost as quietly as he or she came.

We brought them, all of them, to our floors in our evangelical egalitarianism. Most patients are now called clients and soon may be called penitents. Small wonder the medical student asks, Who is the doctor and what does he or she do?

In the past, psychiatrists were distinguished among all physicians by their central interest in the individuality of the patient and the identification and understanding of the patient's disturbances in thinking, feeling, and behavior. With the advent of anxiolytic, neuroleptic, and antidepressant medication, many psychiatrists spend less time listening and more time giving pills. In short, they have become more like other physicians. Our students not only recognized this fact but were puzzled by it.

A ninth factor is the increasing intrusion in our daily practices by governmental and judicial agencies, with consequent erosion and degradation of our traditional discretionary clinical responsibility to the sick patients whose care is entrusted to us.

Tenth is the understandable disappointments when our earlier expectations were not fulfilled. We have awakened to a number of false dawns: the somatic therapies of the 1930s, with the remarkable exception of ECT, which provided relief for psychotically depressed persons; the premature notion of specificity in conditions defined as psychosomatic; the psychotherapeutic exuberance after World War II and the recent exponential increase of psychotherapeutic modes, now 130 in number, some of them defying classification; the bumbling sociopolitical ventures of the community mental health programs, with the good and bad consequences of deinstitutionalization; the mixed blessings of the neuroleptic drugs with their adverse neurological complications; and now, out of the closet, clear and public evidence of the serious problems of chronic mental illness and dependency.

Finally, students observe the difficulties the psychiatric faculty has in accepting, understanding, and using necessary present-day pluralistic approaches to the care of the patients.

What are we to do about all of this? I see no need to seek a wailing wall or to chant a requiem mass for the repose of the soul of psychiatry. Rather, it is time—high time—to sound reveille, to call the profession to rise and fulfill our professional responsibilities more effectively.

Have we fouled our own nest? Have we permitted, even fostered, a teaching program no longer competitive in our students' minds with the excitement and promise of our sister clinical disciplines? Have we uncritically embraced antiauthoritarianism, which has diminished quality in all our undertakings and which has led to breakdown of our previous standards?

Is there not the obvious and urgent need for informed, rigorous minds—both junior and senior—in our profession to serve as examples as we attempt to renew our high standards in presenting substance with clarity and vigor to our students?

If we can re-create the ambiance of the imaginative acquisition of knowledge; if our students see about them residents, interns, and faculty (junior and senior) who exhibit and enjoy the great excitement and richness of our field, which is the most human and the most personal of the medical disciplines; if there are those who retain their curiosity, wish to know more, and wish to apply their knowledge for the benefit of those who seek their help; and if practitioners consider their primary allegiance to be to the problem presented by the patient and the patient's family rather than to their own private ideologies—then, we may not only ensure our survival but actually continue to grow. This growth will require comprehensive understanding of genetic and biological, as well as psychosocial, determinants; the intelligent use of medication when indicated; identification of the type of psychotherapy appropriate to the patient's needs; and the use of community resources beyond the family when indicated. If we can achieve these objectives, we may again earn the respect of our students. If not, there may be no good reason for us to survive as a major medical discipline.

In the intervening years since I wrote my jeremiad, departments of psychiatry have done very little to correct their deficiencies. Small wonder, then, that there continues to be a decline in recruitment of graduates from our medical schools to psychiatry. The number of senior teachers serving as generalists and as good models for students in day-to-day teaching is negligible. It is said by some that recruitment to family medicine programs may reduce the number of students opting for psychiatry, particularly if the government adds financial incentives to primary care medical programs, as these may make family medicine programs more attractive. I have been impressed with the fact that family medicine in its concern for turf has denied any significant relationship to psychiatry and that it chooses psychologists and social scientists, but not psychiatrists, to enhance its programs.

Surely, the psychiatrist of the future is going to be different from the psychiatrist of today. Let us consider the possible reasons.

First, there has been exponential growth in knowledge and information about the anatomy, neurochemistry, and pharmacology of the brain. There has been similar exciting growth in our knowledge and application of genetics. This increased knowledge has led in many instances to a de-emphasis of psychological and social factors as determinants of behavior. The changes have been sufficiently dramatic to warrant the wisdom of Leon Eisenberg's remark that psychiatry, from being brainless, has now become mindless (Eisenberg 1986).

Second, there has been an equally exponential increase in the number of professional and paraprofessional persons performing what psychiatry claimed in the past to be one of its major functions—the systematic use of psychological measures to modify human behavior (i.e., psychotherapy). As mentioned earlier, due to our evangelical egalitarianism, great numbers of psychologists, social workers, nurses, counselors, case managers, and others are engaged in the day-to-day practice of psychotherapy. However, for the most part, most of the patients they see, who are often called "clients" or "consumers," are not traditionally neurotic or psychotic, but rather persons who are classified as having problems in living.

From within medicine, humanistic concerns—once the more or less exclusive concern of the psychiatrist—are now championed by behavioral scientists, family medicine practitioners, and others in internal medicine, pediatrics, obstetrics, gynecology, and even surgery. Can these achievements be considered signs of our success in influencing for the better a wide group of persons who care for the sick?

In addition, there is a flourishing new industry of ethicists. These include militant philosophers, theologians, psychologists, and counselors, whose instant omniscience in matters of privacy, informed consent, and other aspects of medical morality appears to be matched only by their overweening arrogance.

The third factor is a general collapse of the hegemony of psychoanalytic psychology in its influence on both the theory and the practice of the psychiatric profession. Its limited therapeutic usefulness, together with cultist allegiance to beliefs, has reduced its influence. There is little question, however, of its important contributions to the notions about the significance of the life cycle, about transference and countertransference, and about the origins of anxiety. Much of the useful psychoanalytic theory has been woven into general psychiatric thought and practice.

A fourth factor may be economic in terms of affecting reimbursement. Although psychiatrists earn more money today than ever before, they still earn less than physicians in other disciplines, with the exception of general practice and pediatrics. However, I question whether money is a determining factor in recruiting students to the field of psychiatry. Pediatrics, for example, has had no serious difficulty in recruitment.

As a result of these factors, tomorrow's psychiatrists must take care of the most difficult patients. Nonpsychiatric professionals and paraprofessionals, as mentioned earlier, will probably see most patients who have minor degrees of distress or whose distress can be alleviated quickly. Tomorrow's psychiatrists must be medically informed and sophisticated in psychopharmacology. At times, achieving this sophistication may be quite a task because in the recent past many psychiatrists have arrogantly eschewed knowledge of psychopharmacology and have insisted on dealing with behavior only in psychological terms. The psychiatrist of tomorrow must also be attuned to the effects of medication on the nervous system and on the body as a whole.

What are the possible future roles of the psychiatrist? It seems to me that our greatest strength is the breadth as well as the depth of our knowledge and skills. Not only are we students of the human mind and of the relations between persons, but we also study the human body. We are, then, in the highly advantageous position of being able to determine more accurately whether a patient's problem is biological, psychological, or social, or whether it is caused by some combination of those factors. Therefore, we can readily serve as consultants to primary care practitioners, helping them determine the nature of an illness, its course, and treatment.

The psychiatrist of the future may also play an important role as a public health consultant. Duties might include planning diagnostic, therapeutic, and custodial health services and serving as an adviser to political bodies and legislatures concerning the delivery of health services.

Another important function is teaching medical students, psychology and social casework students, law students, and students of divinity and of penology—sharing with them knowledge of the broad range of disturbed human behavior.

Ideally, another role involves collaborating with others in the care of the patient. For example, the psychiatrist might work with the social caseworker, psychologist, and therapist, advising them, examining the patient, prescribing medication, and assisting in follow-up. This collaboration is sometimes called back-up service to nonpsychiatric professionals who conduct psychotherapy with patients. I understand from others that at times psychiatrists prescribe medication for patients they have not seen, which is obvious malpractice.

Despite present-day movements toward increased freedom for the patient, some patients (perhaps a small number) will have to be cared for continuously in intramural settings. We will need psychiatrists to be responsible for the long-term care of patients in hospitals, halfway homes, nursing homes, and so forth. Like other physicians, the psychiatrist of the future must be engaged in research; that is, he or she must look critically at existing knowledge and practice in both the biological and the psychosocial fields and must pursue new ideas, both in theory and in practice. In my opinion, the psychiatrist should not relinquish his or her significant role as a psychotherapist. However, it will be the psychiatrist's task to establish improved methods to obtain detailed knowledge about patients and their families throughout their life cycles.

At the time of this writing (May 1993), there is evidence that mental health professionals across the country have deep fears about the limits that a new national health plan may put on payments for psychotherapy. One psychiatrist commented: "There is a strong preference among managed care companies for therapists who will take a short-term approach to problems. This is especially a threat to psychodynamic therapists who deal with underlying personality patterns that take more time to treat, but if left untreated, can, for example, keep triggering life-long episodes of depression whenever a relationship fails" (Goleman 1993). The article concluded with the statement that the challenge for psychotherapists now seems to be devising more objective guidelines to justify the use of long-term therapy.

The notion that the changes in the role of the psychiatrist will turn him or her into a neurologist is quite disquieting to me. As a young man, I made the deliberate, conscious decision to pursue the profession of psychiatry. I was impressed with the breadth of its concern with genetics, biology, clinical medicine, psychology, the social sciences, and the humanities. Psychiatry is based on the biomedical and social sciences. The contributions made in the past several decades have ensured that our profession will be an advancing clinical discipline. But psychiatry has more—the nonscience factor is greater than it is in any other discipline. Like my British colleague, I have found that psychiatry has to do with humanity (Cawley 1993). As a young man, I thought that psychiatry was by far the most human of the medical disciplines. As an old man, I have found my judgment to be confirmed.

REFERENCES

American Psychiatric Association: One Hundred Years of American Psychiatry. New York, Columbia University Press, 1944

American Psychiatric Association: Psychiatry and Medical Education. Washington, DC, American Psychiatric Association, 1952

American Psychiatric Association: The Psychiatrist, His Training and Development. Washington, DC, American Psychiatric Association, 1953

American Psychiatric Association: Psychiatry and Medical Education. Washington, DC, American Psychiatric Association, 1969

Bakemeier RF, Black GS: Cancer education survey IV. Medical students and cancer education in U.S. medical schools. (Report to the Division of Cancer Control and Rehabilitation of the National Cancer Institute.) Washington, DC, American Association for Cancer Education, 1979

Cawley R: In conversation with Robert Cawley. Psychiatric Bulletin of the Royal College of Psychiatrists 17:260–273, 1993

Cody P: Residency matching in psychiatry continues to decline. Psychiatric News 28:1–20, 1993

Deutsch A: The Shame of the States. New York, Harcourt Brace, 1948

Ebaugh FG: The history of psychiatric education in the U.S., 1844–1944. Am J Psychiatry 100:151–160, 1944

Ebaugh FG, Rymer CA: Psychiatry in Medical Education. New York, The Commonwealth Fund, 1942

Eisenberg L: Mindlessness and brainlessness in psychiatry. Br J Psychiatry 148:497–508, 1986

Goleman D: Mental health professionals worry over coming change in health care. The New York Times, May 10, 1993

Graduate medical education in the changing environment of medicine (editorial). JAMA 268:1097–1105, 1992

Graves WW: Some factors tending toward adequate instruction in nervous and mental diseases. JAMA 63:1707–1713, 1914

Hospitals approved for advanced internships or residencies. JAMA 88:828–834, 1927

Kolb LC, Roizin L: The First Psychiatric Institute. Washington, DC, American Psychiatric Press, 1992

Medalie JH, Goldbourt U: Angina pectoris among 10,000 men. Am J Med 60:910–921, 1976

Noble RA: Psychiatry in Medical Education. New York, National Committee for Mental Hygiene, 1933

Peterson R: Insanity: hospital treatment, in Encyclopedia Britannica, 11th Edition, Vol 14. London, Encyclopedia Britannica, 1911, pp 616–618

Romano J: The elimination of the internship: an act of regression. Am J Psychiatry 116:712–717, 1970

Romano J: On the teaching of psychiatry to medical students: does it have to get worse before it gets better? Psychosom Med 42 (suppl):103–111, 1980

Rond PC: The first professor of psychiatry, Samuel Mitchel Smith. Am J Psychiatry 114:843–844, 1958

Shore JH: Order and chaos: subspecialization and American psychiatry. Academic Psychiatry 17:12–20, Spring 1993

Weissman SH: Report to the National Institute of Mental Health (NIMH) on the May 28 and 29 Conference on Recruitment of U.S. Medical Graduates Into Psychiatry (Organized by the American Association of Directors of Psychiatric Residency Training under contract to NIMH). Washington, DC, July 1992

Chapter 2

Psychiatric Research in America

Heinz E. Lehmann, M.D., and Thomas A. Ban, M.D.

American psychiatric research did not spring full blown, like Pallas Athena from Zeus's head, on this continent. It had its roots in European psychiatry, where research, both theoretical and experimental, had been flourishing for almost a century before the beginnings of serious psychiatric research in North America.

THE BEGINNINGS OF PSYCHIATRIC RESEARCH

Psychiatry was recognized as a medical specialty by the French physician Philippe Pinel (1745–1826) at the time of the French revolution, when he expressly accepted responsibility for the medical profession to care for mentally disturbed patients and devoted his own life to the care and study of these unfortunate people. A few famous clinicians, like Sydenham and Willis in the seventeenth century, had written about a few selected nervous disorders. But until Pinel's time, mentally ill patients had been left in the hands of the church and public authorities. Pinel wrote the first psychiatric textbook and, with his disciple Jean Etienne Esquirol (1772–1840), published the first systematic classification of psychiatric diseases.

The term *psychiatry* was coined in 1803 by the German physician J. C. Reil (1773–1845). Actual research in the new discipline began in 1822, when A. L. Bayle (1799–1858), in France, performed autopsies on the bodies of numerous psychiatric patients. He discovered that the brains of syphilitic patients with mental disorders showed gross pathological changes. After this experimental discovery, an intense, almost passionate, controversy of theoretical paradigms has enlivened, but also created considerable division in, psychiatric research—a controversy that continues to this day.

Two paradigms evolved in early nosological research in psychiatry: the organic and the psychosocial. Fueled by Bayle's discoveries of pathological changes, the battle cry of the organic paradigm was sounded by the German psychiatrist Wilhelm Griesinger (1817–1868), when he stated that there are no psychiatric diseases, only brain diseases. On the psychosocial (or "moral") side were the followers of Johann Christian Heinroth (1773–1843), who contemptuously wrote that the "somaticists" looked on the human mind as "a cadaver which one could cut to pieces with a knife, or as a chemical compound which could be broken down into elements, or as a mechanical contraption, the workings of which one could calculate with the help of mathematics" (Heinroth, quoted in Grulhe 1932, p. 6).

A third nosological paradigm, the agnostic paradigm, was declared by H. Neumann (1814–1884) and his followers in 1859, when he recommended that we "throw overboard the whole business of classifications. . . . There is but one type of mental disturbance and we call it insanity" (Neumann 1859, p. 167).

With the war of the paradigms unresolved, clinical and experimental psychiatric research proceeded at a rapid pace in nineteenth-century Europe. In France, J. P. Falret (1794–1870) discovered the diagnostic category of periodic and bipolar affective disorders (folie circulaire). B. A. Morel (1809–1873) noted genetic factors in the etiology of psychiatric illness. K. L. Kahlbaum (1828–1899), E. Hecker (1843–1909), W. Sander (1838–1922), and S. Korsakoff (1854–1900) described the diagnostic entities of catatonia, hebephrenia, paranoia, and alcoholic amnesia, respectively.

Toward the end of the last century (1896), Emil Kraepelin (1855–1926) presented his nosological tour de force with the creation of the two monolithic diagnoses of dementia praecox and manic-depressive psychosis. He was attacked by his colleagues because no biological causes or consistent correlates of these diseases were known then; of course, they do not exist today either.

During this time, the neuroscientific aspect of psychiatry, in the form of neuroanatomy, was making significant progress with the work of P. Broca (1824–1880), G. Golgi (1843–1926), G. Wernicke (1848–1905), and T. Meynert (1832–1899). In 1870, Fritsch and Hitzig demonstrated cause-effect relationships between electrical stimulation of specific brain areas and motor behavior in animals. Thus, psychiatric nosology, clinical research, neuroanatomy, electroneurophysiology, and animal research were well under way in the last decade of the nineteenth century.

The growing psychiatric research community supported the organic and the clinical agnostic paradigms when, like a historical bombshell, Sigmund Freud's (1856–1939) psychoanalysis exploded within the psychosocial paradigm (1900). Kraepelin and Freud were contemporaries. Almost simultaneously, the 1904 Nobel laureate, Ivan Pavlov (1849–1936), discovered the conditional origins of behavior. Against this lively old-world background, psychiatric research in America was now poised to take off.

CHANGING ATTITUDES TOWARD
RESEARCH IN AMERICA

At the middle of the nineteenth century, American "alienists," as the psychiatric superintendents of mental hospitals were then called, were trying hard to convince themselves and the public with their volumes of statistics that mental disorders were caused by excessive environmental stimulation. But they were soon forced to capitulate to the organic paradigm, which was supported by evidence emerging from neuroanatomical research. By the end of the century, psychiatrists were not interested in research because there was not much they could hope for, as in their view all mental illness was either hereditary or due to brain disease. And of course, there were no cures for these conditions.

John E. Whitehorn, who wrote the chapter on psychiatric research for the centenary of the American Psychiatric Association in 1944, quoted the famous neurologist Weir Mitchell (1830–1914), who 50 years earlier had challenged the members of the American Medico-Psychological Association—now the APA—in this extraordinary manner:

> We, neurologists, think you have fallen behind us, and this opinion is gaining ground outside of our own ranks, and is, in part at least, your own fault.... Where ... are your careful scientific reports? (Mitchell 1894)

This call to arms was heeded by American psychiatrists, who soon unleashed an array of research efforts in many directions. With the Mental Hygiene movement, J. B. Watson's (1878–1958) and B. F. Skinner's (1904–1990) new behaviorism, and most of all, the tidal wave of psychoanalysis that swept in from Europe in the 1930s, they embraced the psychosocial paradigm again—at least in their clinical practice. Adolf Meyer (1866–1950), who may be considered to be the father of modern American psychiatry, was among the powerful leaders in this new orientation. Although his original training was in pathology, he entered the field of psychiatry and emphasized from the beginning the need for careful study of each patient's individuality with what he called the psychobiological approach. However, the almost unopposed reign of the psychosocial paradigm in American clinical practice and academic teaching by the middle of our century was dramatically challenged by the discovery of the new neurotropic drugs in the 1950s.

CATEGORIES OF RESEARCH

Because modern psychiatric research was—and is—taking so many different directions at the same time, the remainder of this chapter is divided into four parts: therapy, nosology, pathology, and epidemiology. It is almost in this chronological order that research in psychiatry has developed. First, there were the clinical needs to develop treatments; next, diagnostic definitions and classifications were needed; then came the need for scientific knowledge; and finally there was the need for statistics and surveys to be used by health services and eventually to shape public policies.

THERAPY

Early Period

Because history has given Benjamin Rush (1745–1813) an unsavory reputation by focusing attention on his aggressive physical treatments (e.g., bloodletting, the revolving chair), it is frequently overlooked that the origin of therapeutic research in American psychiatry is found in his work (Carlson and Simpson 1964). It was Rush (1812) who first employed "moral persuasion" to set the stage for "rational persuasion" by raising emotions in the treatment of "mania." No longer only blindly following past authority, Rush developed rationales based on his own observations. In 1812, he was the first to employ "pain" in the treatment of hypochondriasis on the rationale that there is an incompatibility between physical pain and hypochondriasis (Rush 1812).

After the publication of Rush's treatise, in which he set out a "system of principles" for the treatment of the mind within the "dominion of medicine," bloodletting and the administration of purgatives and emetics, combined with one of several forms of "moral treatment," remained for several decades the prevalent therapy for mental disorders. By the mid-nineteenth century, however, as a result of F. A. F. Sertürner's (1783–1841) isolation of morphine in 1803, bloodletting was replaced by the administration of narcotics such as opium and morphine—at first only in the treatment of acute mental disorders, but later also in the treatment of the chronic stages of these disorders. With the introduction of narcotics, therapeutic research in American psychiatry was ahead of that in Europe for the first time (Allen 1850). Furthermore, because excitement and agitation could now be controlled without extraordinary physical measures, introduction of narcotics opened the door for further research.

Etiological Orientation

Therapeutic research with some of the old remedies, (e.g., laxatives and hydrotherapy) continued, but a second period of therapeutic research in American psychiatry began with a new etiological orientation.

The neurologist Weir Mitchell perceived neurasthenia as the result of rapid urbanization and proposed "altering the moral atmosphere which has been to the patient like the very breathing of the evil," with the hope that it would result in "relief from a host of aches and pains." He referred to his new treatment as "rest cure."

Another harsher, etiology-oriented treatment, akin to the castration and clitorectomy practiced in the past, consisted of the surgical removal of tonsils and teeth. This surgery was done on the basis of Cotton, Draper, and Lynch's (1920) postulation that the cause of mental illness was focal (often hidden) infection. Although it was clearly shown by Kopeloff and Kirby in 1923 that this was not the case, surgical removal of tonsils and even large tracts of the colon continued for several years.

An entirely different series of clinical investigations was triggered by the original reports of Loevenhart et al. (1929) in the *Journal of the American Medical Association* and of Lindemann (1932) in the *Journal of the American Psychiatric Association*. Both dealt with the transient removal of catatonic symptoms, one by carbon dioxide (30% carbon dioxide with 70% oxygen) inhalation and the other by intravenous administration of sodium amobarbital. Follow-up research with carbon dioxide later led to biological approaches to the treatment of anxiety neurosis by L. von Meduna (1896–1964) in Chicago. Further research with amobarbital led to narcotherapy, such as Horsley's (1943) narcoanalysis and Grinker and Spiegel's (1945) narcosynthesis in the treatment of psychoneuroses. These treatments seemed to provide a bridge between the psychological and the somatic aspects of mental illness; however, neither of these therapies is used any longer within the mainstream of practice in American psychiatry.

Major Physical Therapies

Two major physical treatments were imported from Europe in the late 1930s: insulin coma therapy and electroconvulsive therapy (ECT). Insulin treatment was first used by Steck as a special form of the American "rest cure." M. Sakel (1900–1957), in Austria, developed insulin coma therapy in the 1930s. It became one of the most extensively used treatment modalities for schizophrenia during the 1940s. Insulin coma therapy was widely used and systematically studied for two decades, especially in the United States, with regard to its effects on brain metabolism (Wortis and Lambert 1942). By the 1960s, however, hypoglycemic insulin coma therapy had been virtually abandoned by American psychiatry because it eventually proved to be costly, cumbersome, hazardous, and not effective over the long term.

In contrast, ECT, which was introduced by the Italians U. Cerletti (1877–1963) and L. Bini (1908–1964) in 1938 for the treatment of schizophrenia, has remained a major form of treatment in the United States. It has continued to receive strong support in recent years, particularly as a result of the research of Max Fink (1979).

However, the primary clinical indication for ECT today is no longer schizophrenia but depression, an indication based on the original research of the American A. E. Bennett (1940). Bennett was also the first to administer a muscle-relaxing compound, curare, for the prevention of fractures, a frequent complication of ECT (Bennett 1940; Bennett and Wilbur 1944).

During the later 1950s, an alternative to electrically induced convulsions—convulsions induced by the administration of flurothyl—was developed in the United States by Krantz and co-workers (1957). But because this treatment did not offer any advantages over ECT, clinical research with flurothyl was terminated during the 1970s.

Simultaneously with insulin coma and ECT, psychosurgery was introduced. Prompted by Jacobsen's (1935) demonstration at Yale that frontal lobe ablation in a monkey had a calming effect, the first successful lobotomies—severing the connection between the thalamus and frontal lobe—were performed in Portugal by Moniz and Lima in the mid 1930s. Subsequently, a wide variety of psychosurgical techniques and procedures were developed in the United States. They included the bilateral closed operation (Freeman and Watts 1936), open procedures, cortical undercutting, topectomy, thalamotomy, the bimedial operation, and several others. During the 1960s, increasing public concern about the ethics of psychosurgery and questions about its effectiveness led to virtual abandonment of research in this field. Nevertheless, renewed demonstration of its effectiveness and safety, together with improvement of stereotactic techniques, led to a revival of psychosurgery in disabling obsessive-compulsive disorder. Today, at least two procedures are used successfully in obsessive-compulsive disorder: one of these is cingulotomy and the other is anterior capsulotomy, based on cutting the direct interconnections between the frontal lobes and the limbic system (Ballantine et al. 1987; Mindus et al. 1991).

Psychological Treatments

North American contributions to both individual and group psychotherapy are immense. They include the introduction of Rogers's client-centered counseling (Rogers 1959), transactional analysis developed by Berne (1966), short-term anxiety-provoking psychotherapy developed at Harvard University by Sifneos (1972), short-term dynamic psychotherapy developed at McGill University in Canada by Davanloo (1978), time-limited psychotherapy developed at Boston University by Mann (1973), and short-term interpersonal psychotherapy developed in New York by Weissman and Klerman, among many others (Weissman and Klerman 1973). Although research in the dynamic psychotherapies often operated without consideration of the boundaries of diagnostic groups delineated in current classifications, cognitive therapy, which was developed in the United States by Aaron Beck (1976), offers a treatment modality that can be used as an alternative or as a supplementary therapy to other treatments in patients with emotional disorders, especially the anxiety disorders, phobias, and depressions.

Similarly, behavior therapy, deeply rooted in the research (operant conditioning) of Skinner and his associates at Harvard University, can be used as an alternative or as a supplementary therapy to other treatments in patients with a variety of psychiatric disorders (e.g., alcoholism, sexual dysfunctions, phobias, and even psychoses).

The research of Wolpe (1973) and his associates at Temple University in Philadelphia led to the development of several behavior therapy techniques especially relevant to the treatment of anxiety disorders and the modification of numerous behavioral anomalies.

Introduction of Psychotropics

Another period of therapeutic research in American psychiatry began in the early 1950s with the introduction of new psychotropic drugs. Because of their selective action on different brain structures, they yielded treatments with increasing specificity. Furthermore, because pharmacotherapy was more readily accessible than any of the previous treatments, the introduction of psychotropics led to therapeutic research in American psychiatry on an unprecedented scale.

In historical sequence, first came clinical studies with chlorpromazine, the first phenothiazine neuroleptic. They were triggered by Delay and Deniker's (1952) recognition, in France, of the drug's antipsychotic effects. Although Delay and Deniker's observations were confirmed within a year by Staehelin (1954) and Kielholz (1954) in Switzerland and subsequently by Lehmann and Hanrahan (1954) in Canada, it was not until the early 1960s that the therapeutic effects of chlorpromazine on schizophrenia patients were established beyond reasonable doubt by the U.S. Veterans Administration Collaborative Studies (Casey et al. 1960).

The isolation of reserpine from a medicinal plant, *Rauwolfia serpentina*, by Bein et al. (1953) was followed by the clinical trials of Kline (1954) at Rockland State Hospital in New York. Despite the favorable therapeutic effects of reserpine in schizophrenic patients, its use in the treatment of schizophrenia has been virtually abandoned because of its mood depressant and other side effects.

Research on meprobamate, an analog of the muscle relaxant mephenesin, ran parallel with the research on chlorpromazine and reserpine unleashed by Berger's (1954) report on its pharmacological properties. Within a short time, meprobamate became one of the most extensively used drugs for the treatment of anxiety. Although the use of meprobamate has been virtually abandoned today, in a historical perspective, meprobamate played an important role; it provided a bridge between the sedative barbiturates and the anxiolytic benzodiazepines. Probably even more important is that meprobamate extended the scope of pharmacological treatment from the psychoses to the neuroses.

Research on meprobamate was followed by research leading to the clinical development of iproniazid, the first monoamine oxidase inhibitor (MAOI) antidepressant. Although the findings of Crane (1957) and, independently, of Loomer et al. (1957) were supportive of antidepressant effects, research with iproniazid was terminated because of the hepatotoxicity of the drug. But research with other MAOIs, such as phenelzine and tranylcypromine, continued and indicated that MAOIs have a place in the treatment of anxious depression.

At the same time, the clinical development of imipramine, the first tricyclic antidepressant, was under way. It was sparked by the recognition of the antidepressant effect of the drug by Kuhn in Switzerland (1957). Although Kuhn's observations were confirmed within a year by Kielholz and Battegay (1958) in Europe and Lehmann et al. (1958) in Canada, it was not until the mid-1960s that the antidepressant effects of imipramine were established beyond a reasonable doubt in the United States by Klerman and Cole (1965).

Research with tricyclic antidepressants was followed by research on the clinical development of chlordiazepoxide, the first benzodiazepine anxiolytic drug. It was triggered by Randall's (1960) demonstration that, like meprobamate, chlordiazepoxide has "hypnotic, sedative and antistrychnine effects in mice." In later clinical studies, the anxiolytic effects of chlordiazepoxide were borne out.

Research with chlordiazepoxide was followed by research on lithium, the first mood-stabilizing drug, after the demonstration of the mood-stabilizing effects of lithium in manic-depressive psychosis by Schou in Denmark (1959). Schou's consistent findings were substantiated by the results of a large-scale clinical investigation conducted by Prien et al. (1972) in the United States.

With the substantiation of lithium's effectiveness in patients with bipolar illness, therapeutic research in American psychiatry had succeeded in developing pharmacological treatment for the anxiety disorders, unipolar and bipolar affective illness, and schizophrenia.

Centrally Conducted Clinical Investigations

A good case could be made that centrally (and multicentrally) conducted clinical drug development—resembling centrally coordinated nosological development—is one of the most important recent contributions to therapeutic research by American psychiatry.

The Psychopharmacology Service Center was created by the National Institute of Mental Health (NIMH) during the late 1950s. It was the Psychopharmacology Service Center, directed by Jonathan Cole, that developed the necessary machinery—in the form of Early Clinical Drug Evaluation Units—to render the new drugs available for safe and effective clinical use within a short period and to create the necessary methodology for the clinical development and evaluation of new psychotropic drugs. Implementation of this methodology is intimately linked to the establishment of the Biometric Laboratory Information Processing System, which included a standardized assessment battery and data base.

NOSOLOGY

First Period

The roots of nosological research in American psychiatry are again found in the work of Benjamin Rush, the first American physician to write about mental illness. His book, *Medical Inquiries and Observations Upon the Diseases of the Mind,* published in 1812, was to remain the only original American textbook of psychiatry for about 70 years.

Born in Philadelphia, in the same year as Philippe Pinel (born 1745), Rush studied medicine in Edinburgh, where he was exposed to the teachings of William Cullen (1712–1790). Although sharing Cullen's view that "diseases of the mind" are biological (organic), he was at variance with Cullen's all-embracing diagnostic concept of "neurosis" and elaborate classifications of illness.

There was an intimate relationship between the conceptual frameworks of Rush and Pinel in that both perceived "diseases of the mind" or "mental derangements" as an integral part of medicine. Nevertheless, for Rush the boundaries of diseases of the mind extended far beyond Pinel's scope of medical madness and included conditions such as hysteria and hypochondriasis.

Rush also perceived alcoholism as a medical disease—an unprecedented view in the late eighteenth and early nineteenth centuries. Rush's influence was so strong that by 1841 the first institution specializing in the treatment and study of alcoholism was opened in Boston. And in 1876, *The Journal of Inebriety* promoted Rush's contention that "inebriety is a neurosis and a psychosis." Nevertheless, it was not until the end of the 1950s that the disease concept of alcoholism received substantial support from Jellinek's (1960) work.

Rush (1812) also recognized that "derangement of moral faculties" may be present in individuals "with good intellect and sound reason." Rush's text, in which such cases of derangement were discussed, was published more than two decades before Pritchard described and coined the term "moral insanity." Thus, it is reasonable to assume that it was the work of Rush (1812) and not of J.-C. Pritchard (1786–1848), as is commonly believed, that led to our current diagnostic concept of sociopathy or antisocial personality (Craft 1965).

Second Period

Although Benjamin Rush set the stage for the development of nosological research in American psychiatry, the contribution of George Miller Beard (1839–1883) to American nosological research was in focusing attention on a possible relationship between adverse life circumstances and mental illness.

The great frequency of "nostalgia" as a medical diagnosis was noted during the Civil War by many physicians in the Union army. They observed the symptoms of sadness and grief in young soldiers separated from their homes and families. Da Costa (1871) reported a condition he referred to as the "irritable heart syndrome" among the military personnel. Nevertheless, it was Beard's (1869) paper "Neurasthenia and Nervous Exhaustion," published in the *Boston Medical and Surgical Journal* and his "Practical Treatise on Nervous Exhaustion," which appeared in 1880, that focused attention on the possibility that environmental factors may play a role in the development of mental disease.

The perception that neurasthenia was a disease of American civilization and the belief that rapid urbanization brought about the epidemic of fatigue and weakness by "exhausting the nervous system" and causing "weak nerves" hit the foundation of European psychiatry—still excessively preoccupied with constitution, predisposition, heredity, and degeneration—like a bombshell. Nevertheless, Beard's concept of neurasthenia became popular in Europe because it offered an apparent neurological explanation for many bodily and psychological complaints. It was especially appealing to the pragmatists because it was packaged with a seemingly rational treatment: rest cure. American neurology's rest cure, proposed by Weir Mitchell, consisted of the removal of the patient from the family, usually to an isolated rural setting where rest and rich foods were prescribed to bolster an assumedly "weak" nervous system.

Despite its great popularity and wide acceptance, the diagnostic concept of neurasthenia could not be verified by subsequent American nosological research. Therefore, neurasthenia was assimilated into the more clearly defined diagnostic concept of anxiety neurosis in Woodruff et al.'s (1974) monograph "Psychiatric Diagnosis," the first American text focused on nosological issues, and into the American diagnostic concept of dysthymia in DSM-III and DSM-III-R (American Psychiatric Association 1980, 1987). Paradoxically, the old American concept of neurasthenia was retained with its definition virtually unchanged in ICD-9 and ICD-10 (World Health Organization 1975, 1992).

Third Period

The third period of nosological research in American psychiatry was triggered by the discovery of relatively specific drug therapies during the 1950s and 1960s and the recognition that "with the availability of lithium and neuroleptic drugs, distinguishing between mania and schizophrenia—once an interesting academic exercise—might now determine how a patient was treated" (Goodwin and Guze 1989, p. 1). It was this recognition that led to the emergence of neo-Kraepelinian activity in the Department of Psychiatry of Washington University in St. Louis during the 1970s. The St. Louis group recognized that one of the essential prerequisites for achieving their purpose was the development of a methodology for the validation of psychiatric diagnosis. They were also aware that another prerequisite was the development of a methodology that could facilitate consistent diagnostic definitions.

In one of their classic articles, "Establishment of Diagnostic Validity in Psychiatric Illness: Its Application to Schizophrenia," Robins and Guze (1970) emphasized the importance of using external validators in confirming psychiatric diagnoses: correlations between the disease and findings in laboratory testing, follow-up clinical investigations in terms of course and outcome of the illness, family and genetic studies, and response to treatment and social and economic factors. In another article, "Diagnostic Criteria for Use in Psychiatric Research," Feighner et al. (1972) described criteria for the identification of clinically more homogeneous psychiatric populations.

The Biometric Research Department of the New York State Psychiatric Institute was opened in 1956. Under the brilliant leadership of its first director, Joseph Zubin, who served as director from 1956 to 1976, it has become an important force in the facilitation of nosological research in American psychiatry by rendering accessible existing psychometric methods and new statistical techniques, including factor and cluster analyses.

By making it possible to apply many multivariate statistical procedures that could not have been undertaken manually, the introduction of electronic computers in the 1960s stimulated research to classify various dimensional personality traits into patterns and to construct "empirical psychopathologic systems" (Pichot 1983). Although this new quantitative psychopathological approach has inspired a large number of research projects in American psychiatry, it has so far contributed little to progress in psychiatric nosology. However, the psychometric method and biostatistical techniques have opened new perspectives in the study of the reliability of categorical nosological concepts.

An important contribution to this area of research was the introduction of kappa statistics by Fleiss et al. (1972). Kappa is an intraclass correlation coefficient that is corrected for chance and has become essential in the measurement of the degree of concordance and reliability of diagnoses among diagnosticians. By the 1980s, kappa statistics had become one of the most important tools in the detection of reliability problems relevant to psychiatric diagnoses.

Collaboration between the St. Louis group, which was focused on validity, and the New York group, which was focused on reliability, led to the development of the Research Diagnostic Criteria by Spitzer et al. (1975) and the construction of the Schedule for Affective Disorders and Schizophrenia—useful in accessing the diagnostic criteria—by Spitzer and Endicott (1978). This collaboration opened the path for the development of DSM-III, the most important single contribution to nosological progress made by American psychiatrists.

American Psychiatric Association: The New DSM System

By using a multiaxial operational evaluation, DSM-III has the unique capability to combine the two major ancient traditions of medicine. The first is the tradition of Galen (131–201 A.D.), which focused on the study of disease. Disease is evaluated in DSM-III on the basis of categorical judgments and is recorded on Axes I, II, and III of DSM-III, which deal with clinical psychiatric syndromes, personality disorders, and medical illness, respectively. The second is the tradition of Hippocrates, which focused on the treatment of individual patients. Treatment of individual patients is evaluated in DSM-III on the basis of dimensional ratings and recorded on Axes IV and V, which deal with psychosocial stressors and level of adaptive functioning (Mezzich 1980).

Although DSM-III and DSM-III-R are not perfect, it is difficult to deny that American research has provided a nosology for the reliable identification of mental disorders and, thereby, for the selection of suitable populations for the validation of nosological concepts and for the testing of research hypotheses generated by the rapidly advancing basic sciences (e.g., molecular biology and genetics).

PATHOLOGY

Progress in modern psychiatric research in America has occurred at such an extraordinary rate during the last three decades that it is difficult to give even a thumbnail sketch of it in a brief chapter. Fortunately, in the centenary publication of the American Psychiatric Association, J. C. Whitehorn (1944) covered this subject to some extent until 1944. In their book *The First Psychiatric Institute*, L. C. Kolb and L. Roizin (1993) provide further admirable source material on psychiatric research. The development of psychiatric research in Canada until the 1960s recently was covered by R. A. Cleghorn (1984).

The New York State Psychiatric Institute must be viewed as the cradle of systematic psychiatric research in America. Founded in 1895 as the Pathological Institute of the New York State Hospitals (renamed the New York State Psychiatric Institute in 1906), it was certainly the first institute dedicated primarily to psychiatric research in America— probably the first American institute dedicated mainly to any medical research. Its first director, Ira Van Gieson, was a pathologist of international reputation who had the vision that psychiatric research would have to be a "correlation of sciences" (Van Gieson 1898). He recruited a team of excellent researchers in anthropology, bacteriology, neurology, pathology, physiological chemistry, psychology, and cellular biology. Unfortunately, he was forced to resign within 5 years because of an ugly political controversy involving the new president of the New York State Commission on Lunacy. The arguments had been initiated by a group of narrow-minded mental hospital superintendents who insisted that basic research was a luxury and demanded that the institute's main function should be teaching medical staff who were entering the state hospitals (Wise 1900). Only after the governor of the state (then Theodore Roosevelt) had dismissed the man responsible for this attack and had appointed Frederick Peterson, a progressive psychiatrist who had studied widely in Europe, to take charge of the Commission on Lunacy was the new institute given the high sign for its future brilliant development.

Peterson recruited Adolf Meyer from Worcester State Hospital in Massachusetts to be the new director of the Psychiatric Institute. Meyer insisted that the institute be relocated near the Manhattan State Hospital because he was convinced that any valid research in psychiatry must be carried out in close contact with patients. However, the first significant discovery at the Psychiatric Institute, which immediately drew the whole scientific world's attention to it, was made in 1905 by pathologists. J. W. Moore, a staff member of the institute, who was working with H. Noguchi from the Rockefeller Institute, demonstrated the presence of *Treponema pallidum* in the brains of patients with syphilitic general paresis (Noguchi and Moore 1913). This was the first discovery of the causative agent of a mental disease (Figure 2–1). Some 20 years later this discovery was followed by Joseph Goldberger's discovery of the nutritional deficiency that causes pellagra. No new causes of important mental diseases–other than some secondary to gross toxic,

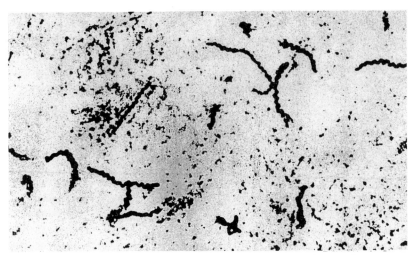

Figure 2–1. Noguchi and Moore's discovery of the cause of general paresis. Reprinted from Kolb LC, Roizin L: *The First Psychiatric Institute: How Research and Education Changed Practice.* Washington, DC, American Psychiatric Press, 1993, p. 31. Used with permission. Copyright 1993 American Psychiatric Press.

metabolic, or organic factors that are of no major significance for public health–have been discovered since then. We have not yet found definitive causal factors for the major functional mental diseases: affective disorders and schizophrenia. However, we have some new knowledge about genetic, neuropsychological, and personal history criteria that, in many cases, indicate vulnerability to these disorders.

The Search for the Causes of Schizophrenia

In 1923, C. B. Dunlap, who worked at the Psychiatric Institute, concluded after a careful review of all published data and a controlled study that there was no basis for the statements by Alzheimer and other European researchers that schizophrenia was an organic brain disease. It gradually became generally accepted that schizophrenia was entirely functional (at least, that it was not associated with any anatomical abnormality in the brain). However, in the 1970s, the new techniques of computed tomography, positron-emission tomography, single photon emission computed tomography, and magnetic resonance imaging revealed structural and functional characteristics in the brain that seemed to be associated with schizophrenia. Andreasen et al. (1982), Buchsbaum et al. (1984), Weinberger (1987), and many others have been working in this area with schizophrenic patients during the last two decades. It should be noted here that two American investigators, L. Sokoloff at NIMH and P. C. Lautebur at New York's Stonybrook

University, played significant roles in the development of some of these sophisticated new research tools in the 1970s—the former with positron-emission tomography (Sokoloff et al. 1977), and the latter with magnetic resonance imaging (Lautebur 1979).

The academic teaching in most American universities in the 1940s considered schizophrenia to be a functional disease without any organic substrate. This concept had to be modified after the therapeutic breakthrough that came with the discovery of the antipsychotic drugs. It was now clear that there were physical factors involved in the etiology of schizophrenia. Because chemical substances could suppress specific psychotic symptoms, an intensive search for the drugs' mechanisms of action and for biochemical causal factors was begun in many laboratories.

After the various unspecific shock therapies for schizophrenia in the 1930s and 1940s, H. E. Himwich and other investigators (1938) held the theory that schizophrenia was due to general hypoxic functioning of the organism. Before this time, endocrinological theories (in particular hypogonadism) had been proposed; however, in 1952, a systematic study of biopsies of the testes of the entire male population of the research ward of Worcester State Hospital in Massachusetts refuted this hypothesis. Still earlier, in the 1920s, Lewis (1925) had looked for thyroid and adrenal disorders and also at primary hypoplasia of the cardiovascular system as etiological factors in dementia praecox. His report was based on 4,800 autopsies. In 1950, after the discovery of the adrenocortical hormones, Hoagland and Pincus (1950) proposed adrenocortical dysfunction as an important etiological factor in schizophrenia. None of these theories would prevail.

In the late 1950s, A. Hoffer and H. Osmond (1959), working in Canada, postulated that schizophrenia was caused by faulty methylation of adrenaline, resulting in production of the hallucinogenic substance adrenochrome. However, the presence of this substance could never be demonstrated in schizophrenic patients. A few years later, J. J. Friedhoff and E. Van Winkel (1963) drew attention to another transmethylation product that manifested its presence as a "pink spot" in the chromatograms of schizophrenic patients. However, in the end the transmethylation theory found little support.

Also in the late 1950s and early 1960s, R. G. Heath caused a stir with his claim that he had isolated from schizophrenic patients a protein that he called taraxein, which, he reported, could temporarily produce schizophrenic symptoms when administered to healthy subjects. His results could not be confirmed (Heath et al. 1957).

About the time that antipsychotic drug treatment was introduced, D. W. Woolley and E. Shaw (1954) suggested that the recently discovered neurotransmitter serotonin might be responsible for schizophrenia symptoms. However, some 10 years later, A. Carlsson, who had worked in B. B. Brodie's laboratory at NIMH, proposed that the dopaminergic theory was more convincing for the pathogenesis of schizophrenia (Carlsson and Lindqvist 1963). This is still the most widely accepted theory today.

Brain Physiology

In 1937, J. W. Papez published an intriguing hypothesis: emotions are not only intangible experiences, they are processed through a circuit in the brain—now called the Papez circuit—that involves the limbic lobe, septal region, amygdala, and hippocampus before they reach the cortex and actual awareness (Papez 1937). P. D. MacLean (1952) expanded this theory and referred to the relevant brain structures as the limbic system or the visceral brain, because of the many autonomic connections. Kety and Schmidt (1948) opened an important scientific window on the metabolism of the human brain when they developed the first reliable method of measuring cerebral blood flow. Experimental evidence provided by Moruzzi and Magoun (1949) threw light on the functions of the reticular activating system in the brain, a system that plays an essential role in regulating and maintaining the states of arousal, wakefulness, and sleep.

Systematic studies of the electroencephalogram as a tool for the diagnosis of psychiatric disorders were started by Charles Shagass in the early 1950s in Canada. Penfield and Jasper's (1954) classic experiments with electrical stimulation of limbic structures during neurosurgery were also undertaken in Canada in the early 1950s. They demonstrated that such stimulation could elicit déjà vu experiences and evoke old memories. The separate functions of the human hemispheres when their integration is disrupted by lesions were studied during these decades by Sperry (1982), who received the Nobel prize in 1981 for his ground-breaking work. Neuroscience was now prepared for the advent of the new drugs and the development of psychopharmacology.

Neurochemistry

A major breakthrough was made by G. A. Jervis in the late 1930s when he identified phenylketonuria as the cause of a special type of mental retardation. Persons with this genetic disorder are unable to metabolize phenylalanine in their food (Jervis et al. 1940). This discovery made it possible later to detect the defect in newborns and to develop preventive measures.

The enormous amount of research on neurotransmitters in the 1950s, 1960s, and 1970s was foreshadowed by the work of H. Waelsh, who in the 1940s laid a solid foundation for this research with his work on glutamic acid and γ-aminobutyric acid (GABA), methionine, glutathione, and protein metabolism (Waelsh and Rittenberg 1942). M. M. Rapport et al. isolated serotonin in 1948, recognizing it at that time mainly as a "serum vasoconstrictor."

In the late 1960s, "orthomolecular psychiatry" represented a temporary, but strange, invasion into psychiatry by Linus Pauling, who received two Nobel prizes in 1954 and 1963 but who was certainly not an expert in the field of mental science. Pauling, a chemist, postulated that mental disorders were caused by a wrong mixture or balance of molecules in the brain. He elaborated his theory with speculations about vitamin deficiencies (Pauling 1968).

The Neurotransmitters

During the 1920s and 1930s, a heated scientific battle was fought on the international scene between those researchers who were convinced that interneuronal communication was electrical and those who believed that chemical transmitters were the principal actors in the process. In the 1920s, W. B. Cannon at Harvard University was the American protagonist for the chemical transmission of nervous excitation to the effector cells. He developed the now popular fight-flight notion based on the action of "sympathin," a mixture of epinephrine and norepinephrine, and created the famous concept of homeostasis. In the late 1950s, B. B. Brodie at NIMH discovered that the behavioral and chemical actions of reserpine could serve as a model for depression and explained the mechanism of action of antidepressant drugs with regard to their effects on serotonin. Julius Axelrod, a 1970 Nobel laureate also at NIMH, elucidated their effects on the catecholamines (Axelrod and Udenfriend 1970).

Many neuropeptides were soon added to the monoamines as chemical modifiers, messengers, and transmitters in the central nervous system. The often subtle—and sometimes dramatic—dynamics of chemical receptors on brain cell membranes, coupled with complex feedback mechanisms, elucidated synaptic transmission.

Pioneering work during the 1970s on the effects of psychopharmacological agents on neurons included S. H. Snyder's work with opiate receptors; R. F. Squires's discovery of benzodiazepine receptors; P. Seeman's studies of neuroleptic receptors; and the work of G. K. Aghajanian, B. S. and W. E. Bunney, F. Sulser, J. J. Schildkraut, J. Maas, and many others.

Psychology

Psychologists have left their imprint on American psychiatry, both in therapy and research. During the early part of the century, J. B. Watson's behaviorism tried to link the continuous search for the origins of mental functioning and illness almost exclusively to the environment. Under Adolf Meyer's directorship at Johns Hopkins Hospital, Watson was the head of the psychological laboratory until 1920.

In the 1940s and 1950s, B. F. Skinner's experiments and theories on the application of animal operant conditioning to the motivation of human behavior started to influence psychiatric thinking, and his stimulus-response, operational approach contributed to the development of new behavioral and cognitive therapies. It also led to the weakening of the dominance of the psychoanalytic perspective for the explanation of mental phenomena.

Experimental evidence and theoretical elaborations on motivation, attachment, and neurosis in primates that had potential application to humans were developed during the 1940s by D. O. Hebb in Canada and in the 1960s by H. F. Harlow in the United States. J. Olds experimentally discovered a "pleasure center" in the septal region of animals in the 1960s, and other neuroscientists thought that because the septal region is part of the limbic system, this finding may be applied to humans (Olds and Travis 1960).

Psychodynamics

In the 1930s, many psychoanalysts immigrated to the United States, and theoretical psychodynamics flourished. But largely independent of the European influence, H. Stack Sullivan became one of the most original American-born psychiatric theorists at that time. He collaborated with the political scientist Harold Lasswell and accepted the philosophy of the physicist P. W. Bridgman. Stack Sullivan defined psychiatry as the study of interpersonal relations and developed his own theory of personality development (Perry 1982). R. Schilder, one of the early immigrant analysts, is best known for coining the term "body image," a concept that has acquired particular importance in today's epidemic of eating disorders. In the 1960s, H. Hartmann (1964) drew the attention of analysts to the autonomy of the ego. E. H. Erikson (1959) noted the various stages of maturing identity. K. Horney (1937) stressed the influence of culture and environment on the development of neurosis. F. Alexander (1950) believed that psychosomatic illness was connected with the autonomic nervous system and chronic psychological stress. F. Dunbar (1954) postulated that different personality types were characteristic of specific psychosomatic diseases. In the 1970s and 1980s, with increasing psychiatric interest in borderline and narcissistic personality disorders, the differences in the theories of Kohut (1971) and Kernberg (1975) were—and still are—widely discussed.

Genetics

Clinicians have known for more than 200 years that major mental illness often runs in families. Scientists have consolidated this clinical knowledge into systematically confirmed observations but had to contend with the doubt that these might be due to environmental factors. In the 1940s, F. J. Kallmann started hereditary twin studies of the functional mental disorders. He continued his work over several decades and showed that if a major functional mental disorder occurred in twins, there was a very significant difference between the concordance in monozygotic twins and that in dizygotic twins, thus clearly proving a strong hereditary component of functional mental disorders (Kallmann 1953). One of his co-workers, N. Erlenmeyer-Kimling, established at the New York State Psychiatric Institute a cohort of children from high-risk families to study early signs of future psychosis. This longitudinal study is still going on.

Even more convincing with respect to the genetic component of schizophrenia were studies in Oregon and Denmark of children from high-risk families who were raised in foster homes or adopted (Heston 1966; Kety et al. 1968). Compared with adopted children of nonschizophrenic biological parents, children adopted away from schizophrenic mothers were significantly more likely to develop schizophrenia and other mental disorders that the investigators called schizophrenia spectrum diseases. Using a similar method later in another Danish study, Goodwin et al. (1977) found that the incidence of psychopathology in adopted-away daughters of alcoholic biological parents was greater than that in the general population.

It was now clear that the etiology of many mental disorders involved both genetic and environmental factors. With the recent emergence of sophisticated molecular biology, the search has now begun in earnest for the genes associated with major mental diseases. A promising start was made when J. F. Gusella and his co-workers (1983) were able to localize, and later to isolate, the gene for Huntington's disease on the short arm of chromosome 4. This discovery allowed for the development of a genetic test that is useful for genetic counseling.

Linkage studies for the genes of more complex diseases, like schizophrenia and affective disorders, have so far been more frustrating, probably because their pathology is not traceable to a single gene. In the late 1980s, the Canadian researcher A. Bassett and co-workers (1988) studied a schizophrenic family with a chromosome anomaly and reported linkage with chromosome 5. But several attempts by others to replicate these results have failed. At Harvard, J. A. Egeland's group (1987), in an interesting study of an Amish community, thought that they had localized a gene for bipolar affective disorder on chromosome 11, but recently they had to reevaluate their results and there is now some doubt about their original findings. About the same time, M. Baron (1992) reported linkage of an affective disorder gene to the X chromosome. However, again, other researchers could not reproduce their results. Definitive answers to the questions of the genetic etiology of mental disorders may well have to wait until we have a more complete knowledge of the human genome.

EPIDEMIOLOGY

Statistics fascinated American psychiatrists—or alienists, as they were called during the nineteenth century when most psychiatrists were enthusiastic collectors of data about patients residing in their hospitals. The numbers they collected were to support administrative and policy-making procedures and to produce proof of the curability of mental patients and of the legitimacy of public mental hospitals. Statistics were also gathered to support the solid belief that mental disease was caused not only by organic factors, but also by a morbid environment from which the patients had to be temporarily liberated to the sane environment of hospitals where they received "moral treatment" (Grob 1985). In the halls of history, we can thus hear harbingers of the antipsychiatrists' voices of the 1960s that said that "normal" civilization was really pathogenic.

The question of whether the incidence of mental illness was increasing tantalized the psychiatric community. In the 1850s, the Massachusetts legislature had become concerned about an unexpectedly rapid growth of populations in mental hospitals. A Commission on Lunacy was set up. Edward Jarvis, a physician who had published a paper on the subject, was put in charge of it, and he produced a long report on the size of mental hospitals and the sex, race, and economic status of their patients. But the report was of little epidemiological value. Jarvis rightly pointed out that institutional data could not prove that there was a real increase in the incidence of insanity in the population, but he still accepted the increase as a fact and tried to explain it by blaming the noxious changes in the environment caused by urbanization, which resulted in "more opportunities and rewards for great and excessive mental action, more uncertain and hazardous employments and consequently more disappointments, more means and provocations for sensual indulgence" (Jarvis 1852, p. 365).

Today, we seek to explain the recent epidemiological enigma of an unprecedented rise of the incidence of depression and suicide in the young population (Klerman and Weissman 1989). This rise has been seen as possibly being related to the increased promises and expectations arising from the iconoclastic atmosphere of the 1960s and greater frustrations and disappointments encountered in the real world of the

1980s and 1990s. A recent publication reports on 12 different studies carried out in six different geographical areas covering several continents. These studies demonstrated a worldwide increase of the incidence and prevalence of depression, which, speculatively, may be related to varying marital stability and fragmented family structure, as well as to large-scale stressful events in some countries (Cross-National Collaborative Group 1992).

Starting in 1840, the federal government regularly undertook a census of mentally afflicted persons, and for three decades Jarvis served as an adviser to the census. In 1870, Francis A. Walker was appointed superintendent of the census. Walker was an economist and later became president of the Massachusetts Institute of Technology. He gave the task of preparing a report on the "defective, dependent and delinquent classes" to Frederick H. Wines, also a nonphysician, as part of the 10th census (U.S. Bureau of the Census 1888). The next census was prepared by John Shav Billings, who was a physician and had been the seventh president of the American Public Health Association. Billings's report was no longer focused on dependency, but was more clinical, presenting data on the "Insane, Feeble Minded, Deaf and Dumb and Blind."

By the time of the next census in 1904, the waves of immigrants from Europe had aroused concerns about the purity (and, presumably, sanity?) of the American population. That led to widespread preoccupation with eugenic theory and even to legislation involving involuntary sterilization laws for mentally retarded and ill persons in some states. (Three decades later, Hitler used such pseudoscience as justification for the Nazi laws that ordered involuntary sterilization and killing of such individuals.) However, the census of 1910 was organized by Joseph A. Hill, a political economist who had studied abroad. He concluded that there was little evidence of an increase of insanity and no evidence that immigration had any bearing on its incidence.

With Clifford W. Beer's (1876–1943) publication in 1908 of his own story, *A Mind That Found Itself*, the attention of psychiatrists began to move to mental health in the community.

Interest in a more sophisticated use of statistics in the field of mental health led to a growing desire for a more reliable classification of mental diseases. A new leader in the field was Horatio M. Pollock, who held the position of director of mental hygiene statistics at the New York State Department of Mental Hygiene. Interestingly, the father of modern American psychiatry, Adolf Meyer (1866–1950), was opposed to general classifications because he was convinced that each psychiatric patient required individual evaluation of his or her history.

Nevertheless, by 1920 the Census Bureau had established a new system of classification of mental disorders, although the architects of this system remained well aware of the difficulties of distinguishing between symptoms and diseases.

Also in the 1920s, epidemiological researchers in American psychiatry began using scientific methodology and the data provided by the U.S. Bureau of the Census, the New York State Office of Mental Hygiene, and the Massachusetts Commission of Mental Diseases. Benjamin Malzberg followed Pollock in 1944 as the chief of the statistical department at the New York State Office of Mental Hygiene. He published widely on the relationship of variables such as age, sex, religion, economic status, and literacy with mental illness. He is best known for his study of migration and mental illness (Malzberg and Lee 1956).

In Massachusetts, Neil A. Dayton obtained grant support from the Rockefeller Foundation for a longitudinal study of admission rates, and in 1940, he published "New Facts on Mental Disorders: Study of 89,190 Cases." His study used data on patients in Massachusetts mental hospitals between 1917 and 1933 (Dayton 1940).

The special problems of psychiatric epidemiology were by then fully recognized: unknown etiology of most mental disorders; subjective data; different nosologies (e.g., of followers of Kraepelin, Meyer, and Freud); and changing descriptive classifications.

Moving from mental hospital data to community studies for a truer evaluation of incidence and prevalence of mental disorders presented new methodological problems. As early as 1916, Aaron Rosanoff had made an attempt in this direction in Nassau County, New York. Robert and Helen Lynd's seminal study, "Middletown" (Lynd and Lynd 1929), and R. E. L. Farris and H. W. Dunham's ground-breaking work, *Mental Disorders in Urban Areas* (1939), spawned the controversial theories that migration or sociogenic factors could account for the accumulation of schizophrenic patients in disadvantaged areas of large cities.

The Bureau of the Census issued its last report in 1948. After that, NIMH took over the task with the National Reporting Program in its Division of Biometry and Epidemiology. Outstanding among the many postwar studies was Hollingshead and Redlich's (1958) *Social Class and Mental Illness: A Community Study.* Covering five distinct social classes, it found an 8 in 1,000 prevalence rate of treated mental patients for a 6-month period. H. Goldhamer and A. W. Marshall (1953) revisited a theme that Jarvis had examined a hundred years earlier with their work on "Psychosis and Civilization." Dohrenwend et al. (1980) published a survey of 16 epidemiological studies before World War II and more than 60 postwar studies. They found consistently significant relationships between mental disorders and social class, gender, and urban versus rural residence.

Alexander Leighton and co-workers (1963) undertook a long-term study of a rural community in Canada, covering 20,000 people. However, their diagnoses were based on the old criteria of DSM-I (American Psychiatric Association 1952), as was the Baltimore Morbidity Study by P. V. Lemkau.

The Midtown Manhattan Study was based on a population of 1,660 Manhattan residents. It was performed by using a structured psychiatric interview and revealed that 23.4% of the sampled population suffered from significant mental impairment (Srole et al. 1962).

The need for reliable tools to identify and diagnose mental disorders had become more and more pressing and led to the construction of the Present State Examination in England in the early 1960s. It was used in the International Pilot Study of Schizophrenia (1965), which was sponsored by the World Health Organization, and in the U.S.–U.K. Diagnostic Project. The latter was initiated and organized by the New York State Office of Mental Health, mainly by Joseph Zubin, in the 1960s. Its impetus had come from a puzzling observation by Morton Kramer at NIMH, to the effect that there seemed to be a significantly greater incidence and prevalence of schizophrenia, with corresponding smaller ratios of affective disorders, in the United States compared with the United Kingdom. The important results of this project showed that this epidemiological discrepancy was not true, but was mainly due to a generalized diagnostic error committed by most American psychiatrists at that time.

The Present State Examination, as a diagnostic instrument, was followed by the Schedule for Affective Disorders and Schizophrenia, a structured interview based on the Research Diagnostic Criteria. The Lifetime Version of the Schedule for Affective Disorders and Schizophrenia was used to diagnose more than 500 residents of the community of New Haven, Connecticut.

With the development of DSM-III by Robert Spitzer and his co-workers at the New York State Psychiatric Institute during the 1970s, a new diagnostic classification of unprecedented reliability had appeared. It soon found international acceptance and has served as a boost to clinical and nosological, as well as epidemiological, research.

In 1981, NIMH developed the Diagnostic Interview Schedule, which requires less training of the interviewer, to be employed in the Epidemiological Catchment Area program, which covers 20,000 counties in the United States. This study has revealed an annual or period incidence rate of 5% and a prevalence rate of 15% of mental disorders diagnosable by DSM-III-R at the present time. One of the still-puzzling findings of this program is the increase of depression in progressively younger generations over the years, a trend that had been noted for some time but has now been confirmed and appears to be present also in several countries outside the United States (Cross-National Collaborative Group 1992; Klerman and Weissman 1989).

In summary, epidemiological researchers today have fine-tuned their instruments and methodology and may be expected to contribute substantially to virtually all other arenas of psychiatric research in the years directly ahead.

REFERENCES

Alexander F: Psychosomatic Medicine: Its Principles and Application. New York, WW Norton, 1950

Allen R: On the treatment of insanity. American Journal of Insanity 6:263–283, 1850

American Psychiatric Association: Diagnostic and Statistical Manual: Mental Disorders. Washington, DC, American Psychiatric Association, 1952

American Psychiatric Association: Diagnostic and Statistical Manual of Mental Disorders, 3rd Edition. Washington, DC, American Psychiatric Association, 1980

American Psychiatric Association: Diagnostic and Statistical Manual of Mental Disorders, 3rd Edition, Revised. Washington, DC, American Psychiatric Association, 1987

Andreasen NC, Olsen SA, Dennert JW, et al: Ventricular enlargement in schizophrenia: relationship to positive and negative symptoms. Am J Psychiatry 139:297–302, 1982

Axelrod J, Udenfriend S: Nobel prize: Three share 1970 award for medical research, I: Von Euler and Axelrod. Science October 23, 1970, pp 422–423

Ballantine HT, Bouckoms AJ, Thomas EL, et al: Treatment of psychiatric illness by stereotactic cingulotomy. Biol Psychiatry 22:807–819, 1987

Baron M: Molecular genetics of affective psychoses, in Genetic Research in Psychiatry. Edited by Mendelwicz J, Hippuns H. New York, Springer-Verlag, 1992

Bassett A, McGillivray BC, Jones BD, et al: Partial trisomy chromosome 5 cosegregating with schizophrenia. Lancet 1:799–780, 1988

Beard GM: Neurasthenia and nervous exhaustion.Boston Medical and Surgical Journal 3:217–221, 1869

Beck AT: Cognitive Therapy and the Emotional Disorders. New York, International Universities Press, 1976

Bein HJ, Gross F, Tripod J, et al: Experimentelle Untersuchungen über "Serpasil" (Reserpin) ein nenes, sehr wirksames Rauwolfia Alkaloid mit neuartiger Zentraler Wirkung. Schweiz Med Wochenschr 83:1007–1012, 1953

Bennett AE: Preventing traumatic complications in convulsive shock therapy by curare. JAMA 141:322–324, 1940

Bennett AE, Wilbur CB: Convulsive shock therapy in involutional states after complete failure with previous estrogen treatment. American Journal of Medical Science 208:170–176, 1944

Berger FM: The pharmacological properties of 2-methyl-2-N-propyl-1,3 propanediol bicarbamate (Miltown), a new interneuronal blocking agent. J Pharmacol Exp Ther 112:413–423, 1954

Berne E: Principles of Group Treatment. New York, Oxford University Press, 1966

Buchsbaum MS, DeLisi LE, Holcomb HH, et al: Anteroposterior gradients in cerebral glucose use in schizophrenia and affective disorders. Arch Gen Psychiatry 41:1154–1166, 1984

Carlson ET, Simpson MM: Moral persuasion therapy, in Current Psychiatric Therapies, Vol 4. Edited by Masserman JM. New York, Grune & Stratton, 1964, pp 13–24

Carlsson A, Lindqvist M: Effect of chlorpromazine or haloperidol on formation of 3-methoxytryamine and normetanephrine in mouse brain. Acta Pharmacol 20:140–144, 1963

Casey JF, Bennett LF, Lindley CJ, et al: Drug therapy in schizophrenia: a controlled study of the relative effectiveness of chlorpromazine, promazine, phenobarbital and placebo. Arch Gen Psychiatry 2:210–220, 1960

Cleghorn RA: The development of psychiatric research in Canada up to 1964. Can J Psychiatry 7:551–556, 1984

Cotton HA, Draper JW, Lynch JM: Internal pathology in the functional psychoses. Medical Record (New York) 97:719–725, 1920

Craft M: Ten Studies into Psychopathic Personalities. Bristol, England, Wright & Sons, 1965

Crane JE: Iproniazid (Marsilid) phosphate, a therapeutic agent for mental disorders and debilitating disease. Psychiatric Research Reports 8:142, 1957

Cross-National Collaborative Group: The changing rate of major depression: cross-national comparisons. JAMA 268:3098–3105, 1992

Da Costa JM: On irritable heart, a chronic form of functional cardiac disorder and its consequences. American Journal of Medical Science 61:2–52, 1871

Davanloo H (ed): Basic Principles and Technique of Short-Term Dynamic Psychotherapy. New York, Spectrum, 1978

Dayton NA: New Facts on Mental Disorders: Study of 89,190 Cases. Springfield, IL, Charles C Thomas, 1940

Delay J, Deniker P: Le traitement des psychoses par une méthode neurolytique dérivée de l'hibernothérapie, in Congrès des Médicins Aliénistes et Neurologistes de France, Vol 50. Luxembourg, 1952

Dohrenwend BP, Dohrenwend BS, Gould MS, et al: Mental Illness in the United States. New York, Praeger, 1980

Dunbar F: Emotions and Bodily Changes. New York, Columbia University Press, 1954

Egeland JA, Gerhardt DS, Pauls D, et al: Bipolar affective disorders linked to DNA markers on chromosome 11. Nature 325:393–399, 1987

Erikson EH: Identity and the life cycle, in Psychological Issues (Monograph 1). Edited by Klein GS. New York, International Universities Press, 1959

Farris REL, Dunham HW: Mental Disorders in Urban Areas: An Ecological Study of Schizophrenia and Other Psychoses. Chicago, IL, University of Chicago Press, 1939

Feighner JP, Robins E, Guze SB, et al: Diagnostic criteria for use in psychiatric research. Arch Gen Psychiatry 26:57–63, 1972

Fink M: Convulsive Therapy—Theory and Practice. New York, Raven, 1979

Fleiss JL, Spitzer RL, Endicott J, et al: Quantification of agreement in multiple psychiatric diagnosis. Arch Gen Psychiatry 26:168–171, 1972

Freeman W, Watts JW: Prefrontal lobotomy in agitated depression: report of a case. Medical Annals: District of Columbia 5:326–328, 1936

Friedhoff JJ, Van Winkel E: Conversion of dopamine to 3,4-dimethoxyphenylacetic acid in schizophrenia patients. Nature 199:1271–1272, 1963

Goldhamer H, Marshall AW: Psychosis and Civilization: Two Studies in the Frequency of Mental Disease. Glencoe, IL, Free Press, 1953

Goodwin DW, Guze SB: Psychiatric Diagnosis, 4th Edition. New York, Oxford University Press, 1989

Goodwin DW, Schulsinger F, Knop J, et al: Psychopathology in adopted and nonadopted daughters of alcoholics. Arch Gen Psychiatry 34:1005, 1977

Grinker RR, Spiegel JP: Men Under Stress. Philadelphia, PA, Blakiston, 1945

Grob GN: The origins of American psychiatric epidemiology. Am J Public Health, March 1975 3:229–236, 1985

Gusella JF, Wexler NS, Conneally PM et al: A polymorphic DNA marker genetically linked to Huntington's disease. Nature 306:234–238, 1983

Hartmann H: Essays on Ego Psychology. New York, International Universities Press, 1964

Heath RG, Martens S, Leach BE, et al: Effect on behavior in humans with the administration of taraxein. Am J Psychiatry 114:14–24, 1957

Heinroth JC, quoted in Geschichtliches by Grulhe HW, in Bumke's Handbuch der Geisteskrankheiten, Vol 12, Part 5. Berlin, 1932

Heston L: Psychiatric disorders in foster home reared children of schizophrenic mothers. Br J Psychiatry 112:819–825, 1966

Himwich HE, Alexander FAD, Lipetz B: Effect of acute anoxia produced by breathing nitrogen, on course of schizophrenia. Proc Soc Exp Biol Med 39:367–369, 1938

Hoagland H, Pincus G: The nature of the adrenal stress response failure in schizophrenic man. J Nerv Ment Dis 111:434–439, 1950

Hoffer A, Osmond H.: The adrenochrome model and schizophrenia. J Nerv Ment Dis 123:18–35, 1959

Hollingshead AB, Redlich FC (eds): Social Class and Mental Illness: A Community Study. New York, Wiley, 1958

Horney K: The Neurotic Personality of Our Time. New York, WW Norton, 1937

Horsley JP: Narco-Analysis. London, Oxford University Press, 1943

Jacobsen CF: Functions of frontal association area in primates. Archives of Neurology and Psychiatry 33:558–569, 1935

Jarvis E: On the supposed increase in insanity. American Journal of Insanity 8:333–365, 1852

Jellinek EM: Alcoholism, a genus and some of its species. Can Med Assoc J 83:1341–1345, 1960

Jervis GA, Block RJ, Bolling D et al: Chemical and metabolic studies on phenylalanine, II: the phenylalanine content of the blood and spinal fluid in phenylpyruvic schizophrenia. J Biol Chem 134:105–113, 1940

Kallmann FJ: Heredity in Health and Mental Disorders: Principles of Psychiatric Genetics in the Light of Comparative Twin Studies. New York, WW Norton, 1953

Kernberg O: Borderline Conditions and Pathological Narcissism. New York, Jason Aronson, 1975

Kety S, Schmidt C: The nitrous oxide method for quantitative determination of cerebral blood flow in man: theory, procedure, and normal values. J Clin Invest 27:475–483, 1948

Kety SS, Rosenthal D, Wender PH, et al: The types and prevalence of mental illness in the biological and adoptive families of adopted schizophrenics. J Psychiatr Res 6 (suppl 1):345–362, 1968

Kielholz P: Über die Largactilwirkung bei depressiven Zusfünden und Manien soire bei der Entziehung von Morphin—und Barbitursüchtigen. Schweiz Arch Neurol Psychiatr 73:291–308, 1954

Kielholz P, Battegay R: Treatment of depressive states with special consideration of Toframil, a new antidepressant. Schweiz Med Wochenschr 88:763–767, 1958

Klerman GL, Cole J: Clinical pharmacology of imipramine and related antidepressant compounds. Pharmacol Rev 17:101–141, 1965

Klerman GL, Weissman MM: Increasing rates of depression. JAMA 261:2229–2235, 1989

Kline NS: Use of Rauwolfia serpentina Benth. in neuropsychiatric conditions. Ann N Y Acad Sci 59:107–132, 1954

Kohut H: The Analysis of the Self. New York, International Universities Press, 1971

Kolb LC, Roizin L: The First Psychiatric Institute: How Research and Education Changed Practice. Washington, DC, American Psychiatric Press, 1993

Kopeloff N, Kirby GH: Focal infection and mental disease. Am J Psychiatry 3:149–197, 1923

Krantz JG Jr, Truitt EB, Spears L, et al: New pharmacoconvulsive agent. Science 126:353, 1957

Kuhn R: Über die Behandlung depressiver Zustände mit einem Iminodibenzylderivat (G22355). Schweiz Med Wochenschr 35/36:1135–1140, 1957

Lautebur PC: Medical imaging by nuclear magnetic resonance. Transactions of Nuclear Science NS 26:2808–2811, 1979

Lehmann HE, Hanrahan GE: Chlorpromazine, new inhibiting agent for psychomotor excitement and manic states. Archives of Neurology and Psychiatry 71:227–237, 1954

Lehmann HE, Cohn GH, De Verteuil KL: The treatment of depressive conditions with imipramine (G22355). Canadian Psychiatric Association Journal 1(4), October 1958

Leighton DC, Harding JS, Macklin DB, et al: Psychiatric findings of the Sterling County study. Am J Psychiatry 119:1021–1026, 1963

Lewis NDC: Pathology of dementia precox. J Nerv Ment Dis 62:225–260, 1925

Lindemann E: Psychological changes in normal and abnormal individuals under the influence of sodium Amytal. Am J Psychiatry 11:1083–1091, 1932

Loevenhart AS, Lorenz WF, Waters RM: Cerebral stimulation. JAMA 92:880–883, 1929

Loomer HP, Saunders JC, Kline NS: A clinical and pharmacological evaluation of iproniazid as a psychic energizer. Psychiatric Research Reports of the American Psychiatric Association 8:129–141, 1957

Lynd RS, Lynd HM: Middletown: A Study in Contemporary American Culture. New York, Harcourt Brace, 1929

MacLean PD: Some psychiatric implications of physiological studies on frontotemporal portion of limbic system (visceral brain). Electroencephalogr Clin Neurophysiol 4:407, 1952

Malzberg B, Lee ES: Migration and Mental Disease: A Study of First Admissions to Hospitals for Mental Disease, New York, 1939–1941. New York, Social Science Research Council, 1956

Mann J: Time-Limited Psychotherapy. Cambridge, MA, Harvard University Press, 1973

Mezzich J: Multiaxial diagnostic systems in psychiatry, in Comprehensive Textbook of Psychiatry, 3rd Edition, Vol 1. Edited by Kaplan HI, Freedman AM, Sadock BJ. Baltimore, MD, Williams & Wilkins, 1980

Mindus P, Nyman H, Mogard J, et al: Orbital and caudate glucose metabolites studied by positron emission tomography (PET) in patients undergoing capsulotomy for obsessive-compulsive disorder, in Understanding Obsessive-Compulsive Disorder (OCD). Edited by Jenick MA, Asberg M. Toronto, Canada, Hogrefe & Huber, 1991

Mitchell SW: Fat and Blood and How to Make Them. Philadelphia, PA, Lippincott, 1877

Mitchell SW: Address delivered to the American Medico-Psychological Association on May 16, 1894. Journal of Mental and Nervous Disease 21:413–438, 1894

Moruzzi S, Magoun HW: Brain stem reticular formation and activation of EEG. Electroencephalogr Clin Neurophysiol 1:455–473, 1949

Neumann H: Lehrbuch der Psychiatrie. Erlangen, Germany, 1859

Noguchi H, Moore JW: A demonstration of Treponema pallidum in the brain of cases of general paresis. J Exp Med 17:232–238, 1913

Olds J, Travis RP: Effects of chlorpromazine, meprobamate, pentobarbital and morphine on self-stimulation. J Pharmacol Exp Ther 128:397, 1960

Papez JW: A proposed mechanism of emotion. Archives of Neurology and Psychiatry 38:725–748, 1937

Pauling L: Orthomolecular psychiatry. Science 160:265–271, 1968

Penfield W, Jasper HM: Epilepsy and the Functional Anatomy of the Human Brain. Boston, MA, Little, Brown, 1954

Perry HS: Psychiatrist of America: The Life of Harry Stack Sullivan. Cambridge, MA, The Belknap Press of Harvard University Press, 1982

Pichot P: A Century of Psychiatry. Paris, France, Roger Dacosta, 1983

Prien RF, Caffey EM Jr, Klett CJ: Comparison of lithium carbonate and chlorpromazine in the treatment of mania. Report of the Veterans Administration and National Institute of Mental Health Collaborative Study Group. Arch Gen Psychiatry 26:146–153, 1972

Randall LO: Pharmacology of methaminodiazepoxide. Diseases of the Nervous System 21 (suppl):7–10, 1960

Rapport MM, Green AA, Page IH: Serum vasoconstrictor (serotonin), IV: isolation and characterization. J Biol Chem 176:1243–1251, 1948

Robins E, Guze SB: Establishment of diagnostic validity in psychiatric illness: its application to schizophrenia. Am J Psychiatry 126:983–987, 1970

Rogers CR: A theory of therapy, personality and interpersonal relationships as developed in the client-centered framework, in Psychology: A Study of Science, Vol 3. Formulations of the Person and Their Social Context. Edited by Koch S. New York, McGraw-Hill, 1959, pp 184–256

Rush B: Medical Inquiries and Observations Upon the Diseases of the Mind. Philadelphia, PA, Kimber & Richardson, 1812

Schou M: Lithium in psychiatric therapy: stock taking after 10 years. Psychopharmacologia 1:65–78, 1959

Sifneos PE: Short-Term Psychotherapy and Emotional Crisis. Cambridge, MA, Harvard University Press, 1972

Sokoloff L, Reivich M, Kennedy C, et al: The (14C) deoxyglucose method for the measurement of local cerebral glucose utilization theory, procedure, and normal values in the conscious and anesthetized albino rat. J Neurochem 28:897–916, 1977

Sperry R: Some effects of discontinuing the cerebral hemispheres. Nobel Lecture, 8 December 1981. Biosci Rep 2:265–276, 1982

Spitzer RL, Endicott J: Schedules for Affective Disorders and Schizophrenia. New York, New York State Psychiatric Institute, 1978

Spitzer RL, Endicott J, Robins E: Research Diagnostic Criteria (RDC) for a Selected Group of Functional Disorders. New York, New York State Psychiatric Institute, 1975

Srole L, Langner TS, Michael ST, et al: Mental Health in the Metropolis: The Midtown Manhattan Study. New York, McGraw-Hill, 1962

Staehelin JE: Einige allgemeine Bemerkungen über die Largactiltherapie in der psychiatrischen Universitätsklinik Basel. Schweiz Arch Neurol Pyschiatr 73:288–291, 1954

U.S. Bureau of the Census: Report on the Defective, Dependent, and Delinquent Classes . . . as Returned at the Tenth Census (June 1, 1880). Washington, DC, U.S. Government Printing Office, 1888

Van Gieson I: The correlation of sciences in psychiatric and neurological research. Journal of Mental Science 44:754–811, 1898

Waelsh H, Rittenberg D: Glutathione, II: the metabolism of glutathione studied with isotopic ammonia and glutamic acid. J Biol Chem 144:53–58, 1942

Weinberger DR: Implications of normal brain development for pathogenesis of schizophrenia. Arch Gen Psychiatry 44:660–669, 1987

Weissman MM, Klerman GL: Psychotherapy with depressed women: an empirical study of content, themes and reflections. Br J Psychiatry 123:55–61, 1973

Whitehorn JC: A century of psychiatric research in America, in One Hundred Years of American Psychiatry. New York, Columbia University Press, 1944, pp 178–193

Wise PM: The State of New York and the pathology of insanity. Medical News 86:862–868, 1900

Wolpe J: The Practice of Behavior Therapy, 2nd Edition. New York, Pergamon, 1973

Woodruff RA Jr, Goodwin DW, Guze SB: Psychiatric Diagnosis. London, Oxford University Press, 1974

Woolley DW, Shaw E: Some neurophysiological aspects of serotonin. Br Med J 2:122–126, 1954

World Health Organization: The ICD-9 Classification of Mental and Behavioural Disorders: Clinical Descriptions and Diagnostic Guidelines. Geneva, World Health Organization, 1975

World Health Organization: The ICD-10 Classification of Mental and Behavioural Disorders: Clinical Descriptions and Diagnostic Guidelines. Geneva, World Health Organization, 1992

Wortis J, Lambert RM: Schizophrenic brain metabolism in the course of insulin shock treatment. New York State J Med 42:1053–1059, 1942

Chapter 3

Psychotherapy 1945–1995

Kenneth Z. Altshuler, M.D.

The year 1945 saw the end of World War II and a glorious victory for freedom and American idealism. Freedom's ideal carried with it the notion of man's limitless reach and certainly the idea that the mind has the power to liberate itself from illness, the tyranny within.

Psychoanalysis also triumphed. Battlefield abreactions had demonstrated the power of the unconscious, and analysis was welcomed as an instrument to free and soothe the individual spirit. Psychoanalysis quickly established itself as sovereign among psychotherapies. Being "in analysis" became a status symbol, and analytic practitioners—nearly always M.D.s who specialized in psychiatry—became the butt of ambivalently tinged humor. Psychoanalysts preferred to see their patients at least four times a week, but financial or other reasons made lesser frequencies acceptable when the treatment was designated as "analytically oriented." Therapies were long and often endured for many years.

As we approach 1995, psychoanalysis casts a smaller shadow. Genetic vulnerabilities and limits to our freedom are recognized. There has been a continuously accelerating search for the physical bases of emotional problems and for chemical means of relieving them. In the psychological arena, there is an emphasis on newer, briefer therapies that are touted as widely effective. These therapies are practiced by M.D.s, Ph.D.s, master's-level practitioners, and self-designated therapists. The therapies themselves have been abbreviated from thousands of hours to 20 hours or so (the number of hours textbooks advocate) and often to 4 or 5 hours (the number of hours pressed for by managed care case managers).

In this chapter, I trace these changes, sketching the role of social factors and medical advances, the emphasis on scientific method, and the concern with costs. I also try to order what common elements can be discerned among the competing voices and what harmonies may blend in psychotherapy's future. The chapter touches on a few specific therapies as illustrations, but it is not a compendious review of each approach alleged to be new. That the chapter is written from the perspective of one person living through the second half of this century is also relevant. Another's life, or the perspective of a social historian looking back, could yield a different view.

BACKGROUND

In propounding his new science, Freud sensibly avoided exaggerated claims. To be analyzed, he said, required the ability to form a transference, a maturity of ego, and a flexibility of mind (S. Freud 1904/1950). Psychotic patients and children, therefore, were excluded, as were the elderly—though, sad to say, he considered 45 years to be the rough cutoff point. His disciples, flush with the excitement of discovery, trod the excluded paths anyway: led by his daughter, Anna, analysts treated children with success in the 1920s (A. Freud 1926–1927), claimed good outcomes with psychotic patients in the 1930s and 1940s (Bychowski 1952; Rosen 1947), and used or modified the classical approach with gratifying results for patients as old as 80 years in the 1950s (Grotjahn 1955; Meerloo 1955). In addition, analytic theory was invaluable in informing studies of child development, was applied widely in sociological and literary research, and promised much in the area of illness prevention (Erikson 1952; Kardiner et al. 1945; Linton 1956).

Shortly after midcentury, then, psychoanalysis had extended its purview to include men, women, and children—from the cradle to the grave. But in the midst of the enthusiasm, there was concern about the cost, length, and effectiveness of the treatment. Claims of impressive results were anecdotal, convincing to those who experienced therapy but not backed by large numbers or case series. Some, like Eysenck, even questioned whether psychotherapy and psychoanalysis were any more effective than simple support and placebo (Eysenck 1965). And despite the claims of a few, analysis was neither widely effective with severely ill patients, nor widely available to them. For these poor individuals, about 100,000 in New York's state hospital system alone, little could be done but to provide support, restraint, or coma treatments of one kind or another.

Cade's rediscovery of lithium in 1949 was an important harbinger of change, but it would take more than 15 years for lithium to gain respectability (Segal 1990). More immediately, the introduction and widespread use of chlorpromazine in the early 1950s signaled that the biological revolution was beginning to gather momentum (Klein and Davis 1969).

THE BEGINNINGS OF CHANGE

As early as the late 1940s, Rogers had begun to experiment with abbreviated therapy, as well as a change of viewpoint. Rogers felt that genuineness, positive regard, and a close attunement of empathy were what made treatment move. Therapists were to interpretively reflect ever more clearly what the patients were feeling, enabling the patients thereby to become aware of their feelings more accurately. The goal was to help patients recognize what they had kept hidden, and so to help them to change. An inner drive to self-actualization was postulated (Rogers 1952).

At first, Rogers recommended only several sessions as necessary for change, but over time the length of treatment increased. He and his followers reported excellent results in patients with a wide variety of conditions, and his method attracted a large following. He also pioneered in bringing psychologists to the practice of psychotherapy; and because his method was relatively atheoretical, he even advocated that nonprofessionals could become adept, with relatively modest training, if they had the right character traits (Altshuler, in press; Gendlin 1988).

Others joined the effort to reduce the time and cost of therapy in the 1950s, although these individuals were mostly apart from what was then the mainstream. Leuner, for example, introduced guided affective imagery, an amalgam of relaxation therapy larded with bits of analytic theory. For example, patients would relax, visualize a meadow, and then traverse it. In the course of the journey, obstacles would arise, symbolically representative of particular conflicts. Resolving the symbolic problem with the help of the therapist presumably resolved, or at least diminished, the conflict it represented (Leuner 1984). Milton Erickson began to become well known for what was subsequently to develop into paradoxical therapy. Paradoxical therapy was active and brief. A prime technique was to prescribe evocation of the symptom, yet cause behavior that led to its surrender. A man fearful of driving beyond the city limits, for example, would be told to dress in his best suit and drive to the edge of town. Once there, he was to get out of the car and lie in the ditch. Then he was to reenter the car, drive the distance between two telephone poles, and repeat the process seriatim. In the illustration, the patient did as he was told once or twice and then got so mad that he just drove on and on (Haley 1973).

Rational emotive therapy was started in 1955 and grew rapidly. Developed by Albert Ellis, a psychologist, it combined cognitive confrontation and behavioral methods as primary techniques. It posited that people held irrational beliefs that influenced their perception of events and their emotional reaction to those events. The irrational beliefs consisted of "musts" and "shoulds" around areas such as "I must be competent in everything and win the approval of all, or I'm rotten," "Others must treat me kindly and as I want, or it's terrible and they are unfair," and "Everything should be just as I want, or it's intolerable and I can't stand it." Tactics were to identify the irrational beliefs and their derivatives; to confront the patient with their inaccuracy and cost; and to find and practice alternative, more realistic reactions and behaviors. Behavioral methods of desensitization, instrumental conditioning, behavior contracts, and modeling were employed to these ends, as were education, recording a diary of pleasures and the frequency of self-sabotaging thoughts, cognitive monitoring and thought-stopping, skills and assertiveness training, and the like (Ellis 1958; Ellis and Grieger 1977). The method also adopted Rogers' principles of unconditional positive regard and full acceptance.

The reader will recognize that these terms have a certain similarity to those used today in cognitive therapy, interpersonal therapy, and others. The similarity is worth keeping in mind, because it bears on questions of progress and an overall understanding of how the field of psychotherapy developed.

Behavioral treatments warrant a final word. Developing from the work of Dollard and Miller (1950), Wolpe (1958) introduced and popularized behavior therapy in the mid-1950s for treatment of phobias. With reports of success, desensitization, flooding, and the principles of operant conditioning soon became widely accepted, and applications for the method spread. Because behavior therapy aimed at symptoms, their removal was an acceptable demonstration of effectiveness; because behavior therapy was brief, numbers of cases could be gathered and compared. Behavior therapy, then, can be credited with several emphases: scientific study of case series, brevity, and symptom relief as a measure of success.

PSYCHOANALYSIS AND BRIEF THERAPY

Psychoanalytic students took longer to begin to shorten treatments. Alexander and French (1946) raised pioneering questions about brief therapy and received the opprobrium of the psychoanalytic field. Among their ideas were role-playing when the treatment strategy suggested it, an emphasis on problem solving, and the view of therapy as a corrective emotional experience. Goldfarb (1955), a psychoanalyst and early geriatric psychiatrist, extended and applied these ideas. Working with institutionalized elderly patients, he derived a brief treatment, a series of 15- to 20-minute sessions aimed at providing insight and support and enhancing adaptation. Using the positive aspects of the transference, he would actively respect, or appear to be manipulated by, a man's display of power or a woman's need to be protected (then the ethos of the time), so as to provide a supportive, ancillary ego in an environment that was already protective. Others, also, made an occasional effort to abbreviate treatment with analytic methods (Castelnuovo-Tedesco 1965), but the idea did not at first catch on.

Two factors acted as impediments to the early development of brief psychoanalytic treatments. The respect analysts had for their method meant that psychoanalysis was the gold standard. Panels that aimed at distinguishing analytic psychotherapy from analysis inevitably defined psychotherapy, therefore, as something less deep that aimed at lesser change—to be used as a second choice when real analysis was not possible (Adler 1970; Rangell 1954). Senior analysts modeled this sentiment yet seemed unaware of the dilemma it posed:

> There is no question but that reconstructive psychoanalytic therapy is the highest and most advanced form of psychiatric treatment, with goals for the individual patient that would not be attempted in psychotherapy. However, there is a limitation as to the type of cases suitable for analysis, and practical considerations prevent most who could use it from getting it. With such a need for effective psychotherapy, it is a matter of concern that there is a widespread attitude of disdain toward psychotherapy as compared with psychoanalysis. (Goldman 1956, p. 111)

A second problem preventing psychoanalysis from getting on the bandwagon for psychotherapy was the theory itself. Freud had developed a theory of instinctual development rather than a theory of emotions and behavior. By the 1940s and 1950s, theoreticians also faced the need to recognize adaptational pressures and to distinguish conflict-resolving and conflict-free aspects of development. Freud's theory required the translation of psychological events into terms of instinctual metapsychology. That meant moving from raw emotions and the behavior they dictated to their redescription in terms of dynamics (the forces involved), economics (the course of the libidinal or aggressive energies involved), and structure (the relation of the forces and their energies to the id, ego, and superego) (Moore and Fine 1990). The fact that both energy and structures were metaphorical, handy constructions to aid in conceptualization often got lost. The prose in theoretical papers became turgid, and efforts to seriously trace the intricacies of "delibidinized" or "deaggressivized" libido as it fused, bifurcated, became "aim-inhibited" or "reinstinctualized," or otherwise transformed itself were frequent and nearly unreadable (Gill 1963; Rapaport 1945; White 1963).

A consequence of these preoccupations was that symptom change as a measure of outcome in psychotherapy was not much respected. Such positive changes would often occur early in therapy, would not be thought to hold, and would be attributed to transference or suggestion. The real gold—and the goal of treatment—was structural change, alterations whereby ego expanded its domain to cover what had previously been repressed, defenses and their libidinal cathexes were yielded or exchanged for those of greater maturity, and function overall reached what was called "genital" levels of adaptation. The fact that such internal changes could not be measured made outcome a matter of agreement (or disagreement) between the therapist and the patient and barred the objective study of treatment efficacy.

The need to free therapy from the burdens of instinct and energetics and from the excessive emphasis on the past that instinctual theory sometimes generated was recognized. Critical voices taught that psychoanalysis was in fact a treatment of current value aimed at current adaptation (Kardiner et al. 1959a, 1959b, 1959c). Ovesey and Jameson (1956) summarized:

> Classical technique emphasized the developmental past and all efforts in therapy were bent at a meticulous reconstruction of the infantile neurosis. The present, it was believed, would take care of itself, once the patient had sufficient insight into the past. [In adaptational technique] the therapist is concerned with failures in adaptation today, how they arose and what the patient must do to overcome them. At all times the patient's adaptation here and now is kept in the foreground. Interpretations begin and end with the present. As quickly as insight is achieved it is used as leverage to help him make required adaptive change. (p. 165)

That such awareness was propounded in midcentury and fought for as the proper approach for psychoanalysis should give us pause when newer therapies claim that one of their distinguishing features is a focus on the present.

THE 1960s AND 1970s

The 1960s began with both pride in and disaffection toward psychoanalysis, an increasingly clear demonstration of the effectiveness of neuroleptics in psychotic patients, several splinter therapies claiming success with brief application, and behavioral methods justifying and demonstrating the importance of description and a focus on symptoms. Analysis was still the most highly regarded psychotherapy. Leuner and Erickson, while attracting a following, were on the fringe. Rogers's and Ellis's therapies commanded a larger number of followers. Both leaders, however, were psychologists, and their efforts and reputation only penetrated slightly what was then the larger domain of psychiatric medicine. Behavior therapy, having developed from the discipline of academic psychology and a Skinnerian learning model that disregarded motivation, similarly claimed only a few adherents in centers for psychiatric residency training.

Efforts to demonstrate whether psychoanalysis was effective had also commenced. Primitive and rather overambitious by today's standards, the 1956 Menninger Foundation Psychotherapy Research Project promised to investigate every aspect imaginable of the psychoanalytic process, using tools not yet developed (Wallerstein et al. 1956). The 1959 Columbia Psychoanalytic Center Research Project and the 1960 Boston Psychoanalytic Project reported improved function after psychoanalysis or analytic psychotherapy, according to self-report, to the therapist, or to other objective raters (Knapp et al. 1960; Weber et al. 1967).

In biological psychiatry, the emphasis was shifting to a greater enthusiasm and excitement for the tools of medicine. The change was barely perceptible at first, but by the late 1960s tricyclics were in widespread use for depression and for panic with agoraphobia, monoamine oxidase inhibitors had been rediscovered, benzodiazepines' utility in anxious states had been discovered, and lithium was beginning to be considered safe (Klein and Davis 1980).

Socially, the Kennedy era of "Camelot" had come and gone, but its legacy included the community psychiatry movement (The President's Commission on Mental Health 1978)—supported by the success of medical treatment—and an overvaluation of what youth could do. The coming of age of the postwar baby boomers made a national focus on youth inevitable. Youthful idealism infused our hopes of community accomplishment. Youthful omnipotence also supported an emphasis on self-realization and self-actualization, which enhanced the national interest in psychotherapy. Later, the disaffection of youths with their elders over the Vietnam War brought an antipathy to authority that contributed to blurring the lines and professional roles in community centers and to a tendency to believe that training was not as important as attitude and heart.

OTHER BRIEF METHODS IN THE 1960s AND 1970s

In 1961, Eric Berne's *Transactional Analysis* was published, followed in 1964 by his *Games People Play* (Berne 1961, 1964). The latter, especially, was a huge success. Selling over 2.5 million copies, it popularized brief psychotherapy as never before. Berne, an analytically trained psychiatrist with an interest in sociology, focused on cognitive activities and their psychological functions. He posited the idea that all of us have a stimulus hunger for affection and recognition. Longing for the original stroking of childhood, we seek and accept symbolic "strokes" in their place as adults. Even painful strokes are theorized to be better than none at all, because they at least carry recognition. Social and interpersonal interchanges are engaged in by the child, parent, or adult in all of us as a series of strokes, a game whereby we elicit the responses we want.

Transactional analysis was a brief treatment, at least at first. Moreover, it was especially practicable with groups—making it cheap as well as fast. And it was thoroughly understandable. Technically, it aimed at confronting the "player" with his or her moves and their effects and purpose and then searching for and supporting alternative means and satisfactions by using modeling, practice, homework contracts, and the like. The method's weakness was its assumption that whatever eventuates from a series of interactions is, in fact, the goal of the participants' behavior. This idea of motivation can trivialize neurotic pain as an end sought after, when it might equally be an undesired yet unavoidable result of maladaptation.

The swollen ranks of a young population, the success of pharmacotherapy, the demands for rapid satisfaction, the nirvana promise of a growing drug culture, and a sense that innovative efforts inevitably win out stimulated analytic therapists to find new ways as well (Wolberg 1965, 1980). In addition, the methods used to test drug efficacy led psychotherapy researchers to a new emphasis on the scientific method. This emphasis was not entirely new, because workers like Knapp in the 1950s and Fisher in the early 1960s had tried to trace the carryforward effects of interventions in one session to the following sessions or to dreams in between sessions (Fisher 1960; Knapp 1957). But although behaviorists and founders of other therapies had used case series designs, analytically trained investigators generally had not.

The result was the publication of several serious efforts to study the outcome of abbreviated psychoanalytic therapy, limited to either about 20 sessions or 6 months (Davanloo 1978; Malan 1976; Mann 1973; Sifneos 1972). The studies can be criticized on the basis of selection criteria so narrow as to bias samples by self-selection and because of difficulties in objectifying change, but they did affirm that improvement was possible, that analytic methods could be flexibly applied; they were science, of a sort.

The late 1960s and 1970s also were a time when many therapies were being devised, from rolfing to humanistically "being" together to nude conjoint bathing, and all were hailed as successful by their founders or the small but vocal schools that formed about them.

CONSOLIDATION AND METHOD

In the field of general psychiatry, efforts were being made to deal with pharmacotherapy without displacing psychotherapy. The report on psychotherapy and pharmacotherapy by the Group for the Advancement of Psychiatry (1975) reflects the conflicting currents of the time. In one section of the report it is noted that "the psychoanalytic, dynamic emphasis in our training programs leads to psychopharmacology being considered a second rate form of treatment, viewed with some disdain" (p. 27). Another section refers to efforts (e.g., Ostow 1962) to recast the success of psychopharmacological tools in terms of their influence on the libidinal energy available to the ego for drive discharge (p. 112). It noted that although drugs "are now prescribed for depression by psychiatrists of all persuasions," the dynamic psychiatrist saw the medications as "adjunctive, reducing symptoms which interfere with achieving insight" into the conflicts that were the real cause of the disease (p. 77). At the same time, it reports the importance of neurochemical theories of depression and takes note of the increasingly strident voices favoring psychopharmacology over psychotherapy almost entirely (Klein and Davis 1969). It also reports efforts to study interactions and differential effects of one or the other interventions (Klerman et al. 1974; Lorr et al. 1961; Prange 1973).

By the later 1970s, several elements were at work. First the Feighner criteria (Feighner et al. 1972) and then the Research Diagnostic Criteria (RDC; Spitzer et al. 1978) were designed. Both enumerated stringent lists of symptoms and their descriptions so as to denote specific illness categories. They were designed to enable researchers to develop samples that would be inclusive yet rigorous, as well as comparable across studies. They were an important strut in the bridgework from a diagnostic system based on conflict theory—with symptoms, therefore, being relative epiphenomena—to a system based on description, in which accretions of symptoms were the illness and relieving them was the aim of treatment. The RDC paved the way for and were a forerunner of DSM-III (American Psychiatric Association 1980). Without them, acceptance of DSM-III, published in 1980, would have been even more difficult than it was for the body of general, practicing psychiatrists—who mostly subscribed to the analytic orientation of their training.

With the RDC, and still further with DSM-III, symptoms became respectable, and curing them became an acceptable measure of a method's success. Behavior therapies were indirect beneficiaries because they had long used symptom relief as an outcome measure, and the effectiveness of these therapies was quietly acknowledged. A new age of psychotherapy research was also heralded, because therapists of every stripe could now work with and compare outcomes in samples defined by similar symptoms and symptom intensities.

Psychopharmacology had pointed the way to science by using case series and symptom scales to document the power of medication. That path was now available to psychotherapy research. However, specifiable therapies were needed—with rules teachable enough to be verified in the course of treatment—so that therapies administered in a case series could be considered comparable. The field of psychotherapy obliged, with Beck et al. (1979) delivering cognitive therapy; Klerman et al. (1974, 1984) codifying interpersonal therapy in 1984, after practicing and testing it even earlier; and others following closely behind (Barlow 1988; Luborsky 1984; Strupp and Binder 1984; Werman 1984).

Testing a therapy requires a treatment paradigm that is itself replicable, as well as inexpensive enough to be tried with different illnesses and at different centers. One reason that analysis had never been tested in case series was that the treatment lasted so long and cost so much. Not even the federal government would support a case series in which each patient was seen four times a week for 4 years—with the study then needing replication to avoid an idiosyncratic result!

Even the earliest efforts in psychotherapy research had abbreviated the time over which treatment was studied; for example, Lorr et al. (1961) followed patients in once-a-week therapy for 8 weeks, following up again after 4 more weeks. By quiet consensus rather than any particular debate, the model generally adopted in studies during the 1980s became one of about weekly sessions for about 20 weeks. This choice was not without consequence (Altshuler 1989b).

The factor of cost was a matter of concern not only to researchers. Because therapies, in practice, went on indefinitely and because both diagnoses and results had had uncertain measures, insurance companies had grappled with reimbursement for mental health services from the time health coverage was introduced. The problem was amplified by the number and variety of mental health practitioners who claimed access to the health care dollar. The scope of license to practice became the definer, and therapists with a master's degree or better (and in substance abuse treatment, those with less) became eligible by the late 1980s.

Insurance companies responded with questions of whether psychotherapy was really helpful and with restriction of benefits—especially those for outpatient psychotherapy. Countering this response, practitioners in the field pressed for parity in coverage, a battle that is still being waged.

The study by Smith et al. provided important evidence justifying psychotherapy (Altshuler 1993; Smith et al. 1980). Using the new technique of meta-analysis, Smith et al. compared the nature and extent of the results in 475 controlled therapy studies. Each study had to pass screening criteria (e.g., accurate description of the sample, scaled measures of symptoms and results) to ensure that only scientifically acceptable studies would be included. The results were a rousing endorsement that psychotherapy was helpful. The average improvement added by psychotherapy (compared with the untreated condition) amounted to a treatment effect of 0.85 standard deviation units (i.e., patients receiving psychotherapy were better off at its conclusion than 80% of the control subjects who received no psychotherapy).

UP TO THE PRESENT

In our enthusiasm for the powerful support for psychotherapy provided by the Smith et al. (1980) study, we did not take much notice of the fact that the data failed to distinguish one treatment from another in terms of effectiveness and suggested that all did equally well in all patient groups. We also de-emphasized the facts that the majority of studies reported on were of behavioral treatments and that most of the therapists were relatively untrained, residents, or students. Unmentioned anywhere was the fact that not a single study had been included in which the treatment had been administered twice a week or more for at least a year (Altshuler 1989b, 1993).

Payers of insurance benefits did take notice, however.

The report by Smith et al., DSM-III, and the manual-based therapies of Beck, Klerman, and others led to an explosion in the number of studies of psychotherapeutic effectiveness. Different psychotherapeutic methods were compared; psychotherapy was compared with drug therapy, combination therapy, and placebo; therapy outcomes in different illnesses were measured; and a number of additional meta-analyses of the new data were done (Barlow 1992; Beutler and Crago 1991; Crits-Christoph 1992; Elkin et al. 1989; Jarrett, in press; Klerman et al. 1987; Kupfer 1989; Robinson et al. 1990; Waldinger and Gunderson 1987). In general, all studies tended to confirm that psychotherapy of whatever stripe was noticeably effective in all conditions for which it was tried, and although the immediate effects of psychotherapy were not particularly distinguished in relation to those of drugs, longer-term effects—for example, in terms of better social adjustment or longer delay to the next episode—were affirmed (Barlow 1992; Beck and Emery 1985; Beck and Freeman 1990; Jarrett, in press; Kupfer 1989).

A reader of history is not surprised by this wide confirmation of the value of psychotherapy, because reports of the effectiveness of psychotherapeutic treatments are not new. Virtually every "new" therapy developed was found to be successful—generally in an ever-more-inclusive circle of diagnoses. Client-centered therapy, for example, was claimed to be efficacious in children and adults with neurotic problems, speech problems, psychosomatic problems, and situational difficulties (Altshuler, in press; Gendlin 1988; Rogers 1952). Guided affective imagery has also had a large range of applications, including use in pain control, holistic medicine, and incurable illness (Altshuler, in press; Leuner 1984). Transactional analysis was held to be effective in patients with neurosis, psychosis, character disorders, sexual psychopathology, and mental retardation (Berne 1964).

Struck by the widespread apparent efficacy of what were claimed to be disparate methods, thinkers such as Strupp, Frank, and Garfield in the late 1970s and early 1980s focused on the question of whether the various therapies were as different as they were claimed to be, or whether instead their power rested in elements common to all. The common elements could be summarized as follows: a healer-patient relationship, acceptance and support, the opportunity to express emotions, rituals of treatment to be observed, and a system of explanation (Altshuler 1989b; Frank 1982; Garfield 1983; Strupp 1977). Taken together, these are potent forces. Arrayed against the usual complaints brought by most patients—feelings of demoralization, anxiety, depression, and low self-esteem—these elements and the common behaviors derived from them could well be more important than the distinguishing factors asserted by the different theories. These common elements could become all the more important when the therapy or therapeutic trial is brief.

A look at cognitive therapy and interpersonal therapy—the two most widely popularized brief therapies in current use—might clarify these issues. Cognitive therapy focuses on cognitions (thoughts or feelings of a given moment) so as to define negative underlying schema (assumptions that organize and guide behavior); these, by their unrealistic and negative bias, support a disturbed emotional state. Identification of the schema is followed by practice, modeling, education, and homework aimed at developing more realistic schema, emotional responses, and behavior (Beck et al. 1979).

Interpersonal therapy focuses on grief (in depression), interpersonal disputes and nonreciprocal expectations, role transitions, and inadequate or unsustaining relationships. Recognition of one's feelings and current role relationships helps alter those that are unrealistic for the better. Emphasis is on empathy, understanding the patient, and interpreting unrealistic expectations or behavior, followed by modeling, contracts, support, and practice of alternatives (Klerman et al. 1984).

Both cognitive and interpersonal therapies were first developed for depression, but cognitive therapy has also been reported to be successful in patients with phobias, eating disorders, obsessive-compulsive disorder, and most recently, personality disorders (Barlow 1988; Beck and Emery 1985; Beck and Freeman 1990). Interpersonal therapy has also been extended to elderly patients and to patients in stressful situations (Klerman et al. 1987; Reynolds et al. 1992). Manuals for the two therapies show a considerable overlap in tactics. Both are prescribed for about 20 weeks on about a once-a-week schedule, and therapists with a master's degree or doctorate were trained to administer the treatments in comparative (or stand-alone) studies.

Even this cursory review should make it unsurprising that research comparing the two therapies rarely and barely distinguishes their results (Elkin et al. 1989). The similarities of these therapies to client-centered therapy, rational emotive therapy, and transactional therapy are also striking and raise three interesting and important questions.

One question is whether the newer therapies are either different from or better than the old ones. Although the newer texts are more organized and directly instructive, it is highly likely that both new and older therapies are powered by the common elements described above and that the major difference may be in the scientific method used now to judge them. Having passed the new scrutiny, the methods are agreed to be helpful. A related, but uninvestigated, part of this question is whether differences might emerge between the methods if they were subjected to longer tests, for example, tests that covered a year of continuous treatment.

A second question has to do with the issue facing third-party payers and the field of psychiatry. If the differences between the treatments are small, and if it doesn't matter who does what to whom (in terms of the therapy administered, the training level of the therapist, or the patient's diagnosis), what arguments can be advanced to pay psychiatrists more—or to pay them preferentially—for psychotherapy compared with master's level experts trained in a particular technique? A related question is whether psychotherapy should be paid for at all if the additive effects of psychotherapy are modest in illnesses for which medication is highly effective.

The third question is a bit more complicated. If the older therapies were similar and equal to the new ones, if both old and new therapies were designed as brief alternatives to analysis, and if their power is limited by the 20-visit frame (although amplified in newer studies by monthly "booster" visits) (Kupfer 1989), where does that leave analysis? Psychoanalysis is the one treatment with a potentially meaningful theoretical difference: its emphasis on the unconscious, resistance, and transference. (Although eschewing transference as a concept, interpersonal therapy and cognitive therapy do take some account of it in practice.) Although efforts under way to test analysis with modern criteria and rigorousness may give it a thin patina of acceptability under the new scientific standards (Beutler and Crago 1991), large-scale or replicated studies, or studies of effect in a variety of disorders, will probably remain elusive (Altshuler 1989b, 1993). Yet if reports of the success of other, earlier therapies were largely correct, with claims for therapies closely related to them now more dignified by the scientific method, should not we extend the same courteous view to the long and consistent clinical lore associated with psychoanalysis?

A VIEW TOWARD THE FUTURE

These questions bring us to the dilemmas that currently confront us. What psychotherapy(ies) will be taught? Who will administer and be paid for them? How much and for how long will these practitioners be paid in an individual case? What more can we expect testing in clinical trials to show? Where and what is the role of psychoanalysis?

The psychiatric profession appears to have spoken with regard to the teaching of psychotherapy, because only a third of residency programs currently require a training experience of more than once-a-week therapy, and long-term treatment is diminishing in popularity (Altshuler 1989a; Verhuist 1991). To me it appears self-evident that short-term, once-a-week treatment provides acceptance, ventilation, a confrontation with distorted thinking patterns, and a supportive structure for efforts to change those patterns. Although manual-based treatments may organize the therapist's activities better, it is unlikely that one manual will give a better result than another or that any manual will be better than other eclectic approaches. Therefore, it seems probable that third-party payers will find no reason to pay differentially for a psychiatrist's psychotherapeutic efforts unless a parallel saving is obtained because the psychiatrist can also administer medications and track their use. It is uncertain whether this situation will result in a further diminishment of psychiatrists' interest in psychotherapy or in psychiatrists lowering their fees to parity with those of therapists having lesser degrees.

Competing currents now roil regarding the conditions under which therapy will be prescribed, how long it will endure, and how frequently it will be administered. The psychiatric profession, the government, and managed-care organizations are all developing guidelines for practice. Those of the profession are permissive: taking account of long clinical experience, they allow psychotherapy of various kinds, including psychoanalysis, for a wide variety of conditions (American Psychiatric Association 1993a, 1993b). The government's guidelines are more narrow, relying on scientific studies of randomized and comparable samples and recommending only therapies that have demonstrated efficacy (Depression Guideline Panel 1993). Managed-care groups tread a different path, with tight control, demands for detailed plans, authorization of only a few sessions at a time, and a close eye on the bottom line; health maintenance organizations press for therapies consisting of five sessions.

Applications to psychoanalytic training centers decreased markedly for several years in the 1980s. With several years of training required, a huge expenditure of time and money, and no premium paid for their services on graduation, students of analysis require a dedication bordering on masochism. Nevertheless, aided perhaps by legal action that opened the doors to nonmedical applicants, class ranks are filled once more. It is unlikely, though, that analyses will be paid for to any considerable extent by insuring groups.

Medications, at first useful only in patients with psychoses and major depressive episodes, now yield excellent results in patients with phobias, panic and other anxious states, eating disorders, and obsessive-compulsive disorders. We can expect medical advances to continue—and to continue eroding what was once the province of psychotherapy.

This success, the pressures of managed care and cost containment, and the likely reduction of medical fees for psychotherapy will tend to reduce further the interest of psychiatrists in psychotherapy and reduce the coverage for it as well—despite the best lobbying efforts. What one can guess will eventuate is a two-track system. Insurance benefits will cover brief counseling and therapy that are absolutely necessary as a part of the medical treatment of illness, whereas persons needing or wanting more extensive introspective assistance or help with unconscious conflicts will pay for it separately, get it at a discount at analytic training centers, or do without it.

Psychotherapy practitioners will no longer be distinguished by their disciplines, only by their special training. Whether the majority of the public will be sophisticated enough to distinguish one type of practitioner from another is questionable. But in any event, psychotherapy will continue to be necessary and practiced.

The next 50 years will be interesting.

REFERENCES

Adler M (reporter): Panel discussion: psychoanalysis and psychotherapy. Int J Psychoanal 51:219–232, 1970

Alexander F, French TM: Psychoanalytic Therapy. New York, Ronald Press, 1946

Altshuler KZ: Whatever happened to intensive psychotherapy? Am J Psychiatry 147:428–430, 1989a

Altshuler KZ: Will the psychotherapies yield differential results? A look at assumptions in therapy trials. Am J Psychother 63:310–320, 1989b

Altshuler KZ: Research and the future of intensive psychotherapy: a commentary. Journal of Psychotherapy Practice and Research 2 (Winter):1–3, 1993

Altshuler KZ: Other methods of psychotherapy, in Comprehensive Textbook of Psychiatry, 6th Edition, Vol 2. Edited by Kaplan HI, Sadock BJ. Baltimore, MD, Williams & Wilkins (in press)

American Psychiatric Association: Diagnostic and Statistical Manual of Mental Disorders, 3rd Edition. Washington, DC, American Psychiatric Association, 1980

American Psychiatric Association: Practice guideline for eating disorders. Am J Psychiatry 150:207–228, 1993a

American Psychiatric Association: Practice guideline for depression. Am J Psychiatry 150 (suppl):1–26, 1993b

Barlow DH: Anxiety and Its Disorders: The Nature and Treatment of Anxiety and Panic. New York, Guilford, 1988

Barlow DH: Cognitive-behavioral approaches to panic disorder and social phobia. Bull Menninger Clin 56:A14–A28, 1992

Beck AT, Emery G: Anxiety Disorders and Phobias: A Cognitive Perspective. New York, Basic Books, 1985

Beck AT, Freeman A: Cognitive Therapy of Personality Disorders. New York, Guilford, 1990

Beck AT, Rush AJ, Shaw DF, et al: Cognitive Therapy of Depression. New York, Guilford, 1979

Berne E: Transactional Analysis in Psychotherapy. New York, Grove Press, 1961

Berne E: Games People Play: The Psychology of Human Relationships. New York, Castle Books, 1964

Beutler LB, Crago M: Psychotherapy Research: An International Review of Programmatic Studies. Washington, DC, American Psychological Association, 1991

Bychowski G: Psychotherapy of Psychosis. New York, Grune & Stratton, 1952

Castelnuovo-Tedesco P: The Twenty-Minute Hour: A Guide to Brief Psychotherapy for the Physician. Boston, MA, Little, Brown, 1965

Crits-Christoph P: The efficacy of brief dynamic psychotherapy: a meta-analysis. Am J Psychiatry 149:151–158, 1992

Davanloo H (ed): Basic Principles and Techniques in Short-Term Dynamic Psychotherapy. New York, Spectrum, 1978

Depression Guideline Panel: Guideline report on the diagnosis and treatment of depression in primary care (AHCPR Publ No 93-0550,0551). Washington, DC, Agency for Health Care Policy and Research, Public Health Service, U.S. Department of Health and Human Services, 1993

Dollard J, Miller NE: Personality and Psychotherapy. New York, McGraw-Hill, 1950

Elkin I, Shea MT, Watkins JT, et al: NIMH treatment of depression collaborative research program: general effectiveness of treatments. Arch Gen Psychiatry 46:971–982, 1989

Ellis A: Rational psychotherapy. J Gen Psychol 59:35–49, 1958

Ellis A, Grieger R: Handbook of Rational-Emotive Therapy. New York, Springer, 1977

Erikson E: Young Man Luther: A Study in Psychoanalysis and History. New York, WW Norton, 1952

Eysenck HJ: The effects of psychotherapy. International Journal of Psychiatry 1:99–144, 1965

Feighner JP, Robins E, Guze SB, et al: Diagnostic criteria for use in psychiatric research. Arch Gen Psychiatry 26:57–63, 1972

Fisher C: Subliminal and supraliminal influences on dreams. Am J Psychiatry 116:1009–1017, 1960

Frank JD: Therapeutic components shared by all psychotherapies, in Psychotherapy Research and Behavior Change. Edited by Harvey JH, Parks MM. Washington, DC, American Psychological Association, 1982

Freud A: The Psycho-Analytical Treatment of Children. London, Imago Publishing, 1926–1927

Freud S: On psychotherapy (1904), in Collected Papers, Vol I. London, Hogarth Press, 1950, p 249

Garfield S: Clinical Psychology: The Study of Personality and Behavior. New York, Aldine Publishing, 1983

Gendlin ET: Carl Rogers (1902–1987). Am Psychol 43:127–128,1988

Gill M: Topography and Systems in Psychoanalytic Theory (Psychological Issues Monograph 10). New York, International Universities Press, 1963

Goldfarb AI: Psychotherapy of aged persons, IV: one aspect of the psychodynamics of the therapeutic situation with aged patients. Psychoanal Rev 42:180–187, 1955

Goldman G: Reparative psychotherapy, in Changing Concepts of Psychoanalytic Medicine. Edited by Rado S, Daniels G. New York, Grune & Stratton, 1956, pp 101–113

Grotjahn M: Analytic psychotherapy with the elderly. Psychoanal Rev 42:419–427, 1955

Group for the Advancement of Psychiatry: Pharmacotherapy and Psychotherapy: Paradoxes, Problems and Progress (Report 93), Vol 9. New York, Mental Health Materials Center, 1975

Haley J: The Uncommon Therapy. New York, WW Norton, 1973

Jarrett RB: Comparing and combining short-term psychotherapy and pharmacotherapy for depression, in Handbook of Depression: Treatment, Assessment and Research. Edited by Beckman EE, Leber WR. Homewood, IL, Dorsey Press (in press)

Kardiner A, with the collaboration of Linton R, DuBois C, West J: The Psychological Frontiers of Society. New York, Columbia University Press, 1945

Kardiner A, Karush A, Ovesey L: A methodological study of Freudian theory, I: basic concepts. J Nerv Ment Dis 129:11–19, 1959a

Kardiner A, Karush A, Ovesey L: A methodological study of Freudian theory, II: the libido theory. J Nerv Ment Dis 129:133–143, 1959b

Kardiner A, Karush A, Ovesey L: A methodological study of Freudian theory, III: narcissism, bisexuality and the dual instinct theory. J Nerv Ment Dis 129:207–221, 1959c

Klein DF, Davis JM: Diagnosis and Treatment of Psychiatric Disorders, Baltimore, MD, Williams & Wilkins, 1969

Klein DF, Davis JM: Diagnosis and Treatment of Psychiatric Disorders, 2nd Edition. Baltimore, MD, Williams & Wilkins, 1980

Klerman GL, DiMascio A, Weissman M, et al: Treatment of depression by drugs and psychotherapy. Am J Psychiatry 131:186–191, 1974

Klerman GL, Weissman MM, Rousavill BJ, et al: Interpersonal Psychotherapy Of Depression. New York, Basic Books, 1984

Klerman GL, Budman S, Berwick D, et al: Efficacy of a brief psychosocial intervention for symptoms of stress and distress among patients in primary care. Med Care 25:1078–1088, 1987

Knapp PH: Conscious and unconscious affects: a preliminary approach to concepts and methods of study. Psychiatry Research Reports 8:55–74, 1957

Knapp PH, Levin S, McCarter RH, et al: Suitability for psychoanalysis: a review of 100 supervised analytic cases. Psychoanal Q 29:459–477, 1960

Kupfer DJ: Maintenance Therapies in Recurrent Depression: New Findings (Strecker Monograph Series #26). Philadelphia, PA, Pennsylvania Hospital, 1989

Leuner H: Guided Affective Imagery: Mental Imagery in Short-Term Psychotherapy. Edited by Richards WA. Translated by Lochman E. New York, Thieme-Stratton, 1984

Linton R: The Tree of Culture. New York, Alfred Knopf, 1956

Lorr M, McNair DM, Weinstein GJ, et al: Meprobamate and chlorpromazine in psychotherapy: some effects on anxiety and hostility of outpatients. Arch Gen Psychiatry 4:381–389, 1961

Luborsky L: Principals of Psychoanalytic Psychotherapy: A Manual for Supportive-Expressive Treatment (SE). New York, Basic Books, 1984

Malan DH: The Frontier of Brief Psychotherapy. New York, Plenum, 1976

Mann J: Time-Limited Psychotherapy. Cambridge, MA, Harvard University Press, 1973

Meerloo JAM: Psychotherapy with elderly people. Geriatrics 10:583–587, 1955

Moore BE, Fine BD: Psychoanalytic Terms and Concepts. New Haven, CT, Yale University Press, 1990

Ostow M: Drugs in Psychoanalysis and Psychotherapy. New York, Basic Books, 1962

Ovesey L, Jameson J: The adaptational technique of psychoanalytic therapy, in Changing Concepts of Psychoanalytic Medicine. Edited by Rado S, Daniels G. New York, Grune & Stratton, 1956, pp 165–179

President's Commission on Mental Health, Thomas E. Bryant, Chairperson: Report to the President From The President's Commission on Mental Health, Vol I (Publ No 040-000-00390-8). Washington, DC, U.S. Government Printing Office, 1978, pp 2–94

Prange AJ: The use of drugs in depression: its theoretical and practical basis. Psychiatric Annals 3(2):56–75, 1973

Rangell L: Panel report: psychoanalysis and dynamic psychotherapy: similarities and differences. Journal of the American Psychiatric Association 2:152–166, 1954

Rapaport D: Organization and Pathology of Thought: Selected Sources. New York, Columbia University Press, 1945.

Reynolds CF III, Frank E, Perel JM, et al: Combined pharmacotherapy and psychotherapy in the acute and continuation treatment of elderly patients with recurrent major depression: a preliminary report. Am J Psychiatry 149:1687–1692, 1992

Robinson LA, Berman JS, Neimeyer RA: Psychotherapy for the treatment of depression: a comprehensive review of controlled outcome research. Psychol Bull 108:30–49, 1990

Rogers C: Client Centered Therapy. Boston, MA, Houghton-Mifflin, 1952

Rosen JN: The treatment of schizophrenia psychosis by direct analytical therapy. Psychiatr Q 21:3–25, 1947

Segal J: Lithium in the treatment of mood disorders (National Clearing House for Mental Health Information, National Institute of Mental Health Publ No 5033). Washington, DC, U.S. Government Printing Office, 1990

Sifneos PE: Short-Term Psychotherapy and Emotional Crisis. Cambridge, MA, Harvard University Press, 1972

Smith ML, Glass GV, Miller TI: The Benefits of Psychotherapy. Baltimore, MD, Johns Hopkins University Press, 1980

Spitzer RL, Endicott J, Robins E: Research diagnostic criteria: rationale and reliability. Arch Gen Psychiatry 35:773–782, 1978

Strupp HH: A reformulation of the dynamics of the therapist's contribution, in Effective Psychotherapy. Edited by Gurman AS, Kazin AM. Elmsford, NY, Pergamon, 1977, pp 3–22

Strupp HH, Binder JL: Psychotherapy in a New Key: A Guide to Time-Limited Dynamic Psychotherapy. New York, Basic Books, 1984

Verhuist J: The psychotherapy curriculum in the age of biological psychiatry: mixing oil with water? Academic Psychiatry 15:120–131, 1991

Waldinger RJ, Gunderson JG: Effective Psychotherapy With Borderline Patients: Case Studies. New York, Macmillan, 1987

Wallerstein RS, Robbins LL, Sargent HD, et al: The psychotherapy research project of the Menninger Foundation. Bull Menninger Clin 20:221–278, 1956

Weber JJ, Elinson J, Moss LM: Psychoanalysis and change: a study of psychoanalytic clinic records utilizing electronic data-processing techniques. Arch Gen Psychiatry 17:687–709, 1967

Werman DS: The Practice of Supportive Psychotherapy. New York, Brunner/Mazel, 1984

White RW: Ego and Reality in Psychoanalytic Theory (Psychological Issues Monograph 11). New York, International Universities Press, 1963

Wolberg LR: Short-Term Psychotherapy. New York, Grune & Stratton, 1965

Wolberg LR: Handbook of Short-Term Psychotherapy. New York, Thieme-Stratton, 1980

Wolpe J: Psychotherapy by Reciprocal Inhibition. Palo Alto, CA, Stanford University Press, 1958

Chapter 4

Women and Psychiatry

Judith H. Gold, M.D., F.R.C.P.C.

Gender is certainly not the only determinant of the mode of expression of an individual's capacities.

V. L. Clower (1991)

During the discussions surrounding the recent development of DSM-IV (American Psychiatric Association 1994), emphasis was placed by the media on the diagnostic categories related to women. For example, as the chairperson of the DSM-IV Work Group on Late Luteal Phase Dysphoric Disorder, I was asked numerous times about the social effects of, and the scientific basis for, the existence of a disorder (late luteal phase dysphoric disorder) that can be diagnosed only in women. In this chapter, I outline and discuss the biological and sociocultural data and theories related to gender differences in the diagnosis and treatment of mental disorders. I describe the data underlying the knowledge of such differences and the controversies and concerns surrounding them that lead to such questioning of psychiatric diagnosis and treatments, not only by the media but also by those concerned for the welfare of women.

The interested reader is referred to Volume 10 of the *American Psychiatric Press Review of Psychiatry* for an excellent and detailed summary of the current knowledge of the psychological and psychodynamic aspects of gender as related to the life cycle and to psychotherapy (Nadelson and Notman 1991; Notman et al. 1991). In contrast, and also in addition to this previous approach to the subject of gender and mental disorders, the focus in this chapter is on a review of the following topics: the recognition and treatments of gender differences in mental disorders in the last part of this century; the recognition of seemingly gender-specific disorders (e.g., late luteal phase dysphoric disorder and self-defeating personality disorder) and the controversies involved; the perceptions of women as patients and their treatment by the profession of psychiatry; and, finally, in this 150th anniversary year of the American Psychiatric Association, the status of women psychiatrists within the profession.

GENDER DIFFERENCES IN
MENTAL DISORDERS

As discussed in detail in other chapters in this section, after World War II, an active group of young, newly trained psychiatrists, full of the energy and enthusiasm of a generation released from the dreadfulness of war and destruction, set out to change and reorganize American psychiatry (R. O. Jones, personal communication).[1] New departments of psychiatry were founded, psychiatry was established as a medical specialty, and changes were demanded and made in many psychiatric organizations. Along with all of this came an interest in psychiatric epidemiology, originating in the studies of cultural influences on behavior that had been used by the Allies during the war in planning strategy against Japan and Germany (A. H. Leighton, personal communication).[1] Although it was well recognized that culture had an influence on behavior, the effect of culture on psychiatric illness was not then known. Furthermore, the actual numbers of people with mental disorders also were unknown, as was the actual effect of gender on both the numbers and the etiology of these disorders. These questions led to studies of the prevalence of disorders by gender. A long-standing clinical impression, bolstered by statistics, was that women seek psychiatric treatment or are hospitalized more frequently than are men (Gove 1979). History has shown that by the seventeenth century there were twice as many cases of mental disorder among women than men; by the nineteenth century, most of the patients in mental institutions were women from all classes and social circumstances (Showalter 1985).

The studies initially did not focus on gender, but their findings must be mentioned as background to this discussion. Among the earliest studies of communities, one of the most influential was the Hollingshead and Redlich (1958) investigation of patients in all types of mental health facilities in New Haven, Connecticut, in the 1950s. Their results documented the rate of mental illness by social class. In the 1960s, Leighton et al. (1963) published results of a large study, which is still ongoing, in which they detailed the prevalence of mental illness in the inhabitants of a rural population. About the same time, Srole et al. (1962) looked at a selected sample of people in midtown Manhattan. These studies together led to conclusions that approximately 20% of

---

[1]These communications occurred over many years of discussion with these two psychiatrists, each of whom participated actively in both academic and organizational psychiatry during these important years in the development of North American psychiatry. R. O. Jones was a founder of the Canadian Psychiatric Association, and its first president. A. H. Leighton is one of the world's foremost epidemiological researchers and teachers.

people required psychiatric care at any time in a community, whereas somewhere between 60% and 80% had some symptoms of mental distress. Factors influencing these rates of illness included the presence of rapid social change and social disintegration in a community.

In 1979, Gove pointed out that, in these and other studies, higher rates of mental illness were found in women, especially "the neurotic and psychophysiologic disorders" (p. 54). He also wrote that this rate of mental disorders was found whether researchers studied women in mental hospitals, in treatment by general physicians, or in community samples. Also, as Weissman (1987) later noted, these studies "demonstrated the importance of poverty, urban anomie, social stress, and rapid social change in the development of impairment" (p. 582). In his discussion of these earlier studies, Robins (1987) stated that the highest rates of mental disorder in these studies were found in elderly people, women, poor people, people who were divorced or separated, and people living in urban areas.

Weissman and Klerman (1979), who summarized data from community surveys, concluded that women were diagnosed with depression more frequently than men. They also examined whether these figures were due to women seeking help or reporting symptoms more easily than men. They considered the possibility that women's lives are more stressful than men's, basing this hypothesis on studies done in the 1960s by Holmes and Rahe (1967) and others that related stress to depression and other mental disorders. "At the same levels of stress, women reported symptom intensities about 25% higher than men" (Weissman and Klerman 1979, p. 393). They summarized studies that showed that women also visit doctors and use more psychotropic drugs than do men. It was noted that although women seek treatment more often for depression, the suicide rate in men is higher. Nevertheless, community studies revealed more depression in women, including those who have never been treated, and that men who are depressed use alcohol instead of complaining of depression.

In the 1970s, researchers had become even more rigorous in their attempts to assess the prevalence of mental disorders by developing standardized interviews and criteria for diagnosis. These tools in turn enabled the National Institute of Mental Health Epidemiologic Catchment Area (ECA) studies to begin in 1980.

These multisite studies have led to more precise information about the actual occurrence of mental disorders in women and men.

Unlike the earlier work, the ECA studies showed little difference overall between men and women in rates of illness, but they did show differences for particular mental disorders (Robins et al. 1984). Major depressive disorder, agoraphobia, and simple phobia were more common in women; alcohol and substance abuse and antisocial personality disorders were more common in men. All of these disorders were found more frequently in people under age 45 years (Regier and Burke 1987). The gender differences in mental illness in the general population were found to be similar to those in clinic samples (Cameron and Hill 1989). These figures echoed hospital data on admissions that had been collected for decades (Gove 1979). Why did these differences exist?

Speculation about the causes of these disorders in women resulted in a number of research studies. In the 1970s and 1980s, the examination of life stressors as etiological factors was popular. The work of G. W. Brown and T. Harris (1978) and Harris et al. (1987) indicated that lack of adequate social supports for women who had stressful life events was associated with a higher incidence of depression. Using the Present State Examination to diagnose unipolar, nonpsychotic depression, they found several significant stressors in the lives of these women compared with nondepressed women: loss of a parent, particularly the mother before age 11; lack of a confiding relationship with a spouse; no employment outside of the home; and three or more children under age 15 at home. An unhappy marriage also contributed to depression in these women.

Other researchers looked at the effects of marriage, divorce, and being single on rates of illness and concluded that the healthiest women were single and childless, and those most likely to become depressed or anxious were young, married women with children. Gove (1979) further stated that "the data on mental illness . . . clearly suggest that in modern Western industrial society marriage is more beneficial to men than women, whereas being single is, if anything, more stressful for men than for women. . . . Sex differences in mental illness are largely a product of societal roles" (p. 57). These findings relate to the predominance among women of the anxiety and depressive disorders and the fact (well known to clinicians) that women are seen more often than men by physicians and psychiatrists for treatment.

In contrast to earlier epidemiological findings that schizophrenia occurred at equal rates in men and women, more recent studies (Castle et al. 1993; Iacono and Beiser 1992; Lewine et al. 1984) demonstrated that schizophrenia occurs more frequently in men and is more debilitating and begins at a younger age in men than in women. Similarly, men have higher rates of psychotic affective disorders. Iacono and Beiser wrote:

> The sexes differ in their anatomy and physiology, processes of biological maturation, social status, occupational attainment, and duration and types of psychosocial experiences encountered. Examining variables related to such factors may provide valuable clues to understanding how schizophrenia develops. (p. 1074)

Seeman (1992) discussed the later age at onset and better outcome for schizophrenic women compared with schizophrenic men. She noted that although women with schizophrenia are more likely to be depressed, to attempt suicide, and to die from accidental and other causes, women are more cooperative with treatment, have more family supports, and respond better to medication. Men tend to be more aggressive, to abuse alcohol and drugs, to be jailed more, and to relapse more frequently. Women with schizophrenia are also victimized more than men. Unlike the previous discussion about depressed and anxious women, Seeman wrote that schizophrenic women seem to benefit from having a spouse and children.

Gender-Specific Disorders: Research and Controversies

The rise of feminism in the 1970s coincided with the growth of epidemiological studies and exacting techniques and with the continuing development of the *Diagnostic and Statistical Manual of Mental Disorders* in North American psychiatry. For DSM-III (American Psychiatric Association 1980), strict criteria for diagnosis were demanded, unlike the merely clinical descriptions accepted previously. The work of the ECA studies and others enabled the development of these criteria and their validation in the population. Thus, diagnosis became standardized, and research into mental disorders became more systematic and replicable than it had been in the past. Researchers could study communities and find rates for disorders rather than just reporting degrees of symptomatology and disability. Still, as noted above, women had higher rates than men for some disorders. Discussion continued as to whether the etiological basis was stress, biology, or social roles—or perhaps a combination of all three.

The antipsychiatry movement in the 1970s and early 1980s also added to this debate. Psychiatric theories were challenged and psychodynamic discussions were modified by consideration of women's roles in society (Nadelson and Notman 1991; Notman et al. 1991; Seiden 1976). An interesting chapter by Bart and Scully (1979) is representative of the period: the authors discussed the history of "hysteria" and its treatment, drawing on centuries of medical literature up to the present day to illustrate how women's symptoms were denigrated and blamed on physiology, inability to accept social roles and patriarchy, and repressed sexuality.

Examination of women's roles in society led some to the conclusion that women are more depressed because of the pressures of their lives and their subordinate position to men; these authors postulated that being depressed is a socially acceptable method of protesting these circumstances for the individual woman (Ussher 1992; Walsh 1987; Williams 1977). Therefore, it was argued by these and numerous other feminist writers that depression in women is not biological or genetic in origin, but rather is socially determined. By this reasoning, women then are given more medication to tranquilize them, dull their complaints, and render them amenable to continuing in their oppressed environments. This theory concludes that women are thus mislabeled as mentally ill. Physicians and society in general fail to address the legitimate anger behind the symptoms, anger generated by oppression (Smith and David 1975). Studies of rates of mental disorders and of etiologies of disorders have been cited by such authors only as proof of women's suffering and secondary social position vis-à-vis men.

In numerous papers, books, and public forums, the theories of Freud and his followers were debated, put into sociocultural context, and revised or rejected. The findings of Masters and Johnson (1966) laid to rest the theory of vaginal orgasm and negated scientifically the theory that a girl needs to give up clitoral satisfaction to become a mature woman. Further research into gender aspects of embryology, developmental physiology, and brain functions added to the scientific knowledge of the development and maturation of males and females (Fausto-Sterling 1985; McEwan 1991). These findings necessitated a revision of the teachings of the analysts about human psychological growth. We now know that human behavior is influenced by both social interactional experiences and by biological factors such as hormones, neurotransmitters, and genetics. As Notman and Nadelson (1991) wrote:

> The intricate blend of gender differences in responsiveness, differential parental encouragement of certain behaviors and responses according to culturally stereotyped concepts of male and female, and expectations of appropriate styles of each gender thus results in early gender role differences with important developmental implications. (p. 32)

Raphael (1992), in discussing women and mental health, also noted "at the outset it must be recognized that socio-demographic factors may place women at greater risk of mental health problems. These include poverty, single parenthood, educational and work inequities" (p. 2).

In summary, the research findings of the past 50 years related to gender and mental disorders have necessitated a change in our thinking about the relationship of gender and illness and gender and health (Anderson and Holder 1989). Centuries-old myths about hysteria and other "female" ailments and theories of psychosexual development from earlier in this century have all been refuted by scientific investigation (Bart and Scully 1979). Biochemical and neurological studies have added to our understanding of the similarities and differences in male and female brains and bodies (Fausto-Sterling 1985). Research methodologies have become more precise, enabling more accurate assessment and diagnosis. The task for the future will be to formulate a scientifically based approach to understanding the differences in the rates of illness by gender.

Treatment

Differences also exist in the responses of men and of women to treatment, especially to pharmacological interventions. These differences are not yet well understood or documented. Often they are not taught to students, and many physicians and patients remain unaware of the variances in drug responses and side effects between the sexes. For example, Seeman (1992) pointed out that because women with schizophrenia often have depressive symptoms, they may require antidepressants rather than neuroleptics for psychosis. She also noted the possibility that the monthly alterations in hormones in women may act on dopamine receptors in a protective manner much like the neuroleptics: "Antipsychotics, because they are antidopaminergic, enhance the effects of naturally occurring estrogens in women. . . . Women require lower doses both in the acute and in the maintenance and prophylactic phases of therapy" (p. 7). Finally, she stated that women have fewer side effects and experience acute dystonia less often because of these lower dosages.

McEwan (1991) added that antidepressants and neuroleptics have differing actions in men and women due to the effects of estrogen and testosterone in the brain. Furthermore, these medications act differently in women before and after menopause. It is also known that the amount of adipose tissue and body fluid affects drug dosage and rate of metabolism and that these should be considered in the prescription of drug treatments. Other treatments vary in effectiveness between men and women as well. Additionally, women respond more favorably to family therapy (Seeman 1992).

Unfortunately, many reports of studies still do not differentiate between males and females in their outcomes, despite all of the evidence of differences in responses to medications and in courses of illness. A recent report by Elkin et al. (1989) on the effectiveness of psychotherapy in patients with major depression noted that 70% of the sample was female, but did not mention any investigation of sex as a response variable. In a recent randomly chosen issue of *Archives of General Psychiatry*, reports of several studies make no distinction between the males and females in the samples in either the statement of findings or in the discussion of results (Hollon et al. 1992; Keller et al. 1992; Kupfer et al. 1992; Shea et al. 1992). Such omissions are widespread, make studies difficult to interpret meaningfully, and are hard to explain after 50 years of verification of gender differences in the prevalence and treatment responses of certain mental disorders. Thus, researchers sometimes ignore differentiation by sex in their study findings and, instead, concentrate on the other variables in interpreting their studies (McBride and McBride 1993). In view of the findings of hormonal, neuroanatomical, and brain function differences between men and women (including differences in responses to stress), as well as sociocultural and political roles, such oversights can invalidate the conclusions of otherwise carefully done research.

GENDER-RELATED DISORDERS

Gender differences have also been noted in the underlying psychodynamics of mental disorders. As stated at the beginning of this chapter, this topic has been discussed in detail by Notman et al. (1991) in an earlier volume of the *American Psychiatric Press Review of Psychiatry.* In the present historical overview it is important at least to summarize a few salient points related specifically to the changes in our understanding of gender differences and psychodynamics over the last 50 years. Although earlier analysts had theorized about women's psychological development, they based their discussions mainly on Freud's teachings.

During the 1940s, Horney (unlike her colleagues) was working with and writing and teaching about women's anger, anger at the expectations placed on them by their social roles (Westkott 1986). Later, Symonds (1971) expanded on this theory in her important article on phobias, describing symptoms of anxiety and phobic reactions as conflicts between autonomy and dependency. Women in the latter half of this century have had to contend with this conflict on a daily basis. As noted above, the feminist literature of the 1970s and 1980s continued this theory. Meanwhile, biological and genetic research have added new dimensions to our understanding of the underlying pathology of these disorders. However, the effects of environment and social stressors are also recognized as catalysts for the emergence of symptoms in susceptible individuals (Gabbard 1992). Why do symptoms begin at a particular time and not earlier in a woman's life? Why can the regulatory physiological mechanisms no longer cope with and contain the symptoms? These questions remain to be answered, as noted in several recent papers discussing research data (Cameron and Hill 1989; Kendler et al. 1992a, 1992b; Rubinow 1992). Hopefully, these and other investigators will continue to search for the answers.

Years ago, such women were called hysterical or neurasthenic and kept to their beds (Bart and Scully 1979). Today, such women would be treated with medications for their disorder, but the precipitant may still be overlooked unless the clinician is also sensitive to the effects of women's social milieu on their mental health, as well as to the effects of biological factors on symptomatology.

Anxiety has long been viewed in psychodynamic terms as a response to an external or internal threat (Beck and Emery, with Greenberg 1985; Cameron and Hill 1989; Lerner 1982; Symonds 1971). Although the physiological results were useful in physical defense, when the threat comes from within, the symptoms themselves become the problem. Thus, the woman focuses on the physical symptoms: her rapid heartbeat, difficult respiration, perspiration, and so on, rather than on the underlying conflicts in her life and social circumstances. Her concern then centers on a possible physical illness, and out of fear that the symptoms will return, she restricts her activities to places and people that feel safe.

During the last century, women—in particular, middle-class white women in North America—have experienced great changes in their social circumstances. As Chafe (1991) stated in his book summarizing social research, women have been given permission by the male power base to work outside their homes in, to some extent, jobs of their choice. Although acceptance of women doing paid outside work came after much struggle and animosity, there are many problems associated with working outside the home (Rothman 1978; Woloch 1984). There are conflicts over family and work demands and how to balance them or even deal with them, conflicts over social roles between men and women, conflicts over appropriate sexual behavior, conflicts over appearance, conflicts over career aspirations, and so on. These were well outlined almost 20 years ago in the Group for the Advancement of Psychiatry's report (1975) titled *The Educated Woman: Prospects and Problems*. These ideas continue to appear in both the popular press and scientific publications.

With these external or societal conflicts come internal ones as well: those of autonomy and dependency augmented by problems of assertion and fear of change and the expression of anger and guilt over being angry (Nadelson and Notman 1991; Notman 1989; Notman et al. 1991; Ussher 1992). These intrapsychic conflicts are perceived as threatening to the woman's customary relationship with the world and to her self-perception. As these authors pointed out, expression of anger leads to anxiety. The original problem is repressed or denied, and the symptoms become all-encompassing. Panic can then occur. If the woman sequesters herself to avoid symptoms, she loses more autonomy and thus more self-esteem. She is more dependent, more trapped, more not in control. Soon she will feel incapable of change. However, her increasing dependency on others remains annoying to her, and her symptoms escalate. Those on whom she leans may become overly protective, authoritarian, and even belittling. The result is a diminution of her self-esteem and a loss of autonomy due to an underlying sense that she could be handling the situation differently if only she knew how (Beck and Emery, with Greenberg 1985).

In today's world, women demand the right of choice. Having struggled for decades to achieve this right to varying degrees, North American women, particularly, face many dilemmas. A large number work outside their homes for purely economic reasons. Of these women, some can choose what kind of work they do, but many cannot. As mothers, they may be torn between demands of the job and demands for child care. Plagued by the lack of adequate day care and after-school care and by household chores, they in fact have several full-time jobs, although only one is a "paying" job. Many studies have shown that women still spend more hours than men doing housework. At the same time, the expectation that both marriage and work should be rewarding and fulfilling has grown, and so have the rate of divorce and the number of single-parent families (Bernard 1991; Chafe 1991; Holder and Anderson 1989). How many things can or should a woman juggle simultaneously?

Friedan (1981) wrote of this second stage of women's emancipation. In her view, the problems women face today are more complicated than balancing career and motherhood and go beyond dependency and traditional feminine roles, evoking conflicts throughout daily life. In North America today, the right to autonomy clashes with the preexisting and still prevailing themes of a woman's role as caretaker, nurturer, and all-accepting and deferential mother who is also youthful and attractive (Anderson and Holder 1989). Faced with these swirling, intertwined ropes of expectations, what is a woman to do?

Some women find the answer, as did their great-grandmothers, in debilitating symptoms. Unable to deal with all of these demands, they become fearful and freeze into psychological inaction (Barnett and Baruch 1987). However, passivity and inactivity are no longer acceptable in the modern woman, who has been taught to be otherwise, but who has not yet always mastered the necessary skills or been given the training. The solution in some women—symptoms of psychological distress—is not in the end a solution, but rather an exacerbation of the problems. Thus, there are increased rates of depressive, anxiety, and somatic disorders in women (Anderson and Holder 1989). In addition, several new disorders have been proposed to define women's symptoms.

In DSM-III-R (American Psychiatric Association 1987), two of these disorders were placed in an appendix for further research: late luteal phase dysphoric disorder and self-defeating personality disorder. Another group of disorders, the eating disorders, which have been diagnosed most prominently in women, have increased in prevalence in the female population since the end of World War II. Furthermore, recognition has grown of the frequency of the incidence of incest and the resultant psychopathology in the victims and of sexual abuse and rape; a diagnosis of posttraumatic stress disorder is made frequently in these women (T. A. Brown et al. 1992; Coons et al. 1989; Spiegel and Cardena 1990). Also, concern has grown publicly over the new visibility of battered women. All of these are "new" disorders in the past 50 years in that now they are being discussed and investigated extensively for the first time.

Books and articles on aspects of women's health are now too numerous to cite. They occupy entire sections of libraries and book stores; courses are given on the subject; a journal is devoted to it (*Journal of Women's Health*); a specialty has been proposed in the field (Harrison 1993). However, the controversies remain as well. Some in the women's movements continue to decry diagnosing mental disorders in women, believing instead that the unequal role of women in society should be addressed. They argue that women are not ill, just angry or frustrated by their insubordinate social position and by the injustices visited on them (Tavris 1992). Treatment, they feel, should center on the expression of these inequities and on teaching the woman how to overcome them. Mental disorder is a stigmatizing diagnosis in this theoretical framework, but one that many women find comfort in, preferring to have a disorder rather than to deal with their sociopolitical reality. This medicalization of women's roles in our society is seen by authors such as Tavris as another example of male dominance and patriarchy (Sherwin 1992).

The alternative view is that women have disabling psychological symptoms that can and should be treated. The current DSM system allows symptoms to be categorized into criteria to form a consistent and reliable diagnosis. Thus, research can be replicated by others because the disorder is well defined and similar populations can be studied. This systematic approach to diagnosis is far more precise than the previous psychodynamic descriptions of illnesses, which lead to great variations in the criteria for various disorders. Only with precise diagnosis can effective treatments be found. In many instances, it may be that social factors are the main causes of the symptoms. This circumstance does not invalidate the description of the symptoms and categorization of them into a diagnostic entity. After all, psychiatric diagnosis currently is a description of signs and symptoms, not a designation of the pathogen or the pathogenic mechanism.

As an example of the discussions related to etiology, let us look at the diagnostic category of the eating disorders. Speculation about the social etiology of these disorders is widespread, whereas researchers have examined the biochemical, as well as the sociocultural, basis of the disorders (Emmett 1985; Garner and Garfinkel 1985; Halmi 1992; Hudson and Pope 1987; Johnson 1991; Orbach 1986; Waller 1993). Both scientific studies and popular literature in this area are legion. Books such as the recently popular *The Beauty Myth* (Wolf 1991) explore women's obsession with thinness and youthfulness. Gone is the emphasis of earlier decades on the girl's refusal to grow up or denial of sexuality. Instead, the emphasis is on her need to fulfill the male image of the eternally adolescent, sexually attractive, thin woman. Additionally, clinical researchers are examining the role of sexual abuse in the bulimic patient's abuse of her body's physiology. Therapy includes psychotherapy, family therapy, group therapy, medications, behavior modification, and so on—that is, a range of techniques to enable the woman to accept herself and assert herself in her society. Treatment, as outlined by the above authors, has moved beyond theory alone and into recognition of the individual and the interactions that led her to these symptoms: sociocultural as well as psychodynamic and biological causes.

DSM-IV

The proposals in 1986 that two new diagnoses be added to the DSM nomenclature brought forth much controversy. It was argued that late luteal phase dysphoric disorder was a discriminatory diagnosis based on the centuries-old myths that menstruation was unclean and rendered a woman susceptible to madness. Opponents of the diagnosis stated that the research into the disorder generally was methodologically unsound. However, clinical experience showed that some women were severely disabled by depressive symptoms related temporally to menstruation. Thus, the disorder was placed into an appendix to DSM-III-R in the hope that this would catalyze more research based on standardized criteria (Spitzer et al. 1989). As a result, in recent years, more systematic research has been carried out. In fact, it is one of the few disorders of women that actually is being studied. The review of that research done by a work group of the Task Force on DSM-IV indicated that there is a substantive body of findings related to the disorder. Based on these findings, the criteria for the disorder were redefined, the dysphoric nature of the symptoms was recognized, and the name was changed to premenstrual dysphoric disorder to reflect the research findings (American Psychiatric Association, in press).

Another proposed diagnosis also placed in the same DSM appendix was self-defeating personality disorder. This disorder was based on psychodynamic understandings of the behavior of some individuals. However, the diagnosis was controversial because it appeared to be related primarily to women who were labeled masochistic. Critics pointed out that women were socialized to accept their subservient role in relationships and to tolerate abuse. Furthermore, it was argued that the self-esteem–destroying effects of continuous abuse were well known; and it had been demonstrated that victims of abuse were not masochistic, but rather were too defeated by the abuse to rescue themselves. This was far different from encouraging or even enjoying the abuse. In the subsequent years, there has been little research into this area, and no biological factors have emerged (A. Frances, personal communication, March 1993). Today, purely social factors are thought to explain the symptomatology, which is now believed to be part of other disorders rather than composing a separate mental disorder. Thus, the proposed diagnosis was dropped from DSM-IV.

The proposal of these two diagnoses illustrates the problems of gender-related diagnosis. First, there must be good epidemiological data on the rates of occurrence in the population. Strict criteria are required to make the diagnosis and thus obtain these data. Then, the etiology must be investigated. The last 50 years have taught us that there is a broad basis to etiology that must include attention to social variables. Gender studies must include an examination of the sociocultural and political milieu of the current society and the effects of that milieu on psychological development and functioning.

CHANGING PERCEPTIONS

As already mentioned, researchers often neglect to consider sex as a variable in interpreting their results; also, others have pointed out the need for more examination of the onset of a disorder to determine what role social stressors play as precipitants of symptoms. Those concerned about social roles are certain that learned responses play a great part in determining the ways in which a woman approaches and deals with conflict in her life. Far more research is needed before these etiological questions can be answered (Geller and Munetz 1988).

Women still make up the majority of patients. It is curious that so little research can be found into the reasons for this fact. In 1992, the National Institutes of Health announced a program dedicated to research into women's health. Hopefully, work under this auspice also will include mental disorders. Meanwhile, the public perception of psychiatry has deteriorated, if the view of the profession as put forward in films and television is an example. No longer is the psychiatrist portrayed as kindly and wise as in the 1950s, but rather as rapacious or mentally ill. The scandals in the last few years surrounding prominent male psychiatrists who have abused their women patients have added to this negative image (APA resource document, "Legal Sanctions for Mental Health Professional–Patient Sex," March 1993; Nadelson 1993). These ethical violations have increased the feeling that psychiatrists are paternalistic and unable to appreciate or assist women with their symptoms or relationships ("Debate on Punishing Patient-Therapist Sex: Not Whether, but How" 1993). The view of psychiatrists as traditional chauvinists (Stephenson and Walker 1981; Ussher 1992) has thus been reinforced. Clinicians are often told by many women that they will only go to a psychiatrist who is female, and then only after inquiring as to her theoretical and treatment orientation. At the same time, the number of women entering psychiatry training programs compared with men is increasing.

In general, women are not in the forefront of the field (APA Official Actions 1993). Like the women who are patients, women who are psychiatrists appear not to be thought of separately or specifically for academic or organizational appointments according to the experience of many (Nadelson 1989). Few women psychiatrists are in senior academic positions, a fact that has not changed over recent decades (APA Official Actions 1993). Training programs overall do not include courses for residents in the psychology of women or in gender differences. Supervision of residents and their treatment of patients does not usually emphasize ethical aspects of the psychiatrist-patient relationship. However, recent newspaper reports and books about prominent therapists have brought about some discussion. Until more women are in leadership positions in psychiatry departments, it is probable that none of the above are likely to change.

If men and women do not work together as equals in a department or obtain equal recognition for their work, then it is not surprising that the effects of social attitudes and roles of women and men are not taught to trainees or considered in case discussions, treatment plans, medication dosages, or research designs. Attitudes toward women as peers in a profession are bound to influence how a man treats his female patients. Similarly, the woman who is experiencing discrimination or lack of recognition from her male peers will no doubt bring her resultant attitude into her conduct of therapy.

Thus, this discussion of the history of gender issues in psychiatry has led from the patient to the therapist. We know that therapy is influenced not only by the personalities of both patient and therapist but also by events and circumstances in the therapist's life (Gold and Nemiah 1992). Women are only well represented in the lower levels of psychiatric academia; there are two women holding chairs in departments of psychiatry in the United States and none in Canada. This picture has not changed in 30 years. Nevertheless, as a result of the decades of women's struggle for equality, women now study in most fields and work in most jobs. Young women believe the battle is over and then are rudely surprised when they apply for promotions (Schaller 1990).

Discussion groups at the annual meeting of the American Psychiatric Association on the difficulties of a career in psychiatry for women always take place in full rooms, and they are repeated by request yearly. Similarly, women are not represented in the higher ranks of the National Institute of Mental Health, and, in fact, charges of discrimination and harassment have been laid against that institution (Garnett 1992; "Women to Get Boost at NIMH" 1992). Women, whether psychiatrists or not, are growing increasingly angry at these injustices ("Forum Examines Obstacles to Women in Medical Research, Teaching Careers" 1993). How can the profession promise patients empathic, knowledgeable care if women are not treated well within the profession itself?

CONCLUSION

At this point in the century, women psychiatrists have the potential to influence the future course of the field as their numbers increase. But numbers do not give power and influence. Although we have learned a great deal about the etiologies of mental disorders over the past 50 years, within the entire profession a great deal remains to be done in implementing that knowledge for both male and female psychiatrists. Further research is also necessary in all the areas that have an impact on the person. The past five decades have demonstrated that biological and genetic influences are of great importance in the genesis of mental disorders; additionally, it has been shown that the impact of the environment in which the person lives must be equally considered. The discussion in this chapter has pointed to the various research findings and theories that demonstrate the special importance of environmental factors in the etiology of symptoms in women patients—particularly at this time in our culture. The insistence of women therapists—and of women theorists and activists—that gender issues are relevant to the elucidation and treatment of mental disorders is one of the accomplishments of the latter part of the twentieth century.

REFERENCES

American Psychiatric Association: Diagnostic and Statistical Manual of Mental Disorders, 3rd Edition. Washington, DC, American Psychiatric Association, 1980
American Psychiatric Association: Diagnostic and Statistical Manual of Mental Disorders, 3rd Edition, Revised. Washington, DC, American Psychiatric Association, 1987
American Psychiatric Association: Diagnostic and Statistical Manual of Mental Disorders, 4th Edition. Washington, DC, American Psychiatric Association, 1994
American Psychiatric Association: DSM-IV Sourcebook, Vol 2. Washington, DC, American Psychiatric Association (in press)
Anderson CM, Holder DP: Women and serious mental disorders, in Women in Families. Edited by McGoldrick M, Anderson CM, Walsh F. New York, WW Norton, 1989, pp 381–405
APA Official Actions: Women in academic psychiatry and research. Am J Psychiatry 150:849, 1993

Barnett RC, Baruch GK: Social roles, gender, and psychological distress, in Gender and Stress. Edited by Barnett RC, Biener L, Baruch GK. New York, Free Press, 1987, pp 122–143

Bart PB, Scully DH: The politics of hysteria: the case of the wandering womb, in Gender and Disordered Behavior. Edited by Gomberg ES, Franks V. New York, Brunner/Mazel, 1979, pp 354–380

Beck AT, Emery G, with Greenberg R: Anxiety Disorders and Phobias: A Cognitive Perspective. New York, Basic Books, 1985

Bernard J: Ground rules for marriage: perspectives on the pattern of an era, in Women and Men. Edited by Notman MT, Nadelson CC. Washington, DC, American Psychiatric Press, 1991, pp 89–115

Brown GW, Harris T: Social Origins of Depression: A Study of Psychiatric Disorder in Women. New York, The Free Press, 1978

Brown TA, Hertz RM, Barlow DH: New developments in cognitive-behavioral treatment of anxiety disorders, in American Psychiatric Press Review of Psychiatry, Vol 11. Edited by Tasman A, Riba MB. Washington, DC, American Psychiatric Press, 1992, pp 285–306

Cameron OG, Hill EM: Women and anxiety, in Women's Disorders. Edited by Parry B. Philadelphia, PA, WB Saunders, 1989, pp 175–186

Castle DJ, Wessely S, Murray RM: Sex and schizophrenia: effects of diagnostic stringency, and associations with premorbid variables. Br J Psychiatry 162:658–664, 1993

Chafe WH: The Paradox of Change: American Women in the 20th Century. New York, Oxford University Press, 1991

Clower VL: The acquisition of mature femininity, in Women and Men: New Perspectives in Gender Differences. Edited by Notman MT, Nadelson CC. Washington, DC, American Psychiatric Press, 1991, pp 75–88

Coons PM, Bowman ES, Pellow TA, et al: Post-traumatic aspects of the treatment of victims of sexual abuse and incest, in Treatment of Victims of Sexual Abuse. Edited by Kluft RP. Philadelphia, PA, WB Saunders, 1989, pp 325–335

Debate on punishing patient-therapist sex: not whether, but how. Psychiatric News, July 2, 1993, pp 5, 14

Elkin I, Shea T, Watkins JT, et al: NIMH treatment of depression collaborative research program: general effectiveness of treatments. Arch Gen Psychiatry 46:971–982, 1989

Emmett SW (ed): Theory and Treatment of Anorexia and Bulimia: Biomedical, Sociocultural, and Psychological Perspectives. New York, Brunner/Mazel, 1985

Fausto-Sterling A: Myths of Gender: Biological Theories About Women and Men, 2nd Edition. New York, Basic Books, 1985

Forum examines obstacles to women in medical research, teaching careers. Psychiatric News, July 2, 1993, pp 2, 20

Friedan B: The Second Stage. New York, Summit, 1981

Gabbard G: Psychodynamic psychiatry in the "decade of the brain." Am J Psychiatry 149:991–998, 1992

Garner DM, Garfinkel PE (eds): Handbook of Psychotherapy for Anorexia Nervosa and Bulimia. New York, Guilford, 1985

Garnett C: Intramural women scientists speak out on status at NIH. NIHAA Update, The Newsletter of the NIH Alumni Association 4:1, 22–24, 1992

Geller JL, Munetz MR: The iatrogenic creation of psychiatric chronicity in women, in Treating Chronically Mentally Ill Women. Edited by Bachrach LL, Nadelson CC. Washington, DC, American Psychiatric Press, 1988, pp 143–177

Gold JH, Nemiah JC (eds): Beyond Transference: When the Therapist's Real Life Intrudes. Washington, DC, American Psychiatric Press, 1992

Gove WR: Sex differences in the epidemiology of mental disorder: evidence and explanations, in Gender and Disordered Behavior. Edited by Gomberg ES, Franks V. New York, Brunner/Mazel, 1979, pp 23–68

Group for the Advancement of Psychiatry: The Educated Woman: Prospects and Problems (GAP Report 92). New York, Group for the Advancement of Psychiatry, 1975

Halmi KA (ed): Psychobiology and Treatment of Anorexia Nervosa and Bulimia. Washington, DC, American Psychiatric Press, 1992

Harris T, Brown GW, Bifulco A: Loss of parent in childhood and adult psychiatric disorder: the role of social class position and premarital pregnancy. Psychol Med 17:163–183, 1987

Harrison M: Women's health: new models of care and a new academic discipline. Journal of Women's Health 2:61–66, 1993

Holder DP, Anderson CM: Women, work, and the family, in Women in Families. Edited by McGoldrick M, Anderson CM, Walsh F. New York, WW Norton, 1989, pp 358–380

Hollingshead AB, Redlich FD: Social Class and Mental Illness. New York, Wiley, 1958

Hollon SD, DeRubeis RJ, Evans MD, et al: Cognitive therapy and pharmacotherapy for depression. Arch Gen Psychiatry 49:774–781, 1992

Holmes TH, Rahe RH: The social readjustment rating scale. J Psychosom Res 11:213–218, 1967

Hudson JI, Pope HG (eds): The Psychobiology of Bulimia. Washington, DC, American Psychiatric Press, 1987

Iacono WG, Beiser M: Are males more likely than females to develop schizophrenia? Am J Psychiatry 149:1070–1074, 1992

Johnson C (ed): Psychodynamic Treatment of Anorexia Nervosa and Bulimia. New York, Guilford, 1991

Keller MB, Lavori PW, Mueller TI, et al: Time to recovery, chronicity, and levels of psychopathology in major depression. Arch Gen Psychiatry 49:809–816, 1992

Kendler KS, Silberg SL, Neale MC, et al: Genetic and environmental factors in the aetiology of menstrual, premenstrual and neurotic symptoms: a population-based twin study. Psychol Med 22:85–100, 1992a

Kendler KS, Neale MC, Kessler RC, et al: Major depression and generalized anxiety disorder: same genes, (partly) different environments? Arch Gen Psychiatry 49:716–721, 1992b

Kupfer DJ, Frank E, Perel JM, et al: Five-year outcome for maintenance therapies in recurrent depression. Arch Gen Psychiatry 49:769–773, 1992

Leighton DC, Harding JS, Macklin DB, et al: The Character of Danger: Psychiatric Symptoms in Selected Communities. New York, Basic Books, 1963

Lerner HE: Special issues for women in psychotherapy, in The Women Patient, Vol 3. Edited by Notman MT, Nadelson CC. New York, Plenum, 1982, pp 273–286

Lewine R, Burbach D, Meltzer HY: Effect of diagnostic criteria on the rates of male to female schizophrenic patients. Am J Psychiatry 141:84–87, 1984

Masters WH, Johnson VE: Human Sexual Response. Boston, MA, Little, Brown, 1966

McBride AB, McBride WL: Women's health scholarship: from critique to assertion. Journal of Women's Health 2:43–47, 1993

McEwan BS: Sex differences in the brain: what they are and how they arise, in Women and Men: New Perspectives in Gender Differences. Edited by Notman MT, Nadelson CC. Washington, DC, American Psychiatric Press, 1991, pp 35–41

Nadelson CC: Professional issues for women. Psychiatr Clin North Am 12:25–33, 1989

Nadelson CC: Emerging issues in medical ethics, in Psychological Aspects of Women's Health Care: The Interface Between Psychiatry and Obstetrics and Gynecology. Edited by Stewart DE, Stotland NL. Washington, DC, American Psychiatric Press, 1993, pp 485–503

Nadelson CC, Notman MT: The impact of the new psychology of men and women on psychotherapy, in American Psychiatric Press Review of Psychiatry, Vol 10. Edited by Tasman A, Goldfinger SM. Washington, DC, American Psychiatric Press, 1991, pp 608–626

Notman MT: Depression in women, in Women's Disorders. Edited by Parry B. Philadelphia, PA, WB Saunders, 1989, pp 221–230

Notman MT, Nadelson CC: A review of gender differences in brain and behavior, in Women and Men: New Perspectives in Gender Differences. Edited by Notman MT, Nadelson CC. Washington, DC, American Psychiatric Press, 1991, pp 23–34

Notman MT, Klein R, Jordan JV, et al: Women's unique developmental issues across the life cycle, in American Psychiatric Press Review of Psychiatry, Vol 10. Edited by Tasman A, Goldfinger SM. Washington, DC, American Psychiatric Press, 1991, pp 556–577

Orbach S: Hunger Strike: The Anorectic's Struggle as a Metaphor for Our Age. New York, WW Norton, 1986

Raphael B: Women and Mental Health (Monograph Series No 1). National Health and Medical Research Council. Canberra, Australian Government Publishing Service, 1992

Regier DA, Burke JD: Psychiatric disorders in the community, in American Psychiatric Association Annual Review, Vol 6. Edited by Hales RE, Frances AJ. Washington, DC, American Psychiatric Press, 1987, pp 610–646

Robins LN: The assessment of psychiatric diagnosis in epidemiological studies, in American Psychiatric Association Annual Review, Vol 6. Edited by Hales RE, Frances AJ. Washington, DC, American Psychiatric Press, 1987, pp 589–609

Robins LN, Helzer JE, Weissman MM, et al: Lifetime prevalence of specific psychiatric disorders in three sites. Arch Gen Psychiatry 41:949–958, 1984

Rothman SM: Woman's Proper Place: A History of Changing Ideals and Practices, 1870 to the Present. New York, Basic Books, 1978

Rubinow DR: The premenstrual syndrome: new views. JAMA 268:1908–1912, 1992

Schaller JG: Commentary: the advancement of women in academic medicine. JAMA 264:1854–1855, 1990

Seeman MV: Addressing gender differences of schizophrenia and its treatment. Contemporary Psychiatry, November–December 1992, pp 4–8

Seiden AM: Overview: research on the psychology of women. Am J Psychiatry 133:995–1007; 1111–1123, 1976

Shea MT, Elkin I, Imber SD, et al: Course of depressive symptoms over follow-up. Arch Gen Psychiatry 49:782–787, 1992

Sherwin S: No Longer Patient: Feminist Ethics and Health Care. Philadelphia, PA, Temple University Press, 1992

Showalter E: The Female Malady: Women, Madness, and English Culture, 1830–1980. New York, Basic Books, 1985

Smith DE, David SJ (eds): Women Look at Psychiatry. Vancouver, Canada, Press Gang Publishers, 1975

Spiegel D, Cardena E: Dissociative mechanisms in posttraumatic stress disorder, in Posttraumatic Stress Disorder. Edited by Wolf M, Mosnaim AD. Washington, DC, American Psychiatric Press, 1990, pp 22–34

Spitzer RL, Severino S, Williams JBW, et al: Late luteal phase dysphoric disorder and DSM-III-R. Am J Psychiatry 146:892–897, 1989

Srole L, Langner TS, Michael ST, et al: Mental Health in the Metropolis: The Midtown Manhattan Study, Vol 1. New York, McGraw-Hill, 1962

Stephenson PS, Walker GA: The psychiatrist-woman patient relationship, in Women and Mental Health. Edited by Howell E, Bayes M. New York, Basic Books, 1981, pp 113–130

Symonds A: Phobias after marriage: a woman's declaration of dependence. Am J Psychoanal 31:144–152, 1971

Tavris C: The Mismeasure of Woman. New York, Simon & Schuster, 1992

Ussher J: Women's Madness: Misogyny or Mental Illness? Amherst, MA, University of Massachusetts Press, 1992

Waller G: Sexual abuse and eating disorders: borderline personality disorder as a mediating factor. Br J Psychiatry 162:771–775, 1993

Walsh MR (ed): The Psychology of Women: Ongoing Debates. New Haven, CT, Yale University Press, 1987

Weissman MM: Epidemiology overview, in American Psychiatric Association Annual Review, Vol 6. Edited by Hales RE, Frances AJ. Washington, DC, American Psychiatric Press, 1987, pp 574–588

Weissman MM, Klerman GL: Sex differences and the epidemiology of depression, in Gender and Disordered Behavior. Edited by Gomberg ES, Franks V. New York, Brunner/Mazel, 1979, pp 381–425

Westkott M: The Feminist Legacy of Karen Horney. New Haven, CT, Yale University Press, 1986

Williams JH: Psychology of Women: Behavior in a Biosocial Context. New York, WW Norton, 1977

Wolf N: The Beauty Myth. New York, Doubleday, 1991

Woloch N: Women and the American Experience. New York, Knopf, 1984

Women to get boost at NIMH, Goodwin promises APA Committee, Psychiatric News, November 6, 1992, pp 2, 15

Chapter 5

Fifty Years of Psychiatric Services: Changes in Treatment of Chronically Mentally Ill Patients

John A. Talbott, M.D.

In the past 50 years, we have seen enormous changes in the delivery of psychiatric services in America, especially those targeted to severely and chronically mentally ill patients. In this chapter, I review the past history of services that set the stage for these more contemporary changes, describe the introduction of services during each decade since 1945, and conclude with some speculation about what changes we can expect in the future.

EARLY HISTORY: 1492–1945

Evolution of the Institution: 1492–1854

In our earliest colonial days, there was no such profession as psychiatry, nor were there any psychiatric services. Mentally ill persons, if they were lucky, were housed at home, in detached buildings, or with sympathetic physicians; if unlucky or oppositional, they were often found wandering around the countryside, the earliest result of "dumping" in America (Dain 1976).

The earliest "institutions" in America were established by various county authorities and consisted of three general categories: poorhouses and almshouses for the destitute, jails for criminals, and workhouses for "rogues, vagabonds, the idle and disorderly" (Maxmen et al. 1974; Quen 1974, 1975; Rothman 1971). All became unwitting repositories for mentally ill persons. Excepting the notable example of witches, who were persecuted, most mentally ill persons were more the cause of community aggravation than concerted treatment.

In 1772, however, the Pennsylvania Hospital in Philadelphia opened as a general hospital with a separate unit for mentally ill patients. Soon after, in 1773, the first hospital devoted solely to mentally ill patients, called the "Publick Hospital," opened in Williamsburg, Virginia. The first private psychiatric hospital, the Friend's Hospital, opened in 1817 in Philadelphia.

In response to the scandalous conditions found in local, largely county facilities, advocates such as Dorothea Dix lobbied the federal government to establish a network of humane psychiatric hospitals. The resultant state mental hospital, now so reviled as a horrible institution, was actually seen as a positive solution to these preceding institutions.

The state hospitals' growth into huge systems, led by New York and Massachusetts, began during the 1800s and continued until 1955. During this entire period, the focus of both private and public asylums was on containment and treatment, specifically "moral treatment," that derived from the work of Pinel in France and the Tukes in the United Kingdom. Although hydrotherapy, activities, and some medication were provided, treatment, in our more modern sense of the word, did not occur.

Devolution of the Institution: 1855 Onward

Although the community developed in Gheel, Belgium, probably represents the first large-scale example of an alternative to psychiatric hospitalization, it was not until the mid-nineteenth century that American psychiatry followed suit. In 1855, a farm program was begun in Williamsburg, Virginia, by J. M. Galt (one of the original 13 founding members of the American Psychiatric Association [APA]); a cottage plan was initiated in Kankakee, Illinois, in 1877; and a boarding-out program was developed in the Commonwealth of Massachusetts in 1885 (Copp 1907; Deutsch 1937; Galt 1855). All, it must be noted, were intended to provide posthospital care rather than an optional treatment avenue at the start of the patient's illness.

Although the development of "aftercare" and other outpatient programs at the turn of the twentieth century was intended primarily to provide follow-up treatment for patients returning to their home environments after discharge from hospitals, eventually these programs began to provide outpatient care to newly identified patients ("A Century of Debate Surrounds Community Care" 1976). The development of these services was soon followed by the creation throughout the country of "mental clinics," university-sponsored "satellite clinics," and "traveling clinics" (the first was established in 1909, with the number growing to over 400 by 1927) (Ewalt 1975; Jarrett 1927).

In addition, the turn of the century saw the beginning of the proliferation of several new types of hospitals. "Psychopathic hospitals" such as the Boston Psychopathic Hospital (1912), now the Massachusetts Mental Health Center, were intended to provide active treatment—rather than custodial care—nearer to families, friends, and community (Hurd 1946; Rossi 1962). Psychiatric units in general hospitals, often run by universities, grew greatly in number. Even the federal government built veterans hospitals, armed forces institutions, and public health service facilities.

Several developments in Europe in the twentieth century pushed to the forefront the implementation of alternatives to traditional hospitals: specific examples include the opening of the first day hospital in Moscow in the 1930s; the development by Querido of a mobile home-care program in Amsterdam; and the establishment by Bierer of a therapeutic social club in England (Bierer 1964; Querido 1956). By the 1950s, partial hospitalization programs (Hoge et al. 1992), home-care programs (Becker et al. 1965), and psychosocial programs were commonplace and had demonstrated their usefulness (H. Modlin, personal communication, November 1981). In addition, the 1950s saw the introduction of several new service elements: halfway houses (Golomb and Kocsis 1988), vocational rehabilitation programs, and 24-hour walk-in services (Becker et al. 1965; Bellak 1964; Black 1964) (Figure 5–1).

Setting the Stage for Change

With the advantage of hindsight, it seems obvious that despite the steady and staggering growth of psychiatric hospitals, the introduc-

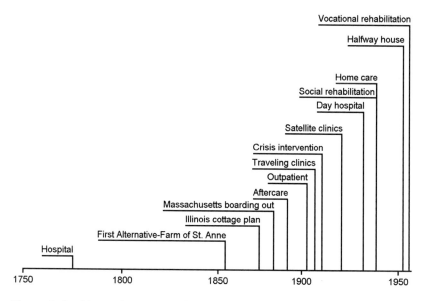

Figure 5–1. Alternatives to state hospitals. Starting in 1855, a number of alternative programs to state hospitals were established in the United States. *Source.* Reprinted from Talbott JA: "Current Perspectives in the United States on the Chronically Mentally Ill," in *Recent Advances in Schizophrenia.* Edited by Kales A, Stefanis CN, Talbott JA. New York, Springer-Verlag, 1990, pp. 279–295. Used with permission.

tion of ambulatory alternatives to hospitals would result in a similar growth spurt. Although such alternatives were widespread, no one community ever had an adequate number and range of these newer services. Dramatic changes in thinking and action were needed to bring about true changes in the systems established to care for mentally ill patients. World War II provided an impetus for just such changes.

PLANNING FOR CHANGE: 1945–1954

Following World War II

World War II provided an unwitting stimulus to change. First, previously civilian armed forces physicians, the government, and eventually the American public were shocked by the numbers of discharges from the military for reasons of mental illness. During the period of the war, 1.8 million Americans were found unfit for service on induction and 850,000 were discharged for reasons of mental illness, a figure that comprised 40% of all discharges (Mora 1959; Whittington 1966). During one period, more soldiers were discharged for psychiatric reasons than were inducted. Second, state mental hospitals were drained of their physician staffs, and conditions there were found to be "shocking" by "naive" conscientious objectors performing alternative service (Joint Commission on Mental Health and Illness 1961; Musto 1975). Third, nonpsychiatric military physicians became increasingly interested in psychiatry because 1) psychiatric treatment was such an integral component of armed forces medicine, 2) psychiatrists were routinely performing consultations on nonpsychiatric wards, 3) it was evident that conditions such as "war neurosis" could be effectively treated using short-term techniques and principles (Salmon 1917), and 4) some physicians who were pressed into psychiatric duty decided to remain in the field (Linn 1964; Zusman 1961).

Finally, after the war, psychiatry itself was reinvigorated when a group of "young turks" founded the Group for the Advancement of Psychiatry as an alternative organization to the APA, which they perceived as more stodgy.

The Federal Scene

In 1930, the U.S. Public Health Service established a Division of Mental Hygiene (Rossi 1962). It was not until after World War II, however, that Congress, concerned about the deplorable conditions in the state hospitals and the incidence of mental illness among soldiers in the armed forces, passed the visionary Mental Health Act of 1946. It renamed the Division of Mental Hygiene as the National Institute of Mental Health (NIMH); increased its funding; and charged it with conducting research and demonstration projects as well as providing coordination, training, and assistance to states for community programs (Mechanic 1969; Musto 1975). The first director of NIMH, Robert Felix (1947), then proceeded to promote psychiatric screening, prevention, and outpatient treatment with the hope that eventually there would be one outpatient clinic for every 100,000 Americans. Thus, this first federal initiative to provide psychiatric services was clearly intended to strengthen the capacity for providing services not in hospitals but in ambulatory settings.

Developments Both Abroad and at Home

It should be noted that developments in Europe were also proceeding along noninstitutional lines; in the United Kingdom, wards were opened (Glasscote et al. 1964), Maxwell Jones (1953) introduced his innovative "therapeutic community," and the National Health Act of 1948 ensured that the relatives of patients could obtain their discharge unless the patients were dangerous. In France, Paul Sividon was an early proponent of sociotherapy, resocialization, and a unit system for psychiatric hospitals (Caplan and Caplan 1967; Symposium on Preventive and Social Psychiatry 1958).

Ironically, in this country, it took the Korean War (1950–1953) to cause us to remember Salmon's (1917) lessons on treating psychiatric casualties (e.g., posttraumatic stress disorder) learned years before in World War I—the lessons of immediacy, proximity, and expectancy. In addition, hundreds of military psychiatrists were trained (Glass 1958; Talbott 1969) to practice "command consultation," a form of community consultation and community psychiatry that helped provide psychiatric treatment to soldiers nearer the lines. Also during this decade, Lindeman's pioneering work with disaster victims focused attention on short-term crisis intervention (Lindeman 1944); the first day hospital in the United States was started at the Menninger Clinic in Topeka, Kansas (H. Modlin, personal communication, November 1981); and group therapy techniques were becoming increasingly popular (Mechanic 1969).

Also during this decade, the numbers of psychiatric units in general hospitals continued to grow. These units often found it easier to provide aftercare and involve families than did state facilities (Linn 1964). The Veterans Administration increased its psychiatric services to care for the huge influx of mentally disabled dischargees (Glasscote et al. 1964). Because society valued outpatient rather than inpatient care, the number of outpatient clinics rapidly proliferated; therapeutic communities were becoming more common, as were community education efforts, consultation to community agencies, attempts to avoid hospitalization, and increased interest in developing alternatives to hospitalization (Hunt 1956; Joint Commission on Mental Health and Illness 1961).

Finally, in the United States, shortly after World War II, the first well-known, organized psychiatric rehabilitation program was founded in New York City at Fountain House (Glasscote et al. 1971). Fountain House offered patients discharged from state hospitals housing, vocational rehabilitation, and social rehabilitation using a "clubhouse model"; that is, afflicted persons were members of a social club, not patients in a medical setting.

However, despite this decade of incredible innovation and promise, we still lacked a plan for a true systems change. In 1952, though, a World Health Organization committee chaired by Daniel Blain, a former president and medical director of the APA, formulated just such a plan (Table 5–1). This plan was for a "community mental hospital" that would provide outpatient, partial hospitalization, and rehabilitation services, as well as conduct research and community education (Glasscote et al. 1964).

In 1953, in his presidential address, Kenneth Appel—then president of the APA—called for a new and critical examination of state mental hospitals. He and subsequent APA President Harry Solomon called for "an organized plan for growth" and an end to state hospitals as we knew them, respectively, to be replaced by community treatment and rehabilitation.

The states were listening. In 1954, the first state legislation was passed in New York to implement a plan not unlike that proposed by Blain's World Health Organization committee (Glasscote et al. 1964), but that one included inpatient care and community consultation as well (Table 5–1).

So, entering 1955, psychiatric services were at a critical point. State mental hospitals had grown steadily to accommodate a staggering number (almost 560,000) of persons (Figure 5–2) in antiquated, overcrowded asylums. Alternatives to traditional institutions had sprung up all over the globe, albeit in inadequate numbers. There were now international and state plans for a balanced service system incorporating inpatient, outpatient, community, and rehabilitation services. Enter a new phenomenon—deinstitutionalization.

DEINSTITUTIONALIZATION AND COMMUNITY MENTAL HEALTH CENTERS: 1955–1964

The Pharmacological Revolution

Quite unbeknownst to mental health planners and legislators, psychopharmacological researchers had discovered new and powerful medications that in many instances could control what we now call the

Table 5–1.   Components of community mental health centers

World Health Organization Committee (1954)	New York State (1954)	Regulations	
		CMHC (1965)	CMHC Amendment (1975)
	Inpatient	Inpatient	Inpatient
Outpatient	Outpatient	Outpatient	Outpatient
Partial hospitalization		Partial hospitalization	Partial hospitalization
		Emergency (24 hour)	Emergency (24 hour)
Community education	Consultation and education	Consultation and education	Consultation and education
		Diagnostic	
		Precare and aftercare	Screening patients for courts and agencies before commitment to state hospital
			Follow-up care
Rehabilitation	Rehabilitation	Rehabilitation	
Research		Research and evaluation	
			Transitional housing
			Services for elderly patients
			Services for children
			Services for alcoholic patients
			Services for patients with drug problems

Note.   CMHC = community mental health center.
Source.   Reprinted from Talbott JA: "Trends in the Delivery of Psychiatric Services," in *Psychiatric Administration: A Comprehensive Text for the Clinician-Executive.* Edited by Talbott JA, Kaplan SR. New York, Grune & Stratton, 1983, p. 12. Used with permission.

"positive symptoms" of schizophrenia (Carpenter et al. 1988). By 1955, chlorpromazine had been introduced into most state hospital system formularies. Its impact was dramatic; it is hard for those trained since 1955 to really appreciate what the treatment of individuals with psychoses was like before.

Shortly after 1955, antidepressants were introduced in teaching and research institutions, and within the decade lithium was introduced as well. To this day, experts argue about the contributing factors behind deinstitutionalization; but surely the foremost factor was psychotropic medication.

Deinstitutionalization: The Early Phase

The first phase of deinstitutionalization was ushered in rather quietly—without planning, without warning, and without even a name. The earliest definition in the literature of the term "deinstitutionalization" was in a speech by then-NIMH Director Bertram Brown two decades later (Bachrach 1976). I mention this fact to bring home the point that although we were poised in 1955 for major changes in the treatment and care of chronically mentally ill patients—hospitals were deplorable and overcrowded, alternatives to hospitals had been found to be valuable, social and community psychiatric theories abounded, and two plans for a more "community-based" care system had been formulated—no one yelled "charge!" We did not set a public policy to move patients from hospital to community settings; rather, it happened due to a confluence of events (Talbott 1985).

These events included 1) the presence of an ideological and philosophical base (e.g., community psychiatric care); 2) the introduction of a new technology (e.g., chlorpromazine); 3) the legal advocacy pressures to decrease involuntary commitment and later to ensure patients' rights to refuse treatment, be treated in the "least restrictive environment," and so forth; and 4) even later, the economic push to treat patients in "community" settings where they were eligible for the new federal entitlements of the 1960s—Medicaid, Medicare, Supplemental Security Income, and Social Security disability income.

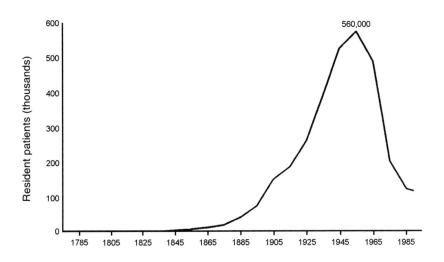

Figure 5–2. State hospital population. After a peak in 1955, deinstitutionalization resulted in an 80% decrease over the next three decades.
Source. Adapted from Stroup and Manderscheid 1988.

In this early phase (1955–1964), the total state hospital census fell relatively slowly, because despite the pace of discharge, total admissions kept rising (Figure 5–3). However, these discharges included those patients who were least ill and disabled, with families who could be located and who would take them. The sicker and tougher-to-place patients would come later.

Programmatic and Research Developments

During the decade of 1955–1964, several new programmatic elements appeared on the landscape of psychiatric services. These included home-care programs (Becker et al. 1965); a new variety of traveling clinic (Brown et al. 1957); troubleshooting clinics (e.g., 24-hour emergency walk-in clinics) (Bellak 1964); suicide prevention centers (Kiev 1963); and community clinics for state hospital patients (Sampson et al. 1958). In addition, during this period, Altro Workshops was established in the Bronx, New York, as a therapeutic workshop for chronically mentally ill patients and served as a model for vocational rehabilitation efforts elsewhere (Black 1986).

Even the state hospitals were influenced by these new programmatic elements. Large state hospitals in Kansas and New York were broken up into smaller, decentralized, and subsequently geographically related "units"; satellite hospitals in the community were established in Connecticut and Massachusetts; and the first attempt to integrate

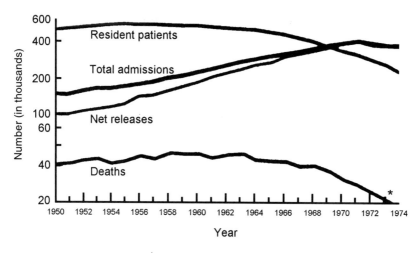

Figure **5–3.** Patient statistics for state and county hospitals, United States 1950–1974. *There were 19,899 deaths in 1973 and 16,597 deaths in 1974. *Source.* Published and unpublished data of the National Institute of Mental Health.

county and state services to provide precare, inpatient care, and after-care was pioneered in Dutchess County, New York, followed by attempts to provide continuity of care (Milbank Memorial Fund 1956, 1960, 1962).

In the United Kingdom, the Mental Health Act of 1959 ended the legal distinction between mental hospitals and general hospitals and established community-care facilities such as hostels, clubs, sheltered workshops, and "retraining" units (Mechanic 1969). In this country, superintendents of state facilities discovered the "open-door" movement pioneered in the United Kingdom.

Finally, reflecting the fervor felt by those in psychiatric services, the research community was focusing on treatment of victims of disasters, individual stress, and brainwashing. It also began to examine the impact of "total institutions" (Goffman 1961) and the startling incidence and prevalence of mental disorders (Symposium on Preventive and Social Psychiatry 1958). Others areas of focus were the maldistribution of psychiatrists and the differential treatment of illnesses according to socioeconomic status (Hollingshead and Redlich 1958), as well as the effect of community disorganization on psychiatric morbidity (Leighton 1959).

Prevention

Although at first blush prevention does not seem to fit in a chapter on the history of services for chronically mentally ill patients, its prominence in the discussions about community psychiatry make it relevant. Soon after the turn of the century, Adolf Meyer (1915) was the first American psychiatrist to advocate a public health approach to psychiatry and the importance of prevention of mental illness, as well as the *integration* of prevention, treatment, and aftercare. Clifford Beers (1908), a layperson, conceived and brought to life the "mental health movement" that stressed mental health rather than mental illness. A third influence was the "child guidance movement," which also began shortly after the turn of the century and also stressed prevention (Caplan and Caplan 1967).

A change in social attitudes had also taken place in the United States—from social Darwinism to progressivism. Thus, rather than viewing mental illness as the result of biological and hereditary factors, prompting treatment, people viewed mental illness as the result of environmental conditions (e.g., inadequate child rearing, slum conditions, and poor family background), prompting attempts at social engineering (Caplan and Caplan 1967; Musto 1975). Throughout the first half of the twentieth century, many psychiatrists called for increased involvement with other mental health professionals, lawyers, teachers, clergy, business executives, and recreation leaders (Bassett 1933).

Gerald Caplan brought together the existing knowledge and sys-temized the concept of prevention in the 1950s and 1960s (Caplan 1961, 1964; Caplan and Caplan 1967) (Table 5–2). Caplan was the first Amer-ican psychiatrist to devote his life to the pursuit of primary prevention. He advocated working with social workers, child care workers, teach-ers, and other professionals in settings such as public health clinics, schools, and businesses. His advocacy for primary, rather than second-ary or tertiary, preventive activities in community mental health was a critical influence at this time.

In retrospect, it is clear to most experts that tertiary prevention was getting short shrift as deinstitutionalization began in earnest in the United States (Talbott 1983). For those of us who embraced Caplan's direction, the 1960s were heady times, but consulting with community agencies and lecturing to the police never came close to meeting the real problem that was facing us (Talbott and Talbott 1971; Talbott 1977).

Action for Mental Health

The federal Mental Health Study Act of 1955 created a Joint Commis-sion on Mental Health and Illness whose final report, *Action for Mental Health* (1961), constituted another step in the formation of a blueprint for what was later enacted in law as the community mental health cen-ter. The report called for more money to be spent on mental health ser-

Table 5–2.   Caplan's schema for prevention of mental illness

Type of prevention	Goal	Methods
Primary	Reduction in the incidence of all mental disorders	1. Consultation to caregivers 2. Education of community leaders 3. Social action
Secondary	Reduction in the duration of those incidents of mental illness that do occur	1. Early detection and screening 2. Early diagnosis and referral 3. Prompt and effective treat-ment
Tertiary	Reduction in impair-ment resulting from mental illness	1. Education to eliminate prejudice 2. Communication with social networks 3. Avoidance of hospitalization 4. Hospital-community proximity

Source.   Reprinted from Talbott JA: "Trends in the Delivery of Psychiatric Services," in *Psychiatric Administration: A Comprehensive Text for the Clinician-Executive.* Edited by Talbott JA, Kaplan SR. New York, Grune & Stratton, 1983, pp. 3–19. Used with permission.

vices, more research, community clinics connected with general hospitals to serve populations of 50,000, rehabilitation, community services, community education to foster prevention, care nearer patients' homes, more nonprofessional mental health workers, and an end to any new state hospitals housing over 1,000 patients.

This dramatic statement from a high-level commission, calling for what President Kennedy later termed a "bold new approach," was in keeping with the other attempts at social change during this decade. Indeed, at the same time the federal government launched the "hunger program," the "Great Society," neighborhood health centers, model cities, and the Elementary and Secondary Education Act of 1964 (Chu and Trotter 1974).

It is perhaps worthwhile at this point to recapitulate the state of knowledge and the values held at this unique point in our history. For 100 years, psychiatric services in the United States had evolved from a single monolithic institution, the mental hospital, to encompass multiple programmatic elements. These elements were found at times in single programs (e.g., hostels) and at times in a combined delivery entity (e.g., crisis intervention, 24-hour emergency treatment, walk-in clinics) (Table 5–3).

In addition, at least since the turn of the twentieth century, new values and philosophies had replaced the former institutional ones, ranging from a preference for primary prevention to a concept of geographic responsibility (Table 5–4). Both the programmatic elements and the concepts, evolved over 100 years of progress and experimentation with services, found expression in the new, dominant mental health service—the community mental health center (CMHC).

The CMHC

Between the time that *Action for Mental Health* (Joint Commission on Mental Health and Illness 1961) was published and John Fitzgerald Kennedy signed The Mental Retardation Facilities and Community Mental Health Centers Construction Act of 1963, the blueprint for building this embodiment of the programmatic elements and concepts composing community psychiatry underwent some changes (Connery 1968, Foley 1975). Principally, mental retardation services were introduced as a separate act.

However, for the most part, the CMHC act spelled out a "center" that followed the line of development of the past 100 years, providing services to all, accountability to the community, ease of information exchange and referral, and overall an emphasis on *comprehensive services and continuity of care* (Kennedy 1964; Public Law 88-164 1963). The key elements, following the World Health Organization and New York State precedents (Table 5–1), were to be inpatient care; outpatient care;

Table 5–3.   Program elements in community psychiatry

Aftercare	Hostels
Alternatives to asylums (psychopathic and general hospitals)	Indirect services (consultation and education)
Alternatives to hospitalization	Integrated programs of prevention, treatment, and aftercare
Brief treatment	Integration of state and county programs
Citizen participation	
Clinics (outpatient, traveling, and satellite)	Interdisciplinary teams and training
Community education	Nonmedical personnel (e.g., social workers, nurses)
Community consultation	
Community participation	Open wards
Crisis intervention	Paraprofessionals
Emergency treatment (24 hour)	Partial hospitalization (day, night, weekend)
Family care	Prevention (primary, secondary, and tertiary)
Family orientation	
Foster care	Rehabilitation (social and vocational)
General practitioners	Therapeutic community
Halfway houses	Unitization
Home care	Walk-in clinics

Source.   Reprinted from Talbott JA: "Twentieth-Century Developments in American Psychiatry." *Psychiatric Quarterly* 54:215–216, 1982. Used with permission.

partial hospitalization; 24-hour emergency care; community consultation and education; diagnostic, precare, and aftercare services; rehabilitation; and research and evaluation. This model was to set the thinking on delivery of psychiatric services to severely mentally ill patients for the next two decades.

THE IMPACT OF DEINSTITUTIONALIZATION: 1965–1974

The Middle Phase of Deinstitutionalization

During this decade, the pace of deinstitutionalization picked up, and state hospital censuses began to drop more dramatically (Figure 5–2). However, there remained an optimism that CMHCs would take over the state facilities' burden.

One downside of the enthusiasm of the 1960s—at least for chronically mentally ill patients—was the belief that mental hospitals caused mental illness and that care in the community would decrease total

Table 5–4. Concepts of community psychiatry

Accessibility	Integration of state and local services
Accountability to the community	Interdisciplinary collaboration
Active treatment	Linkages between human services network
All ages served	
Availability	Live in community
Alternatives to hospitalization	Mental disorder as only one part of life
Avoidance of hospitalization	Minimal interventions
Catchment areas (districts)	Multidisciplinary
Citizen participation	Planning for gaps in service
Communication between workers and agencies	Poor, care for
	Prevention (primary, secondary, and tertiary)
Community care better	
Community participation	Proximity
Community ties retained	Public health
Comprehensive treatment	Rehabilitation
Continuity of care	Reintegration into the community
Coordination among agencies	Responsible person enters other systems when patient goes (e.g., hospital)
Early detection and treatment	
Environmental influence	
Expectancy	Segmental treatment
Geographic responsibility	Social engineering
Health more important than illness	Sociocultural influence
Immediacy	Transfer easy among elements
Indirect services	Written agreements
Information exchange easy	

Source. Reprinted from Talbott JA: "Twentieth-Century Developments in American Psychiatry." *Psychiatric Quarterly* 54:215–216, 1982. Used with permission.

morbidity. At some point, however, it became obvious that mental illness was *not* less evident in the community; instead, it was more so. In addition, the prevailing enthusiasm for unsubstantiated primary prevention services (which were intended to bring about elimination of all mental illness)—with inadequate attention to tertiary prevention (prevention of future or further disability)—led to de facto neglect of chronically ill patients in favor of less psychiatrically impaired populations.

Despite this situation, however, most professionals attempted valiantly to cope with the increasingly chronic discharged population rather than condemning deinstitutionalization (Shapiro 1971). However, professional and lay publications began to mention the problem. *The NYSDB Bulletin* published a series of critical articles titled "Who Will Care for the Patients?" (Talbott 1972). *The New York Times* also published a series on the problem in 1974 (Schumach 1974).

After a decade of deinstitutionalization, the consequences of its total lack of planning, inadequate funding of community care, and naive implementation were beginning to become obvious. Seedy hotels became "community residences" for discharged patients, emergency rooms of general hospitals were flooded with patients with chronic illnesses, and no one seemed responsible for severely and chronically ill patients anymore (Talbott 1979). In addition, one survey conducted in 1975 revealed an absolute paucity of community care, housing, jobs, and rehabilitation services to serve those patients now deinstitutionalized (Talbott 1978b).

In examining the 1970 census data compared with the data of 1950, Morton Kramer (1975), a leading NIMH epidemiologist, pointed out that in fact the total percentage of Americans in institutions had not changed since 1955. What had changed was the number of people in each type of institution; Kramer noted that the number of persons in state hospitals had decreased by two-thirds, compensated for by those who were now in nursing homes and jails (Figure 5–4). This phenomenon became known as transinstitutionalization, and its implications were disturbing to health policy experts (Talbott 1979).

CMHC Development

Despite the beginning awareness that deinstitutionalization was not proceeding without hitches, the enthusiasm for CMHCs was high during this period. Several important books (Beigel and Levenson 1972; Bindman and Spiegel 1969; Whittington 1966) appeared and shaped the thinking of those who were planning and implementing psychiatric services. In addition, the zeitgeist of the time was embodied in "movements": the civil rights movement, the student movement, the free speech movement, and the women's movement. The cry of the day was community control, and CMHCs became caught up in issues (e.g., rats, lead paint, racism) that psychiatrists knew little about, at the expense of severe and chronic mental illnesses, which they knew much more about.

In addition, the vision of a network of CMHCs spanning the country turned illusory, with inadequate federal funding for all 750 catchment areas, inadequate support from all states for this new allocation from state tax levies, and wariness on the part of some local hospitals and governments about establishing new services.

General Hospitals

It was hoped that general hospitals would "pick up some of the slack" created by state hospital downsizing, and that happened to some ex-

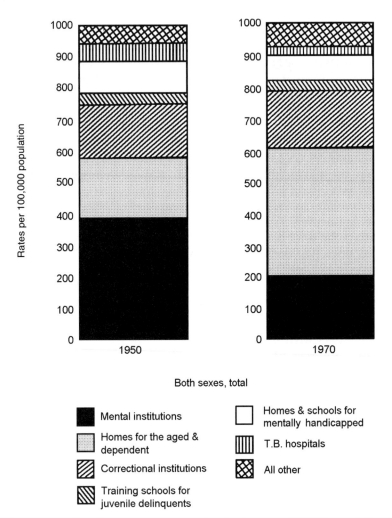

Figure 5–4. Distribution of persons in institutions per 100,000 population by type of institution, United States, 1950 and 1970.
Source. Reprinted from Talbott JA: "The Chronic Adult Mental Patient: An Overview," in *Chronic Mental Illness in Children and Adolescents.* Edited by Looney J. Washington, DC, American Psychiatric Press, 1988, pp. 19–37. Used with permission. Data from U.S. Bureau of the Census: *Persons in Institutions, 1950 and 1970.* Washington, DC, U.S. Bureau of the Census.

tent. However, Bachrach (1979) showed that at least during one 4-year period, this effort on the part of the general hospitals was insufficient.

The country was now at another critical point—one that would lead to a reexamination of deinstitutionalization and the capacity of CMHCs and general hospitals to ever pick up the slack created by deinstitutionalization of patients in the state facilities.

FIXING THE SYSTEM: 1975–1984

The Later Phase of Deinstitutionalization

It was in these years that the drop in state hospital censuses became precipitous. Between 1955 and 1976, the census in state hospitals dropped from 558,992 to 193,436 persons—a net loss of 365,556 patients. Where had they gone? State governments pointed out that many had died.

But by this point, many other victims of deinstitutionalization were beginning to be seen on our cities' streets, in what would become a legion of homeless mentally ill persons (Lamb 1984). In addition, there were demonstrable numbers of severely and chronically mentally ill patients in other institutions such as jails, nursing homes, and deplorable "community residences." The press, the government, and organized psychiatry began to propose solutions.

The Community Mental Health Center Amendment of 1975

Realizing that CMHCs were not adequately serving many mentally ill persons, Congress passed the Community Mental Health Center Amendment of 1975 (Public Law 94-63 1975), which called for services to screen patients for courts and agencies; follow-up care; transitional housing; and services for specialized populations: elderly persons, children, and persons with alcohol and drug abuse (Table 5–1). The services mandated by this legislation make it obvious which patients were falling through the cracks.

The Critical Reports

Within the same time frame, three prestigious groups—the General Accounting Office (1977), the Group for the Advancement of Psychiatry (1978), and the APA (Talbott 1978a)—issued reports critical of the role of both federally sponsored CMHCs and state-run mental hospitals in caring for severely and chronically mentally ill patients. They agreed that, in the General Accounting Office's words, "more needs to be done" and that patients could not simply be discharged to unprepared communities, with no training in everyday living skills and too few supportive housing situations, community treatment facilities, rehabilitation opportunities, and social supports.

These groups also stressed the need for formalized community support programs (Turner 1977) that would provide all the services needed by mentally ill patients in the community, including escort services, advocacy and support for families, and 24-hour crisis assistance and case management that would enable patients to make use of existing services. The groups also appreciated the need for a continuum of housing and treatment opportunities available in each community to enable patients to achieve their maximum level of functioning (Figure 5–5).

They also stressed the need for fiscal and administrative reform that would operationalize the above recommendations, as well as repair the fragmentation and dysfunction of the service systems. President Jimmy Carter's Commission on Mental Health (1978) not only agreed with the recommendations of these groups, it also set in motion a new federal initiative, the Mental Health Systems Act of 1980 (Public Law 96-398 1980), which was never fully realized due to Carter's defeat in the presidential election of 1980. There was also to be a large federal initiative in housing and community support programs, which was blunted by the new conservatism of President Ronald Reagan.

The Carter commission and the Group for the Advancement of Psychiatry also examined the state of CMHCs at this point (Group for the Advancement of Psychiatry 1983). Reports such as the one by Windle et al. (1978) demonstrated that many CMHCs had not fulfilled their requirement for comprehensive services (e.g., no 24-hour emergency service) and that some CMHCs were "skimming off" better-paying patients and thus not serving their entire catchment area. These facts, coupled with the dawning realization that the ambitious goal of establishing 750 new CMHCs would never be realized, prompted a reappraisal of the central role of the CMHC as a model for future services.

In addition, President Reagan's move to shift from categorical funding (e.g., funds designated solely for prenatal care or mental health) to "block grants" (wherein all monies were placed in 25 huge groupings

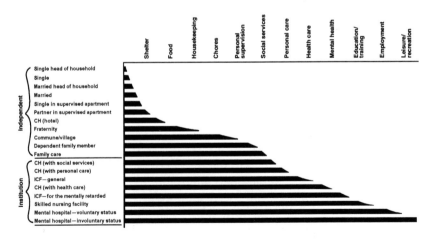

Figure 5–5. Needs and settings for chronically mentally ill persons.
CH = congregate housing. ICF = intermediate care facility.
Source. Elizabeth Boggs, Ph.D., personal communication, August 1980.

that the state governments could allocate in turn) changed the venue in planning and implementing psychiatric services back to the states, from which it had been taken 16 years before. Ironically, we moved from 150 years of largely state-dominated planning and implementation to only 16 years when the federal CMHC was in ascendance, at which point control was once again assigned to the states.

Assertive Community Treatment

In 1980, Leonard Stein and associates (Stein and Test 1980; Test and Stein 1980; Weisbrod et al. 1980) published a landmark series of articles that detailed their success in Madison, Wisconsin, in treating severely and chronically mentally ill persons in the community with slightly more resources than they would have received if they had been treated in a state hospital. The principles and elements of the service delivery developed by Stein et al. were consonant with the recommendations stated above. In many instances, Stein and Test's work strongly influenced services later developed by others.

These elements included individualized treatment, aggressivity and assertiveness in reaching out to patients, community supports, and mobility—all of which have become the means we use to treat the casualties encountered in the nation's unsuccessful attempt to shift the care of mentally ill patients from institutional to community auspices.

Rehabilitation

Despite the examples cited earlier, widespread adoption of both social and vocational rehabilitation did not come to pass until relatively recently. Through the work of pioneers such as William Anthony (1979), Robert Liberman and associates (1987, 1989), and John Strauss and Will Carpenter (1978), the principles underlying this critical element in tertiary prevention were articulated and disseminated based on experience and research.

By this decade (1975–1984), rehabilitation programs had become widespread in community and institutional settings (Farkas and Anthony 1989; Liberman 1992; Talbott 1981). By 1985 in Maryland, for example, almost 40 psychosocial rehabilitation programs—some freestanding and others affiliated with hospitals or CMHCs—had been developed.

Consumer-Parent Movements

In the not-too-distant past, psychiatric services encountered parents largely around grievances they had about care of their afflicted children. In 1978, however, disparate parent groups across the nation banded together into the National Alliance for the Mentally Ill (NAMI), with local and state chapters (Hatfield 1981). One of the purposes of NAMI is to advocate for better services for the members' relatives, as well as to educate parents of mentally ill individuals about the nature, treatment, and course of the disease and to advocate for research. NAMI's presence on the services landscape has forced the field to address issues of concern to parents and other relatives rather than only those issues that professionals deem important or see as doable.

Likewise, consumer groups were largely concerned in the past with abuses and grievances, but they also have moved into alliances with professional efforts, as well as running alternatives or adjuncts to other psychiatric services. Consumer-run services now number in the hundreds.

THE WORST AND BEST OF TIMES: 1985–1994

During the decade 1985–1994, the worst of times came in the form of increasing problems with persons whose plight was worse because of deinstitutionalization—homeless mentally ill persons and those with drug and alcohol abuse and mental illness (e.g., the dually diagnosed)—and in the form of new economic forces, principally managed care. However, the decade brought out the best in some individuals and organizations, with new forms of services, experiments in mental health services, and the hope at the end of the decade for a new national health plan.

Increasingly Difficult-to-Treat Populations

There were numerous attempts, first by the private sector (principally churches, soup kitchens, and community groups) and later by medical and governmental agencies, to deal with the growing numbers of mentally ill persons who were also homeless (Lamb et al. 1992). However, their numbers grew throughout the decade.

The plight of these persons and the systems that serve them was highlighted nationally after publicity that began in the New York newspapers surrounding two infamous cases. The first involved Billie Boggs, who was living, washing, and defecating, as well as shouting obscenities at passersby, on the city's streets. The second involved Larry Hogue, who was repeatedly admitted and discharged from hospitals attempting to treat his coincident mental illness and substance abuse and who lived on one corner, chronically threatened passersby, scratched neighbors' cars, and was a fearsome menace.

A second patient group that became more of a problem were those with severe mental illness who also abused drugs and alcohol. Again, there were numerous publications detailing how best to deal with the problem (Ridgely 1989; Ridgely et al. 1986, 1987), but the problem persisted.

A third infamous case became the symbol for our difficulty in treating this group: the patient was Mr. Battiste, a dually diagnosed man who killed an 83-year-old woman neighbor while he was intoxicated and apparently psychotic. To prevent such incidents in the future, New York State's commissioner, for the first time in 38 years, called for evaluation of the shelter population, and some persons were sent to state hospitals.

New Services

One new service was the Inn at the Massachusetts Mental Health Center (Gudeman et al. 1983). The authors converted an underutilized gymnasium and other available space into a massive day and night center for those persons who could not live easily in the community in existing residences but who did not need the acuity of inpatient treatment.

Another new service was represented by the mobile treatment unit, a traveling form of crisis intervention, which was able to deliver and direct services during crises to patients wherever they were. Attributed to Querido (1956) as a means of treating patients before and during World War II in Amsterdam, mobile treatment has been extended now to deal with the overwhelming numbers of deinstitutionalized patients in various community residences (Cohen 1990) and the streets themselves (Cohen et al. 1984).

The proliferation of assertive community treatment programs, mentioned above, is probably the most recent development. These programs combine many different elements into an aggressive approach that seeks to give each patient the precise sorts of treatment and rehabilitation needed—whether pharmacological, psychotherapeutic, or other—while the patient resides in the community (Stein and Test 1980).

For a decade after publication of the results obtained with the "Madison model" for assertive community treatment programs, very few other programs adopted the model. But with the increasing difficulty in dealing with homeless mentally ill and dually diagnosed patients, assertive community treatment teams have become commonplace (Dixon et al. 1993).

The New Economics

For much of this decade we have been more influenced by political and economic pressures than by clinical and scientific ones. Indeed, a great deal of what has occurred in U.S. medicine in the recent past has been the result of economic concerns about the growing size of our medical expenditures rather than of our scientific advances; in fact, many policymakers link the two.

To stem the growth of medical expenses, U.S. medical practitioners—often beginning with those in the field of psychiatry—have had a number of initiatives thrust upon them. These initiatives include the following:

1. Promotion of competition and competitive bidding for care contracts among provider groups (e.g., health maintenance organizations, preferred provider organizations, independent practice associations)
2. Promotion of private corporations (the so-called investor-owned or chain hospitals) to run medical services
3. Payment to hospitals based on diagnostic-related groups rather than actual costs (termed prospective pricing or prospective payment)
4. Managed care, the establishment of corporations that attempt to monitor care and control costs for insurance companies and government by providing services more cheaply; directing patients to providers who, in their opinion, are "less costly"; and indicating how much care and how many services or days or visits they will pay for (Sharfstein 1990)

All of these new economic realities began in the private sector but have now moved into the public arena. Indeed, without a new national health plan, we can expect to see all services to chronically mentally ill patients put under the knife of cost cutting, competitive provision, and managed care. Even public services are now being "privatized" in Massachusetts and Florida: psychiatric treatment of Medicaid patients is being put out for competitive bidding, and public health maintenance organizations are seen as a solution to controlling the states' economic and patient care problems.

Experiments in Mental Health Services

Almost 40 years after deinstitutionalization began, research on health services is beginning to bear fruit. As a result, we may design public policies for the betterment of patients rather than let untried ideologies, economics, and politics batter patients. The results of two large-scale research efforts are at various stages of publication and influence.

The first effort is an extension of Leonard Stein's work using capitated funding to improve and unify services in one county in Wisconsin, one in Arizona, and two in New York State (Lehman 1987).

The second is an attempt, sponsored by the Robert Wood Johnson

Foundation, to use quasi-public authorities to bring together mental health services provided by various entities in nine large U.S. cities (Austin, Texas; Baltimore, Maryland; Charlotte, North Carolina; Cincinnati, Ohio; Columbus, Ohio; Dayton, Ohio; Denver, Colorado; Honolulu, Hawaii; and Philadelphia, Pennsylvania). These "authorities" are separate from local and state governments but are accountable to them. This model is based to some extent on the successes of other quasi-public authorities that built bridges and tunnels in New York City and revitalized the inner-city area in Baltimore (Goldman et al. 1990).

In addition, there are several proposals that have not yet been funded. The first was initiated by the Institute of Medicine, an arm of the National Academy of Sciences, and was instigated and funded by Congress. It proposed creating a new comprehensive care system for all those persons in need of ongoing support services—whether they be frail elderly patients, chronically mentally ill patients, or mentally retarded persons over age 21, the age at which most state responsibility for their comprehensive care ceases.

The second proposal is a revision of an idea initially proposed by Milton Friedman, an economist, for the educational system: provision of vouchers for services required by mentally ill patients, one voucher for housing and the other for psychiatric services (Talbott and Sharfstein 1986). Thus, the system would not only be driven by the market but also would be driven by the consumers (with advice from bank trust officers about housing and from case managers about services)—rather than being driven, as it is now, by the providers.

The third proposal is for a new federal entitlement program for all chronically mentally ill patients that would combine at a federal level all funding streams that the population *is currently eligible for* but rarely uses effectively (Talbott and Sharfstein 1986). If state, local, and private monies were added to this entitlement program, it might also provide comprehensive care.

Last, a federal inter-Cabinet–level task force recommended several innovative sorts of care and service for homeless mentally ill persons ("Federal Task Force Develops National Strategy to Improve Services to Homeless Mentally Ill" 1992). These include a holding environment, more enforced care, and better housing opportunities.

THE FUTURE: 1994 ONWARD

Summary

In a mere half century, the mental health system serving chronically mentally ill patients in the United States has evolved from a largely monolithic one seated in state hospitals to a complex series of alternatives, a bewildering array of programs and services, and an overlapping and yet fragmented group of service systems. Of course, the bottom line is patient care, and in that, the services are as wanting now as they were 50 years ago.

Picking Up the Pieces

It is clear from an examination of the history of services for chronically mentally ill patients over the past 50 years that there have been tremendous changes in treatment, programs, and populations served. Predicting the future is always chancy (Talbott 1989), but in this case it would appear that we have much to do in simply picking up the pieces of our previous policies (e.g., deinstitutionalization and CMHCs) before moving on to new services.

The Future

Undoubtedly, the changes we are undergoing in the area of health care and health care financing reform will have the most impact on the treatment, rehabilitation, and care of chronically mentally ill patients. But assuredly we can state that the next 50 years will be as difficult and unpredictable as the past, as we face new dilemmas, patient illnesses, and complicated political-economic realities.

REFERENCES

A century of debate surrounds community care. Hosp Community Psychiatry 27:490, 1976

Anthony WA (ed): The Principles of Psychiatric Rehabilitation. Baltimore, MD, University Park Press, 1979

Bachrach LL: Deinstitutionalization: An Analytical Review and Sociological Perspective. Rockville, MD, U.S. Department of Health, Education, and Welfare, 1976

Bachrach LL: General hospitals taking greater role in providing services for chronic patients. Hosp Community Psychiatry 30:488, 1979

Bassett C (ed): Mental Hygiene in the Community. New York, Macmillan, 1933

Becker A, Murphy M, Greenblatt M: Recent advances in community psychiatry. N Engl J Med 272:621–626, 1965

Beers C: A Mind that Found Itself. Garden City, NY, Doubleday, 1908

Beigel A, Levenson AI (ed): The Community Mental Health Center: Strategies and Programs. New York, Basic Books, 1972

Bellak L: The comprehensive community psychiatry program at city hospital, in Handbook of Community Psychiatry and Community Mental Health. Edited by Bellak L. New York, Grune & Stratton, 1964, pp 144–165

Bierer J: The Marlborough experiment, in Handbook of Community Psychiatry and Community Mental Health. Edited by Bellak L. New York, Grune & Stratton, 1964, pp 221–247

Bindman AJ, Spiegel AD (ed): Perspectives in Community Mental Health. Chicago, IL, Aldine Publishing, 1969

Black B: Psychiatric rehabilitation in the community, in Handbook of Community Psychiatry and Community Mental Health. Edited by Bellak L. New York, Grune & Stratton, 1964, pp 248–264

Black B: Work as Therapy and Rehabilitation for the Mentally Ill. New York, Altro Institute for Rehabilitation Services, 1986

Brown WH, Takraff LH, Gostes BH, et al: Using community agencies in the treatment program of a travelling child guidance clinic. Mental Hygiene 41:372–377, 1957

Caplan G (ed): An Approach to Community Mental Health. New York, Grune & Stratton, 1961

Caplan G (ed): Principles of Preventive Psychiatry. New York, Basic Books, 1964

Caplan G, Caplan RB: Development of community psychiatry concepts, in Comprehensive Textbook of Psychiatry. Edited by Freedman AM, Kaplan HI. Baltimore, MD, William & Wilkins, 1967, pp 1499–1515

Carpenter WT, Heinrichs DW, Wagman AMI: Deficit and non-deficit forms of schizophrenia: the concept. Am J Psychiatry 145:578–583, 1988

Chu FD, Trotter S (eds): The Madness Establishment. New York, Grossman, 1974

Cohen NL (ed): Psychiatry Takes to the Streets: Outreach and Crisis Intervention for the Mentally Ill. New York, Guilford, 1990

Cohen NL, Putnam JF, Sullivan AM: The mentally ill homeless: isolation and adaptation. Hosp Community Psychiatry 35:922–924, 1984

Connery RH (ed): The Politics of Mental Health. New York, Columbia University Press, 1968

Copp O: Further experience in family care of the insane in Massachusetts. American Journal of Insanity 53:361–365, 1907

Dain N: From colonial America to bicentennial American: two centuries of vicissitudes in the institutional care of mental patients. Bull N Y Acad Med 52:1179–1197, 1976

Deutsch A (ed): The Mentally Ill in America: A History of Their Care and Treatment from Colonial Times. Garden City, New York, Doubleday, 1937

Dixon LB, Friedman N, Lehman AH: Housing patterns of homeless mentally ill persons receiving assertive treatment services. Hosp Community Psychiatry 44:286–288, 1993

Ewalt JR: The birth of the community mental health movement, in An Assessment of the Community Mental Health Movement. Edited by Barton WE, Sanborn JC. Lexington, MA, Lexington Books, 1975, pp 13–20

Farkas MD, Anthony, WA (eds): Psychiatric Rehabilitation Programs: Putting Theory Into Practice. Baltimore, MD, Johns Hopkins University Press, 1989

Federal task force develops national strategy to improve services to homeless mentally ill. Hosp Community Psychiatry 43:523–524, 1992

Felix RH: Psychiatry in prospect. Am J Psychiatry 103:600–604, 1947

Foley H (ed): Community Mental Health. Lexington, MA, Lexington Books, 1975

Galt JM: The farm of St. Anne. American Journal of Insanity 11:352–357, 1855

General Accounting Office, Comptroller General of the United States: Report to the Congress, Returning the Mentally Disabled to the Community: Government Needs to Do More (HRD 76-152). Washington, DC, U.S. General Accounting Office, 1977

Glass AJ: Observations upon the epidemiology of mental illness in troops during warfare, in Symposium on Preventive and Social Psychiatry. Washington, DC, Walter Reed Army Institute of Research, U.S. Government Printing Office, 1958, pp 185–198

Glasscote RM, Sanders DS, Forstenzer HM, et al (eds): The Community Mental Health Center: An Analysis of Existing Models. Washington, DC, American Psychiatric Association, 1964

Glasscote RM, Cumming E, Rutman I, et al. (eds): Rehabilitating the Mentally Ill in the Community. Washington, DC, American Psychiatric Association, 1971

Goffman E: On the characteristics of total institutions, in Asylums. Edited by Goffman E, Garden City, NY, Doubleday, 1961

Goldman HH, Lehman AF, Morrissey JP, et al: Design for the national evaluation of the Robert Wood Johnson Foundation program on chronic mental illness. Hosp Community Psychiatry 41:1217–1221, 1990

Golomb S, Kocsis A (eds): The Halfway House: On the Road to Independence. New York, Brunner/Mazel, 1988

Group for the Advancement of Psychiatry: The Chronic Mental Patient in the Community. New York, Group for the Advancement of Psychiatry, 1978

Group for the Advancement of Psychiatry: Community Psychiatry: A Reappraisal. New York, Mental Health Materials Center, 1983

Gudeman JE, Shore MF, Dickey B: Day hospitalization and an inn instead of inpatient care for psychiatric patients. N Engl J Med 308:749–753, 1983

Hatfield A: Families as advocates for the mentally ill: a growing movement. Hosp Community Psychiatry 32:641–642, 1981

Hoge MA, Davidson L, Hill WL, et al: The promise of partial hospitalization: a reassessment. Hosp Community Psychiatry 43:345–354, 1992

Hollingshead AB, Redlich CF (ed): Social Class and Mental Illness: A Community Study. New York, Wiley, 1958

Hunt RC: Community responsibility for mental health in Britain, the Netherlands and New York State. Psychiatr Q 30:684–697, 1956

Hurd HM (ed): The Institutional Care of the Insane in the United States and Canada, Vol 1. Baltimore, MD, Johns Hopkins University Press, 1946

Jarrett MC: Mental clinics, in Clinics, Hospitals and Health Centers. Edited by Davis MM. New York, Harper, 1927, pp 426–452

Joint Commission on Mental Health and Illness: Action for Mental Health: Final Report of the Joint Commission on Mental Health and Illness. New York, Basic Books, 1961

Jones M: The Therapeutic Community. New York, Basic Books, 1953

Kennedy JF: Message from the President of the United States relative to mental illness and mental retardation. Am J Psychiatry 120:729–737, 1964

Kiev A: Some background factors in recent English psychiatric programs. Am J Psychiatry 119:851–856, 1963

Kramer J: Psychiatric Services and the Changing Institutional Scene. Bethesda, MD, National Institute of Mental Health, 1975

Lamb HR (ed): The Homeless Mentally Ill: A Task Force Report of the American Psychiatric Association. Washington, DC, American Psychiatric Association, 1984

Lamb HR, Bachrach LL, Kass FI (eds): Treating the Homeless Mentally Ill: A Task Force Report of the American Psychiatric Association. Washington, DC, American Psychiatric Association, 1992

Lehman AF: Capitation payment and mental health care: a review of the opportunities and risks. Hosp Community Psychiatry 38:31–38, 1987

Leighton AH (ed): My Name is Legion. New York, Basic Books, 1959

Liberman RP: Skills training for community adaptation of chronic mental patients. Community Psychiatrist 2(3):5, 17, 1987

Liberman RP: Effective Psychiatric Rehabilitation (New Directions for Mental Health Services, No 53). Edited by Lamb HR. San Francisco, CA, Jossey-Bass, 1992, pp 1–123

Liberman RP, DiRisi WJ, Mueser KT (eds): Social Skills Training for Psychiatric Patients. New York, Pergamon Press, 1989

Lindeman E: Symptomatology and management of acute grief. Am J Psychiatry 104:141–148, 1944

Linn L: Some aspects of a psychiatry program in a voluntary general hospital, in Handbook of Community Psychiatry and Community Mental Health. Edited by Bellak L. New York, Grune & Stratton, 1964, pp 126–143

Maxmen J, Tucker GJ, Lebow M (eds): Rational Hospital Psychiatry: The Reactive Environment. New York, Brunner/Mazel, 1974

Mechanic D (ed): Mental Health and Social Policy. Englewood Cliffs, NJ, Prentice-Hall, 1969

Meyer A: Organizing the community for the protections of its mental life. Survey 34:557–560, 1915

Milbank Memorial Fund: The Elements of a Community Mental Health Program. New York, Milbank Memorial Fund, 1956

Milbank Memorial Fund: Steps in the Development of Integrated Psychiatric Services. New York, Milbank Memorial Fund, 1960

Milbank Memorial Fund: Decentralization of Psychiatric Services and Continuity of Care. New York, Milbank Memorial Fund, 1962

Mora G: Recent American psychiatric developments (since 1939), in Handbook of American Psychiatry. Edited by Arieti S. New York, Basic Books, 1959, pp 18–57

Musto D: The community mental health center movement in historical perspective, in An Assessment of Community Mental Health Movement. Edited by Barton WE, Sanborn JC. Lexington, MA, Lexington Books, 1975, pp 1–11

President's Commission on Mental Health: Report to the President From the President's Commission on Mental Health. Washington, DC, U.S. Government Printing Office, 1978

Public Law 88-164: The Mental Retardation Facilities and Community Mental Health Centers Construction Act of 1963. Washington, DC, U.S. Government Printing Office, 1963

Public Law 94-63: The Community Mental Health Center Amendment of 1975. Washington, DC, U.S. Government Printing Office, 1975

Public Law 96-398: Mental Health Systems Act of 1980. Washington, DC, U.S. Government Printing Office, 1980

Quen J: Review of *The Discovery of the Asylum: Social Order and Disorder in the New Republic,* by Rothman DJ. Journal of Psychiatric Law 2:105–122, 1974

Quen J: Learning from history. Psychiatric Annals 5:15–31, 1975

Querido A: Early diagnosis and treatment services, in Milbank Memorial Fund: The Elements of a Community Mental Health Program. New York, Milbank Memorial Fund, 1956

Ridgely MS (ed): Special issue on dual diagnosis. Hosp Community Psychiatry 40:985–1104, October 1989

Ridgely MS, Goldman HH, Talbott JA: Chronic Mentally Ill Young Adults With Substance Abuse Problems: A Review of Relevant Literature and Creation of a Research Agenda. Mental Health Policy Studies. Baltimore, MD, University of Maryland, 1986

Ridgely MS, Osher FC, Talbott JA: Chronic Mentally Ill Young Adults With Substance Abuse Problems: Treatment and Training Issues. Mental Health Policy Studies. Baltimore, MD, University of Maryland, 1987

Rossi A: Some pre-World II antecedents of community mental health theory and practice. Mental Hygiene 46:78–98, 1962

Rothman DJ: The Discovery of the Asylum: Social Order and Disorder in the New Republic. Boston, MA, Little, Brown, 1971

Salmon T: War neuroses: "shell shock." Military Surgery 41:674–694, 1917

Sampson H, Ross D, Engle B, et al: Feasibility of community clinic treatment for state mental hospital patients. AMA Archives of Neurology and Psychiatry 80:71–77, 1958

Schumach M: The New York Times, January–April 1974

Shapiro JH (ed): Communities of the Alone: Working With Single-Room Occupants in the City. New York, Association Press, 1971

Sharfstein SS (ed): Special issue on managed care. Hosp Community Psychiatry 41:1–63, October 1990

Stein LI, Test MA: Alternative to mental hospital treatment: conceptual model, treatment program, and clinical evaluation. Arch Gen Psychiatry 37:392–397, 1980.

Strauss J, Carpenter WT: The prognosis of schizophrenia: rational for a multidimensional concept. Schizophr Bull 4(1):56–67, 1978

Stroup AL, Manderscheid RW: The development of the state mental hospital system in the United States: 1840–1980. Journal of the Washington Academy of Sciences 78:59–68, 1988

Symposium on Preventive and Social Psychiatry. Washington, DC, Walter Reed Army Institute of Research, U.S. Government Printing Office, 1958

Talbott JA: Community psychiatry in the army: history, practice and applications to civilian psychiatry. JAMA 210:1233–1237, 1969

Talbott JA (ed): Who will care for the patients? (continued in subsequent issues). NYSDB Bulletin 14(5):1–9, 1972

Talbott JA: The elements of community consultation. Psychiatr Q 29:273–290, 1977

Talbott JA: Report to the President for the President's Commission of Mental Health (Stock No 040-000-00390-8). Washington DC, U.S. Government Printing Office, 1978a

Talbott JA (ed): The Chronic Mental Patient: Problems, Solutions, and Recommendations for a Public Policy. Washington, DC, American Psychiatric Association, 1978b

Talbott JA: Deinstitutionalization: avoiding the disasters of the past. Hosp Community Psychiatry 30:621–624, 1979

Talbott JA (ed): The Chronic Mentally Ill: Treatment, Programs, Systems. New York, Human Sciences Press, 1981

Talbott JA: Trends in the delivery of psychiatric services, in Psychiatric Administration: A Comprehensive Text for the Clinician-Executive. Edited by Talbott JA, Kaplan SR. New York, Grune & Stratton, 1983, pp 3–19

Talbott JA: Presidential address: our patients' future in a changing world: the imperative for psychiatric involvement in public policy. Am J Psychiatry 142:1003–1008, 1985

Talbott JA (ed): Future Directions for Psychiatry. Washington, DC, American Psychiatric Association, 1989

Talbott JA, Sharfstein SS: A proposal for future funding of chronic and episodic mental illness. Hosp Community Psychiatry 37:1126–1130, 1986

Talbott JA, Talbott SW: Training police in community relations and urban problems. Am J Psychiatry 127:894–900, 1971

Test MA, Stein LI: Alternative to mental hospital treatment, III: social cost. Arch Gen Psychiatry 37:409–412, 1980

Turner JE: Comprehensive community support systems for adults with seriously disabling mental health problems. Psychosocial Rehabilitation Journal 1(3):39–47, 1977

Weisbrod BA, Stein LI, Test MA: Alternative to mental hospital treatment, II: economic benefit-cost analysis. Arch Gen Psychiatry 37:400–405, 1980

Whittington HG (ed): Psychiatry in the American Community. New York, International Universities Press, 1966

Windle C, Albert MB, Sharfstein SS: Collaborative program evaluation to improve emergency services in community mental health centers. Hosp Community Psychiatry 29:708–710, 1978

Zusman J: The philosophic basis for a community and social psychiatry, in An Assessment of the Community Mental Health Movement. Edited by Barton WE, Sanborn CJ, Lexington, MA, Lexington Books, 1961, pp 21–34

Afterword to Section I

Michael J. Vergare, M.D., and John S. McIntyre, M.D.,
Section Editors

A knowledge of the past enriches our understanding of the present and helps us plan for the future. This section has actualized that statement and brings meaning to the current American Psychiatric Association presidential theme—"Our Heritage Our Future."

The authors of the five chapters have summarized in a thorough and scholarly manner five major aspects of the development of psychiatry in this country: education, research, psychotherapy, gender issues, and the treatment of patients with chronic mental illness.

Each of the authors has been a central figure in the unfolding drama of the growth of our profession and has made field-defining contributions in the areas each chapter describes.

Dr. Romano's masterful chapter not only provided a rich and scholarly account of the development of psychiatric education, but also identified key issues currently facing our profession, including subspecialization, recruitment, boundary issues with other mental health professions, and our relationship with the rest of medicine. Dr. Romano did not avoid discussing some of our failings as professionals and mistakes as an association. An awareness of these errors is crucial to our continued growth. He closed the chapter with a powerful and effective plea to preserve the humanness of our work.

The exponential growth of knowledge about mental illnesses and their treatments was documented by Drs. Lehmann and Ban in a deceptively simple style. They systematically described how scientific progress at times built slowly on the past as information accumulated and at times occurred more rapidly with major paradigm shifts. Throughout the chapter, the reader was reminded of the central role of research in our profession. Research is also one of the prime objectives of our association. In the words of Dr. Pliny Earle, one of the founders of the American Psychiatric Association, members "should cooperate in collecting statistical information relating to insanity and above all should assist each other in improving the treatment of [patients with mental illness]."

Dr. Altshuler, in a succinct and convincing manner, examined the effect of four major factors in the practice of psychotherapy: social issues, medical advances (especially pharmacology), emphasis on the scientific method, and concern with cost. His exploration of the common element among many psychotherapies was clear and historically accurate; it not only reflected Dr. Altshuler's breadth of scholarship but also provided an integrating paradigm that will be useful for future practice and research.

Dr. Gold's lively and informative chapter has summarized some of the "biological and sociocultural data and theories related to gender differences in the diagnosis and treatment of mental disorders." Using the recent controversies concerning the diagnoses of late luteal phase dysphoric disorder and self-defeating personality disorder, Dr. Gold described in an insightful and thoughtful manner how such issues are viewed by many women and more specifically by women as patients. Dr. Gold appropriately challenged the profession and the American Psychiatric Association to face the issue of the status of women in our field and respond accordingly.

Dr. Talbott's chapter, which described the evolution of psychiatric services for patients with severe and chronic mental illness, dealt in a very comprehensive and clarifying manner with one of our field's most important challenges. After touching on the approach to these patients in the colonial era, the nineteenth century, and the first half of this century, Dr. Talbott then focused on the profound changes in psychiatric services that have occurred in the past 50 years. The realities of deinstitutionalization were highlighted, as were the factors that led to these policies and the subsequent attempts to "pick up the pieces." Talbott closed by challenging the field, noting that despite the significant changes that have occurred, unfortunately with respect to patient care "the services are as wanting now as they were 50 years ago."

These five chapters have provided us with a wealth of insights and challenges. Learning about our past is both invigorating and inspiring. It is also crucial to our planning for a more enriched future. Each of the chapters identifies the challenges that lie ahead and the great amount of work yet to be done. As Dr. Romano states, it is "time—high time—to sound reveille, to call the profession to rise and fulfill our professional responsibilities more effectively."

II

Biological Markers

Section II

Biological Markers

Foreword

Jack M. Gorman, M.D., and Laszlo A. Papp, M.D.,
Section Editors

Finding biological markers for psychiatric disease has been, and likely will continue to be, one of the most difficult enterprises in medical research. There are at least three reasons for this: one scientific, one clinical, and one sociological.

Unlike all other organs, the brain lies encased behind a shield, called the blood-brain barrier, that has seemed nearly impenetrable to researchers. Although cardiologists, nephrologists, and endocrinologists can assay relevant parameters in the body fluids of their patients, almost nothing that goes on in the human brain has thus far been accurately reflected in any peripherally measurable factor. Nor can psychiatrists, unlike their colleagues in other specialties, readily pass angiographically guided catheters into or obtain biopsy samples of the organ of interest. Hence, it has been a great scientific challenge to figure out how to gain access to the billions of cells and synapses that make up the system that controls human behavior.

Clinically, we face the problem of diagnosis. Although diagnosis is a problem for other medical specialties, we have particular difficulties in psychiatry being sure that we have selected a relatively homogeneous clinical entity for biological study. Should there be, for example, unique biological markers for schizophrenia and bipolar affective disorder or a single marker for psychotic illness? Are we to be dismayed when a group of panic disorder patients and a group of depressed patients share a common biological finding, or intrigued that we have found a common biological underpinning? How do we know when someone has passed the age of risk for a particular psychiatric disorder and therefore may be counted as "normal" for the purposes of genetic studies? Even with the substantial advances in psychiatric diagnosis made in the last decade with the establishment of the *Diagnostic and Statistical Manual of Mental Disorders* system, we still face important diagnostic problems that make the location of biological markers for psychiatric illness especially hard.

Finally, there is a sociological, or perhaps more properly, a philosophical resistance to looking for and accepting biological markers in the first place. Some mistakenly believe that the search for biological markers of psychiatric disorders implies a conviction that the disorders are fundamentally "biological" as opposed to "psychological" or "experiential." The idea that depression, anxiety, alcoholism, or borderline personality disorder might be associated with unique biological findings strikes some as reductionistic. Nowadays, fortunately, many clinicians and scientists alike take a broader view, recognizing that even complex behavior is ultimately mediated by discrete, albeit highly obscure, neuronal processes. Disorders of these processes may well be reflected in measurable factors without implying that the causes are entirely "biological."

For all three of the above reasons, and undoubtedly many more, we do not yet have in psychiatry a laboratory test that helps us make diagnoses. Yet, as one reads the subsequent chapters, it is apparent that biological research has now produced a series of near-startling discoveries in psychiatry that tell us a great deal about likely etiology.

The pace of biological research in schizophrenia has recently been dazzling. As Jeffrey A. Lieberman, M.D., Alan S. Brown, M.D., and Jack M. Gorman, M.D., note in Chapter 6, it is now possible to say with some certainty that, on the basis of sophisticated structural and functional brain imaging studies and neuropathological studies, at least a subgroup of patients with schizophrenia have reduced temporal and limbic lobe mass and decreased functional capacity of the prefrontal cortex. Further, more recent evidence strongly suggests that the insult to the temporal region occurs in patients with schizophrenia during the early part of gestation, probably in the first and second trimesters. Investigators are now pursuing a variety of genetic and epigenetic factors that may be responsible for this neurodevelopmental abnormality.

In Chapter 7, on mood disorders, Kalpana I. Nathan, M.D., and Alan F. Schatzberg, M.D., leave us with little doubt that at least some forms of depression involve hyperactivity of the hypothalamic-pituitary-adrenal (HPA) axis. Although the dexamethasone suppression test never entirely made good on its original promise, abundant further research clearly implicates HPA axis dysfunction at least in the most severe forms of depression. Further, these authors show us the impressive evidence that diminished serotonergic function, along with alteration of the adrenergic-cholinergic balance, must be involved in mood regulation. In this area, then, a series of neuroendocrine challenge, cerebrospinal fluid, and neuropathological studies have given us two likely foci of pathology for depression.

Similarly, in Chapter 8, on anxiety disorders, Laszlo A. Papp, M.D., Jeremy Coplan, M.D., and Jack M. Gorman, M.D., present evidence to implicate a triad of possible brain stem abnormalities associated with panic disorder. Here, the classic work of Redmond, Charney, and others from Yale University implicating noradrenergic and locus coeruleus hyperactivity is joined by other work indicating decreased serotonergic function and hyperactive respiratory control. Hence, a cogent and testable biological theory for panic disorder that exists in perfect harmony with cognitive and behavior theories has now emerged.

In Chapter 9, Marc A. Schuckit, M.D., reviews impressive long-term work that has revolutionized our thinking about alcoholism. His own group has followed cohorts not only of alcoholic patients but also of the nonalcoholic sons of alcoholic fathers. A series of replicated biological findings makes clear that a biological and heritable abnormality is associated with some forms of alcoholism. It is not at all beyond the realm of possibility that this kind of testing may sooner than later lead to screening techniques that will enable physicians to warn individuals who are at high risk for developing addiction to alcohol.

Although many psychiatrists tend to think of the personality or Axis II disorders as "nonbiological," Larry J. Siever, M.D., Bonnie J. Steinberg, M.D., Robert L. Trestman, Ph.D., M.D., and Joanne Intrator, M.D., put forth cogent arguments in Chapter 11 that even these conditions may be susceptible to biological investigation. It may be that here we will learn the most about how early life experience permanently alters basic neurobiological processes and how these alterations ultimately become associated with enduring personality dysfunction.

In similar fashion, Chapter 10 on eating disorders by Denise M. Heebink, M.D., and Katherine A. Halmi, M.D., and Chapter 12 on childhood psychiatric illness by Dorothy E. Grice, M.D., Ann M. Rasmusson, M.D., and James F. Leckman, M.D., review the painstaking work of many investigators to find replicable biological markers for complex behavioral problems. In each case it is impressive to see the systematic, almost dogged, approach that investigators have taken to assess each neurotransmitter and neuroendocrine system. As the technical capacity to measure receptor function improves, we will undoubtedly see further such attempts.

One theme emerges prominently from the seven chapters on biological markers: the need to apply sophisticated technology to the study of the brain. Without the ability to perform high-resolution magnetic resonance imaging, for example, we could not possibly be certain that the temporal lobe of the schizophrenic brain is reduced in size. Without the ability to identify, synthesize, and infuse corticotropin-releasing hormone, the idea that HPA axis overactivity is a part of depression would have been left dormant. Because the human brain is by far the most complex biological system in nature, it will take the most intricate technology to study it properly. Hence, as biomedical technology advances, so will research identifying biological markers of psychiatric disease. All of us, therefore, should become informed about and highly supportive of the efforts outlined in the chapters in this section.

Chapter 6

Schizophrenia

Jeffrey A. Lieberman, M.D., Alan S. Brown, M.D., and Jack M. Gorman, M.D.

Numerous investigators have conducted extensive investigations in the search for biological markers in schizophrenia. These studies have attempted to identify specific, sensitive, and replicable physiological and anatomical measures that can be obtained relatively noninvasively. The search for biological markers has extended through a wide range of disciplines, including psychophysiology, neurochemistry, neuroendocrinology, neuroimmunology, and brain imaging, and it has yielded a number of putative trait markers and state markers for schizophrenia (see Table 6–1). In this chapter we describe the putative markers that have been found in each of these research areas, evaluate both their promise and their limitations, and discuss their potential utility in clarifying diagnostic, genetic, therapeutic, and prognostic issues in schizophrenia.

PSYCHOPHYSIOLOGY

Eye-Movement Dysfunction

Eye-movement dysfunction (EMD) is generally considered one of the most promising biological markers for schizophrenia (Clementz and Sweeney 1990; Holzman 1985, 1991; Iacono 1988; Szymanski et al. 1991). Numerous independent investigations have reported a prevalence of EMD ranging from 50% to more than 85% in schizophrenic patients compared to 22% of nonschizophrenic psychotic patients and only 8% of healthy control subjects (Holzman 1991). The two eye-movement functions that have been studied most are smooth pursuit eye movement (SPEM)—consisting of horizontal following movements—and saccadic, or rapid fixation, movements. These eye movements are examined by having the subject follow a target that slowly moves sinusoidally as either a triangular wave (constant velocity) or a

This work was supported by a Research Scientist Development Award (MH00537) to J.A.L. and the Mental Health Clinical Research Center for the Study of Schizophrenia (MH41960) at Hillside Hospital. We thank Anne Brown for her assistance in preparing the table.

Table 6–1. Summary of biological markers in schizophrenia

Type of study	Markers	Advantages	Disadvantages
Psychophysiology			
Eye movements	Abnormalities of SPEM and saccades	Present in 50%–85% of sz patients, 8% of controls Relatively stable Noninvasive, relatively easy to measure	Lack of specificity for sz: reported in bipolar disorder
Event-related potentials	Reduced auditory P300 amplitude	82% sensitive, 91% specific in differentiating sz patients from controls May be correlated with positive/negative symptoms	Lack of specificity: found in affective disorders and neurological conditions
	Diminished P50 suppression	Present in 80%–90% of sz patients Both measures obtained noninvasively, relatively inexpensively	Nonspecific: reported in bipolar mania, adjustment disorders, substance abuse
	Mismatched negativity		Requires further replication
Neuroimmunology	Increased autoantibodies, including heat shock protein antibody; increased interleukin-2, and soluble interleukin-2 receptors in sz patients versus controls	Heat shock protein antibody present in 44% of sz patients, 8% of controls Relatively noninvasive and inexpensive	Considerable overlap of most measures between sz and control groups Lack of specificity Conflicting findings among studies
Neuroendocrinology			
GH	Blunted GH response to apomorphine in chronic sz patients versus controls	Can be obtained routinely, inexpensively	Inconsistent findings in GH studies; substantial overlap between patient and control values

	Findings	Advantages	Comments
TSH	Increased basal GH levels in sz patients versus controls Less blunted TSH response to TRH in sz patients compared with schizoaffective, bipolar patients	Can be obtained routinely, inexpensively	No difference in TSH response among sz patients, healthy controls, depressed patients
LH, FSH	Decreased basal LH and FSH; decreased LH response to GnRH in sz patients versus controls	Can be obtained routinely, inexpensively	LH and FSH abnormalities found in other psychiatric disorders
PRL	Increased secretory amplitude before and after sleep	Can be obtained routinely, inexpensively	Probably more valuable as a neuro-endocrinological-clinical correlate of treatment outcome than as a biological marker
Neurochemistry HVA	Basal pretreatment levels of plasma HVA are correlated with therapeutic response	Peripheral measures easy to obtain, relatively inexpensive	Peripheral measures (plasma, urine) derived only in part from brain Numerous potential confounding variables CSF and plasma HVA levels do not discriminate sz patients from controls Significant overlap in values between patients and controls
NE and MHPG	Increased CSF NE in sz patients versus controls CSF NE level is predictive of psychotic relapse CSF NE and MHPG are correlated with positive and negative symptoms	Peripheral measures easy to obtain, relatively inexpensive	CSF measures require lumbar puncture NE/MHPG abnormalities also found in affective disorders

continued

Table 6–1. Summary of biological markers in schizophrenia (*continued*)

Type of study	Markers	Advantages	Disadvantages
Neurochemistry			
Serotonin and 5-HIAA	Decreased CSF 5-HIAA correlated with brain atrophy and suicidal behavior in sz patients Increased serotonin levels in platelets and whole blood in sz patients versus controls		Most studies show no difference in CSF 5-HIAA levels between sz patients and controls Decreased CSF 5-HIAA found in patients with affective and personality disorders Inconsistent findings in platelet and blood studies
Pharmacological challenges			
Psychostimulants	Clinical worsening in 40%–60% of sz patients, 2% of non-sz controls	Represent potential pharmacological models	Underrepresentation of acutely psychotic non-sz patients studied to determine specificity
m-Chlorophenyl-piperazine	Psychotogenic effect in sz patients in some studies	Represent potential pharmacological models	Behavioral effects may be nonspecific No direction comparison of sz patients and healthy controls
Ketamine	Psychotogenic effect in sz patients and controls	Represent potential pharmacological models	Potential toxicity
Neuroimaging			
Structural (CT, MRI)	Enlargement of lateral/third ventricles	Noninvasive techniques Well-replicated findings Correlates with negative symptoms, poor treatment response and outcome	Substantial variation and overlap in values for patients and controls May be present only in subgroup (20%–40%) of sz patients Not specific to sz

	Decreased area and volume of mesiotemporal structures (amygdala, hippocampus, parahippocampal gyrus) Increased size of temporal horns in sz patients Corpus callosum abnormalities Decreased frontal and prefrontal cortical size	Well-replicated findings Correlates with positive symptoms	Inconsistent findings among studies
Functional blood flow studies (rCBF, PET, SPECT)	Hypofrontality	Well replicated May correlate with negative symptom severity	Considerable overlap between sz patients and controls May be identifiable in only a minority of patients Complex methodology, expensive Not specific to sz
Neuroreceptor studies	Increased D_2 receptor density in caudate nuclei	In vivo quantitation of neurotransmitter receptors	Conflicting findings Potential confounding factors
MRS	Decreased phosphomonoesters; increased phosphodiesters; decreased adenosine triphosphate; decreased inorganic phosphate	Direct assessment of brain metabolism Findings have been replicated May be specific to sz	Technique still relatively new Expensive, not yet practical for routine assessment

Note. CSF = cerebrospinal fluid. CT = computed tomography. FSH = follicle-stimulating hormone. GH = growth hormone. GnRH = gonadotropin-releasing hormone. 5-HIAA = 5-hydroxyindoleacetic acid. HVA = homovanillic acid. LH = luteinizing hormone. MHPG = 3-methoxy-4-hydroxyphenylglycol. MRI = magnetic resonance imaging. MRS = magnetic resonance spectroscopy. NE = norepinephrine. PET = positron-emission tomography. PRL = prolactin. rCBF = regional cerebral blood flow. SPEM = smooth pursuit eye movement. SPECT = single photon emission computed tomography. sz = schizophrenia. TRH = thyroid-releasing hormone. TSH = thyroid-stimulating hormone.

linear ramp. The eye-movement abnormalities most frequently observed in patients with schizophrenia are low-gain pursuit (the ratio of eye-movement velocity to target velocity) and two types of saccadic interruptions of smooth pursuit: saccadic tracking (compensatory eye movements that correct for low-gain pursuit) and saccadic intrusions (eye movements with no corrective function).

EMD appears to be potentially a trait marker rather than a state marker for schizophrenia. This conclusion is supported by several lines of evidence. First, most studies have demonstrated that treatment with and withdrawal from antipsychotic medications do not affect EMD (Shagass et al. 1974), although EMD can be induced by sedatives, hypnotics, and lithium. Second, EMD does not appear to change with alterations in the patient's clinical state (Holzman 1991). Third, there is evidence of a genetic component of EMD. A higher prevalence of a biological marker in family members of patients than in the general population is an important criterion for a trait marker (Garver 1987; Szymanski et al. 1991). Holzman et al. (1974) reported that 40% of first-degree relatives of schizophrenic patients had EMD that was indistinguishable from that of schizophrenic patients, compared to only 10% of the relatives of nonschizophrenic patients. In addition, monozygotic twin pairs discordant for schizophrenia had greater eye-tracking similarity ($r = .77$) than clinically discordant dizygotic pairs ($r = .39$) (Holzman et al. 1980). These concordance rates for EMD are about 80% of the theoretically predicted values for a trait under polygenic control. Matthysse et al. (1986) proposed that there is a "latent trait" determined by a single major locus, which can be expressed as schizophrenia, as EMD, or as both disorders. Finally, EMD does not appear to be related to recording artifacts or subject variables such as motivation, comprehension of the task, or sustained attention during the test period (Holzman 1991). Although Clementz and Sweeney (1990) have challenged each of these lines of evidence, even these authors comment that EMD is "undoubtedly one of the most promising biological markers for schizophrenia" (p. 81).

In evaluating EMD as a putative biological marker, its specificity to schizophrenia must be considered. Previous studies have suggested that EMD may be associated with functional psychosis and not specifically with schizophrenia (Lipton et al. 1980; Shagass et al. 1974). Although higher rates of SPEM abnormalities have been found in schizophrenic patients compared with patients who have unipolar depression (Iacono et al. 1982; Shagass et al. 1974), several studies did not demonstrate differences in the rate of SPEM anomalies between schizophrenic and bipolar subjects (Iacono et al. 1982; Lipton et al. 1980; Shagass et al. 1974). However, this apparent nonspecificity may be secondary to the effects of lithium carbonate, which appears to disrupt SPEM (Levy et al. 1985). Indeed, Levy et al. (1985) found that eight of nine acutely psychotic manic patients who were free of lithium and sedative-hypnotic medications performed normally on an eye-tracking task; however, most of these subjects' test results were abnormal after they were treated with lithium. More recently, Amador et al. (1992) demonstrated that on an attention-enhancing sinusoidal target motion condition (monitor-sinusoidal), 60% of the schizophrenic patients performed abnormally compared to only 25% of the manic patients and 5% of healthy control subjects. Another task assessed in this study was visual fixation, a measure of the subjects' capacity to maintain fixation on a stationary object. Visual fixation scores differed significantly between the schizophrenic and bipolar groups. Thus, the use of particular conditions, such as monitor-sinusoidal and visual fixation, may offer promise in differentiating patients with schizophrenia from those with bipolar disorder.

Further evidence for the specificity of EMD to schizophrenia is derived from family studies. Holzman et al. (1984) found that 34% of the parents (or 55% of the parental pairs) of schizophrenic patients showed EMD compared to 10% of the parents (or 17% of the parental pairs) of bipolar patients. These data have been replicated (Siegel et al. 1984); overall, EMD has been demonstrated in 34%–58% of the first-degree relatives of patients with schizophrenia compared to 5%–13% of first-degree relatives of individuals with other psychiatric diagnoses (Clementz and Sweeney 1990).

In conclusion, EMD appears to be a potential biological trait marker for schizophrenia for three major reasons. First, EMD is present in a substantial number of patients with schizophrenia, and it has a low base rate in the general population. Second, there is sufficient evidence to qualify EMD as a relatively stable measure. Global pursuit, saccadic reaction time, and saccadic frequency have high retest reliability, which may be stable for as long as 2 years (Clementz and Sweeney 1990). EMD does not appear to be altered by antipsychotic medications and may represent a genetic vulnerability marker for schizophrenia. Third, EMD assessment can be accomplished noninvasively and expediently. Although the lack of demonstration of specificity is a concern, the future application and development of specific eye-movement tasks have a strong potential to help to improve the capacity to differentiate schizophrenia from other psychiatric and neurological disorders.

Event-Related Potentials

P300 waveform.   Several event-related brain potentials (ERPs) have been investigated in schizophrenia. Perhaps the best studied of these is the auditory P300 wave, a brain potential that occurs when subjects detect and process infrequent and meaningful changes in the auditory environment. This potential typically reaches a poststimulus peak between 300 and 400 ms after presentation of a task-relevant, infrequent auditory stimulus. Medial temporal lobe limbic structures, particularly the hippocampus, are proposed to be the generators for the P300 wave (McCarley et al. 1991). The P300 wave is believed to reflect, physiologically, the subjects' updating of what is expected in the environment, an important cognitive function that may be impaired in patients with schizophrenia (Donchin 1979).

Reduced P300 amplitude in patients with schizophrenia compared with healthy control subjects is a replicated finding (McCarley et al. 1991; St. Clair et al. 1989). The largest difference in P300 waves between groups has occurred at the left temporal (T3) electrode site in several studies (Faux et al. 1988; McCarley et al. 1991). A mean integrated P300 amplitude of 2 mV differentiated patients with schizophrenia from healthy control subjects with a sensitivity of 82% and a selectivity of 91%, values comparable to those in previous studies (McCarley et al. 1991). These findings could not be explained by the effects of antipsychotic medications, because the P300 amplitude reduction was present regardless of neuroleptic treatment (Faux et al. 1988); however, other studies of P300 amplitude present conflicting data on medication effects (Blackwood et al. 1987; Pfefferbaum et al. 1989; St. Clair et al. 1989).

Evidence also suggests that the P300 deficit may represent a potential trait marker or vulnerability marker for schizophrenia. Reduced P300 amplitude persists despite antipsychotic treatment and overall clinical improvement (Blackwood et al. 1987; Pfefferbaum et al. 1989). In addition, prolonged auditory P300 latencies were demonstrated in 12 children with schizophrenic parents compared with healthy control subjects (Schreiber et al. 1989).

Given that the P300 waveform at the T3 site is proposed to reflect temporal lobe functioning, investigators have attempted to correlate P300 amplitude with brain morphology, clinical symptomatology, and diagnosis. Investigators found significant negative correlations between P300 amplitude in the left temporal region and left Sylvian fissure widening in computed tomographic (CT) scans (McCarley et al. 1989) and positive correlations between P300 amplitude and volume reduction in the left posterior superior temporal gyrus (O'Donnell et al. 1992). Auditory P300 amplitude at the T3 site has also been positively correlated with positive symptoms of schizophrenia (Shenton et al. 1989), and P300 amplitudes evoked by auditory and visual means have been negatively correlated with negative symptoms in unmedicated schizophrenic patients (Pfefferbaum et al. 1989). Although little attention has been paid to the question of ERPs and diagnostic subtypes, patients with paranoid and nonparanoid schizophrenia are reported to have a similar frequency of P300 abnormalities (St. Clair et al. 1989).

There are limitations to the use of the P300 waveform as a biological marker in schizophrenia. Reduced P300 amplitude has also been reported in other psychiatric and neurological conditions, including the major affective disorders, Alzheimer's disease, and multiple sclerosis. Although this finding appears to be state related in patients with affective disorders (in contrast to patients with schizophrenia), patients with affective disorders generally cannot be distinguished from those with schizophrenia in cross-sectional studies using P300 amplitude alone (Javitt 1993). In addition, because P300 generation is highly dependent on attention, motivation, and level of arousal, the P300 deficit in schizophrenic patients might be related to generalized attentional disturbance, despite attempts to control for these factors (Javitt 1993).

Sensory gating. Sensory gating defects are another frequently reported abnormality in schizophrenia. These result from difficulties in filtering or gating sensory afferent input, potentially causing hyperalertness and stimulus discrimination problems (Baker et al. 1987). Testing for these defects involves a conditioning-testing paradigm in which paired stimuli are presented to the subject and evoked potential responses are recorded. The P50 auditory evoked response has been the most studied of the early cortical waves. In this paradigm, the subjects are first given a "conditioning" stimulus, followed 0.5 seconds later by a "test" stimulus, and the cortical waves elicited by each stimulus are recorded. Normally, there is a substantial decrement in the amplitude of the P50 cortical wave elicited by the test stimulus, reflecting the activation of gating mechanisms. Compared with healthy control subjects, patients with schizophrenia have significantly less suppression of the amplitude of the second P50 wave (Adler et al. 1982), a finding that is not correlated with clinical state (Baker et al. 1987) and is unaffected by treatment with antipsychotic medications (Freedman et al. 1983). Diminished gating has been observed in approximately 80%–90% of patients with schizophrenia. However, lack of P50 suppression has also been demonstrated in patients with other psychiatric diagnoses, including bipolar mania (Franks et al. 1983), adjustment disorder, and substance abuse (Baker et al. 1987). Nevertheless, this abnormality appears to be trait related rather than state related in patients with schizophrenia, in contrast to patients with mania and other nonschizophrenic psychiatric illnesses, in whom anomalies of P50 suppression appear to be correlated with worsening of clinical state (Baker et al. 1987; Franks et al. 1983). Another finding supporting P50 nonsuppression as a potential trait marker in schizophrenia is decreased auditory P50 wave suppression in more than 50% of first-degree relatives of schizophrenic patients (Siegel et al. 1984).

Other ERPs. Other ERPs that have been examined in schizophrenia include mismatch negativity and the N200 wave, which precede the

P300 wave. These ERPs reflect earlier stages of information processing involved in the detection, classification, and analysis of deviant stimuli. These ERPs are not as well studied as the P50 or P300 wave, but preliminary studies suggest diminished amplitude of mismatch negativity and the N200 wave in patients with schizophrenia compared with healthy control subjects (Javitt 1993).

Thus, there is considerable evidence supporting ERPs, particularly the P300 and the P50 waveforms, as potential biological markers in schizophrenia. Several issues must be resolved before marker status can be conferred on these cortical waves. These include the clarification of medication effects, improvement in our understanding of the correlations between clinical variables (e.g., symptomatology, treatment response) and the ERP waveforms, the significance of differences in task requirements between studies, and more precise determination of the specificity of these ERPs to schizophrenia. Finally, each of these tests, like SPEM, offers the advantage of being noninvasive, an important feature for the utility of a biological marker.

NEUROIMMUNOLOGY

The suggestion that schizophrenia shares clinical, epidemiological, and genetic characteristics with diseases of known autoimmune pathogenesis (Knight 1985) has stimulated investigations of potential autoimmune factors in schizophrenia. Higher levels of serum and cerebrospinal fluid (CSF) autoantibodies (DeLisi 1986; Rabin et al. 1989), interleukin-2 (Sharief et al. 1991), and soluble interleukin-2 receptors (Rapaport et al. 1989) have been demonstrated in patients with schizophrenia compared with healthy control subjects. Although these studies have yielded important results in terms of elucidating a theory of autoimmune pathogenesis in schizophrenia, there are several reasons why their usefulness as biological markers may be limited. The considerable overlap in these immunological values between schizophrenic and control groups markedly reduces their specificity. Moreover, some of these autoimmune findings have also been reported in patients with other psychiatric diagnoses and neurological disorders (DeLisi 1986; Ganguli and Rabin 1989; Sharief et al. 1991). Another problem with these studies has been their frequent lack of replicability. For example, Dalgalarrondo et al. (1992) was unable to find differences in serum interleukin-2 receptor levels between schizophrenic patients and healthy control subjects, in contrast to the results of Sharief et al. (1991), whereas results of studies of serum antibrain autoantibodies in schizophrenia have been inconsistent and often controversial (Knight 1985).

Recent findings by Kilidireas et al. (1992) offer a promising direction in the search for an autoimmune marker in schizophrenia. These investigators found that 14 of 32 (44%) otherwise healthy patients with schizophrenia—compared to only 8% of control subjects (including healthy subjects and patients with a variety of neurological and autoimmune diseases, tuberculosis, and acquired immunodeficiency syndrome)—had serum immunoglobulin G antibodies to the 60-kilodalton human heat shock protein, also known as the P1 mitochondrial protein. Although the pathophysiological significance of antibodies to 60-kilodalton human heat shock protein is currently unclear, if these results are confirmed they provide a promising line of investigation in the pathophysiology of schizophrenia, as well as a potential biological marker.

NEUROENDOCRINOLOGY

Several neuroendocrine abnormalities that may reflect brain pathology have been reported in schizophrenic patients. Because of the large number of studies in this area, we focus on only the most promising findings.

Growth hormone (GH) secretion has been extensively studied in schizophrenia, largely because dopamine input to the hypothalamus leads to phasic stimulation of GH release from the anterior pituitary (Rivier et al. 1982). Most pharmacological challenge studies with apomorphine, a dopamine agonist that stimulates GH release, have demonstrated an increased range and overall blunted GH responses in chronically psychotic and neuroleptic-naive schizophrenic patients compared with control subjects (reviewed by Garver 1988), although two studies did not differentiate patients from control subjects on the basis of their initial GH response (Brown et al. 1988; Zemlan et al. 1986). In contrast, fewer long-term patients appear to have either a greater GH response (Zemlan et al. 1986) or a bimodal response (Garver 1988) to apomorphine. Increased GH response was positively correlated with severity of thought disorder (Zemlan et al. 1986) and positive symptoms (Brown et al. 1988), and blunted GH response may be associated with negative symptoms (Garver 1988). In studies of basal GH secretion, Lieberman et al. (1992a, 1993a) demonstrated that acutely ill, first-episode schizophrenic patients had higher basal GH levels than control subjects, in contrast to a prior study (Brown et al. 1988) that found no differences between patients and control subjects. In addition, increased basal GH was associated with a longer time to remission and worse outcomes (Lieberman et al. 1992a, 1993b).

Other pharmacological probes that have been used in GH challenge paradigms are bromocriptine and methylphenidate, direct and indirect dopamine agonists, respectively. Blunted GH response to methylphenidate has been observed in schizophrenic patients versus control subjects (Janowsky et al. 1978; Pandey et al. 1977), although more recent studies of methylphenidate challenge did not differentiate schizophrenic from nonschizophrenic patients on the basis of GH response (Lieberman et al. 1993a; Sharma et al. 1990, 1991). Studies with bromocriptine showed that the GH response in schizophrenic patients was blocked by haloperidol at the minimum effective antipsychotic dose (Hirschowitz et al. 1991). The GH response to growth hormone–releasing factor (GHRF) has also been examined in patients with schizophrenia. Two studies (Mayerhoff et al. 1990; Nerozzi et al. 1990) found no difference in GH response to GHRF between patients and control subjects, whereas Peabody et al. (1990) observed that schizophrenic patients had a significantly lower GH response than nonschizophrenic and control groups; the conflicting findings could be due to small sample sizes.

Clonidine, an α-adrenergic agonist that stimulates GH release, has been used to test the noradrenergic system of patients with schizophrenia. Van Kammen et al. (1989a), in a double-blind, placebo-controlled clonidine challenge study, demonstrated that treatment response was correlated with GH response to clonidine before treatment and with spontaneous GH peaks after administration of placebo. Patients with mostly positive symptoms were reported to have an elevated GH response to clonidine, whereas those with mainly negative symptoms were shown to have diminished responses (Garver 1988).

Studies that measured the response of thyroid-stimulating hormone (TSH) to thyrotropin-releasing hormone (TRH) challenge have shown no significant differences in the TSH response between patients with schizophrenia and healthy control subjects (Baumgartner et al. 1988; Roy et al. 1989). Patients with major depression and schizophrenic patients had similar TSH responses after stimulation by TRH in two studies (Baumgartner et al. 1988; Siris et al. 1991). However, compared with schizoaffective and bipolar patients, schizophrenic patients had a TSH response that was significantly less blunted (Kiriike et al. 1988). No relationship has been found between psychopathology or treatment response and levels of TSH after injection of TRH (Baumgartner et al. 1988; Keshavan et al. 1988; Kiriike et al. 1988; Siris et al. 1991).

Studies using the dexamethasone suppression test indicate that nonsuppression of plasma cortisol, although observed in 11%–33% of patients with schizophrenia, is much more prevalent in patients with affective disorders (Garver 1988). However, Coppen et al. (1983) suggested some potential value for the dexamethasone suppression test in patients with schizophrenia, because suppression was demonstrated in 32% of the patients with predominantly negative symptoms but in only 10% of those with predominantly positive symptoms.

A small number of investigations of gonadal hormone function in patients with schizophrenia have demonstrated relatively consistent abnormalities that may further our understanding of gender differences in this illness. Lower basal levels of the pituitary gonadotropins luteinizing hormone and follicle-stimulating hormone (Brambilla et al. 1977) and reduced spontaneous fluctuations in secretion of luteinizing hormone (Ferrier et al. 1983) have been found in unmedicated male patients with chronic schizophrenia. Studies involving stimulation with gonadotropin-releasing hormone have revealed blunted responses of luteinizing hormone and follicle-stimulating hormone in patients with schizophrenia compared with psychiatric control subjects (Brambilla 1980; Ferrier et al. 1983).

Because of its regulation by dopamine, prolactin has been extensively studied in patients with schizophrenia. Compared with healthy control subjects, patients with schizophrenia were shown to have a markedly increased secretory amplitude of prolactin immediately before and after sleep, and there was an increased frequency of prolactin pulses in patients versus control subjects, leading the authors to suggest that increased prolactin responsiveness to sleep could be a biological marker for schizophrenia (van Cauter et al. 1991). However, prolactin has proved to be more valuable as a measure of pathophysiology and as a correlate of treatment response and illness course than as a biological marker of the illness. In a study of male schizophrenic patients receiving haloperidol maintenance treatment, Newcomer et al. (1992) reported inverse correlations between plasma prolactin and tardive dyskinesia and between plasma prolactin and positive and negative symptoms, suggesting that plasma prolactin may serve as a peripheral marker of dopamine activity in the nigrostriatal and mesolimbic pathways. A positive correlation was found between plasma prolactin levels and clinical response to haloperidol, which was strongest at the 5-mg dosage (van Putten et al. 1991). Lieberman et al. (1990) demonstrated that lower peak prolactin responses to acute administration of haloperidol were associated with an increased risk of relapse.

Although neuroendocrine findings in schizophrenia have helped to elucidate pathophysiological mechanisms, they have yet to provide us with a suitable biological marker. There are no consistent findings for any of the hormones that we have discussed in terms of their value in differentiating patients with schizophrenia from healthy control subjects or patients with other psychiatric disorders. However, studies do indicate that some neuroendocrine findings—particularly the basal GH levels and response to challenges with dopamine agonists and the prolactin levels in patients receiving maintenance antipsychotics and in response to neuroleptic challenges—may have promise in predicting treatment response and in serving as correlates of symptomatology. The development of challenge agents with more specific pharmacological effects may help considerably in the future identification of neuro-endocrine markers in patients with schizophrenia.

NEUROCHEMISTRY

The theory that schizophrenia results from dysfunction of key neuro-chemical systems has prompted numerous investigations of neuro-transmitters and their metabolites in body fluids of patients with this illness. Although several neurotransmitters have been identified as playing potentially important roles in the pathophysiology of schizo-phrenia, three major neurotransmitters have emerged as the most plausible candidates: dopamine, serotonin (5-hydroxytryptamine; 5-HT), and norepinephrine. Because accurate measurements of each of these neurochemicals and their metabolites in body fluids can be obtained, it is not surprising that each of them has been examined as a potential biological marker for this illness.

Dopamine and Homovanillic Acid

Despite its inconsistencies and limitations, the dopamine hypothesis remains the most enduring and viable pathophysiological theory of schizophrenia (Davis et al. 1991). The best studied measure of dopa-mine as a potential biological marker is its major metabolite homo-vanillic acid (HVA). Investigations of this metabolite have included measurements of CSF, plasma, and urinary HVA levels.

Studies of CSF HVA in schizophrenic patients have yielded inconsis-tent results. CSF HVA levels have not been found to differentiate schizophrenic patients from healthy control subjects, and associations between CSF HVA and symptomatology or diagnostic subtypes have not been demonstrated (Widerlov 1988). Antipsychotic treatment was associated with increases in CSF HVA, but these increases were not re-lated to treatment response (reviewed in Kahn et al. 1993). However, some studies have shown that the more acute and severe the psychosis, the higher the CSF HVA level (Bowers 1978).

Plasma HVA (pHVA) has also been explored as a potential biological marker. Basal levels of pHVA in drug-free patients discriminated be-tween schizophrenic and control subjects in only a few studies (re-viewed by Davis et al. 1991; Kahn and Davidson 1993), while studies that examined the correlations between pHVA levels and severity of illness have also found inconsistent results (reviewed by Davis et al. 1991). Notably, Koreen et al. (in press) found no correlation between pHVA and symptom severity in first-episode schizophrenic patients despite the fact that multiple pHVA samples were taken, one method-ological issue raised by Davis et al. (1991) to explain discrepancies in the findings among studies. This finding might suggest that chronic neuroleptic treatment may alter dopamine neuronal activity such that the correlation between psychopathology and pHVA is enhanced (Koreen et al., in press). A more consistent finding, however, has been the association between pretreatment basal pHVA levels and change in pHVA values with antipsychotic treatment, and therapeutic response (reviewed by Davis et al. 1991; Koreen et al., in press). Thus, pHVA may potentially be used as a marker of neuroleptic response.

There are several limitations to the use of pHVA and CSF HVA as biological markers. It is unclear whether and to what extent HVA from these sources reflects dopamine activity in brain regions that are relevant to schizophrenia. Of the total body HVA synthesized, only 11%–35% comes from the brain (Maas et al. 1993). The use of agents like debrisoquine, a monoamine oxidase inhibitor that does not penetrate the central nervous system, may yield HVA measurements that more specifically reflect dopamine function in the brain rather than being influenced by peripheral dopamine activity (Maas et al. 1993). It has been suggested that CSF HVA reflects dopamine activity in the cerebral cortex, whereas pHVA more closely reflects subcortical dopamine activity (Kahn and Davidson 1993); however, further research is needed to confirm this hypothesis. Finally, HVA levels are affected by age, sex, height, diet, motor activity, time of day, and season, factors that often were not adequately controlled for in studies of this metabolite (Davis et al. 1991).

Another peripheral measurement of dopamine activity previously reported as a potential biological marker of schizophrenia is spiroperidol-labeled dopamine receptors on circulating lymphocytes (Bondy and Ackenheil 1987; Bondy et al. 1984). Although this marker clearly would be promising, these results have not been replicated and may have been due to methodological factors (Wodarz et al. 1992).

Norepinephrine and 3-Methoxy-4-Hydroxyphenylglycol

A substantial amount of evidence implicating norepinephrine in the pathogenesis of schizophrenia has emerged (reviewed by van Kammen and Kelley 1991). Van Kammen and Kelley (1991) proposed that norepinephrine activity, although not necessarily of etiological importance, appears to regulate symptomatology, course, outcome, and medication response, perhaps in part through interactions of norepinephrine with dopamine. Studies of norepinephrine in medication-free patients with schizophrenia consistently demonstrate that CSF norepinephrine is elevated compared with that in control subjects (Maas et al. 1993; van Kammen et al. 1989a, 1989b). CSF norepinephrine has been shown to increase prodromally before relapse or exacerbations of psychotic symptoms (van Kammen 1991). Van Kammen et al. (1989b) found that CSF norepinephrine was increased during halo-peridol maintenance treatment in patients who relapsed after haloper-idol withdrawal, despite similar psychosis ratings during treatment for the relapsing and nonrelapsing groups. After haloperidol with-drawal, only nonrelapsing patients showed a decrease in norepineph-rine levels.

Despite these interesting results, there are limitations to the use of norepinephrine and 3-methoxy-4-hydroxyphenylglycol (MHPG) as bi-ological markers. As is true with HVA, significant overlap is present in norepinephrine and MHPG levels between drug-free patients with schizophrenia and control subjects. Most studies that showed positive associations between norepinephrine and features of schizophrenia in-volved CSF measurements (which require a lumbar puncture) rather than blood or urine measurements, thus making it more difficult to rou-tinely measure norepinephrine and MHPG as a part of diagnosis or treatment planning. As is likely true for other neurochemicals, the ef-fects of norepinephrine in schizophrenia either may be direct or may involve complex interactions with dopamine and other neurotransmit-ters (van Kammen 1991). In addition, abnormalities of norepinephrine are not specific to schizophrenia, as they have been also associated with affective disorders (Preskorn et al. 1992).

5-HT and 5-Hydroxyindoleacetic Acid

The recent success of clozapine in the treatment of schizophrenia has contributed to a rekindled interest in the role of 5-HT. Meltzer (1989) hypothesized that the unique mechanism of action of clozapine in schizophrenia is due to its antagonism of 5-HT_2 receptors along with D_2 receptors. Preclinical and clinical evidence suggests that clozapine blocks functional effects of 5-HT and downregulates 5-HT_2 receptors (Meltzer 1989, 1990). In addition, the ratio of 5-HT_2 to D_2 receptor affin-ities is higher for the atypical antipsychotic agents than for the typical agents (Meltzer 1991); based in part on these neurochemical effects, Meltzer (1989) proposed that dysregulation of the interaction between 5-HT and dopamine may be involved in the pathophysiology of schizophrenia. Consistent with this hypothesis, Pickar et al. (1992)—in a crossover, double-blind, placebo-controlled comparison of clozapine and fluphenazine—demonstrated that a low ratio of CSF HVA to 5-hydroxyindoleacetic acid (5-HIAA) during each phase of treatment predicted superior response to clozapine. Similar findings were seen in subsequent studies (Hsiao et al. 1993; Kahn et al. 1993; Szymanski et al. 1993).

Studies in which 5-HIAA has been measured in the CSF and platelets of patients with schizophrenia have produced mixed results. Although some studies have shown diminished CSF 5-HIAA levels, most investigators have not detected any differences in levels of this metabolite between schizophrenic and control subjects (for a review, see Bleich et al. 1988). In addition, treatment neither with typical antipsychotics (van Kammen et al. 1986) nor with clozapine (Hsiao et al. 1993; Kahn et al. 1993; Pickar et al. 1992; Szymanski et al. 1993) appears to change CSF 5-HIAA concentrations. There are, however, two major findings from CSF studies that indicate serotonergic involvement in schizophrenia: correlations between diminished CSF 5-HIAA and brain atrophy and between low CSF 5-HIAA and suicidal behavior in schizophrenic patients. With respect to the former finding, Bleich et al. (1988) argued that patients with chronic schizophrenia with predominant type II symptomatology (more negative symptoms) (Crow 1980) may have abnormal serotonergic activity based in part on the link between neuroanatomical abnormalities and negative symptoms. However, caution must be used in interpreting these reports. First, given the positive correlation between HVA and 5-HIAA (van Kammen et al. 1986), it is possible that diminished 5-HIAA in patients with brain atrophy may be a function of low HVA, which has also been linked to similar neuroanatomical anomalies (Bleich et al. 1988). Second, low CSF 5-HIAA is probably more specific to suicidality than to schizophrenia, because it has also been demonstrated in suicidal patients with affective and personality disorders; in fact, it is actually a more prominent finding in patients with affective and personality disorders than in patients with schizophrenia (L. S. Cohen et al. 1988).

A number of studies have examined 5-HT levels in platelets and whole blood in patients with schizophrenia. A majority of these studies found that 5-HT in platelets and whole blood is elevated in patients with schizophrenia and that these findings are unrelated to age, sex, or medication status. However, inconsistency in these results (Bleich et al. 1988) indicates that further investigation is warranted to determine further the potential of this measurement as a biological marker.

Thus, although there are no clear indications at present that 5-HT or 5-HIAA is particularly useful as a biological marker in schizophrenia, future studies of the balance between serotonergic and dopaminergic function may suggest that the combined use of 5-HT and dopamine measures may be more advantageous than either one alone. In addition, the possibility exists that serotonergic abnormalities are associated with specific characteristics of schizophrenia, such as negative symptomatology.

Psychostimulant Challenge Studies

The induction of psychotic symptoms resembling schizophrenia after psychostimulant administration is one of the strongest lines of evidence implicating dopamine and other biogenic amines in schizophrenia, because these medications increase catecholaminergic neuro-transmission (Angrist and van Kammen 1984). The mechanism by which this increase occurs involves the stimulation of catecholamine release from presynaptic nerve terminals and blockade of cate-cholamine reuptake (Moore 1978). Thus, it has been proposed that psychostimulant-induced psychotic symptoms represent a valid pharmacological model for schizophrenia (Snyder 1973). As a result, numerous studies of schizophrenia have used psychostimulants as pharmacological probes for diagnosis, prediction of treatment re-sponse, and exploration of pathophysiology (for reviews, see Lieber-man et al. 1987b and Robinson et al. 1991) based on the rationale that schizophrenic patients have an increased vulnerability to the psy-chotogenic effects of psychostimulants. In these investigations, sub-jects receive an acute dose of a psychostimulant that would not induce psychotic symptoms in subjects without schizophrenia to maximize the differential responsiveness between patients and control subjects (Robinson et al. 1991).

In a review of 36 psychostimulant studies in schizophrenic patients, Lieberman et al. (1987b) found that challenge with these agents in-duced a heterogeneous response in the activation of psychotic symp-tomatology. Among patients with schizophrenia, 40% worsened, 19% improved, and 41% were unchanged; among nonschizophrenic sub-jects, who were diagnostically heterogeneous, 18% worsened, 2% worsened with psychotic symptoms, 40% improved, and 40% were un-changed. In 7 of 11 studies that compared the response rates of schizo-phrenic and nonschizophrenic subjects, the rate of symptom activation was considerably higher in the schizophrenic group. Although the rates of behavioral worsening in nonschizophrenic subjects within in-dividual studies were highly variable (0%–50%), psychotic symptoms occurred very rarely in these groups. However, few of these non-schizophrenic subjects had psychotic symptoms at the time of testing, and they were diagnostically heterogeneous. It is thus premature to conclude that a psychotogenic response is specific to schizophrenia, be-cause actively psychotic nonschizophrenic patients (such as those with affective psychoses) were underrepresented in these studies (Lieber-man et al. 1987b).

The marked variability in these 36 studies indicates that the psy-chotogenic response to psychostimulants is influenced by numerous factors that differed among studies (Lieberman et al. 1987b). There are differences in potency between the three psychotogens (methylpheni-date, D-ephedrine, and amphetamine) that were used. Interestingly, methylphenidate, a nonamphetamine cocainelike psychostimulant, produced the highest rate of worsening (74%) and the lowest rates of improvement (0%) and no change (26%). However, the differences in potency may be at least partially confounded by other factors, such as dose and route of administration. Stage of illness and presence of neuroleptic treatment may also affect the psychotogenic response.

Janowsky et al. (1973), in a test-retest paradigm, found that patients who were challenged with psychostimulants during an acute psychotic episode experienced worsening of symptoms, but they did not demonstrate any symptomatic exacerbation when the challenge was repeated after they were treated with neuroleptics and were in remission. This study suggests that the response to psychostimulant challenge may be state related, as was subsequently demonstrated by van Kammen et al. (1982). However, a review by Lieberman et al. (1987b) reported little difference in the rates of worsening between patients with active versus inactive symptoms (43% versus 35%), although higher rates of improvement (21% versus 6%) and lower rates of no change (36% versus 59%) were demonstrated in patients with active symptoms. These treatment-related differences in the response to psychostimulants appear to reflect changes in the clinical state but may also reflect the influence of neuroleptic effects. In more recent work, Lieberman et al. (1993a) found that 60% of first-episode schizophrenic patients experienced activation of psychotic symptoms in response to methylphenidate. This result suggests that clinical state and stage of illness are factors that influence the response to psychostimulants.

Apart from their potential utility as a diagnostic test for schizophrenia, psychostimulant challenge tests have shown promise as a method to identify which patients are most prone to relapse. Several investigators have found that positive symptom activation in response to a challenge with an indirect-acting dopamine agonist was associated with a higher likelihood of relapse after medication withdrawal (Angrist et al. 1985; Lieberman et al. 1987a; van Kammen et al. 1982).

In conclusion, psychostimulant challenge studies have yielded promising leads toward detecting vulnerability to psychosis and have provided a means by which to investigate the dopamine hypothesis of schizophrenia. However, the present lack of sensitivity and the unproven specificity of psychotogenic responses to psychostimulant challenge, as well as continuing questions regarding variations in psychostimulant administration and effects of the clinical state and neuroleptics, limit the practical utility of this measure as a biological marker. Nevertheless, in the future, psychostimulant challenges could prove to be of clinical value in the prediction of outcome and illness course.

Other Pharmacological Probes in Challenge Studies

***m*-Chlorophenylpiperazine.** The behavioral response of schizophrenic patients after challenge with *m*-chlorophenylpiperazine (m-CPP), a selective 5-HT receptor agonist, has been investigated. Some studies have shown that m-CPP has a psychotogenic effect in schizophrenia (Iqbal et al. 1991; Krystal et al. 1991), which is antagonized by ritanserin and clozapine (Krystal et al. 1991). These studies support the serotonergic hypothesis of schizophrenia. However, two other m-CPP studies showed a worsening of anxiety and somatic symptoms but no change in psychotic symptoms (Kahn et al. 1992, 1993; S. Szymanski, D. Mayerhoff, A. Koreen, J. M. J. Alvir, R. Munne, D. Umbricht, J. M. Kane, C. Lemus, and J. A. Lieberman, "The Behavioral Effect of IV M-CPP in First Episode and Chronic Schizophrenia and Schizoaffective Disorder," submitted for publication, July 1993), suggesting that the behavioral effects of m-CPP may be nonspecific (Lieberman and Koreen 1993).

Ketamine. The phencyclidine/N-methyl-D-aspartate (NMDA) hypothesis of schizophrenia (Javitt and Zukin 1991) has been investigated with ketamine challenge studies. Krystal et al. (1992, 1993) demonstrated in healthy subjects dose-related psychotogenic effects of ketamine, including thought disorder, illusions (but not hallucinations), alterations in time and body perception, and derealization. In addition, social withdrawal and psychomotor retardation, two negative symptoms, were observed. Lahti et al. (1993) reported preliminary results from a ketamine challenge study in haloperidol-treated schizophrenic patients, which showed a short-term exacerbation of psychotic symptoms, including delusions, hallucinations, and thought disorder in some patients. A ketamine challenge study comparing schizophrenic patients with healthy control subjects with respect to symptom measures is clearly warranted, particularly in light of the finding (Krystal et al. 1993) that ketamine induced illusions, but not hallucinations, in healthy control subjects.

Other Neurochemical Markers

Several other neurotransmitters have been considered as potential candidates for biological markers in schizophrenia. The evidence is weaker for these substances than it is for dopamine, norepinephrine, and 5-HT. We focus on the most promising candidates.

The induction of symptoms similar to those of schizophrenia after phencyclidine administration and the link between this drug and the NMDA system have stimulated interest in the role of glutamate and related excitatory amino acids in schizophrenia. In the only recent clinical investigation of an excitatory amino acid in schizophrenia, no difference in CSF N-acetyl-L-aspartic acid levels was found between schizophrenic patients and healthy control subjects, although CSF HVA and MHPG levels were negatively correlated with N-acetyl-L-aspartic acid levels in control subjects but not in patients (Swahn 1990). Several postmortem studies of glutamate and phencyclidine-NMDA binding sites demonstrated differences in glutamate and phencyclidine-NMDA binding between schizophrenic patients and control subjects, although these findings have not been consistent (Deakin et al. 1989; Kerwin et al. 1988, 1990; Simpson et al. 1992). Clearly, more direct neurochemical studies of excitatory amino acids in schizophrenia are necessary to clarify their potential as biological markers in schizophrenia.

Several neuropeptides have been studied in schizophrenia. Neurotensin, an endogenous tridecapeptide that is colocalized with dopaminergic neurons and appears to modulate dopamine functioning, may have relevance to schizophrenia. A few clinical studies of neurotensin have demonstrated diminished CSF neurotensin concentrations in patients with schizophrenia compared with healthy control subjects (Garver et al. 1991; Nemeroff et al. 1989). Although there was a large degree of overlap in neurotensin levels between these two groups, there appears to be some diagnostic specificity, as patients with depression, patients with anorexia nervosa or bulimia, and healthy control groups did not differ with respect to levels of neurotensin (Nemeroff et al. 1989). Neurotensin concentration seems to be state related, as levels of this neurotransmitter have been found to increase with antipsychotic treatment (Garver et al. 1991). There are suggestions that low neurotensin levels are correlated with increased severity of symptomatology in schizophrenia (Garver et al. 1991). Studies of CSF somatostatin, a substance that functions as a hypothalamic releasing factor, have yielded conflicting results in schizophrenic patients; somatostatin abnormalities appear to be seen more consistently in patients with affective disorders (Vecsei and Widerlov 1988). Other neuropeptides that have been studied in schizophrenia include cholecystokinin and β-endorphin, although there is insufficient evidence to suggest them as possible biological markers (reviewed by Lieberman and Koreen 1993).

Phospholipids

Membrane phospholipids in plasma, platelets, and lymphocytes offer yet another possible direction in the search for biochemical markers in schizophrenia. In one study of phospholipase A_2, a key enzyme involved in phospholipid metabolism, increased plasma phospholipase A_2 was observed in schizophrenic patients compared with nonschizophrenic psychiatric patients and healthy control subjects; phospholipase A_2 levels declined with treatment (Gattaz et al. 1990). However, a replication study found no difference in phospholipase A_2 levels between patients with schizophrenia and control subjects (Bennett et al. 1991). Lysophosphatidylcholine, a toxic substance that is a product of phospholipase A_2–mediated metabolism of phosphatidylcholine, was found to be significantly elevated in the platelets of schizophrenic patients compared with that in platelets of control subjects (Pangerl et al. 1991). Three studies of essential fatty acids, which may be involved in dopamine release (Horrobin et al. 1989), have consistently demonstrated diminished platelet linoleic acid in schizophrenic patients versus control subjects (Bates et al. 1992; Horrobin et al. 1989; Kaiya et al. 1991). In studies of the phosphoinositide system, increased turnover of phosphatidylinositol was found in the platelets of patients who were on and off medications, but not in medication-naive patients (Das et al. 1992; Essali et al. 1990; Yao et al. 1992). However, another study found diminished phosphatidylinositol turnover in patients with acute schizophrenia compared with control subjects (Kaiya et al. 1989). Further studies of membrane phospholipids in schizophrenia are indicated.

NEUROIMAGING

Structural Brain Imaging

Neuropathological alterations have been found consistently in the brains of schizophrenic patients postmortem (Bogerts et al. 1991). CT was the first technique that allowed the human brain to be imaged in vivo in a noninvasive manner. Since the early CT studies in schizophrenia (Johnstone et al. 1976; Weinberger et al. 1980), an array of neuroanatomical abnormalities have been demonstrated in patients with this illness, the most prevalent and replicable of which have been lateral and third ventricular enlargement (Raz and Raz 1990). Despite the initial results with CT, magnetic resonance imaging (MRI) has become the dominant structural neuroimaging technique. MRI offers several advantages over CT, including higher tissue contrast and resolution, the generation of images in all three planes of orientation, and the absence of ionizing radiation (Bogerts et al. 1990; Kelsoe et al. 1988). As a result, MRI has permitted the visualization of specific brain structures in studies that are more detailed and of higher quality than CT studies.

The most consistent finding from MRI studies has been the confirmation of enlargement of the lateral and third ventricles in schizophrenic patients versus control subjects (Andreasen et al. 1989). In one of the most notable MRI studies of schizophrenia to date, ventriculomegaly occurred in almost every affected twin of monozygotic twin pairs discordant for schizophrenia (Suddath et al. 1990). Enlarged lateral ventricles have been demonstrated in first-episode patients with schizophrenia and thus are not due to the effects of medication and disease chronicity (Degreef et al. 1992c). Despite the reproducibility of ventriculomegaly, there are factors that limit the usefulness of this abnormality as a biological marker. First, there is substantial variation in this structure between patients and control subjects, leading to a considerable degree of overlap in the values for both groups. On one hand, it has been claimed that this finding occurs only in a subgroup of between 20% and 40% of the patients with schizophrenia (DeLisi et al. 1991; Suddath et al. 1990). On the other hand, the wide range of normal anatomic variation and the multiple factors that affect it (e.g., sex, body size, age) may require precise parameters that are not yet available for application to schizophrenic patients (Lieberman et al. 1992b, 1992c; Suddath et al. 1990). Second, ventriculomegaly is not specific to schizophrenia: it occurs with normal aging (Pfefferbaum et al. 1986); in patients with bipolar disorder—albeit less prominently (Altshuler et al. 1991; Swayze et al. 1990); and to a greater extent in patients with dementia (Perry and Markowitz 1988).

Other neuroanatomical abnormalities that have been found in neuroimaging studies of schizophrenic patients include diminished area and volume of total and specific cortical regions (Zipursky et al. 1992) and medial temporal lobe structures (Bogerts et al. 1990, 1993) and anomalies of corpus callosa size and shape (Nasrallah et al. 1986). In addition, DeGreef et al. (1992a) found an increased prevalence of cavum septum pellucidum in patients with schizophrenia compared with healthy control subjects and nonschizophrenic patients. This finding has been replicated in a postmortem series and is further evidence of a neurodevelopmental disturbance in schizophrenia (DeGreef et al. 1992b). Reduced frontal cortical size (Andreasen et al. 1986; Zipursky et al. 1992) and prefrontal white matter volume (Breier et al. 1992) have also been reported; these findings conflict with those of other investigators who failed to find diminished frontal cortical volume (Andreasen et al. 1990; Kelsoe et al. 1988; Suddath et al. 1989, 1990).

Recent technological advances in neuroimaging have permitted increasingly precise quantitation of discrete brain regions and structures. These methodological innovations include enhanced magnetic field strength of the scanner; development of pulse sequences to acquire whole-brain images with high resolution that enable three-dimensional reconstruction in multiple planes; and an array of image-analysis techniques, including computer-assisted morphometry, stereology, three-dimensional surface rendering, and shape analysis (Lieberman 1992c). The combination of improved resolution, the use of thinner sections, and increasingly sophisticated methods of determining the volume of brain structures has markedly diminished the measurement error. These improvements have thus enhanced the capacity to detect subtle differences in the size of specific brain structures between groups, an advantage with important implications in the search for a biological marker.

The most intriguing and consistent findings that have emerged from the recent application of these refined imaging and analytic techniques involve the temporolimbic regions. Diminished left temporal gray matter volume has been demonstrated in schizophrenic twins compared with their corresponding unaffected monozygotic twins (Suddath et al. 1990). Studies examining specific structures in schizophrenic patients and control subjects have found that schizophrenic patients have decreased area (DeLisi et al. 1991) and volume (Bogerts et al. 1990; Breier et al. 1992; Johnstone et al. 1989) of the amygdala-hippocampal complex; increased size of the temporal horns (Bogerts et al. 1990; Degreef et al. 1992c; Shenton et al. 1992); diminished area and volume of the hippocampus, bilaterally (Suddath et al. 1990) and on the left side (Bogerts et al. 1990; Breier et al. 1992; Shenton et al. 1992); decreased volume of the amygdala bilaterally (Breier et al. 1992); and smaller volumes of the left parahippocampal gyrus and superior temporal gyrus (Barta et al. 1990; Shenton et al. 1992).

The use of brain pathomorphological findings as biological markers is subject to the same limitations of specificity and overlap in the distribution among patient and healthy populations previously described with ventriculomegaly.

Some investigators have examined the clinical correlates of brain pathomorphology on MRI. Greater severity of negative symptoms has been shown to correlate with enlarged lateral ventricles (Andreasen et al. 1990), increased temporal horn volume (Degreef et al. 1992c), and increased T1 relaxation times in the left frontal lobe (Besson et al. 1987). Greater severity of positive symptoms was associated with reduced hippocampal volume (Bogerts et al. 1993), larger left temporal horn volume (Degreef et al. 1992c), and increased T1 relaxation times in the left medial temporal lobe (Besson et al. 1987). In addition, Barta et al. (1990) reported an association between diminished volume of the left superior temporal gyrus and increased auditory hallucinations, whereas Shenton et al. (1992) found an association between the degree of thought disorder and diminished volume of the left superior temporal gyrus. Despite the pathophysiological link between frontal lobe lesions and negative symptoms, there is little evidence that supports a relationship between reduced frontal or prefrontal cortical volumes and negative symptoms (Bogerts et al. 1991; Buchanan et al. 1993).

Several studies have found a relationship among brain morphological abnormalities, treatment response, and outcome (DeLisi et al. 1983; Kaplan et al. 1990; Lieberman et al. 1993b; Luchins et al. 1984; Schulz et al. 1983; Vita et al. 1988). The specific structures include the lateral and third ventricles; larger ventricular size was associated with poorer treatment response and long-term outcome. Most of the studies mentioned used quantitative morphometric procedures to assess the differences between patient and comparison groups. Although quantitative methods are preferred in the scientific investigations of morphological differences between patient and comparison groups and have yielded meaningful findings, they are not yet practical for assisting in routine patient evaluation, a major reason for seeking biological markers. Lieberman et al. (1992c), using blind qualitative assessment of brain MRI scans, detected rates of abnormal brain morphology that were comparable to rates found in prior studies of similar populations. These findings indicated that, although not scientifically optimal, qualitative assessment can be sensitive enough to detect clinically meaningful differences. Because morphological brain anomalies are associated with poor neuroleptic response and outcome, qualitative assessment may be useful in determining the prognosis and treatment of patients in a clinical setting (Lieberman et al. 1992b).

In conclusion, the use of MRI has great potential in the search for biological markers of schizophrenia, although issues of variability among and within diagnostic groups, conflicting findings among studies, lack of specificity, and potential confounding variables need to be addressed. Future neuroimaging research using increasingly sophisticated techniques may help to define particular anomalies of brain structures that are replicable and highly specific to schizophrenia and that may eventually serve as biological markers of this disorder.

Functional Brain Imaging

The recent application of sophisticated methods of functional brain imaging to psychiatry has substantially advanced our understanding of the pathophysiology of mental illness. Nowhere has this advance been more apparent than in the study of schizophrenia. These techniques have permitted the visualization of the metabolic features of dynamic psychological processes in patients with schizophrenia and comparison subjects.

The predominant functional imaging techniques currently in use are "two-dimensional" xenon-133 inhalation regional cerebral blood flow (2D-rCBF), single photon emission computed tomography (SPECT), and positron-emission tomography (PET). However, functional MRI with magnetic resonance spectroscopy (MRS) and high-speed and echo planar MRI are experimental applications of magnetic resonance that have been used to study schizophrenia. Although these techniques have been used only to a limited extent in schizophrenic patients, they offer great promise for the future.

The common and individual features of radiolabeled tomographic imaging are reviewed by Berman and Weinberger (1991). Each of these techniques is capable of measuring regional cerebral blood flow (rCBF), which can serve as a marker for the quantitation of metabolic activity in the brain. PET can also measure glucose metabolism, and both PET and SPECT can image and quantitate various neuroreceptors, enzymes, and neurotransmitter activity.

All three techniques (2D-rCBF, SPECT, PET) use various radioactive tracers to measure blood flow, metabolic activity, and neuroreceptors, and each has its own advantages and disadvantages. The major advantages of 2D-rCBF are its low expense, technical convenience, and noninvasiveness; these practical features are particularly beneficial in a test for a biological marker. However, 2D-rCBF has poor spatial resolution, and it is primarily used to measure superficial, rather than deep, structures. SPECT offers better spatial resolution than 2D-rCBF, and because the half-lives of the radiotracers used with SPECT are longer than those of the radiotracers used with PET, SPECT scans can be performed several hours after the radiotracers are administered. The major disadvantages of SPECT are attenuation of radiation counts (which can produce artificially lower values for deep brain regions and artificially higher values for superficial regions) and lower spatial resolution than that seen with PET. Because PET uses radioisotopes of elements that are found in organic compounds, this technique is particularly useful in the study of in vivo physiological and biochemical processes. PET's superior spatial resolution (3–6 mm) permits more precise quantitation of metabolic and neurochemical activity in specific brain structures. Nevertheless, the substantial expense and invasiveness of this method will likely prohibit its routine use, at least in its present form.

Numerous functional brain imaging studies have been conducted in schizophrenic patients. Two major paradigms have been used: studies of patients in resting conditions and studies that involve activation or stimulation procedures (Berman and Weinberger 1991). In resting studies, subjects are not asked to perform motor, sensory, cognitive, or other behavioral activities, and attempts are made to control for sensory stimuli. This paradigm has been criticized for two major reasons. First, it has been argued that the mental experience during a "resting state" may vary markedly among individuals. Second, the amount and type of sensory input that are appropriate during the scan have not been clearly defined. The development of activation paradigms has helped to address these limitations. By having each subject serve as his or her own control, interindividual variability in baseline cerebral metabolic activity is minimized. In addition, there is greater standardization and control of sensory, cognitive, and behavioral experiences, thus reducing the degree of measurement "noise" and enhancing the comparability among studies. Finally, a subtle or latent functional disturbance is more likely to become apparent under a condition in which the brain is stressed. The differences in findings among studies may be explained by the large number of inadequately controlled variables that can affect the parameters being measured. These include sex, handedness, age, arterial P_{CO_2}, and the effects of emotional state (Berman and Weinberger 1991).

The most frequently reported and consistent finding in functional brain imaging studies of schizophrenia has been hypofrontality, which was first demonstrated by Ingvar and Franzen (1974a, 1974b). In these landmark studies, which used the intracarotid xenon-133 technique to measure rCBF in the lateral cortex, patients with schizophrenia had diminished blood flow to frontal brain regions (relative hypofrontality), in contrast to healthy subjects, who showed relatively more blood flow to frontal areas (relative hyperfrontality). These investigators found greater hypofrontality in the more apathetic, inactive, and autistic patients. Since these pioneering studies, most researchers in the area of functional brain imaging have demonstrated hypofrontality in the majority of resting and cognitive challenge studies (Buchsbaum et al. 1992). The cognitive challenge that has revealed the most replicable abnormality is the Wisconsin Card Sorting Test, a neuropsychological test that is relatively specific for the dorsolateral prefrontal cortex (Berman and Weinberger 1991). In these studies of rCBF, patients (in contrast to healthy control subjects) did not show prefrontal activation over their baseline blood flow levels while performing the Wisconsin Card Sorting Test. Performance of other neuropsychological tests that are not linked to dorsolateral prefrontal cortex function did not produce this abnormal response pattern. Hypofrontality with performance of other tasks requiring frontal lobe function has also been demonstrated in PET studies (R. M. Cohen et al. 1987; Volkow et al. 1987).

Although the finding of hypofrontality was initially questioned largely on the basis that it might reflect the effects of neuroleptics, chronicity of illness, and brain atrophy, more recent controlled studies of neuroleptic-naive (Andreasen et al. 1992; Buchsbaum et al. 1992) and medication-free (Wolkin et al. 1992) patients still indicate that hypofrontality may be a feature of schizophrenia rather than occurring secondarily to medication treatment or chronicity. However, other studies have failed to find hypofrontality (reviewed by Andreasen et al. 1992) and have shown increased glucose metabolism in the frontal regions of first-episode drug-naive schizophrenic patients (Cleghorn et al. 1989).

It is likely that the potentially confounding factors mentioned above also contribute to differences in findings among these studies. However, even if these factors were controlled, the use of hypofrontality as a biological marker would still be limited. As with other biological measures, considerable overlap in prefrontal metabolic activity exists between groups of patients with schizophrenia and comparison subjects. Although Berman et al. (1992) demonstrated hypofrontality in each schizophrenic twin of discordant twin pairs, suggesting that this abnormality may be characteristic of schizophrenia in general, this phenomenon could be limited to a minority of patients because of the biological heterogeneity of schizophrenia, the regional heterogeneity of the frontal lobe, and variability in measurement of PET indices.

Buchsbaum et al. (1992) pointed out that the hypofrontality effect is moderately sensitive and not very specific. In addition, anatomic registration of functional brain images is methodologically complex and difficult. Finally, hypofrontality may not be specific for schizophrenia, as it has been demonstrated in PET studies of patients with bipolar affective disorder (Baxter et al. 1985; Buchsbaum et al. 1986). Functional imaging studies in patients with unipolar depression also found hyperfrontality (Buchsbaum et al. 1986) and global reductions in cortical blood flow (Sackeim et al. 1990), as well as differences from healthy control subjects (Kling et al. 1986).

Functional brain imaging studies of cerebral laterality in schizophrenic patients have yielded inconsistent results. Left-hemisphere overactivation as indicated by rCBF has been reported in medication-free patients who were challenged with verbal and spatial tasks (Gur et al. 1985). A PET study of medication-free patients under resting conditions showed higher ratios of left-hemisphere to right-hemisphere activation, a condition that was reversed when the patients were placed on medication (Gur et al. 1987). Other studies, however, reported different results or demonstrated greater left-hemisphere rCBF during cognitive tasks (reviewed by Berman and Weinberger 1990).

Despite these limitations, there are indications that functional brain imaging studies may someday be used to define specific diagnostic subgroups or to predict treatment response in patients with schizophrenia. In a SPECT study of neuroleptic-naive and nonnaive patients who were examined with the Tower of London, a standard test of prefrontal function, Andreasen et al. (1992) found diminished activation of the left mesial frontal cortex only in patients with high negative symptom scores. Wolkin et al. (1992) found a strong correlation between negative symptom scores and prefrontal hypometabolism in a study of 20 chronic medication-free patients with schizophrenia. Buchsbaum et al. (1992) reported that a low metabolic rate in the caudate nucleus and putamen predicted a favorable clinical response to haloperidol.

Another exciting application of functional brain imaging is the study of neuroreceptors in vivo. Two major PET studies in this area (Farde et al. 1986; Wong et al. 1986) have been done in neuroleptic-naive patients with schizophrenia. In the study by Wong et al., which used carbon-11–labeled N-methylspiperone, a ligand with high affinity for both D_2 and 5-HT_2 receptors, dopamine receptor density in the caudate nucleus was significantly elevated in patients compared with nonpsychiatric control subjects. The study by Farde et al., which used the selective D_2 receptor antagonist carbon-11 raclopride as a ligand, found no difference in D_2 receptor binding between patients and nonpsychiatric control subjects. This pattern of different degrees of D_2 receptor density was also found in other studies (Hietala et al. 1991; Martinot et al. 1990). These contrasting findings could be due to differences in the choice of radioligand, patient selection, and modeling methods (Seeman et al. 1990). Recently the D_4 receptor was identified and cloned (Van Tol et al. 1992) and found to be present in greater numbers in postmortem brain specimens of schizophrenic patients compared with nonpsychiatric control subjects (Seeman 1992; Seeman et al. 1993). Seeman et al. (Seeman 1992; Seeman et al. 1993) suggest that the differential affinity of ^{11}C-labeled N-methylspiperone and ^{11}C-labeled raclopride for the D_4 receptor may be responsible for the difference in findings of the two approaches. Although this controversy awaits resolution, future studies may eventually permit the identification of neuroreceptor anomalies that are specific to schizophrenia, which then can be used as possible biological markers.

MRS is emerging as a promising technique with which to evaluate in vivo brain chemistry in humans (reviewed by Pettegrew et al. 1993). Unlike PET, SPECT, and rCBF, which indirectly measure brain metabolism by quantitating blood flow or glucose uptake, MRS using phosphorous-31 can directly assess brain membrane phospholipids and high-energy phosphate metabolism. In a phosphorous-31 MRS study of the dorsolateral prefrontal cortex by Pettegrew et al. (1991), patients with schizophrenia had significantly diminished levels of phosphomonoesters, increased phosphodiester levels, increased levels of adenosine triphosphate, and decreased levels of inorganic phosphate. These findings have been generally replicated by other investigators (Fukuzako et al. 1992; O'Callaghan et al. 1991; Williamson et al. 1991) and suggest alterations in membrane phospholipid and energy metabolism that may have pathophysiological significance for schizophrenia (Pettegrew et al. 1993). Phosphorous-31 MRS studies in patients with autism and Alzheimer's disease revealed phosphomonoester and phosphodiester findings different from those in patients with schizophrenia, indicating that particular metabolic changes may be specific to schizophrenia. Clearly, future studies in this exciting area are warranted.

Functional neuroimaging studies may eventually be used to identify biological markers in patients with schizophrenia; however, the methodology (particularly in the case of PET) will need to become less invasive and expensive and the abnormalities will need to be more precisely defined.

CONCLUSION

In the last two decades, we have witnessed rapid growth in our knowledge of the neurobiology of schizophrenia. Recent technological advances have made possible the exploration of numerous aspects of brain function and structure and have permitted the development of biological measures that could potentially serve as markers of schizophrenia. However, despite dramatic progress in these research areas, biological markers with sufficient specificity, sensitivity, and replicability to be used in clinical evaluation have not yet been identified. Nevertheless, there are several promising candidates.

We suggest a strategy that may be useful in future investigations. Because no single measure is capable of serving as a biological marker of schizophrenia, different combinations of measures could be examined. At present, diagnostic laboratory and imaging procedures in psychiatry are used primarily to rule out psychiatric conditions that are secondary to neuromedical illnesses. One could conceive of a battery of studies that could be performed as part of a routine patient evaluation. These studies could complement the information gained from diagnostic interviews, clinical history, physical examination, and psychological-neuropsychological testing and could provide a broader and more objective informational base from which clinicians could determine diagnosis and treatment strategies.

REFERENCES

Adler LE, Pachtman E, Franks RD, et al: Neurophysiological evidence for a defect in neuronal mechanisms involved in sensory gating in schizophrenia. Biol Psychiatry 17:639–654, 1982

Altshuler LL, Conrad A, Hauser P, et al: Reduction of temporal lobe volume in bipolar disorder: a preliminary report of magnetic resonance imaging. Arch Gen Psychiatry 48:482–483, 1991

Amador XF, Sackeim HA, Mukherjee S, et al: Specificity of smooth pursuit eye movement and visual fixation abnormalities in schizophrenia: comparison to mania and normal controls. Schizophr Res 5:135–144, 1992

Andreasen NC, Nasrallah HA, Dunn V, et al: Structural abnormalities in the frontal system in schizophrenia: a magnetic resonance imaging study. Arch Gen Psychiatry 43:136–144, 1986

Andreasen NC, Ehrhardt J, Yuh W, et al: Magnetic resonance imaging in schizophrenia: an update, in Schizophrenia: Scientific Progress. Edited by Schulz SC, Tamminga CA. New York, Oxford University Press, 1989, pp 207–215

Andreasen NC, Ehrhardt JC, Swayze VW, et al: Magnetic resonance imaging of the brain in schizophrenia. Arch Gen Psychiatry 47:35–44, 1990

Andreasen NC, Rezai K, Alliger R, et al: Hypofrontality in neuroleptic-naive patients and in patients with chronic schizophrenia: assessment with xenon 133 single-photon emission computed tomography and the Tower of London. Arch Gen Psychiatry 49:943–958, 1992

Angrist B, van Kammen DP: CNS stimulants as tools in the study of schizophrenia. Trends Neurosci 7:388–390, 1984

Angrist B, Peselow E, Rubinstein M, et al: Amphetamine response and relapse risk after depot neuroleptic discontinuation. Psychopharmacology 85:277–283, 1985

Baker N, Adler LE, Franks RD, et al: Neurophysiological assessment of sensory gating in psychiatric inpatients: comparison between schizophrenia and other diagnoses. Biol Psychiatry 22:603–617, 1987

Barta PE, Pearlson GD, Powers RE, et al: Reduced volume of superior temporal gyrus in schizophrenia: relationship to auditory hallucinations. Am J Psychiatry 147:1457–1462, 1990

Bates C, Horrobin DF, Ells K: Fatty acids in plasma phospholipids and cholesterol esters from identical twins concordant and discordant for schizophrenia. Schizophr Res 6:1–7, 1992

Baumgartner A, Graf KJ, Kurten I, et al: The hypothalamic-pituitary-thyroid axis in psychiatric patients and healthy subjects: parts 1–4. Psychiatry Res 24:271–332, 1988

Baxter LR, Phelps ME, Mazziotta JC, et al: Cerebral metabolic rates for glucose in mood disorders (studies with positron emission tomography and fluorodeoxyglucose F-18). Arch Gen Psychiatry 42:441–447, 1985

Bennett ER, Yedgar S, Lerer B, et al: Phospholipase A2 activity in Epstein-Barr virus transformed lymphoblast cells from schizophrenic patients. Biol Psychiatry 29:1058–1062, 1991

Berman KF, Weinberger DR: Lateralisation of cortical function during cognitive tasks: regional cerebral blood flow studies of normal individuals and patients with schizophrenia. J Neurol Neurosurg Psychiatry 53:150–160, 1990

Berman KF, Weinberger DR: Functional localization in the brain in schizophrenia, in American Psychiatric Press Review of Psychiatry, Vol 10. Edited by Tasman A, Goldfinger SM. Washington, DC, American Psychiatric Press, 1991, pp 24–59

Berman KF, Torrey EF, Daniel DG, et al: Regional cerebral blood flow in monozygotic twins discordant and concordant for schizophrenia. Arch Gen Psychiatry 49:927–934, 1992

Besson JAO, Corrigan FM, Cherryman GR, et al: Nuclear magnetic resonance brain imaging in chronic schizophrenia. Br J Psychiatry 150:161–163, 1987

Blackwood DHR, Walley LJ, Christie JE, et al: Changes in auditory P3 event-related potential in schizophrenia and depression. Br J Psychiatry 150:154–160, 1987

Bleich A, Brown SL, Kahn R, et al: The role of serotonin in schizophrenia. Schizophr Bull 14:297–315, 1988

Bogerts B, Ashtari M, Degreef G, et al: Reduced temporal limbic structure volumes on magnetic resonance images in first episode schizophrenia. Psychiatry Res 35:1–13, 1990

Bogerts B, Falkai P, Degreef G, et al: Neuropathological and brain imaging studies in positive and negative schizophrenia, in Negative Versus Positive Schizophrenia. Edited by Maneros A, Andreasen NC, Tsuang MT. Berlin, Springer, 1991, pp 292–316

Bogerts B, Lieberman JA, Ashtari M, et al: Hippocampal-amygdala volumes and psychopathology in chronic schizophrenia. Biol Psychiatry 33:236–246, 1993

Bondy B, Ackenheil M: ^{3}H-spiroperidol binding sites in lymphocytes as possible vulnerability marker in schizophrenia. J Psychiatr Res 21:521–529, 1987

Bondy B, Ackenheil M, Birzle W, et al: Catecholamines and their receptors in blood: evidence for alterations in schizophrenia. Biol Psychiatry 19:1377–1393, 1984

Bowers MB Jr: CSF monoamine metabolites in psychotic syndromes: what might they signify? Biol Psychiatry 13:375–383, 1978

Brambilla F: Neuroendocrine function in schizophrenia. Acta Psychiatr Belg 80:421–435, 1980

Brambilla F, Rovere C, Guastalla A, et al: Effects of clomiphene citrate administration on the hypothalamo-pituitary-gonadal axis of male chronic schizophrenics. Acta Psychiatr Scand 56:399–406, 1977

Breier A, Buchanan RW, Elkashef A, et al: Brain morphology and schizophrenia: a magnetic resonance imaging study of limbic, prefrontal cortex, and caudate structures. Arch Gen Psychiatry 49:921–926, 1992

Brown G, Cleghorn J, Kaplan R, et al: Longitudinal growth hormone studies in schizophrenia. Psychiatry Res 24:123–136, 1988

Buchanan RW, Breier A, Kirkpatrick B, et al: Structural abnormalities in deficit and nondeficit schizophrenia. Am J Psychiatry 150:59–65, 1993

Buchsbaum MS, Wu J, DeLisi LE, et al: Frontal cortex and basal ganglia metabolic rates assessed by positron emission tomography with F-18-2-deoxyglucose in affective illness. J Affect Disord 10:137–152, 1986

Buchsbaum MS, Haier RJ, Potkin SG, et al: Frontostriatal disorder of cerebral metabolism in never-medicated schizophrenics. Arch Gen Psychiatry 49:935–942, 1992

Cleghorn JM, Garnett ES, Nahmias C, et al: Increased frontal and reduced parietal glucose metabolism in acute untreated schizophrenia. Psychiatry Res 28:119–133, 1989

Clementz BA, Sweeney JA: Is eye movement dysfunction a biological marker for schizophrenia: a methodologic review. Psychol Bull 108:77–92, 1990

Cohen LS, Winchel RM, Stanley M: Biological markers of suicide risk and adolescent suicide. Clin Neuropharmacol 11:423–425, 1988

Cohen RM, Gross M, Nordahl TE, et al: Dysfunction in a prefrontal substrate of sustained attention in schizophrenia. Life Sci 40:2031–2039, 1987

Coppen A, Abou-Saleh P, Metcalfe M, et al: Dexamethasone suppression test in depression and other psychiatric illness. Br J Psychiatry 142:498–504, 1983

Crow TJ: Positive and negative symptoms and the role of dopamine. Br J Psychiatry 137:383–386, 1980

Dalgalarrondo P, Schroder HC, Gattaz WF: Serum concentrations of interleukin-2, interferon-alpha, and interferon-gamma in schizophrenia: failure to detect abnormalities (abstract). Schizophr Res 6:140, 1992

Das I, Essali MA, de Belleroche J, et al: Inositol phospholipid turnover in platelets of schizophrenic patients. Prostaglandins Leukot Essent Fatty Acids 46:39–46, 1992

Davis KL, Kahn RS, Ko G, et al: Dopamine in schizophrenia: a review and reconceptualization. Am J Psychiatry 148:1474–1486, 1991

Deakin JFW, Slater P, Simpson MDC, et al: Frontal cortical and left temporal glutamatergic dysfunction in schizophrenia. J Neurochem 52:1781–1786, 1989

Degreef G, Lantos G, Bogerts B, et al: Abnormalities of the septum pellucidum on MR scans in first-episode schizophrenia. AJNR 13:835–840, 1992a

Degreef G, Bogerts B, Falkai P, et al: Increased prevalence of the cavum septum pellucidum in magnetic resonance scans and post-mortem brains of schizophrenic patients. Psychiatry Res: Neuroimaging 45:1–13, 1992b

Degreef G, Ashtari M, Bogerts B, et al: Volumes of ventricular system subdivisions measured from magnetic resonance images in first-episode schizophrenic patients. Arch Gen Psychiatry 49:531–537, 1992c

DeLisi LE: Neuroimmunology: clinical studies of schizophrenia and other psychiatric disorders, in Handbook of Schizophrenia, Vol 1: The Neurology of Schizophrenia. Edited by Nasrallah HA, Weinberger DR. Amsterdam, Elsevier, 1986, pp 377–396

DeLisi LE, Schwartz CC, Targum SD, et al: Ventricular brain enlargement and outcome of acute schizophreniform disorder. Psychiatry Res 9:169–171, 1983

DeLisi LE, Hoff AL, Schwartz JE, et al: Brain morphology in first-episode schizophrenic-like psychotic patients: a quantitative magnetic resonance imaging study. Biol Psychiatry 29:159–175, 1991

Donchin E: Event-related potentials: a tool in the study of human information processing, in Evoked Brain Potentials and Behavior. Edited by Begleiter H. New York, Plenum, 1979, pp 13–88

Essali MA, Das I, Belleroche J, et al: The platelet phosphoinositide system in schizophrenia: the effects of neuroleptic treatment. Biol Psychiatry 28:475–487, 1990

Farde L, Hall H, Ehrin E, et al: Quantitative analysis of d2 dopamine receptor binding in the living human brain by PET. Science 231:258–261, 1986

Faux SF, Torello MW, McCarley RW, et al: P300 in schizophrenia: confirmation and statistical validation of temporal region deficit in P300 topography. Biol Psychiatry 23:776–790, 1988

Ferrier IN, Johnstone EC, Crown TJ, et al: Anterior pituitary hormone secretion in chronic schizophrenics. Arch Gen Psychiatry 40:755–761, 1983

Franks RD, Adler LE, Waldo MC, et al: Neurophysiological studies of sensory gating in mania: comparison with schizophrenia. Biol Psychiatry 18:989–1005, 1983

Freedman R, Adler LE, Waldo MC, et al: Neurophysiological evidence for a defect in inhibitory pathways in schizophrenia: comparison of medicated and drug-free patients. Biol Psychiatry 18:537–551, 1983

Fukuzako H, Takeuchi K, Fujimoto T, et al: P31 magnetic resonance spectroscopy of schizophrenic patients with neuroleptic resistant positive and negative symptoms. Biol Psychiatry 31 (suppl):204A–205A, 1992

Ganguli R, Rabin BS: Increased serum interleukin-2 receptor concentration in schizophrenic and brain-damaged subjects (letter). Arch Gen Psychiatry 46:292, 1989

Garver DL: Methodological issues facing the interpretation of high-risk studies: biological heterogeneity. Schizophr Bull 13:525–529, 1987

Garver DL: Neuroendocrine findings in the schizophrenias. Endocrinol Metab Clin North Am 17:103–109, 1988

Garver DL, Bissette G, Yao JK, et al: Relation of CSF neurotensin concentrations to symptoms and response of psychotic patients. Am J Psychiatry 148:484–488, 1991

Gattaz WF, Hubner C, Nevalainen T, et al: Increased serum phospholipase A2 activity in schizophrenia: a replication study. Biol Psychiatry 28:495–501, 1990

Gur RE, Gur RC, Skolnik BE, et al: Brain function in psychiatric disorders, III: regional cerebral blood flow in unmedicated schizophrenics. Arch Gen Psychiatry 42:329–334, 1985

Gur RE, Resnick SM, Gur RC, et al: Regional brain function in schizophrenia, II: repeated evaluation with positive emission tomography. Arch Gen Psychiatry 44:126–129, 1987

Hietala J, Syvälahti E, Vuorio K, et al: Striatal dopamine D2 receptor density in neuroleptic-naive schizophrenics studied with positron emission tomography, in Biological Psychiatry, Vol 2. Edited by Racagni G, Brunello N, Fukuda T. Amsterdam, Excerpta Medica, 1991, pp 386–387

Hirschowitz J, Hitzemann R, Burr G, et al: A new approach to dose reduction in chronic schizophrenia. Neuropsychopharmacology 5:103–113, 1991

Holzman PS: Eye movement dysfunctions and psychosis. Int Rev Neurobiol 27:179–205, 1985

Holzman PS: Eye movement dysfunction in schizophrenia, in Handbook of Schizophrenia: Neuropsychology, Psychophysiology and Information Processing. Edited by Steinhauser SR, Grugelier JH, Zubin J. Amsterdam, Elsevier, 1991, pp 129–145

Holzman PS, Proctor LR, Levy DL, et al: Eye-tracking dysfunctions in schizophrenic patients and their relatives. Arch Gen Psychiatry 31:143–151, 1974

Holzman PS, Kringlen E, Levy DL, et al: Deviant eye tracking in twins discordant for psychosis: a replication. Arch Gen Psychiatry 37:627–631, 1980

Holzman PS, Solomon CM, Levin S, et al: Pursuit eye movement dysfunctions in schizophrenia: family evidence for specificity. Arch Gen Psychiatry 41:136–139, 1984

Horrobin DF, Manku MS, Morse-Fisher N, et al: Essential fatty acids in plasma phospholipids in schizophrenics. Biol Psychiatry 25:562–568, 1989

Hsiao JK, Colison J, Bartko JJ, et al: Monoamine neurotransmitter interactions in drug-free and neuroleptic-treated schizophrenics. Arch Gen Psychiatry 50:606–614, 1993

Iacono WG: Eye movement abnormalities in schizophrenic and affective disorders, in Neuropsychology of Eye Movements. Edited by Johnston CW, Pirozzolo FJ. Hillsdale, NJ, Erlbaum, 1988, pp 115–145

Iacono WG, Peloquin WJ, Lumry AE: Eye tracking in patients with unipolar and bipolar affective disorders in remission. J Abnorm Psychol 91:35–44, 1982

Ingvar DH, Franzen G: Abnormalities of cerebral blood flow distribution in patients with chronic schizophrenia. Acta Psychiatr Scand 50:425–462, 1974a

Ingvar DH, Franzen G: Distribution of cerebral activity in chronic schizophrenia. Lancet 2:1484–1486, 1974b

Iqbal N, Asnis GM, Wetzler S, et al: The role of serotonin in schizophrenia: new findings. Schizophr Res 5:181–182, 1991

Janowsky DS, El-Yousef MK, Davis JM, et al: Provocation of schizophrenic symptoms by intravenous administration of methylphenidate. Arch Gen Psychiatry 28:185–191, 1973

Janowsky DS, Leichner P, Parker D, et al: The effect of methylphenidate on serum growth hormone. Arch Gen Psychiatry 35:1384–1389, 1978

Javitt DC: Neurophysiological approaches to analyzing brain dysfunction in schizophrenia. Psychiatric Annals 23:144–150, 1993

Javitt DC, Zukin SR: Recent advances in the phencyclidine model of schizophrenia. Am J Psychiatry 148:1301–1308, 1991

Johnstone EC, Crow TJ, Firth CD, et al: Cerebral ventricular size and cognitive impairment in schizophrenia. Lancet 2:924–926, 1976

Johnstone EC, Owens DG, Crow TJ, et al: Temporal lobe structure as determined by nuclear magnetic resonance in schizophrenia and bipolar affective disorder. J Neurol Neurosurg Psychiatry 52:736–741, 1989

Kahn RS, Davidson M: On the value of measuring dopamine, norepinephrine and their metabolites in schizophrenia. Neuropsychopharmacology 8:93–95, 1993

Kahn RS, Siever LJ, Gabriel S, et al: Serotonin function in schizophrenia: effects of metachlorophenylpiperazine in schizophrenic patients and healthy subjects. Psychiatry Res 43:1–12, 1992

Kahn RS, Davidson M, Knott P, et al: Effect of neuroleptic medication in cerebrospinal fluid monoamine metabolite concentrations in schizophrenia: serotonin-dopamine interactions as a target for treatment. Arch Gen Psychiatry 50:599–605, 1993

Kaiya H, Nishida A, Imai A, et al: Accumulation of diacylglycerol in platelet phosphoinositide turnover in schizophrenia: a biological marker of good prognosis? Biol Psychiatry 26:669–676, 1989

Kaiya H, Horrobin DF, Marku MS, et al: Essential and other fatty acids in plasma in schizophrenics and normal individuals from Japan. Biol Psychiatry 30:357–363, 1991

Kaplan MJ, Lazoff M, Kelly K, et al: Enlargement of cerebral third ventricle in psychotic patients with delayed response to neuroleptics. Biol Psychiatry 27:205–214, 1990

Kelsoe JR Jr, Cadet JL, Pickar D, et al: Quantitative neuroanatomy in schizophrenia. Arch Gen Psychiatry 45:533–541, 1988

Kerwin RW, Patel S, Meldrum BS, et al: Asymmetrical loss of a glutamate receptor subtype in schizophrenia. Lancet 1:583–584, 1988

Kerwin RW, Patel S, Meldrum BS: Quantitative autoradiographic analysis of glutamate binding sites in the hippocampal formation in normal and schizophrenic brain post mortem. Neuroscience 39:25–32, 1990

Keshavan M, Toone BK, Marshall W, et al: Neuroendocrine dysfunction in schizophrenia: a familial perspective. Psychiatry Res 23:345–348, 1988

Kilidireas K, Sadiq SA, Strauss DH, et al: Antibodies to the human P1 mitochondrial heat shock protein in patients with schizophrenia. Lancet 340:569–572, 1992

Kiriike N, Izumiya S, Nishiwaki Y, et al: TRH test and DST in schizoaffective mania, mania and schizophrenia. Biol Psychiatry 24:415–422, 1988

Kling AS, Metter EJ, Riege WH, et al: Comparison of PET measurement of local brain glucose metabolism and CAT measurement of brain atrophy in chronic schizophrenia and depression. Am J Psychiatry 143:175–180, 1986

Knight JG: Possible autoimmune mechanisms in schizophrenia. Integrative Psychiatry 3:134–143, 1985

Koreen AR, Lieberman J, Alvir J, et al: Plasma homovanillic acid in first-episode schizophrenia: psychopathology and treatment response. Arch Gen Psychiatry (in press)

Krystal JH, Seibyl JP, Price LP, et al: M-CPP effects in schizophrenia patients before and after typical and atypical neuroleptic treatment (abstract). Schizophr Res 4:350, 1991

Krystal JH, Karper L, Seibyl JP: Effects of the NMDA antagonist ketamine in humans. Paper presented at the annual meeting of the American Psychiatric Association, Washington, DC, May 1992

Krystal JH, Karper LP, Seibyl JP, et al: Dose-related effects of the NMDA antagonist ketamine in healthy humans. Paper presented at the 4th International Congress on Schizophrenia Research, Colorado Springs, CO, April 1993

Lahti AC, Gao XM, Cascella NG, et al: Can NMDA antagonists help us understand the psychosis mechanism in schizophrenia? Paper presented at the 4th International Congress on Schizophrenia Research, Colorado Springs, CO, April 1993

Levy DL, Dorus E, Shaughnessy R, et al: Pharmacologic evidence for specificity of pursuit dysfunction to schizophrenia. Arch Gen Psychiatry 42:335–341, 1985

Lieberman JA, Koreen A: Neurochemistry and neuroendocrinology of schizophrenia: a selective review. Schizophr Bull 19:371–429, 1993

Lieberman JA, Kane JM, Sarantakos S, et al: Prediction of relapse in schizophrenia. Arch Gen Psychiatry 44:597–603, 1987a

Lieberman JA, Kane JM, Alvir J: Provocative tests with psychostimulant drugs in schizophrenia. Psychopharmacology 91:415–433, 1987b

Lieberman JA, Kane JM, Woerner M, et al: Prediction of relapse in schizophrenia. Clin Neuropharmacol 13:434–435, 1990

Lieberman JA, Alvir JMJ, Woerner M, et al: Prospective study of psychobiology in first-episode schizophrenia at Hillside Hospital. Schizophr Bull 18:351–371, 1992a

Lieberman JA, Bogerts B, Degreef G, et al: Qualitative assessment of brain morphology in acute and chronic schizophrenia. Am J Psychiatry 149:784–794, 1992b

Lieberman JA, Andreasen N, Bilder R, et al: Methodologic issues in quantitative neuroimaging. Paper presented at the annual meeting of the American College of Neuropsychopharmacology, San Juan, Puerto Rico, December 14–18, 1992c

Lieberman JA, Jody D, Alvir JMJ, et al: Brain morphology, dopamine and eye tracking abnormalities in first episode schizophrenia: prevalence and clinical correlates. Arch Gen Psychiatry 50:357–368, 1993a

Lieberman JA, Jody D, Geisler S, et al: Time course and biological correlates of treatment response in first episode schizophrenia. Arch Gen Psychiatry 50:369–376, 1993b

Lipton RB, Levin S, Holzman PS: Horizontal and vertical pursuit eye movements, the oculocephalic reflex, and the functional psychoses. Psychiatry Res 3:193–203, 1980

Luchins DJ, Lewine R, Meltzer H: Lateral ventricular size, psychopathology and medication response in the psychoses. Biol Psychiatry 19:29–44, 1984

Maas JW, Contreras SA, Miller AL, et al: Studies of catecholamine metabolism in schizophrenia/psychosis—I. Neuropsychopharmacology 8:97–109, 1993

Martinot J-L, Peron-Magnan P, Huret J-D, et al: Striatal D2 dopamine receptors assessed with positron emission tomography and [^{76}Br] bromospiperone in untreated schizophrenic patients. Am J Psychiatry 147:44–50, 1990

Matthysse S, Holzman PS, Lange K: The genetic transmission of schizophrenia: application of Mendelian latent structure analysis to eye tracking dysfunctions in schizophrenia and affective disorder. J Psychiatric Res 20:57–76, 1986

Mayerhoff D, Lieberman JA, Lemus C, et al: Growth hormone response to growth hormone–releasing hormone in schizophrenic patients. Am J Psychiatry 147:1072–1074, 1990

McCarley RW, Faux SF, Shenton ME, et al: CT abnormalities in schizophrenia: a preliminary study of their correlations with P300/P200 electro-physiological features and positive/negative symptoms. Arch Gen Psychiatry 46:698–708, 1989

McCarley RW, Faux SF, Shenton ME, et al: Event-related potentials in schizophrenia: their biological and clinical correlates and a new model of schizophrenic pathophysiology. Schizophr Res 4:209–231, 1991

Meltzer HY: Clinical studies on the mechanism of action of clozapine: the dopamine-serotonin hypothesis of schizophrenia. Psychopharmacology 99:S18–S27, 1989

Meltzer HY: The role of serotonin in the action of atypical antipsychotic drugs. Psychiatric Annals 20:571–579, 1990

Meltzer HY: The mechanism of action of novel antipsychotic drugs. Schizophr Bull 17:263–287, 1991

Moore KE: The actions of amphetamine on neurotransmitters: a brief review. Biol Psychiatry 12:451–462, 1978

Nasrallah H, Olson SC, McCalley-Whitters M, et al: Cerebral ventricular enlargement in schizophrenia. Arch Gen Psychiatry 43:157–159, 1986

Nemeroff CB, Bissette G, Widerlov E, et al: Neurotensin-like immunoreactivity in cerebrospinal fluid of patients with schizophrenia, depression, anxiety, nervosa-bulimia, and premenstrual syndrome. J Neuropsychiatry 1:16–20, 1989

Nerozzi D, Antonozzi I, Frajese G: Prolactin and growth hormone responses to growth hormone–releasing hormone in acute schizophrenia. Neuropsychology 23:15–17, 1990

Newcomer JW, Riney SJ, Vinogradov S, et al: Plasma prolactin and homovanillic acid as markers for psychopathology and abnormal movements during maintenance haloperidol treatment in male patients with schizophrenia. Psychiatry Res 41:191–202, 1992

O'Callaghan EO, Redmond O, Ennis R, et al: Initial investigation of the left temporoparietal region in schizophrenia by P31 magnetic resonance spectroscopy. Biol Psychiatry 29:1149–1152, 1991

O'Donnell BF, Shenton ME, McCarley RW, et al: Auditory P300 amplitude and left posterior superior temporal gyrus volume reduction in schizophrenia. Paper presented at the annual meeting of the Society of Biological Psychiatry, Washington, DC, May 1992

Pandey GN, Garver DC, Tamminga C, et al: Postsynaptic supersensitivity in schizophrenia. Am J Psychiatry 134:518–522, 1977

Pangerl AM, Steudk A, Jaroni H, et al: Increased platelet membrane lysophosphatidyl choline in schizophrenia. Biol Psychiatry 30:837–840, 1991

Peabody C, Warner MD, Markoff E, et al: Growth hormone response to growth hormone releasing hormone in depression and schizophrenia. Psychiatry Res 32:269–276, 1990

Perry SW, Markowitz J: Organic mental disorders, in The American Psychiatric Press Textbook of Psychiatry. Edited by Talbott JA, Hales RE, Yudofsky SC. Washington, DC, American Psychiatric Press, 1988, pp 279–311

Pettegrew JW, Keshavan MS, Panchalingam K, et al: Alterations in brain energy phosphate and membrane phospholipid metabolism in first episode drug naive schizophrenics. Arch Gen Psychiatry 48:563–568, 1991

Pettegrew JW, Keshavan MS, Minshew NJ: P31 nuclear magnetic resonance spectroscopy: neurodevelopment and schizophrenia. Schizophr Bull 19:35–53, 1993

Pfefferbaum A, Zatz L, Jernigan TL: Computer-interactive method for quantifying cerebrospinal fluid and tissue in brain CT scans: effects of aging. J Comput Assist Tomogr 10:571–578, 1986

Pfefferbaum A, Ford JM, White PM, et al: P3 in schizophrenia is affected by stimulus modality, response requirements, medication status, and negative symptoms. Arch Gen Psychiatry 46:1035–1044, 1989

Pickar D, Owen RR, Litman RE, et al: Clinical and biologic response to clozapine in patients with schizophrenia: crossover comparison with fluphenazine. Arch Gen Psychiatry 49:345–353, 1992

Preskorn SH, Hughes CW, Bupp SJ: Neurobiological etiology of schizophrenia and affective disorders, in Psychiatry, Vol 1. Edited by Michels R, Cooper AM, Guze SB, et al. Philadelphia, PA, JB Lippincott, 1992, pp 1–23

Rabin BS, Cohen S, Ganguli R, et al: Bidirectional interactions between the central nervous system and the immune system. Crit Rev Immunol 9(4):279–311, 1989

Rapaport MH, McAllister CG: Neuroimmunologic factors in schizophrenia, in Psychoimmunology Update. Edited by Gorman JM, Kertzner RM. Washington, DC, American Psychiatric Press, 1991, pp 31–54

Rapaport MH, McAllister CG, Pickar D, et al: Elevated levels of interleukin-2 receptors in schizophrenia. Arch Gen Psychiatry 46:291–292, 1989

Raz S, Raz N: Structural brain abnormalities in the major psychoses: a quantitative review of the evidence from computerized imaging. Psychol Bull 108:93–108, 1990

Rivier J, Spiess J, Thorner M: Characterization of a growth hormone releasing factor from a pancreatic islet tumor. Nature 300:1321–1328, 1982

Robinson D, Jody D, Lieberman JA: Provocative tests with methylphenidate in schizophrenia and schizophrenia spectrum disorders, in Ritalin: Theory and Patient Management. Edited by Greenhill LL, Osman BB. New York, Mary Ann Liebert, 1991, pp 309–320

Roy A, Wolkowitz OM, Doran A, et al: TRH test in schizophrenic patients and controls. Biol Psychiatry 25:523–526, 1989

Sackeim HA, Prohovnik I, Moeller JR, et al: Regional cerebral blood flow in mood disorders, I: comparison of major depressives and normal controls at rest. Arch Gen Psychiatry 47:60–70, 1990

Schreiber H, Stolz G, Kornhuber HH, et al: Prolonged latencies of the N2 and P3 of the auditory event-related potential in children at risk for schizophrenia. Eur Arch Psychiatry Neurol Science 238:185–188, 1989

Schulz SC, Koller MM, Kishore PR, et al: Ventricular enlargement in teenage patients with schizophrenia spectrum disorder. Am J Psychiatry 140:1592–1595, 1983

Seeman P: Dopamine receptor sequences: therapeutic levels of neuroleptics occupy D_2 receptors, clozapine occupies D_4. Neuropsychopharmacology 7:261–284, 1992

Seeman P, Niznik HB, Guan H-C: Elevation of D2 dopamine receptors in schizophrenia is underestimated by radioactive raclopride. Arch Gen Psychiatry 47:1170–1172, 1990

Seeman P, Guan H-C, Van Tol HHM: Dopamine D4 receptors elevated in schizophrenia. Nature 365:441–445, 1993

Shagass C, Amadeo M, Overton DA: Eye-tracking performance in psychiatric patients. Biol Psychiatry 9:245–260, 1974

Sharief MK, Hentges R, Thompson EJJ: The relationship of interleukin-2 and soluble interleukin-2 receptors to intrathecal immunoglobulin synthesis in patients with multiple sclerosis. J Neuroimmunol 32:43–51, 1991

Sharma R, Javaid JI, Pandey G, et al: Pharmacological effects of methylphenidate in plasma homovanillic acid and growth hormone. Psychiatry Res 32:9–17, 1990

Sharma R, Javaid JI, Pandey G, et al: Behavioral and biochemical effects of methylphenidate in schizophrenic and nonschizophrenic patients. Biol Psychiatry 30:459–466, 1991

Shenton ME, Faux SF, McCarley RW, et al: Correlations between abnormal auditory P300 topography and positive symptoms in schizophrenia: a preliminary report. Biol Psychiatry 25:710–716, 1989

Shenton ME, Kikinis R, Jolesz FA, et al: Abnormalities of the left temporal lobe and thought disorder in schizophrenia: a quantitative magnetic resonance imaging study. N Engl J Med 327:604–612, 1992

Siegel C, Waldo M, Miznor G, et al: Deficits in sensory gating in schizophrenic patients and their relatives. Arch Gen Psychiatry 41:607–612, 1984

Simpson MDC, Slater P, Royston MC, et al: Alterations in phencyclidine and sigma binding sites in schizophrenic brains: effects of disease process and neuroleptic medication. Schizophr Res 6:41–48, 1992

Siris SG, Frechen K, Swahan A, et al: Thyroid releasing-hormone test in schizophrenic patients with post-psychotic depression. Prog Neuropsychopharmacol Biol Psychiatry 15:369–378, 1991

Snyder SH: Amphetamine psychosis: a "model" schizophrenia mediated by catecholamines. Am J Psychiatry 130:61–67, 1973

St. Clair D, Blackwood D, Muir W: P300 abnormality in schizophrenic subtypes. J Psychiatric Res 23:49–55, 1989

Suddath RL, Casanova MF, Goldberg TE, et al: Temporal lobe pathology in schizophrenia: a quantitative magnetic resonance imaging study. Am J Psychiatry 146:464–472, 1989

Suddath RL, Christison GW, Torrey EF, et al: Anatomical abnormalities in the brains of monozygotic twins discordant for schizophrenia. N Engl J Med 322:789–794, 1990

Swahn CG: Determination of N-acetyl-L-aspartic acid in human cerebrospinal fluid by gas chromatography-mass spectrometry. J Neurochem 54:1584–1588, 1990

Swayze VW, Andreasen NC, Alliger RJ, et al: Structural brain abnormalities in bipolar affective disorder: ventricular enlargement and focal signal hyperintensities. Arch Gen Psychiatry 47:1054–1059, 1990

Szymanski S, Kane JM, Lieberman JA: A selective review of biological markers in schizophrenia. Schizophr Bull 17:99–111, 1991

Szymanski S, Lieberman J, Pollack S, et al: The dopamine-serotonin relationship in clozapine response. Psychopharmacology 112:S85–S89, 1993

van Cauter E, Linkowski P, Kerkhofs M, et al: Circadian and sleep-related endocrine rhythms in schizophrenia. Arch Gen Psychiatry 48:343–356, 1991

van Kammen DP: The biochemical basis of relapse and drug response in schizophrenia: review and hypothesis. Psychol Med 21:881–895, 1991

van Kammen DP, Kelley M: Dopamine and norepinephrine activity in schizophrenia: an integrative perspective. Schizophr Res 4:173–191, 1991

van Kammen DP, Docherty J, Bunney W: Prediction of early relapse after pimozide discontinuation by response to D-amphetamine during pimozide treatment. Biol Psychiatry 17:233–242, 1982

van Kammen DP, Peters J, van Kammen WB: Cerebrospinal fluid studies of monoamine metabolism in schizophrenia. Psychiatr Clin North Am 9:81–97, 1986

van Kammen DP, Peters JL, van Kammen WB, et al: Clonidine treatment of schizophrenia: can we predict treatment response? Psychiatry Res 27:297–311, 1989a

van Kammen DP, Peters JL, van Kammen WB, et al: CSF norepinephrine in schizophrenia is elevated prior to relapse after haloperidol withdrawal. Biol Psychiatry 26:176–188, 1989b

van Putten T, Marder SR, Mintz J: Serum prolactin as a correlate of clinical response to haloperidol. J Clin Psychopharmacol 11:357–361, 1991

Vecsei L, Widerlov E: Brain and CSF somatostatin concentrations in patients with psychiatric or neurological illness. Acta Psychiatr Scand 78:657–667, 1988

Vita A, Sacchetti E, Valvoassori G, et al: Brain morphology in schizophrenia: a 2- to 5-year CT scan follow-up study. Acta Psychiatr Scand 78:618–621, 1988

Volkow ND, Wolf AP, Van Gelder P, et al: Phenomenological correlates of metabolic activity in 18 patients with chronic schizophrenia. Am J Psychiatry 144:151–158, 1987

Weinberger DR, Bigelow LB, Kleinman JE, et al: Cerebral ventricular enlargement in chronic schizophrenia. Arch Gen Psychiatry 37:11–13, 1980

Widerlov E: A critical appraisal of CSF monoamine metabolite studies in schizophrenia. Ann N Y Acad Sci 537:309–323, 1988

Williamson P, Drost D, Stanley J, et al: Localized phosphorus 31 magnetic resonance spectroscopy in chronic schizophrenic patients and normal controls (letter). Arch Gen Psychiatry 48:578, 1991

Wodarz N, Fritze J, Kornhuber J, et al: ^{3}H-spiroperidol binding to human peripheral mononuclear cells: methodological aspects. Biol Psychiatry 31:291–303, 1992

Wolkin A, Sanfilipo M, Wolf AP, et al: Negative symptoms and hypofrontality in chronic schizophrenia. Arch Gen Psychiatry 49:959–965, 1992

Wong DF, Wagner HN Jr, Tune LE, et al: Positron emission tomography reveals elevated D2 receptors in drug-naive schizophrenics. Science 234:1558–1563, 1986

Yao JK, Yasaci P, van Kammen DP: Increased turnover of platelet phosphatidylinositol in schizophrenia. Prostaglandins Leukot Essent Fatty Acids 46:39–46, 1992

Zemlan F, Hirschowitz J, Garver D: Relation of clinical symptoms to apomorphine-stimulated growth hormone release in mood-incongruent psychotic patients. Arch Gen Psychiatry 43:1162–1167, 1986

Zipursky RB, Lim KO, Sullivan EV, et al: Widespread cerebral gray matter volume deficits in schizophrenia. Arch Gen Psychiatry 49:195–205, 1992

Chapter 7

Mood Disorders

Kalpana I. Nathan, M.D., and Alan F. Schatzberg, M.D.

Over the years, considerable research has been done in identifying neurotransmitter, neuroendocrine, and other biological measures as potential markers for mood disorders, but their general clinical application has been limited by issues of sensitivity and specificity. Still, these measures have yielded important information regarding the biology of mood disorders and can be useful in certain clinical situations.

Nurnberger (1992) distinguished among three types of biological markers—diagnostic, linkage, and pathophysiological. Diagnostic markers usually connote a specific disease process, and maximum sensitivity and specificity are critical to their usefulness. The limited sensitivity and specificity of many current markers have led to most not being used routinely in patients with mood disorders.

An optimal genetically based biological marker should be more prevalent in individuals with the disorder than in those without; should be more common in family members who are also ill; and should be a trait rather than a state-dependent marker; in other words, it should still be present after recovery from the illness. Unfortunately, research to date in this area has not yielded conclusive data regarding these types of potential markers in mood disorders.

Pathophysiological markers are primarily research tools that are useful in subtyping heterogeneous conditions and have the potential for developing into diagnostic markers. Nonsuppression on the dexamethasone suppression test (DST) is a pathophysiological marker of depression that, although neither very sensitive nor specific, has helped tremendously in understanding the biology of the disorder. Research work in the allied areas of biochemistry, physiology, and endocrinology continues to contribute to a greater knowledge of the biopsychosocial underpinnings of mood disorders.

In this chapter, we review the status of a number of diagnostic and pathophysiological markers. We attempt to provide information about how such markers may be used clinically and what they may tell us about the physiology of mood disorders. We primarily focus on unipolar and bipolar disorders in this chapter, although the broad category

---

We express our appreciation to Randall Weingarten, M.D., for his helpful comments and criticism.

---

of mood disorders includes dysthymia, adjustment disorder with depressed mood, cyclothymia, and organic mood disorder.

NEUROTRANSMITTERS
AND RECEPTORS

Dysregulation of several neurotransmitters, as well as their presynaptic and postsynaptic receptors, has been implicated in the pathogenesis of mood disorders. We have primarily focused on norepinephrine and serotonin (5-hydroxytryptamine; 5-HT), both of which have been studied extensively. Research data on acetylcholine, γ-aminobutyric acid (GABA), and enzymes such as monoamine oxidase (MAO), although thought provoking, are still inconclusive.

A variety of approaches have been applied to the study of neurotransmitters in humans: measurement of levels of neurotransmitters and metabolites in peripheral blood and cerebrospinal fluid (CSF), as well as in postmortem brain tissue; direct investigation of neurotransmitter receptors in platelets and leukocytes, cell cultures of fibroblasts, and postmortem brain tissue; and study of neuroendocrine responses to receptor agonists and antagonists.

Norepinephrine

The catecholamine hypothesis of affective disorders (Schildkraut 1965) proposed that some forms of depression are associated with a deficiency of catecholamine activity, particularly norepinephrine activity, at functionally important adrenergic receptor sites in the brain, whereas mania may be associated with a relative excess of catecholamines.

Early studies reported that urinary levels of 3-methoxy-4-hydroxyphenylglycol (MHPG), the major metabolite of central nervous system (CNS) norepinephrine, were elevated in the manic phase of bipolar and schizoaffective disorders compared with the depressed phase of these disorders. There were also reports of significantly lower 24-hour urinary MHPG levels in bipolar depressed patients compared with unipolar patients or healthy control subjects. The finding of low urinary MHPG in depressed patients with bipolar type I illness appears to be of potential diagnostic use. Some seemingly unipolar patients, however, demonstrate low MHPG values, and the sensitivity and specificity for separating bipolar I patients from those with other types of disorders or from control subjects need to be further elucidated. More recently, the use of discriminant function analysis of urinary catecholamine and metabolite data (so-called D-type scores) appears to provide greater sensitivity and specificity for separating bipolar I from unipolar depressed patients than do MHPG levels alone (Schatzberg et al. 1989). There are limitations to collecting 24-hour urine samples (e.g., missed collections), and the MHPG is highly affected by a variety of medications, requiring patients to be drug free for extensive periods before study. Assays for plasma MHPG are improving and may open an avenue for overcoming the sampling problem.

Patients with unipolar depression are heterogeneous, with some showing high and low MHPG levels. Biochemical subtypes of depression have been proposed based on MHPG levels (Schatzberg et al. 1982; Schildkraut et al. 1981). Patients with the subtype associated with low MHPG levels may have low norepinephrine output or release and are responsive to noradrenergically active antidepressants, such as imipramine. Recent data indicate they also respond to the serotonergic antidepressant fluoxetine. Patients with high MHPG levels may have high norepinephrine output, which may be secondary to cholinergic hyperactivity (Schildkraut et al. 1984). Such patients respond less well to both tricyclic antidepressants and fluoxetine than do patients with low MHPG levels. Mooney et al. (1988) reported that depressed patients with high catecholamine output responded to treatment with alprazolam, a benzodiazepine, which may decrease catecholamine output and correct the desensitization of the adenylate cyclase system as measured in blood components. Here, too, D-type scores may add greater precision vis-à-vis prediction of drug response than do MHPG levels alone (Mooney et al. 1991). The changes in MHPG levels in response to treatment indicate that such levels are state markers.

Adrenergic Receptors

The platelet offers an opportunity to peripherally study adrenergic receptors in the periphery that are akin to those found in the brain. Several studies have demonstrated supersensitivity of platelet α_2-adrenoceptors (presynaptic inhibitory autoreceptors) in depressed patients (Garcia-Sevilla 1989). In addition, treatment with antidepressants has been associated with decreases in the density and sensitivity of these receptors. However, some studies have reported that there is decreased responsivity of α_2 receptors in depression, especially when receptor activation was measured by prostaglandin E_1–stimulated cyclic adenosine monophosphate (cAMP) production. This discrepancy, coupled with the technical difficulties in performing this assay (e.g., preparation of platelets), makes these measures relatively less likely to be used as markers.

An indirect method for studying α_2 receptors is to challenge the patient with the α_2 receptor agonist clonidine. Administration of clonidine induces growth hormone (GH) secretion, primarily via postsynaptic α receptors. Several abnormalities in GH release in depressed patients have been reported, including blunted GH response to growth hormone–releasing hormone, clonidine, desipramine, and thyrotropin-releasing hormone and reduced nocturnal and increased diurnal GH secretion. However, the blunted GH response to clonidine in unipolar depressed patients (Matussek et al. 1982; Siever and Uhde 1984) supports the concept of decreased responsiveness of postsynaptic α_2-adrenergic receptors in depressed patients. Siever et al. (1992) reported that the GH response to clonidine was significantly blunted in both acutely ill and remitted patients compared with control subjects, suggesting that blunted GH response to clonidine may be a trait marker in some forms of depression. Although abnormal GH secretion has been reported in some studies, Rubin et al. (1990) reported that GH secretion in depressed patients was relatively normal, with more severely depressed patients having moderately lower nocturnal GH values.

Alpha-2 receptor studies have been unable to define a consistent pattern of adrenoceptor abnormalities, possibly due to either methodological problems or heterogeneity of depression, despite evidence of underlying noradrenergic dysfunction in mood disorders. These studies are worthy of further investigation, but in their present forms they are not simple to administer in routine clinical practice.

Serotonin

The role of indolamines in the pathogenesis of affective illness was originally hypothesized over two decades ago (Coppen et al. 1972), and there has been a steadily increasing research effort in this area, in part because of the advent of selective serotonergic antidepressants. The permissive hypothesis (Prange et al. 1974) of 5-HT function postulated that a deficit in central serotonergic transmission permits the development of an affective illness, but this deficit is not sufficient to cause it. According to this theory, both the manic and depressive phases are characterized by low central 5-HT function but differ in high versus low norepinephrine activity. In this theory, low 5-HT is thought to be a trait function.

The assessment of serotonergic function in mood disorders involves a series of parameters. There is a reduction in CSF concentrations of 5-hydroxyindoleacetic acid (5-HIAA)—the principle metabolite of 5-HT—in many depressed patients. Asberg et al. (1976) reported that low concentrations of CSF 5-HIAA may be a marker for suicidal behavior and for suicide risk in depressed patients. Several subsequent studies have replicated these observations and have suggested that decreased CSF 5-HIAA may predict suicide, aggression, or poor impulse control (Linnoila and Virkkunen 1992). To date, there have been, at best, limited follow-up data on whether decreased CSF 5-HIAA is trait or state dependent. Again, this test is cumbersome to the patient, and clinical application is thus limited.

Of the several types of 5-HT receptors, investigators have particularly explored 5-HT$_1$ and 5-HT$_2$ receptors in depression. 5-HT$_{1a}$ receptors have been implicated in the physiology of anxiety and depression, and selective 5-HT$_{1a}$ agonists and partial agonists such as buspirone have been shown to have anxiolytic and antidepressant effects (Gonzalez-Heydrich and Peroutka 1990).

Mann et al. (1986) reported an increased number of postsynaptic 5-HT$_2$ receptors in the brains of depressed patients. Thus, there may be a functional deficiency of presynaptic serotonergic neurotransmitter activity in depression that leads to an increased number or up-regulation of postsynaptic 5-HT$_2$ serotonergic receptors (Risch and Nemeroff 1992). Beigon et al. (1990) suggest that 5-HT$_2$ receptor binding on platelets may be viewed as a state-dependent marker in major depression. They measured receptor binding at baseline and after 1 and 3 weeks of treatment with maprotiline in 15 depressed patients. There was a significant decrease in 5-HT$_2$ receptor binding with clinical improvement, whereas there was an increase or no change in receptor binding in the nonresponders. 5-HT$_2$ receptor binding is hence a state phenomenon. This test appears to be promising as a peripheral marker for depression.

5-HT agonists are effective stimulants of prolactin release, and in healthy subjects administration of L-tryptophan, a 5-HT precursor, produces a robust increase in prolactin level. Prolactin response to L-tryptophan and to the 5-HT releasing agent fenfluramine is blunted in depression (Cowen and Charig 1987; Siever et al. 1984). This response may be due to abnormal 5-HT receptors, particularly 5-HT$_{1c}$ and 5-HT$_2$, or it may be mediated by an effect of high cortisol concentrations on 5-HT$_1$ receptor function (Deakin et al. 1990). The specificity and sensitivity of blunted prolactin response in depression need to be further studied before prolactin response can be of clinical use.

[^{3}H]Imipramine binds to the 5-HT transporter on the presynaptic nerve terminal and in the platelet. Several studies have reported that there is a reduction in the number of platelet [^{3}H]imipramine-binding sites in depressed patients (Briley et al. 1980; Langer and Raisman 1983; Lewis and McChesney 1985). Also, Perry et al. (1983) reported that there is decreased density of [^{3}H]imipramine-binding sites in the hippocampus and occipital cortex of depressed patients. Freeman et al. (1993) measured pre- and posttreatment platelet [^{3}H]imipramine-binding in 35 depressed patients. The slow treatment responders demonstrated an increase in the posttreatment density of [^{3}H]imipramine-binding sites, suggesting that this may be a state-dependent marker. However, the report of the World Health Organization multicenter collaborative study (1990) concluded that [^{3}H]imipramine binding is not a valid biological marker of endogenous depression; this study investigated data from 154 depressed patients and 130 control subjects and found no significant difference in [^{3}H]imipramine-binding capacity between depressed patients and control subjects. Nemeroff et al. (1991) reported that there are reduced binding sites for [³H]paroxetine, a more selective ligand for the platelet 5-HT transporter than [³H]imipramine, in depressed patients. This may ultimately prove to be a more useful tool.

NEUROENDOCRINOLOGY

Hypothalamic-Pituitary-Adrenal Axis

There has been considerable research on the relationship between hypothalamic-pituitary-adrenal (HPA) axis activity and depression. About 40%–50% of patients with endogenous depression demonstrate resistance to HPA suppression when challenged with dexamethasone, the so-called DST (Brown et al. 1979; Carroll and Davies 1970). Early studies were often performed in more severely and more endogenously depressed patients. Studies in outpatients with major depression have yielded much lower rates of nonsuppression, often as low as 30%. In a comprehensive review of the literature, Arana et al. (1985) reported that the sensitivity of the DST in major depression is limited (44% in over 5,000 cases), but is higher in psychotic affective disorders and mixed manic-depressive states (67%–78%). The specificity of the DST in manic-depressive patients versus control subjects is high (over 90%), but the specificity is less evident when depressed patients are compared with patients with dysthymic disorder (77%) and other severe psychiatric disorders such as mania and acute psychoses (52%–65%). Thus, the DST cannot be easily applied as a routine screen for depression.

The data suggest that the DST can be used to help address focused clinical diagnostic questions. For example, in patients who present with psychotic thinking, the DST may help separate those with schizophrenia from those with psychosis related to affective illness, because nonsuppression rates are lower in the schizophrenic patients, as are postdexamethasone cortisol levels.

Another focused approach has been to use the DST to predict who will respond to somatic therapy. Here, too, the DST is limited in its ability to help predict treatment response, with 76%–82% of the patients with major depression and a positive DST responding favorably to antidepressants, in contrast to 64%–74% of depressed patients with a negative DST. Still, two useful observations have been made about the DST with respect to treatment. First, DST nonsuppressors generally do not respond to placebo. Second, failure to respond normally to the DST after treatment is associated with increased risk for relapse. Ribiero et al. (1993), in an extensive review of the literature on the DST as a predictor of course and outcome in major depression, concluded that posttreatment nonsuppression of cortisol on the DST is strongly associated with poor outcome, although baseline DST results may be devoid of prognostic value.

Exploring the pathophysiological significance of the DST has led to possible ways of enhancing the test's sensitivity and specificity. Koyama and Meltzer (1986) found the 5-hydroxytryptophan (5-HTP)–induced cortisol response to be enhanced in unmedicated depressed patients and decreased after treatment with antidepressants. They postulated that serotonin may play an important role in the stimulation of basal plasma cortisol secretion.

Maes et al. (1991) studied the effect of L-5-HTP–stimulated DST in 62 depressed patients, 33 of whom met criteria for melancholic depression. In these melancholic patients, L-5-HTP had a significant enhancing effect on the post-dexamethasone cortisol values; six patients converted from the suppressor to the nonsuppressor state (>5 μg/dl), and 11 nonsuppressors exhibited significantly increased cortisol responses to L-5-HTP. The L-5-HTP–stimulated DST results increased the sensitivity for melancholia from 46% to 68%, and the specificity remained unchanged (96%).

Although the DST may be limited as a broad-based biological marker for depression, it has led to detailed study of the HPA axis, providing important pathophysiological and diagnostic information.

Corticotropin-releasing hormone. Despite early thinking that DST nonsuppression may be due to faulty feedback on central corticotropin-releasing hormone (CRH) release, considerable evidence has emerged that hypercortisolemia in depression is caused by excessive hypothalamic CRH drive (Gold 1988). Nemeroff and Krishnan (1992) investigated CSF CRH in several studies and found that patients with major depression had elevated CRH levels; this finding was supported by postmortem studies in depressed patients who committed suicide, in which a decrease in the number of frontal CRH receptors was found, consistent with the hypothesis that chronic hypersecretion of the peptide causes a reduction in CRH receptor density. In depressed patients, there is an attenuated adrenocorticotropic hormone (ACTH) response to CRH administration, which has been thought to reflect increased central CRH activity but which may also be due to feedback inhibition of ACTH by cortisol.

Holsboer-Trachsler et al. (1991) administered human CRH to 14 patients with major depression and 13 age-matched control subjects after premedication with an overnight dose of 1.5 mg of dexamethasone. Cortisol as well as ACTH responses were significantly higher in depressed patients than in control subjects. After treatment with trimipramine for 6 weeks and significant improvement in depression, the challenge test with dexamethasone and human CRH was repeated. The cortisol response appeared to have normalized, whereas ACTH release remained exaggerated.

These studies are quite compelling. Still, CRH is not routinely measured clinically for several reasons. First, sensitivity and specificity data are not available. A reasonable number of depressed patients have CSF CRH values in the range seen for healthy control subjects, and we know little regarding CSF CRH values in patients with other psychiatric disorders. Second, spinal taps are difficult to perform in routine psychiatric practice. CRH measures in blood have been extremely difficult to perform for technical reasons, although improved methods are being worked on. Moreover, the significance of CRH levels in blood is not clear, because the sources of CRH in the periphery may be other than brain.

Adrenocorticotropic hormone. Hypercortisolemia may also result from hyperresponsiveness of the adrenal gland to ACTH (Amsterdam et al. 1987; Gold et al. 1986). Several studies have reported that depressed patients demonstrate an increased cortisol response to supraphysiological doses of ACTH (250 μg), which may not normalize with improvement in mood. However, Krishnan et al. (1990) found no difference in plasma cortisol elevation after administration of a low dose of ACTH (50 μg) in depressed patients compared with control subjects. They suggested that cortisol responses to high doses of ACTH may reflect adrenocortical hypertrophy rather than increased sensitivity of ACTH receptors. Indeed, adrenal enlargement has been reported in depressed patients (Nemeroff et al. 1992). Still, ACTH sensitivity may prove useful clinically. Limitations are its lack of ease of administration in routine psychiatric practice and lack of sensitivity and specificity data.

The occurrence of hypercortisolemia in depression is not unique to the illness and is observed in several medical conditions, such as Cushing's disease. Patients with Cushing's disease often have symptoms of depression, mania, and impaired cognitive function. Administration of corticosteroids has been known to precipitate psychiatric syndromes. However, in depressed patients with hypercortisolemia, there are no significant clinical cushingoid features. It has been postulated that this may be because of 1) lesser degrees of HPA activation in most depressed patients, 2) exposure to increased corticosteroids over a shorter period of time, and 3) defects in peripheral corticosteroid receptor characteristics that lead to relative corticosteroid resistance (Holsboer et al. 1986). Kling et al. (1991) reported that CSF CRH and ACTH concentrations were lower in patients with Cushing's disease, whereas plasma CRH and ACTH concentrations were higher, compared with control subjects and patients with major depression. They suggested that the ratio of plasma ACTH to CSF ACTH may be useful in distinguishing between these two conditions.

HPA Axis Activity and Monoamines

A number of studies have reported positive correlations between measures of cortisol and catecholamines. For example, MHPG has been reported to correlate positively and significantly with cortisol in various tissues. These correlations may reflect simultaneous activation of these two systems or the possible activation of one by the other.

The administration of dexamethasone can significantly increase plasma free dopamine and homovanillic acid (HVA) in healthy control subjects (Rothchild et al. 1984; Wolkowitz et al. 1985). Schatzberg et al. (1985) postulated that glucocorticoid enhancement of dopaminergic activity may explain the development of psychosis and delusion in depression. Compared with nonpsychotic depressed patients, psychotically depressed patients have been reported to have lower levels of serum dopamine–β-hydroxylase activity and higher CSF HVA levels (Schatzberg et al. 1985; Sweeney et al. 1978). This area is worthy of further research.

Hypothalamic-Pituitary-Thyroid Axis

Hypothyroidism has been long associated with depression, although depressed patients as a group are mostly euthyroid. There have also been reports of heightened thyroid activity, but these may reflect temporary increases during initial days of psychiatric hospitalization. The thyrotropin-releasing hormone (TRH) test, which measures the release of pituitary thyroid-stimulating hormone (TSH) after TRH administration, has been studied extensively in mood disorders and appears to have more potential as a biological marker than the measurements of the thyroid hormones alone. However, there are no conclusive data at this time to support the clinical use of these tests as biological markers for mood disorders.

A blunted TSH response to TRH is seen in some 25%–30% of depressed patients (Loosen and Prange 1982). As with the CRH stimulation test, the blunted TSH response may be due to an increase in endogenous central peptide (i.e., TRH) in depressed patients. TSH blunting, however, is not specific for depression. It has also been reported in patients with mania, anorexia nervosa, borderline personality disorder, and alcoholism. It is unclear whether the blunted TSH is a state marker or a trait marker. Several investigations have produced data to support both of these arguments. The use of the TRH test to assess clinical response to antidepressants has been investigated, but here, too, there are no conclusive data.

There appears to be no clear association between measures of HPA axis activity and hypothalamic-pituitary-thyroid (HPT) axis activity. Rubin et al. (1987) measured nocturnal serum TSH concentration, TSH response to TRH administration, and serum triiodothyronine and thyroxine concentrations in depressed patients, and examined the relationships between the HPT measures and the pre-dexamethasone and post-dexamethasone serum and urine cortisol measures. They reported significant reductions in TSH and triiodothyronine concentrations, but measures of HPT axis activity were unrelated to measures of HPA axis activity.

Endocrine and Sleep Activity

Sleep studies in mood disorders are discussed in detail in Chapter 26. Steiger et al. (1993) performed a series of studies to investigate changes in sleep and endocrine activity in depressed patients and control subjects. Normally, the first half of the night is characterized by greater slow-wave sleep activity, GH surges, and low concentrations of cortisol, whereas the second half of the night is characterized by more rapid eye movement (REM) sleep with low concentrations of GH and sharp rises in cortisol levels. Steiger et al. found that patients with depression had enhanced cortisol secretion and blunted release of GH early in the night, as well as decreased slow-wave sleep and disinhibition of REM sleep. There were no differences in nocturnal release of prolactin, but testosterone release was blunted in depressed patients. They suggested that the sleep changes and blunted GH release may be potential trait markers, because these changes persisted in remitted drug-free patients, as opposed to cortisol and testosterone levels, which normalized after recovery.

SECOND-MESSENGER SYSTEMS

Guanine Nucleotide–Binding Proteins

In the past few years, considerable attention has been paid to so-called second-messenger systems in the affective disorders. These studies suggest a variety of possible abnormalities in mood disorders and point to possible drug mechanisms of action.

Avissar and Schreiber (1992) proposed that hyperactivity of guanine nucleotide–binding proteins, either as a trait marker or as a state function, leads to an unstable dynamic system in bipolar disorder. Lithium treatment is hypothesized to attenuate the function of guanine nucleotide–binding proteins, dampen the oscillatory system, and stabilize both manic and depressed mood states.

Adenylate Cyclase System

Mooney et al. (1988) proposed that catecholamines, possibly acting through prostaglandins, may regulate platelet adenylate cyclase enzyme activity by agonist-nonspecific heterologous desensitization. In their study of 17 depressed patients and 10 control subjects, they found significant inverse correlations between 24-hour urinary catecholamine levels and various measures of receptor-mediated (prostaglandin D_2 and α_2-adrenergic) platelet adenylate cyclase activity. Also, depressed patients who had favorable antidepressant responses to alprazolam had significantly higher pretreatment urinary catecholamine output and lower receptor-mediated and non-receptor-mediated platelet adenylate cyclase activities compared with control subjects. Normalization with treatment suggests that the measures are largely state dependent.

Phosphoinositide System and Calcium

Lithium has been found to alter phosphoinositide turnover and metabolism (Baraban et al. 1989). The phosphoinositide turnover system has been shown to be inversely linked to the adenylate cyclase cAMP second-messenger system.

Pandey et al. (1991) examined whether the mode of action of antidepressants is related to their interaction with the phosphoinositide system by studying the effect of tricyclic antidepressants (desipramine, imipramine, and amitriptyline) and iprindole (an atypical antidepressant) on thrombin-stimulated formation of inositol phosphate in human platelets. The antidepressants were found to decrease thrombin-stimulated inositol phosphate formation and increase the level of [^{3}H]inositol-labeled phospholipids, most likely mediated through the inhibition of phospholipase C. Their findings suggest 1) that antidepressants may cause changes in the phosphoinositide signaling system and 2) that changes in receptors caused by antidepressants may be related to the effects of the antidepressants on membrane phospholipids. Those findings are worthy of further investigation.

Within neurons, calcium plays an important role in regulation of neuronal processes such as synthesis and release of neurotransmitters and modulation of ion channels that determine action potentials. Several studies have implicated hyperactivity of calcium in bipolar disorder. Dubovsky et al. (1991) reported that intracellular calcium is significantly higher in untreated depressed bipolar patients than in untreated unipolar depressed patients. They also reported that calcium levels did not differ between euthymic-treated bipolar patients and control subjects. They suggested that calcium hyperactivity may be a state-dependent marker in patients with bipolar disorder. The specificity and sensitivity need to be further elucidated before calcium activity can be of clinical use.

PINEAL FUNCTION AND CIRCADIAN RHYTHM

Alterations in the circadian rhythms of sleep, body temperature, and plasma melatonin, prolactin, and cortisol concentrations have been reported in depressed patients. These may occur due to desynchronization of rhythms or phase advancement of certain rhythms in mood disorders.

Several studies have shown low nocturnal output of melatonin in depressed patients (Boyce 1985; Nair et al. 1984). Beck-Friis et al. (1985) reported that depressed patients with an abnormal DST had lower melatonin concentrations than those with a normal DST, suggesting a low-melatonin syndrome in depressed patients with an abnormal DST and 24-hour cortisol rhythm. However, these data have not been replicated by other studies. Indeed, Rubin et al. (1992), in their study of 38 depressed patients, reported a trend toward elevated average nocturnal melatonin secretion, primarily accounted for by 14 premenopausal women, and no consistent relationship between HPA axis measures and melatonin levels.

SUMMARY

Several hypotheses have been put forward to explain the pathogenesis of mood disorders. There appears to be a disruption in the homeostatic balance, which triggers a cascade of events that give rise to several abnormalities in the interactions of the neurotransmitter and hormonal systems. Tables 7–1 and 7–2 summarize potential state-dependent and trait markers that have been reviewed. However, no single parameter can be solely implicated. Several studies have shown that interactions of catecholamines and corticosteroids play an important role in the biology of mood disorders. Almost all the putative neurotransmitters have been implicated, with 5-HT and norepinephrine apparently playing major roles. Although no particular neurotransmitter can be singled out for pathogenesis of mood disorders, it is possible that each may contribute to a different subgroup of symptomatology.

We have reviewed several biological measures that have been studied as state or trait markers. Most of the neuroendocrinological and neurochemical changes that occur appear to be state dependent, although some indices, such as blunted GH response and cholinergic hypersensitivity, may be potential trait markers. There is a definite need for continuing research in this area, as well as a need to define underlying genetic processes.

Table 7–1. Potential state-dependent biological markers in mood disorders

Alteration in neurotransmitters or receptors
  1. Norepinephrine (MHPG)
  2. Serotonin (5-HIAA)
  3. Dopamine (HVA)
  4. Adrenergic receptor binding
  5. 5-HT$_2$ and 5-HT$_{1c}$ receptor binding
  6. [^{3}H]Imipramine binding
Neuroendocrine measures and challenges in depression
  1. ↑ Cortisol levels
  2. ↑ CRH levels
  3. ↑ Cortisol response to dexamethasone/human CRH
  4. DST nonsuppression
  5. L-5-HTP–induced DST nonsuppression
  6. ↓ TSH response to TRH
  7. ↓ Prolactin response to fenfluramine
  8. ↓ Testosterone levels
  9. ↓ Melatonin levels

Note. CRH = corticotropin-releasing hormone. DST = dexamethasone suppression test. 5-HIAA = 5-hydroxyindoleacetic acid. 5-HT = 5-hydroxytryptamine (serotonin). HVA = homovanillic acid. L-5-HTP = L-5-hydroxytryptophan. MHPG = 3-methoxy-4-hydroxyphenylglycol. TRH = thyrotropin-releasing hormone. TSH = thyroid-stimulating hormone.

Table 7–2. Potential trait markers in mood disorders

Neuroendocrine measures and challenges in depression
  1. ↓ GH release
  2. ↓ GH response to clonidine
  3. ↑ ACTH response to dexamethasone/human CRH
  4. G-protein measures
Other measures
  1. ↓ serum DBH in delusional depression
  2. Disinhibition of REM sleep
  3. ↓ slow-wave sleep

Note. ACTH = adrenocorticotropic hormone. CRH = corticotropin-releasing hormone. DBH = dopamine–β-hydroxylase. GH = growth hormone. G-protein = guanine nucleotide–binding protein. REM = rapid eye movement.

REFERENCES

Amsterdam JD, Maislin G, Winokur A, et al: Pituitary and adrenocortical responses to the ovine corticotropin releasing hormone in depressed patients and healthy volunteers. Arch Gen Psychiatry 44:775–781, 1987

Arana GW, Baldessarini RJ, Ornsteen M: The dexamethasone suppression test for diagnosis and prognosis in psychiatry. Arch Gen Psychiatry 2:1193–1204, 1985

Asberg M, Traskman LM, Thoren P: 5-HIAA in the cerebrospinal fluid: a biochemical suicide predictor? Arch Gen Psychiatry 3:1193–1197, 1976

Avissar S, Schreiber G: The involvement of guanine nucleotide binding proteins in the pathogenesis and treatment of affective disorders. Biol Psychiatry 31:435–459, 1992

Baraban JM, Norley PF, Snyder SH: Second messenger systems and psychoactive drug action: focus on the phosphoinositide system and lithium. Am J Psychiatry 146:1251–1263, 1989

Beck-Friis J, Kjellman BF, Ljunggren J-G, et al: The pineal gland and melatonin in affective disorder, in The Pineal Gland: Endocrine Aspects (Advances in Bioscience, Vol 53). Edited by Brown GM, Wainwright SD. Oxford, England, Pergamon, 1985, pp 313–325

Beigon A, Essar N, Israeli M, et al: Serotonin 5-HT$_2$ receptor binding on blood platelets as a state dependent marker in major affective disorder. Psychopharmacology 102:73–75, 1990

Boyce PM: 6-Sulphatoxy melatonin in melancholia. Am J Psychiatry 42:125–127, 1985

Briley M, Langer SZ, Raisman R, et al: Tritiated imipramine binding sites are decreased in platelets of untreated depressed patients. Science 209:303–305, 1980

Brown WA, Johnson R, Mayfield D: 24-hour dexamethasone suppression test in a clinical setting: relationship to diagnosis, symptoms and responses to treatment. Am J Psychiatry 136:543–547, 1979

Carroll BJ, Davies B: Clinical associations of 11-hydroxy-corticosteroid suppression and non-suppression in severe depressive illness. Br Med J 3:285–287, 1970

Coppen A, Prange AJ Jr, Whybrow PC, et al: Abnormalities of indolamines in affective disorders. Arch Gen Psychiatry 26:474–478, 1972

Cowen PJ, Charig EM: Neuroendocrine responses to tryptophan in major depression. Arch Gen Psychiatry 44:958–966, 1987

Deakin JFW, Pennell I, Upadhyaya AJ, et al: A neuroendocrine study of 5-HT function in depression: evidence for biological mechanisms of endogenous and psychosocial causation. Psychopharmacology 101:85–92, 1990

Dubovsky SL, Lee C, Christiano J, et al: Elevated platelet intracellular calcium concentration in bipolar depression. Biol Psychiatry 29:441–450, 1991

Freeman AM III, Stankovic SMI, Bradley RJ, et al: Tritiated platelet imipramine binding and treatment response in depressed outpatients. Depression 1:20–23, 1993

Garcia-Sevilla JA: The platelet alpha-2 adrenoceptor as a potential biological marker in depression. Br J Psychiatry 154 (suppl 4):67–72, 1989

Gold PW, Loriaux DL, Roy A, et al: Responses to corticotropin releasing hormone in the hypercortisolism of depression and Cushing's disease: pathophysiologic and diagnosis implications. N Engl J Med 314:1329–1335, 1986

Gold PW, Goodwin FK, Chrousos GP: Clinical and biochemical manifestations of depression: relation to the neurobiology of stress. N Engl J Med 319:413–419, 1988

Gonzalez-Heydrich J, Peroutka SJ: Serotonin receptors and reuptake sites: pharmacologic significance. J Clin Psychiatry 51:4 (suppl):5–12, 1990

Holsboer F, Von Bardeleben U, Gerken A: Studies of the hypothalamus-pituitary-adrenocortical system: an example of progress in psychoneuroendocrinology, in New Results in Depression Research. Edited by Hippius H, Klerman GL, Matussek N. New York, Springer-Verlag, 1986, pp 217–249

Holsboer-Trachsler E, Stohler R, Hatzunger M, et al: Repeated administration of the combined dexamethasone-human corticotropin releasing hormone stimulation test during treatment and depression. Psychiatry Res 38:163–171, 1991

Kling MA, Roy A, Doran AR, et al: Cerebrospinal fluid immunoreactive CRH and ACTH secretion in Cushing's disease and major depression: potential clinical implications. J Clin Endocrinol Metab 2:260–271, 1991

Koyama T, Meltzer HY: A biochemical and neuroendocrine study of the serotonergic system in depression, in New Results in Depression Research. Edited by Hippius H, Klerman GL, Matussek N. New York, Springer-Verlag, 1986, pp 169–188

Krishnan KRR, Ritchie JC, Saunders WB, et al: Adrenocortical sensitivity to low dose ACTH administration in depressed patients. Biol Psychiatry 27:930–933, 1990

Langer SZ, Raisman R: Binding of [^{3}H]imipramine and [^{3}H]desipramine as biochemical tools for studies in depression. Neuropharmacology 22:407–413, 1983

Lewis AD, McChesney C: Tritiated imipramine binding distinguishes among subtypes of depression. Arch Gen Psychiatry 42:485–488, 1985

Linnoila VM, Virkkunen M: Aggression, suicidality and serotonin. J Clin Psychiatry 53:10 (suppl):46–51, 1992

Loosen PT, Prange AJ: Serum thyrotropin response to thyrotropin-releasing hormone in psychiatric patients: a review. Am J Psychiatry 139:405–416, 1982

Maes M, D'Hondt P, Martin M, et al: L-5-hydroxytryptophan stimulated cortisol escape from dexamethasone suppression in melancholic patients. Acta Psychiatr Scand 83:302–306, 1991

Mann JJ, Stanley M, McBride PA, et al: Increased 5-HT$_2$ and β-adrenergic receptor binding in the frontal cortices of suicide victims. Arch Gen Psychiatry 43:954–959, 1986

Matussek N, Ackenheil M, Hippius H, et al: Effect of clonidine on growth hormone release in psychiatric patients and controls. Psychiatry Res 7:271–277, 1982

Mooney JJ, Schatzberg AF, Cole JO, et al: Rapid antidepressant response to alprazolam in depressed patients with high catecholamine output and heterologous desensitization of platelet adenyl cyclase. Biol Psychiatry 23:543–559, 1988

Mooney JJ, Schatzberg AF, Cole JO, et al: Urinary 3-methoxy-4-hydroxyphenylglycol and the depression-type score as predictors of differential responses to antidepressants. J Clin Psychopharmacol 11(6):339–344, 1991

Nair PNV, Hariharasubramanian N, Pilapil C: Circadian rhythm of melatonin in endogenous depression. Prog Neuropsychopharmacol Biol Psychiatry 19:1215–1228, 1984

Nemeroff CB, Krishnan KRR: Neuroendocrine alterations in psychiatric disorders. Neuroendocrinology 328–441, 1992

Nemeroff CB, Knight DL, Krishnan KRR: Reduced platelet [3H]-paroxetine and [3H]-imipramine binding in major depression. Society for Neuroscience Abstracts 17:1472, 1991

Nemeroff CB, Krishnan KRR, Reed D, et al: Adrenal gland enlargement in major depression: a computed tomographic study. Arch Gen Psychiatry 9:384–387, 1992

Nurnberger JI Jr: Should a biologic marker be sensitive and specific? Acta Psychiatr Scand 86:1–4, 1992

Pandey SC, Davis JM, Schwertz DW, et al: Effect of antidepressants and neuroleptics on phosphoinositide metabolism in human platelets. J Pharmacol Exp Ther 56:1010–1018, 1991

Perry EK, Marshall EF, Blessed G, et al: Decreased imipramine binding in the brains of patients with depressive illness. Br J Psychiatry 42:188–192, 1983

Prange AJ Jr, Wilson IC, Lynn CW, et al: L-Tryptophan in mania: contribution to a permissive hypothesis of affective disorders. Arch Gen Psychiatry 30:56–62, 1974

Ribiero SCM, Tandon R, Grunhaus L, et al: The DST as a predictor of outcome in depression: a meta-analysis. Am J Psychiatry 150:1618–1629, 1993

Risch SC, Nemeroff CB: Neurochemical alterations of serotonergic neuronal systems in depression. J Clin Psychiatry 53:10 (suppl):3–7, 1992

Rothchild AJ, Langlais PJ, Schatzberg AF, et al: Dexamethasone increases plasma free dopamine in man. J Psychiatr Res 18:217–223, 1984

Rubin RT, Poland RE, Lesser M, et al: Neuroendocrine aspects of primary endogenous depression, IV: pituitary-thyroid axis activity in patients and matched control subjects. Psychoneuroendocrinology 12:333–347, 1987

Rubin RT, Poland RE, Lesser M, et al: Neuroendocrine aspects of primary endogenous depression, V: serum prolactin measures in patients and matched controls. Biol Psychiatry 25:4–21, 1989

Rubin RT, Poland RE, Lesser M: Neuroendocrine aspects of primary endogenous depression, X: serum growth hormone measures in patients and matched control subjects. Biol Psychiatry 27:1065–1082, 1990

Rubin RT, Heist K, McGeoy SS, et al: Neuroendocrine aspects of primary endogenous depression, XI: serum melatonin measures in patients and matched controls. Arch Gen Psychiatry 49:558–567, 1992

Schatzberg AF, Orsulak PJ, Rosenbaum AH, et al: Towards a biochemical classification of depressive disorders, V: biochemical heterogeneity of unipolar depression. Am J Psychiatry 139:471–475, 1982

Schatzberg AF, Rothchild AJ, Langlais PJ, et al: A corticosteroid/dopamine hypothesis for psychotic depression and related states. J Psychiatr Res 19:57–64, 1985

Schatzberg AF, Samson JA, Bloomingdale KL, et al: Toward a biochemical classification of depressive disorders, X: urinary catecholamines, their metabolites, and D-type scores in subgroups of depressive disorders. Arch Gen Psychiatry 46:260–268, 1989

Schildkraut JJ: The catecholamine hypothesis of affective disorders: a review of supporting evidence. Am J Psychiatry 122:509–522, 1965

Schildkraut JJ, Orsulak PJ, Schatzberg AF, et al: Possible pathophysiological mechanisms in subtypes of unipolar depressive disorders based on differences in urinary MHPG levels. Psychopharmacol Bull 17:90–91, 1981

Schildkraut JJ, Orsulak PJ, Schatzberg AF, et al: Urinary MHPG in affective disorders, in Neurobiology of Mood Disorders. Edited by Post RM, Ballenger JC. Baltimore, MD, Williams & Wilkins, 1984, pp 519–528

Siever LJ, Uhde TW: New studies and perspectives on the noradrenergic receptor system in depression: effects of the alpha-adrenergic agonist clonidine. Biol Psychiatry 19:131–156, 1984

Siever LJ, Murphy DL, Slater S, et al: Plasma prolactin change following fenfluramine in depressed patients compared to controls: an evaluation of central serotonergic responsivity in depression. Life Sci 34:1029–1039, 1984

Siever LJ, Trestman RL, Coccaro EF, et al: The growth hormone response to clonidine in acute and remitted depressed male patients. Neuropsychopharmacology 6(3):165–177, 1992

Steiger A, Von Bardeleben U, Guldner J, et al: The sleep EEG and nocturnal hormonal secretion studies on changes during the course of depression and on effects of CNS-active drugs. Prog Neuropsychopharmacol Biol Psychiatry 17:125–137, 1993

Sweeney D, Nelson C, Bowers M, et al: Delusional versus nondelusional depression: neurochemical differences. Lancet 2:100–101, 1978

Wolkowitz OM, Sutton ME, Doran AR, et al: Dexamethasone increases plasma HVA but not MHPG in normal humans. Psychiatry Res 16:101–109, 1985

World Health Organization collaborative study: Validity of imipramine platelet binding sites as a biological marker for depression. Pharmacopsychiatry 23:113–117, 1990

Chapter 8

Anxiety Disorders

Laszlo A. Papp, M.D., Jeremy Coplan, M.D.,
and Jack M. Gorman, M.D.

For the majority of anxiety disorders, successful treatments are currently available. Early therapeutic successes in the 1960s generated a number of biological hypotheses regarding the etiology of anxiety disorders and triggered an unprecedented surge of research. Over the past three decades, research on anxiety disorders has become the testing ground for a number of advanced psychiatric techniques like brain imaging, neurochemistry, pharmacological challenges, and sophisticated psychophysiological monitoring. The resulting rich data base shows that patients with various anxiety disorders differ significantly from one another and from a series of comparison groups on a number of biological measures.

A prominent example is the differential biological response of various diagnostic groups to pharmacological treatments. The finding that the tricyclic antidepressant imipramine selectively blocks panic attacks practically revolutionized research on anxiety disorders (Klein and Fink 1962) and is primarily responsible for the dissection of the formerly homogeneous "anxiety neurosis" category. Selective response to a pharmacological agent is an important biological marker. Treatment studies with more and more specific pharmacological agents continue to be important tools for research into the nature of anxiety disorders.

An important outgrowth of treatment studies are pharmacological challenge studies. Baseline abnormalities may be masked by compensatory mechanisms. An acute pharmacological intervention may disrupt the balance and reveal an abnormality. Pharmacological challenges range from simple prechallenge versus postchallenge behavioral observations to relating the challenge-induced changes to sophisticated brain images and repeating the challenges after treatments. Pharmacological challenges are probably the single richest source of information regarding biological markers.

The main assumption behind the pharmacological challenge strategy is that increasingly specific challenge agents will be identified that

This work was supported by a Scientist Development Award for Clinicians (MH00858) to L.A.P.

in turn will target specific neurotransmitter systems. However, anatomical and functional interactions are numerous among the many neurotransmitter systems in the brain. Therefore, investigation of a particular neurotransmitter system has to take into consideration the possibility of nonspecificity both with regard to the particular anxiety disorder and to the particular neurotransmitter system.

For instance, noradrenergic dysregulation is one of the most frequently reported findings in a number of anxiety and mood disorders. The interpretation of this abnormality is complicated by the fact that most neurotransmitter systems such as serotonin (5-hydroxytryptamine; 5-HT), opiate, glutamate, and γ-aminobutyric acid (GABA) have a direct impact on noradrenergic functions. It is also possible that noradrenergic abnormality is a trait marker indicating a biological predisposition to develop a variety of anxiety or affective disorders depending on environmental factors.

Assumptions made about central neurotransmission are further weakened by the unreliability of the peripheral measures available. The most frequently used parameters—plasma and spinal fluid levels of neurotransmitters, hormones, and breakdown products—are multiply determined and can originate from various parts of the brain as well as from other organs.

Finding biological markers is substantially complicated by comorbidity. Anxiety disorders are frequently comorbid with each other as well as with mood disorders, substance abuse, and personality disorders. Diagnostic homogeneity is, at best, relative.

Abnormalities in physiological functions such as blood pressure, pulse rate, skin conductance, or respiration would be convenient markers of anxiety disorders. Unfortunately, they are almost never specific enough to serve as biological markers. With all these caveats, this chapter is an attempt to summarize the most promising findings, with emphasis on the potential of a biological abnormality or difference to be considered a biological marker.

PANIC DISORDER

Because consistent biological differences have not been identified between panic disorder patients with and without agoraphobia and most relevant studies do not differentiate the two, these diagnostic categories will be discussed together. Panic attacks, the hallmark of panic disorder, are sudden, unexpected, episodic bursts of anxiety accompanied by a series of autonomic and cognitive symptoms such as sweating, hyperventilation, palpitation, light-headedness, and fear of impending doom. Most panic attacks last from 5 to 30 minutes. Anticipatory anxiety (which is the almost constant fear of panic attacks), phobic avoidance of situations associated with panic attacks, and depression occasionally leading to suicidal thoughts frequently complicate the fluctuating course of panic disorder. Without treatment, patients are severely limited in their social and occupational roles: some are completely housebound. Successful treatments, however, dramatically alter the outcome of the disorder; most panic disorder patients can now lead normal lives.

Panic disorder has a strong familial basis: about 50% of panic disorder patients have at least one affected relative. Because of its high degree of familiality and well-defined phenotype, panic disorder is frequently targeted by geneticists. Several marker systems have been suggested as the "panic gene," only to be ruled out later as causally unrelated to panic disorder (reviewed by Crowe 1990).

Panic disorder is probably the best researched of all the anxiety disorders. We believe that pharmacological challenges have provided the most promise in identifying biological markers for panic disorder.

Pharmacological Challenges

The infusion of sodium lactate, the gold standard of laboratory panic induction, identifies up to 80% of patients with panic disorder as lactate sensitive. The lactate sensitivity of psychiatrically healthy control subjects and patients with most other anxiety or mood disorders is below 20% (reviewed by Cowley and Arana 1990). Because lactate sensitivity significantly diminishes after successful treatment, it appears to be a state marker. However, as possible evidence for trait-marker status, lactate sensitivity may identify asymptomatic family members of anxiety disorder patients as well (Balon et al. 1989).

Although similarly high rates of sensitivity have been reported for a number of other panicogenic agents, their specificity is less well established. Carbon dioxide (Gorman et al. 1988), yohimbine (Charney et al. 1989), and cholecystokinin (Bradweyn et al. 1991) are the agents with the most promise both as biological markers and heuristically relevant probes.

A substantial disadvantage of lactate is the complexity of its action. Many years and hundreds of infusions later, its panicogenic effect is still unexplained. Nevertheless, the search for the panicogenic mechanism of lactate produced a whole series of potential biological markers. For instance, the focus on respiratory abnormalities in panic disorder grew out of the finding that patients who panic in response to lactate infusion, defying physiology, almost invariably increase their minute volume. In fact, respiratory stimulation seems to be the common physiological link among the many agents capable of inducing laboratory panic attacks (Papp et al. 1993).

Respiratory Abnormalities

Subsequent research of the respiratory psychophysiology of panic disorder identified serum phosphate (Gorman et al. 1984), inspiratory drive (Gorman et al. 1988), arterial blood gasses (Papp et al. 1989a), carbon dioxide sensitivity (Papp et al. 1989b), and urine pH (Papp and Gorman 1990) as potential biological markers for the disorder. The phosphate, blood gas, and urine pH findings may reflect the tendency of panic disorder patients to hyperventilate, whereas increased inspiratory drive and carbon dioxide hypersensitivity are consistent with an abnormal brain stem response to respiratory stimulation. Although most of these data await replication, they confirm the psychophysiology literature in suggesting that respiratory parameters are the best correlates of subjective anxiety (Grossman 1983) and provide preliminary evidence that panic disorder is a biologically distinct diagnostic category.

Klein (1993) hypothesized that in panic disorder patients a "suffocation false alarm" mechanism is triggered by a rising CO_2 concentration. If hyperventilation fails to lower the CO_2 concentration, the patient's fear of suffocation may lead to panic. Interestingly, the so-called hyperventilation test, long promoted as a diagnostic test of panic disorder (Lum 1976), lacks sensitivity and specificity (Bass et al. 1989; Hibbert and Pilsbury 1989) and thus cannot be considered a biological marker.

Neurotransmitter Abnormalities

Biological markers indicating possible noradrenergic abnormalities include yohimbine-induced increase in 3-methoxy-4-hydroxyphenyl-glycol (MHPG) (Charney et al. 1984), clonidine-induced MHPG reduction (Uhde et al. 1989), and blunted growth hormone response to clonidine administration. This last finding is one of the most consistently reported noradrenergic abnormalities in patients with panic disorder (Nutt 1989). Although its specificity is questionable (Rapaport et al. 1989), this response appears to be a valid biological marker. Because blunted growth hormone response is unaltered by successful pharmacological treatment, it may represent a trait marker (Coplan et al. 1992).

Although serotonergic medications are clearly effective in treating panic disorder patients, decreased platelet 5-HT uptake and low plasma 5-HT levels are the only serotonergic abnormalities reported in panic disorder (Pecknold 1990). Because these findings are not specific to panic disorder, they are not acceptable as biological markers.

Other Abnormalities

In addition to the above-described noradrenergic abnormalities, the involvement of the *hypothalamic-pituitary-adrenal (HPA) axis* in panic disorder is reflected in attenuated corticotropin and cortisol response to corticotropin-releasing factor (Roy-Byrne et al. 1986), and in cortisol hypersecretion (Goldstein et al. 1987). Because uncertainties still remain about the direction of these abnormalities and their trait-versus-state dependence, HPA axis abnormalities cannot be considered reliable biological markers.

Decreased functional *benzodiazepine sensitivity* may explain the reduced saccadic eye-movement velocity in panic disorder patients (Roy-Byrne et al. 1990). If the specificity of this test is confirmed, it could be an easily administered biological marker.

The few available *brain imaging studies* in panic disorder patients report global changes in response to laboratory anxiogenesis, possibly secondary to hyperventilation-induced vasoconstriction. Localized abnormalities in the temporal and frontal lobes and in the hippocampal region have also been reported but not replicated consistently (Kellner and Roy-Byrne 1990; Mathew and Wilson 1990).

SOCIAL PHOBIA

Patients with social phobia experience severe anxiety accompanied by autonomic discharge in social situations. These symptoms will reinforce their fear of embarrassment and humiliation and frequently lead to significant avoidance. Patients with "generalized" social phobia experience anxiety in almost any social situation, whereas "limited" social phobia typically involves one specific situation (e.g., public speech). Most frequently beginning in late adolescence, social phobia often continues as a lifelong disability. Lifetime prevalence rates for social phobia range from 1.8% to 3.2% of the general population (Schneier et al. 1992). Substance abuse as an attempt at self-medication, secondary depression, and suicidal ideation are frequent complications.

Biophysiology and Biochemistry

Social phobia has a relatively short history in American psychiatry. As a result, research data on biological markers are relatively sparse. Until the introduction of the term in 1980, most studies used healthy control subjects in stressful social situations. Although their relevance to social phobia is limited, these studies generally confirm the findings of elevated pulse rate, blood pressure, and plasma catecholamine levels reported in socially anxious patients (Dimsdale and Moss 1980).

On the other hand, during simulated public speech, healthy control subjects actually had greater heart rate increases than patients with social phobia, whereas changes in plasma epinephrine and norepinephrine levels were comparable in the two groups (Levin et al. 1988).

Although not replicated with patients who had social phobia as defined by DSM-III (American Psychiatric Association 1980), more fluctuations in resting spontaneous galvanic skin resistance were demonstrated by socially anxious patients than by control subjects (Lader 1967).

Pharmacological Challenges

Three studies have attempted to apply the biochemical challenge strategy to patients with social phobia. The infusion of sodium lactate, a powerful panicogenic agent in patients with panic disorder, induced panic attacks in only 1 of 15 patients with social phobia (Liebowitz et al. 1985). In response to the intravenous administration of epinephrine, only 1 of 11 patients with social phobia experienced observable anxiety, despite a robust rise in blood pressure and pulse rate (Papp et al. 1988). Similarly, the inhalation of 5% CO_2, a reliable anxiogenic procedure in panic disorder patients, failed to produce significant anxiety in patients with social phobia (Gorman et al. 1988). Thus, patients with social phobia are clearly different from patients with panic disorder in their response to anxiogenic agents.

Neurotransmitter Abnormalities

Unfortunately, tests of specific neurotransmitter function in patients with social phobia have been rare and somewhat contradictory. The prolactin response to levodopa *(dopaminergic function)* appears to be normal in patients with social phobia (Tancer and Golden 1992). Prominent *noradrenergic* abnormality in patients with social phobia is unlikely in view of a normal growth hormone response to clonidine challenge (Tancer and Golden 1992), the absence of consistent noradrenergic hyperactivity, and the lack of response to epinephrine infusions (Papp et al. 1988). *Serotonergic* abnormality may be responsible for increased cortisol response to fenfluramine challenge in patients with social phobia compared with control subjects (Tancer and Golden 1992). However, the prolactin response to m-chlorophenylpiperazine (m-CPP) was found to be normal in this patient population (Hollander et al. 1992). In view of the weak and inconsistent data, the identification of biological markers in social phobia is unlikely.

OBSESSIVE-COMPULSIVE DISORDER

Patients with obsessive-compulsive disorder (OCD) experience repetitive, usually senseless thoughts or impulses (obsessions) and/or repetitive and also senseless behaviors like washing, counting, or checking (compulsions). Spontaneous remissions are rare, and without appropriate treatment most OCD patients will remain symptomatic and impaired. Depression is a common complication. OCD was formerly believed to be a rare disorder; however, recent epidemiological surveys confirm that the lifetime prevalence rate of OCD is among the highest of all anxiety disorders.

OCD runs in families. Twin studies show a higher concordance rate for OCD features among monozygotic twins than among dizygotic twins, suggesting a genetic predisposition for the disorder (Torgersen 1990).

Serotonergic Abnormalities

Medication trials showing the efficacy of 5-HT reuptake inhibitors like clomipramine, fluoxetine, and fluvoxamine in patients with OCD focused attention on a possible serotonergic abnormality in OCD patients. It appears that even though the therapeutic action of these medications may very well be mediated by the 5-HT system, the evidence is far from convincing that OCD is a 5-HT dysregulation disorder. Serotonergic abnormalities in OCD are complicated by the heterogeneity of the 5-HT system (Murphy 1987), the lack of specificity of serotonergic probes (Hamik and Peroutka 1989), and multiple interactions of various neurotransmitter systems. Nevertheless, the 5-HT system still remains the richest source of potential biological markers in OCD.

As an indirect index of brain 5-HT activity, cerebrospinal fluid concentrations of 5-hydroxyindoleacetic acid correlate with OCD symptomatology (Asberg et al. 1982) and with response to treatment with clomipramine (Thoren et al. 1980). The partial 5-HT agonist m-CPP, but not fenfluramine, exacerbates OCD symptoms (Zohar and Insel 1987). Blunted prolactin response to m-CPP may correlate with this behavioral effect. Clomipramine treatment blunts the behavioral effects of m-CPP (Zohar et al. 1988). Exacerbated OCD symptoms seem to be a specific effect of m-CPP because other anxiogenic agents like sodium lactate, carbon dioxide, yohimbine, and caffeine are ineffective in OCD patients. Although the neurochemical effects of m-CPP are contradictory, the behavioral response to this agent may be considered a biological state marker identifying as many as 50% of OCD patients. That is about the percentage of patients who respond to treatment with selective 5-HT reuptake inhibitors.

Other Neurotransmitter Abnormalities

Preliminary investigations of neurotransmitter systems other than 5-HT have not yet resulted in potential biological markers for OCD. Although altered *noradrenergic* activity in OCD patients is suggested by the beneficial behavioral effects of clonidine (Hollander et al. 1988), the accompanying blunted growth hormone response, a commonly reported noradrenergic abnormality in panic disorder and possibly in generalized anxiety disorder (GAD), has not been consistently found in OCD (Lee et al. 1990). No differences between patients and control subjects were found after oral administration of the α_2-adrenergic antagonist yohimbine (Rasmussen et al. 1987).

The involvement of the *dopaminergic* system is suggested by preclinical (Wallach and Gershon 1971) and clinical (Johnson and Lucey 1987) data, whereas cholinergic abnormalities may be responsible for certain memory deficits observed in OCD patients (Reed 1977). However, peripheral markers of dopaminergic function such as sulfotransferase activity have not yet provided consistent data in OCD patients (Marazziti et al. 1992). Amphetamine challenges induced mild improvement or no change in OCD patients (Swinson and Joffe 1988). To our knowledge, the only cholinergic abnormality reported in OCD patients is elevated growth hormone response to the acetylcholinesterase inhibitor pyridostigmine (Lucey et al. 1993).

Brain Imaging

Electroencephalogram abnormalities in OCD patients are nonspecific and inconsistent (Jenike and Brotman 1984), whereas studies of auditory, visual, and somatosensory evoked potentials provide promising leads to identifying biological markers (Beech et al. 1983).

Frontal lobe and basal ganglia abnormalities have been identified in OCD patients by using positron-emission tomography (PET) scans (Nordahl et al. 1989). The high incidence of tics in OCD patients also suggests the involvement of the basal ganglia. Together with decreased caudate volumes and lesions in the striatum, these findings point to a possible neurological basis of OCD. Indeed, neurological soft signs were significantly more common in OCD patients than in a comparison group (Hollander et al. 1990). A cutoff of three or more soft signs seemed to best distinguish patients from control subjects. Because successful behavioral and pharmacological treatments seem to change glucose metabolism in the right head of the caudate nucleus in OCD patients (Baxter et al. 1992), these neurological findings likely represent state rather than trait phenomena.

OCD research targeting this most "biological" of the anxiety disorders is likely to yield reliable biological markers for the disorder in the near future.

POSTTRAUMATIC STRESS DISORDER

The diagnosis of posttraumatic stress disorder (PTSD) is made when an exposure to a severe stressor is followed by continued reexperiencing of the original trauma, avoidance, and hyperarousal. PTSD often becomes a chronic condition with anxiety, depression, and impaired functioning as common complications. Approximately 1% of the general population will suffer from PTSD during their lifetimes. The rate of full or partial PTSD in survivors of war can reach 50% (Kulka et al. 1990). Strong genetic influence on symptom liability has been confirmed in twin studies (True et al. 1993).

Neurotransmitter Abnormalities

The highly variable symptomatology of PTSD—coupled with the finding that a therapeutic effect can be achieved with medications from diverse pharmacological groups—suggests that PTSD involves a number of neurotransmitter systems. Indeed, preclinical and clinical literature reveals multiple neurotransmitter alterations in response to trauma.

Noradrenergic abnormalities in PTSD patients include heightened sympathetic nervous system arousal in response to specifically relevant stimuli (Orr 1990), elevated 24-hour urinary norepinephrine excretion (Kosten et al. 1987), a 40% reduction in platelet α_2-adrenergic binding sites compared with control subjects (Perry et al. 1987), and an exaggerated loss of platelet receptor protein on in vitro exposure to epinephrine (Perry et al. 1990). Simultaneously elevated heart rate, blood pressure, and plasma epinephrine levels have also been recorded in combat veterans with PTSD exposed to a combat film (McFall et al. 1990).

The intravenous administration of the α_2-adrenergic agonist yohimbine induced typical flashbacks in 40% of PTSD patients, along with marked increase in sympathetic activity (Southwick et al. 1993). Approximately 70% of the patients experienced panic attacks during the infusion. The panic attacks were unrelated to comorbid panic disorder. Parameters of noradrenergic reactivity are probably the most promising biological markers in PTSD (Charney et al. 1993).

Investigation of the *opiate* system in PTSD was prompted by the early observation that traumatized soldiers in World War II required fewer narcotics than did civilians (Beecher 1946). The apparent analgesia during self-mutilation that follows a significant trauma in a group of psychiatric patients would also support such an association (Richardson and Zaleski 1983). Indeed, the opiate antagonist naloxone seems to reverse stress-induced analgesia in veterans with PTSD (Pitman et al. 1990). According to the opiate theory of PTSD, the reexperiencing of the original trauma would trigger the release of endogenous opiates.

Serotonergic abnormalities in anxiety and mood disorders—including panic disorder, depression, and OCD—have been subjected to intensive investigations. Because PTSD shares a number of features with these disorders, the application of serotonergic probes in PTSD patients should be revealing.

Substantial evidence points to the involvement of the *dopaminergic* system in schizophrenic psychosis. The dopaminergic system may also play a significant role in stress-induced psychosis in PTSD. Ingestion of amphetamine or cocaine frequently induces typical PTSD symptoms such as paranoia and hypervigilance, probably via dopaminergic mechanisms (Satel et al. 1991).

Similarly, the relevance of the *benzodiazepine-GABA* system in panic disorder has been made obvious. Given the symptomatic overlap between panic disorder and PTSD, the need for assessing GABAergic abnormalities in PTSD is unquestionable. Unfortunately, to our knowledge, there are no clinical studies investigating these last two neurotransmitter systems in PTSD.

Hypothalamic-Pituitary-Adrenal Axis Abnormalities

The preclinical finding that uncontrollable stress precipitates multiple alterations in the functioning of the HPA axis (Sapolsky and Plotsky 1990) has led to a series of clinical investigations in PTSD patients. Traditional wisdom would predict a parallel increase in plasma levels of norepinephrine and cortisol in response to stress. Interestingly, patients with PTSD exposed to chronic stress were shown to have low urinary cortisol levels and increased norepinephrine concentrations (Mason et al. 1988). Perhaps reflective of a deranged HPA axis, the low cortisol response coupled with increased suppression in response to dexamethasone challenge (Yehuda et al. 1991) are some of the most promising biological markers in PTSD.

GENERALIZED ANXIETY DISORDER

GAD patients suffer from "unrealistic or excessive anxiety and worry" for at least 6 months (American Psychiatric Association 1987, p. 251). Their multiple symptoms cluster in three areas: motor tension, autonomic hyperactivity, and vigilance. The course of GAD fluctuates from severe disability with depression as a common complication to periods of complete remission.

GAD is probably the most common anxiety disorder. According to recent epidemiological surveys, the 1-year prevalence of GAD ranges from 2% to 8% in the general population (Meyers et al. 1989). Although most patients with GAD are severely disabled for many years, they are rarely seen by psychiatric clinicians. Rather, the nature of their symptomatology subjects them to a series of medical workups. Even though organic abnormalities are almost never found, GAD patients as a rule resist psychiatric referral. When psychiatric treatment is attempted, response rates are generally lower than those seen with other anxiety disorders. For these reasons, the extent of the biological research into GAD has been somewhat limited.

GAD, like most anxiety disorders, runs in families. Approximately 20% of first-degree relatives of GAD patients suffer from GAD (Noyes et al. 1987). This percentage is between those reported for panic disorder (50%) and social phobia (7%). Twin studies found that monozygotic twins are four times as concordant for "clinical anxiety" than dizygotic twins (Torgersen 1990). However, if those twins with coexisting panic attacks and GAD are excluded from the comparison, the difference in concordance rates disappears (monozygotic = 17%; dizygotic = 20%).

Biophysiology and Biochemistry

Normal stress reaction, which used to serve as the paradigm for studies on generalized anxiety, is usually accompanied by increased blood pressure, heart rate, minute volume, skin conductance, muscle tension, and plasma levels of epinephrine, norepinephrine, growth hormone, cortisol, and prolactin. Unfortunately, none of these findings are replicated in GAD patients with the consistency needed for a biological marker. None of the most frequently recorded psychophysiological parameters (e.g., resting blood pressure, heart rate, minute volume, skin conductance) have proven to be consistently abnormal in GAD patients either.

Similarly weak and inconsistent results have been reported for a series of biological parameters in GAD patients. Both hyperthyroidism and euthyroidism have been found in GAD patients (Munjack and Palmer 1988). Although some studies failed to detect differences between patients and control subjects, others showed resting catecholamine and MHPG levels and platelet monoamine oxidase inhibitor activity to be higher in GAD patients than in control subjects.

Pharmacological Challenges

Sodium lactate infusion, the gold standard for laboratory induction of panic in panic disorder patients, induced more anxiety in GAD patients than it did in healthy control subjects but did not result in panic attacks (Cowley et al. 1988).

Possible postsynaptic α_2-receptor subsensitivity in GAD patients is indicated by decreased platelet α_2-adrenoceptor binding compared with healthy control subjects and patients with depression (Sevy et al. 1989). Blunted growth hormone response to clonidine in GAD patients compared with control subjects (Abelson et al. 1991) is also consistent with adrenergic abnormality. However, the absence of differences between GAD patients and control subjects with respect to clonidine-induced (Abelson et al. 1991) and oral yohimbine-induced (Charney et al. 1989) blood pressure, heart rate, and MHPG changes questions the validity of adrenergic abnormality in GAD patients.

The rate of cortisol nonsuppression in response to the dexamethasone test in GAD patients was comparable to that in depressed patients (Tiller et al. 1988); this finding was unrelated to the presence of depression in GAD patients (Schweizer et al. 1986). Given the lack of specificity, however, the dexamethasone suppression test is an unlikely candidate as a biological marker in GAD.

Sleep Physiology

Sleep electroencephalogram studies in GAD patients, although somewhat contradictory, seem to indicate that GAD patients have longer rapid eye movement latency, less rapid eye movement activity, and less total sleep time than depressed patients (Papadimitriou et al. 1988). Sleep abnormalities in general lack the specificity of biological markers.

Brain Imaging

Although mild to moderate arousal in general produces a significant increase in cerebral blood flow and metabolism, severe anxiety results in cerebral vasoconstriction. Resting measurements of cerebral blood flow revealed no global differences between GAD patients and control subjects, but state anxiety showed a significant inverse correlation with cerebral blood flow in the GAD patients. Inhalation of 5% CO_2 over 30 minutes also produced an inverse relationship between anxiety and cerebral blood flow in nine GAD patients, but again no differences in anxiety levels were found between patients and control subjects (Mathew and Wilson 1990). One PET study of 18 benzodiazepine-treated GAD patients found higher relative metabolic rates in the occipital, temporal, and frontal lobes of the patients compared with control subjects. GAD patients showed reduced metabolism in the basal ganglia. Benzodiazepine treatment resulted in further reduction of basal ganglia metabolism. Benzodiazepine treatment also decreased metabolism in the cortex and limbic system (Wu et al. 1991). The clinical implications of these findings are limited. GAD patients may or may not exhibit cerebral blood flow and cerebral metabolism patterns that are clearly distinct from those of healthy control subjects or patients with other anxiety disorders.

Surprisingly, despite inducing significant anxiety, epinephrine infusions did not result in detectable changes in regional or hemispheric cerebral blood flow in 20 GAD patients (Mathew and Wilson 1990). Electroencephalogram changes induced by ingestion of caffeine may successfully differentiate GAD patients from both healthy control subjects and panic disorder patients (Bruce et al. 1992).

Studies searching for potential biological markers in GAD patients are relatively few and have failed to produce results comparable to those seen in patients with other anxiety disorders. Diagnostic uncertainties, poor treatment results, and few available research patients hinder progress.

SIMPLE PHOBIA

Simple phobia is defined as a persistent, irrational, and excessive fear of an object or situation not associated with agoraphobia or social phobia. The fear and avoidance are markedly stressful and may interfere with role functioning. Lifetime prevalence rates ranging from 4% to 25% have been reported. Approximately 31% of the relatives of patients with simple phobia have a phobic disorder (Fyer et al. 1990). The highest familiality of any anxiety disorder has been reported for blood and injury phobia (68%), whereas the percentages for the two most common simple phobias, dental and animal phobias, have been found to be 25% and 15%, respectively (Ost and Hugdahl 1985). Twin studies estimate the concordance rates of "phobic neurosis" at 88% for monozygotic twins and 38% for dizygotic twins (Carey and Gottesman 1981).

Despite its high familiality and, in the case of blood and injury phobia, unique physiology (vagal response), simple phobia has received almost no attention from biological researchers. There are no data regarding specific neurotransmitter involvement or patient response to biological challenges. Other than elevated heart rate, blood pressure, plasma norepinephrine, epinephrine, insulin, cortisol, and growth hormone in patients with animal phobia (Curtis et al. 1976) and decreased heart rate and blood pressure in patients with blood and injury phobia (Ost et al. 1984) on exposure to the phobic stimulus, biological data are unavailable.

CONCLUSION

Table 8–1 is a summary of potential biological markers in anxiety disorders. Once their specificity and sensitivity are established, these findings can be considered *state* markers. During symptomatic periods of the illness, they are capable of differentiating patients from comparison groups. The most promising biological markers at present are specific behavioral and biophysiological reactions to pharmacological

Table 8–1. Biological markers in anxiety disorders

- **Panic disorder**
  Panic in response to panicogenic agents (e.g., lactate, CO_2, cholecystokinin)
  Respiratory abnormalities (se PO_4, blood gases, CO_2 sensitivity)
  5-HT abnormalities (decreased 5-HT platelet uptake, low plasma 5-HT level)
  Noradrenergic abnormalities (blunted GH response and reduced MHPG
  after administration of clonidine, increased MHPG after administration of
  yohimbine)
  HPA axis abnormalities (blunted cortisol response after administration of
  CRF, cortisol hypersecretion)
  Benzodiazepine abnormalities (reduced saccadic eye-movement velocity)
  Brain imaging (lactate-induced vasoconstriction; temporal, frontal, and
  hippocampal changes)

- **Social phobia**
  Biophysiology and biochemistry (changes in P, BP, catecholamines, and
  galvanic skin response)
  5-HT abnormalities (possible increase in cortisol after administration of
  fenfluramine)

- **Obsessive-compulsive disorder**
  5-HT abnormalities (CSF 5-HIAA correlates with symptoms, symptoms
  increase and prolactin response is blunted after administration of m-CPP)
  Acetylcholinesterase abnormalities (increased GH response after
  administration of pyridostigmine)
  Brain imaging (frontal lobe, basal ganglia, striatum, and caudate changes)
  Neurological soft signs

- **Posttraumatic stress disorder**
  Noradrenergic abnormalities (increased sympathetic arousal and urinary
  norepinephrine excretion, decreased platelet α_2-adrenergic binding,
  increased plasma catecholamine, flashbacks in response to administration
  of yohimbine)
  HPA axis abnormalities (low urinary cortisol, increased suppression in
  response to DST)

- **Generalized anxiety disorder**
  Biophysiology and biochemistry (possibly increased P, BP, minute volume,
  catecholamines, and galvanic skin response)
  Noradrenergic abnormalities (decreased platelet α_2-adrenoceptor binding,
  blunted GH response to clonidine)
  HPA axis abnormalities (possible cortisol nonsuppression in response to
  DST)
  Sleep physiology (longer REM latency, less REM activity, less total sleep
  time)
  Brain imaging (reduced metabolism in basal ganglia, EEG changes after
  caffeine ingestion)

- **Simple phobia**
  Blood and injury phobia
  Vagal response (decreased BP and P)
  Animal phobia
  Biophysiology and biochemistry (increased P, BP, and catecholamine)

Table 8–1. Biological markers in anxiety disorders *(continued)*

Note. BP = blood pressure. CRF = corticotropin-releasing factor. CSF = cerebrospinal fluid. DST = dexamethasone suppression test. EEG = electroencephalogram. GH = growth hormone. 5-HIAA = 5-hydroxyindoleacetic acid. HPA = hypothalamic-pituitary-adrenal. 5-HT = 5-hydroxytryptamine (serotonin). m-CPP = *m*-chlorophenylpiperazine. MHPG = 3-methoxy-4-hydroxyphenylglycol. P = pulse. REM = rapid eye movement.

challenges and peripheral manifestations of neurotransmitter abnormalities. Our next task is to screen for the most consistently identified biological markers and the most conveniently administered tests for those markers in the family members of anxiety disorder patients. We also have to conduct long-term follow-up studies and retest remitted, symptom-free patients. These research strategies will lead to the identification of biological *trait* markers. In the absence of trait markers, our current ability to predict anxiety disorders in asymptomatic carriers is severely limited.

REFERENCES

Abelson JL, Glitz D, Cameron OG, et al: Blunted growth hormone response to clonidine in patients with generalized anxiety disorder. Arch Gen Psychiatry 48:157–162, 1991

American Psychiatric Association: Diagnostic and Statistical Manual of Mental Disorders, 3rd Edition. Washington, DC, American Psychiatric Association, 1980

American Psychiatric Association: Diagnostic and Statistical Manual of Mental Disorders, 3rd Edition, Revised. Washington, DC, American Psychiatric Association, 1987

Asberg M, Thoren P, Bertilsson L: Clomipramine treatment of obsessive disorder: biochemical and clinical aspects. Psychopharmacol Bull 18:13–21, 1982

Balon R, Jordan M, Pohl R: Family history of anxiety disorders in control subjects with lactate induced panic attacks. Am J Psychiatry 146:1304–1306, 1989

Bass C, Lelliot P, Marks I: Fear talk versus voluntary hyperventilation in agoraphobics and normals: a controlled study. Psychol Med 19:669–676, 1989

Baxter LR, Schwartz JM, Bergman KS, et al: Caudate glucose metabolic rate changes with both drug and behavior therapy for obsessive-compulsive disorder. Arch Gen Psychiatry 49:681–689, 1992

Beech HR, Ciesielski KT, Gordon KT: Further observations of evoked potentials in obsessional patients. Br J Psychiatry 142:605–609, 1983

Beecher HK: Pain in men wounded in battle. Ann Surg 123:96–105, 1946

Bradweyn J, Koszicky D, Shriqui C: Enhanced sensitivity to cholecystokinin-tetrapeptide in panic disorder: clinical and behavioural findings. Arch Gen Psychiatry 48:603–607, 1991

Bruce M, Scott N, Shine P, et al: Anxiogenic effects of caffeine in patients with anxiety disorders. Arch Gen Psychiatry 49:867–869, 1992

Carey G, Gottesman II: Twin and family studies of anxiety, phobic and obsessive disorders, in Anxiety: New Research and Changing Concepts. Edited by Klein DF, Rabkin J. New York, Raven, 1981, pp 117–136

Charney DS, Heninger GR, Breier A: Noradrenergic function in panic anxiety. Arch Gen Psychiatry 41:751–763, 1984

Charney DS, Woods SW, Heninger GR: Noradrenergic function in generalized anxiety disorder: effects of yohimbine in healthy subjects and patients with generalized anxiety disorder. Psychiatry Res 27:173–182, 1989

Charney DS, Deutch AY, Krystal JH, et al: Psychobiologic mechanisms of posttraumatic stress disorder. Arch Gen Psychiatry 50:294–305, 1993

Coplan JD, Papp LA, Gorman JM, et al: Persistence of noradrenergic dysregulation in panic disorder following chronic serotonin reuptake blockade with fluoxetine. Proceedings of the Annual Meeting of the American College of Neuropsychopharmacology, Puerto Rico, December 1992. San Juan, Puerto Rico, American College of Neuropsychopharmacology, 1992, pp 117–136

Cowley DS, Arana GW: Diagnostic utility of lactate sensitivity in panic disorder. Arch Gen Psychiatry 47:277–284, 1990

Cowley DS, Dager SR, McClellan J, et al: Response to lactate infusion in generalized anxiety disorder. Biol Psychiatry 24:409–414, 1988

Crowe RR: Molecular genetics and panic disorder, in Neurobiology of Panic Disorder. Edited by Ballenger J. New York, Wiley-Liss, 1990, pp 59–70

Curtis G, Nesse R, Buxton M, et al: Flooding in vivo as a research tool and treatment for phobias. Compr Psychiatry 17:153–160, 1976

Dimsdale JE, Moss J: Plasma catecholamines in stress and exercise. JAMA 243:340–342, 1980

Fyer AJ, Mannuzza S, Gallops MA, et al: Familial transmission of simple phobias and fears. Arch Gen Psychiatry 47:252–256, 1990

Goldstein S, Halbreich V, Ashis G, et al: The hypothalamic pituitary-adrenal system in panic disorder. Am J Psychiatry 144:1320–1323, 1987

Gorman JM, Cohen BS, Liebowitz MA, et al: Blood gas changes and hypophosphatemia in lactate-induced panic. Arch Gen Psychiatry 141:857–861, 1984

Gorman JM, Fyer MR, Goetz R, et al: Ventilatory physiology of patients with panic disorder. Arch Gen Psychiatry 45:31–39, 1988

Grossman P: Respiration, stress and cardiovascular function. Psychophysiology 20(3):284–300, 1983

Hamik A, Peroutka SJ: 1-m-Chlorophenylpiperazine (mCPP) interactions with neurotransmitter receptors in the human brain. Biol Psychiatry 25:569–575, 1989

Hibbert G, Pilsbury D: Hyperventilation: is it a cause of panic attacks? Br J Psychiatry 155:805–809, 1989

Hollander E, Fay M, Cohen B, et al: Serotonergic and noradrenergic function in obsessive compulsive disorder. Am J Psychiatry 145:1015–1017, 1988

Hollander E, Schiffman E, Cohen B, et al: Signs of central nervous system dysfunction in obsessive-compulsive disorder. Arch Gen Psychiatry 47:27–32, 1990

Hollander E, Stein DJ, DeCaria C, et al: Neuropsychiatry and 5-HT function in OCD and social phobia (abstract), in Proceedings of the Annual Meeting of the American College of Neuropsychopharmacology, Puerto Rico, December 1992. San Juan, Puerto Rico, American College of Neuropsychopharmacology, 1992, p 147

Jenike MA, Brotman AW: The EEG in obsessive compulsive disorder. J Clin Psychiatry 45:122–124, 1984

Johnson, Lucey PA: Encephalitis lethargica, a contemporary cause of catatonic stupor: a report of two cases. Br J Psychiatry 151:550–552, 1987

Kellner C, Roy-Byrne PP: Computed tomography and magnetic resonance imaging in panic disorder, in Neurobiology of Panic Disorder. Edited by Ballenger J. New York, Wiley-Liss, 1990, pp 271–280

Klein DF: False suffocation alarms, spontaneous panics, and related conditions: an integrative hypothesis. Arch Gen Psychiatry 50:306–317, 1993

Klein DF, Fink M: Psychiatric reaction patterns to imipramine. Am J Psychiatry 119:432–438, 1962

Kosten TR, Mason JW, Giller EL, et al: Sustained urinary norepinephrine and epinephrine elevation in post-traumatic stress disorder. Psychoneuroendocrinology 12:13–20, 1987

Kulka RA, Schlenger WE, Fairbank JA, et al: The national Vietnam veterans readjustment study: table of findings and appendices, in Trauma and the Vietnam War Generation. New York, Brunner/Mazel, 1990

Lader MH: Palmar skin conductance measures in anxiety and phobic states. J Psychosom Res 11:271–281, 1967

Lee MA, Cameron OG, Gurguis GNM, et al: Alpha2-adrenoreceptor status in obsessive-compulsive patients. Biol Psychiatry 27:1083–1093, 1990

Levin AP, Sandberg D, Stein J, et al: Plasma catecholamines in social phobia, in Proceedings of the Annual Meeting of the American Psychiatric Association, Montreal, Canada, May 1988, p 121

Liebowitz MR, Fyer AJ, Gorman JM, et al: Specificity of lactate infusions in social phobia versus panic disorder. Am J Psychiatry 142:947–950, 1985

Lucey JV, Butcher G, Clare AW, et al: Elevated growth hormone responses to pyridostigmine in obsessive-compulsive disorder: evidence of cholinergic supersensitivity. Am J Psychiatry 150:961–962, 1993

Lum LC: The syndrome of habitual chronic hyperventilation, in Modern Trends in Psychosomatic Medicine, Vol 3. Edited by Hill OW. London, Butterworths, 1976

Marazziti D, Hollander E, Lensi P, et al: Peripheral markers of serotonin and dopamine function in obsessive-compulsive disorder. Psychiatry Res 42:41–51, 1992

Mason JW, Giller EL, Kostin TR, et al: Elevation of urinary norepinephrine/cortisol ratio in post traumatic stress disorder. J Nerv Ment Dis 176:498–502, 1988

Mathew RJ, Wilson WH: Cerebral blood flow in anxiety and panic, in Neurobiology of Panic Disorder. Edited by Ballenger J. New York, Wiley-Liss, 1990, pp 281–312

McFall M, Murburg M, Ko G, et al: Autonomic responses to stress in Vietnam combat veterans with post traumatic stress disorder. Biol Psychiatry 27:1165–1175, 1990

Meyers JK, Weissman MM, Tischkler GL, et al: Six-month prevalence of psychiatric disorders in three communities: 1980–1982. Arch Gen Psychiatry 41:959–967, 1989

Munjack DJ, Palmer R: Thyroid hormones in panic disorder with agoraphobia and generalized anxiety disorder. J Clin Psychiatry 49:229–231, 1988

Murphy DL: Serotonin and anxiety: an overview. Paper presented at the 140th annual meeting of the American Psychiatric Association, Chicago, IL, May 1987

Nordahl TE, Benkelfat C, Semple W, et al: Cerebral glucose metabolic rates in obsessive compulsive disorder. Neuropsychopharmacology 2:23–28, 1989

Noyes R, Clarkson C, Crowe RC, et al: A family study of generalized anxiety disorder. Am J Psychiatry 144:1019–1024, 1987

Nutt DJ: Altered central alpha2 sensitivity in panic disorder. Arch Gen Psychiatry 46:165–169, 1989

Orr SP: Psychophysiologic studies of posttraumatic stress disorder, in Biological Assessment and Treatment of Posttraumatic Stress Disorder. Edited by Giller EL. Washington, DC, American Psychiatric Press, 1990, pp 135–157

Ost L-G, Hugdahl K: Acquisition of blood and dental phobia anxiety response patterns in clinical patients. Behav Res Ther 23:27–31, 1985

Ost L-G, Sterner U, Lindahl IL: Physiological responses in blood phobics. Behav Res Ther 22:109–117, 1984

Papadimitriou GN, Kerkhofs M, Kempenaers C, et al: EEG sleep studies in patients with generalized anxiety disorder. Psychiatry Res 26:183–190, 1988

Papp LA, Gorman JM: Urine pH in panic: a possible screening device (letter). Lancet 335:355, 1990

Papp LA, Gorman JM, Liebowitz MR, et al: Epinephrine infusions in patients with social phobia. Am J Psychiatry 145:733–736, 1988

Papp LA, Martinez JM, Klein DF, et al: Arterial blood gas changes during lactate-induced panic. Psychiatry Res 28:171–180, 1989a

Papp LA, Goetz R, Cole A, et al: Hypersensitivity to carbon dioxide in panic disorder. Am J Psychiatry 146:779–781, 1989b

Papp LA, Klein DF, Gorman JM: Carbon dioxide hypersensitivity, hyperventilation, and panic disorder. Am J Psychiatry 150:1149–1157, 1993

Pecknold JC: Serotonin abnormalities in panic disorder, in Neurobiology of Panic Disorder. Edited by Ballenger JC. New York, Wiley-Liss, 1990, pp 121–141

Perry BD, Giller EL, Southwick SM: Altered platelet alpha-2 adrenergic binding sites in posttraumatic stress disorder. Am J Psychiatry 144:1511, 1987

Perry BD, Southwick SM, Yehuda R, et al: Adrenergic dysregulation in PTSD, in Biological Assessment and Treatment of Posttraumatic Stress Disorder. Edited by Giller EL. Washington, DC, American Psychiatric Press, 1990, pp 87–114

Pitman RK, van der Kolk BA, Orr SP, et al: Naloxone-reversible analgesic response to combat related stimuli in post traumatic stress disorder. Arch Gen Psychiatry 47:541–544, 1990

Rapaport MH, Risch SC, Gillin JC, et al: Blunted growth hormone response to peripheral infusion of human growth hormone releasing factor in patients with panic disorder. Am J Psychiatry 146:92–95, 1989

Rasmussen SA, Goodman WK, Woods SW, et al: Effects of yohimbine in obsessive compulsive disorder. Psychopharmacology 93:308–313, 1987

Reed G: Obsessional personality disorder and remembering. Br J Psychiatry 130:177–183, 1977

Richardson JS, Zaleski WA: Naloxone and self mutilation. Biol Psychiatry 18:99–101, 1983

Roy-Byrne PP, Uhde TW, Post RM, et al: The corticotropin releasing hormone stimulation test in patients with panic disorder. Am J Psychiatry 143:896–899, 1986

Roy-Byrne PP, Cowley DS, Greenblatt D, et al: Reduced benzodiazepine sensitivity in panic disorder. Arch Gen Psychiatry 47:534–538, 1990

Sapolsky RM, Plotsky PM: Hypercortisolism and its possible neural bases. Biol Psychiatry 27:937–952, 1990

Satel SL, Southwick SM, Gawin FM: Clinical features of cocaine-induced paranoia. Am J Psychiatry 148:495–499, 1991

Schneier FR, Johnson J, Hornig CD, et al: Social phobia: comorbidity and morbidity in an epidemiologic sample. Arch Gen Psychiatry 49:282–288, 1992

Schweizer EE, Swenson CM, Winokur A, et al: The dexamethasone suppression test in generalized anxiety disorder. Br J Psychiatry 149:320–322, 1986

Sevy S, Papadimitriou GN, Surmont DW, et al: Noradrenergic function in generalized anxiety disorder, major depressive disorder and healthy subjects. Biol Psychiatry 25:141–152, 1989

Southwick SM, Krystal JH, Morgan A, et al: Abnormal noradrenergic function in posttraumatic stress disorder. Arch Gen Psychiatry 50:266–274, 1993

Swinson RP, Joffe RT: Biological challenges in obsessive compulsive disorder. Prog Neuropsychopharmacol Biol Psychiatry 12:269–275, 1988

Tancer ME, Golden RN: Monoamine neurotransmitter function in social phobia (abstract), in Proceedings of the Annual Meeting of the American College of Neuropsychopharmacology, Puerto Rico, December 1992. San Juan, Puerto Rico, American College of Neuropsychopharmacology, 1992, p 145

Thoren P, Asberg M, Cronholm B, et al: Clomipramine treatment of obsessive-compulsive disorder, II. Arch Gen Psychiatry 37:1286–1294, 1980

Tiller JW, Biddle N, Maguire KP, et al: The dexamethasone suppression test and plasma dexamethasone in generalized anxiety disorder. Biol Psychiatry 23:261–270, 1988

Torgersen S: Twin studies in panic disorder, in Neurobiology of Panic Disorder. Edited by Ballenger JC. New York, Wiley-Liss, 1990, pp 51–58

True WR, Rice J, Eisen SA, et al: A twin study of genetic and environmental contributions to liability for posttraumatic stress symptoms. Arch Gen Psychiatry 50:257–264, 1993

Uhde TW, Stein MB, Vittone BA, et al: Behavioral and physiologic effects of short-term and long-term administration of clonidine in panic disorder. Arch Gen Psychiatry 46:170–177, 1989

Wallach MB, Gershon S: Sensitization to amphetamine. Psychopharmacol Bull 7(4):30–31, 1971

Wu JC, Buchsbaum MS, Hershey TG, et al: PET in generalized anxiety disorder. Biol Psychiatry 29:1181–1199, 1991

Yehuda R, Giller EL, Boisoneau D, et al: Low dose DST in PTSD (144), in New Research Program and Abstracts: American Psychiatric Association 144th Annual Meeting, New Orleans, LA, May 1991

Zohar J, Insel TR: Obsessive-compulsive disorder: psychobiological approaches to diagnosis, treatment and pathophysiology. Biol Psychiatry 22:667–687, 1987

Zohar J, Insel TR, Zohar-Kadouch RC, et al: Serotonergic responsivity in obsessive-compulsive disorder: effects of chronic clomipramine treatment. Arch Gen Psychiatry 45:167–172, 1988

Chapter 9

Alcoholism

Marc A. Schuckit, M.D.

The goal of this chapter is to review biological markers of risk related to alcoholism. The material presented is an attempt to synthesize the complex and sometimes contradictory information that exists in the literature.

As is true with most major psychiatric syndromes, biological markers for alcoholism (alcohol abuse or dependence) fall into the two general categories of state and trait phenomena (Schuckit 1990). There are many state markers associated with the current status of heavy intake of alcohol. This drug is easily absorbed into the body, is widely distributed, and is associated with changes in almost all body systems (Schuckit 1989). Thus, state markers for heavy drinking usually involve relatively straightforward blood tests evaluating changes in enzymes (e.g., γ-glutamyl transferase), characteristics of red blood cells (e.g., mean corpuscular volume and alterations in hemoglobin), and tests that relate to kidney and liver functioning (Schuckit 1989). As the name implies, these state changes are temporary and are likely to return toward normal within days to weeks of abstinence (Irwin et al. 1988). There is no convincing evidence that these same values serve as markers of a predisposition toward alcohol dependence.

The focus here will not be on these tests; rather, it will be on biological attributes of an individual that can be measured with moderate ease, can be observed before the onset of alcohol dependence, and are associated either directly or indirectly with a predisposition toward alcoholism (Begleiter and Porjesz 1988). Most of these tests were originally identified through comparisons of alcoholic patients and control subjects, which were done in an attempt to observe characteristics that do not return to normal with abstinence. Following up on these findings, additional investigations were carried out in individuals felt to be at high risk for the future development of alcoholism, usually children of alcoholic persons (Schuckit 1990). Young relatives of alcoholic persons were selected as the focus in the search for biological markers of risk because of data supporting the importance of genetic factors in this disorder. Studies indicate that alcohol dependence is familial, and the

This work was supported by NIAAA Grants 05526, 08401, and 08403 and the Veterans Affairs Research Service.

majority of the investigations demonstrate that identical twins of alcoholic persons have a much higher level of similarity or concordance for alcoholism than do fraternal twins of alcohol-dependent individuals (Schuckit 1992). Perhaps the most impressive data come from the evaluation of sons and daughters of alcoholic persons who were adopted away early in life and usually raised without knowledge of their biological parents' problems (Goodwin et al. 1974). All of these studies carried out since 1950 have demonstrated a twofold to fourfold increased risk for alcohol dependence in these children, with no commensurate increased risk for severe alcohol problems in adopted-away children of nonalcoholic persons. It does not appear that being raised by an alcoholic person increases the risk for future alcohol dependence beyond the level predicted by an alcoholic biological parent alone (Goodwin et al. 1974; Schuckit et al. 1972).

Thus, there are logical reasons for pursuing investigations of potential biological markers of future risk and for focusing these investigations on close relatives of alcoholic persons. A rapid review of the literature, however, reveals what appear to be contradictory results. It is likely that much of this divergence is a result of methodological issues as well as the very nature of the genetic influences. Reflecting these considerations, the next section presents an overview of methodological issues relevant to studies of biological markers of the risk for alcoholism. This section is followed by an overview of potential markers of risk that have been identified in the literature.

METHODOLOGICAL CONSIDERATIONS

Definitions

The work cited in this section focuses on the general concept of "alcoholism" to allow a synthesis of studies that have been carried on since the 1970s. Technically, the concept under study has evolved through different versions of both American and European diagnostic manuals, coming in the most recent versions to relate to alcohol abuse or dependence (with abuse being the equivalent of hazardous use in the international classification) (Rapaport et al. 1993). As confusing as this array of diagnoses appears at first glance, there is a high level of concordance for the concepts of alcohol dependence across systems, probably reflecting the reliance that each rubric has placed on severe, repetitive alcohol-related problems. In this review, however, whenever possible an emphasis will be placed on studies that actually focus on the concept of alcohol dependence as it relates to biological trait markers, with much less reliance on those studies that appear to focus on less severe problems or drinking practices. Special consideration is given to investigations that demonstrate that the majority of the subjects report alcohol dependence in multiple generations.

Selection of Subjects

In an attempt to avoid confounding influences resulting from the recent effects of alcohol (i.e., state markers), most of the work investigating biological markers of a predisposition toward alcoholism has focused on people who are at high risk for the future development of severe, repetitive alcohol problems. This vulnerability has been defined several different ways, with some studies using a constellation of psychological factors (Sher and Walitzer 1986). However, most investigators believe that such psychological processes are difficult to define as actual predisposing factors, and they have therefore chosen to select their subjects based on the presence of alcoholism in a close relative of the subject.

When observing genetic markers of a predisposition, it seems to make the most sense to emphasize people who have an alcoholic biological parent. To select subjects solely because of alcoholism in a sibling does little to reassure the field that the phenomenon under study is likely to be genetically influenced within that pedigree. An additional methodological consideration relates to the desire to avoid a focus on attributes of an individual that were the result of the fetal alcohol effect (Streissguth et al. 1980), with the result that the majority of investigations select children of alcoholic fathers. If children of alcoholic mothers are included, all possible efforts must be made to delete from the sample those whose mothers were drinking heavily during their period of gestation.

Another consideration of importance is the optimal age at which subjects should be investigated (Schuckit 1992). The selection of prepubertal children has the advantage of being able to determine an individual's attributes before he or she has been exposed to alcohol or other drugs. However, at this young age neither the brain nor the rest of the body has developed to an adult state. Thus, if mature neuronal or hormonal systems are relevant to the marker being investigated, choosing individuals at an exceptionally young age may make it difficult to study some important attributes. In addition, as discussed in the following sections, a number of studies have opted to take advantage of the reaction to alcohol as a potential marker of risk, with the result that ethical considerations argue against the selection of very young subjects. Also, choosing individuals in their late teens as opposed to their prepubertal years has the advantage that prospective investigations can be completed in a shorter period of time (perhaps one or two decades). These studies of older subjects also carry the advantages of body and brain maturity and the ability to gain informed consent for challenges with various substances. However, such investigations must do everything possible to control for the quantity and frequency of alcohol intake before the time of testing for high-risk and low-risk subjects.

Controlling for Additional Genetic Influences

A corollary of the complexity of the genetic data is the need to recognize that severe alcohol-related life problems can appear in the context of a number of major clinical conditions. Thus, there are data to indicate that in the course of the hyperactivity and poor judgment inherent in a *manic* episode, individuals are likely to drink to excess and might at least temporarily fulfill criteria for alcohol dependence (Schuckit 1989). Similarly, men and women with *schizophrenia* have been shown to have higher-than-expected rates of severe alcohol and drug problems that develop in the context of their psychotic illness (Booth et al. 1992). Another complicating factor occurs with those men and women whose severe alcohol-related life problems occur in the context of *antisocial personality disorder* (ASPD), a syndrome characterized by high levels of impulsivity, difficulty learning from mistakes, and problems in establishing close relationships (Hesselbrock et al. 1985). Some of the same attributes are observed with residual *attention-deficit disorder* (Lie 1992). Each of these major preexisting psychiatric syndromes has been shown to exhibit probable genetic influences, but none is observed in the majority of alcohol-dependent individuals. Indeed, many of the twin and adoption studies excluded men and women with obvious preexisting psychiatric disorders. Thus, it is plausible that studies attempting to observe genetic factors that might be uniquely tied to alcoholism should optimally use samples of subjects who lack these additional psychiatric disorders (Schuckit 1992). A corollary is to exclude individuals whose alcoholic relatives only developed their alcohol-related life problems in the context of mania, schizophrenia, ASPD, or another psychiatric disorder.

The Need for Large Samples

The mode of inheritance likely to operate in alcoholism is complex. The best data to date indicate that this disorder is *not* likely to be autosomal dominant or recessive or sex-linked (Chakravarti and Lander 1990; Devor and Cloninger 1989; Schuckit, in press [a]). It is probable that either multiple genes are operating simultaneously (i.e., the inheritance is either oligogenic or polygenic) or that a limited number of dominant genes are involved, but the genetic material does not always express itself as a clinical syndrome (i.e., incomplete penetrance). Further complicating the picture is the probability that environmental factors can increase the chances that an individual will regularly drink heavily, thus increasing the risk of alcoholism. Therefore, even when alcoholism is genetically related, most cases are multifactorial, involving the interaction between genes and the environment. A further implication of the importance of environmental events is the probability that some men and women develop alcoholism solely as a response to environmental influences (i.e., the cases of alcoholism are phenocopies). Finally, regarding genetic complexities, it is possible that the mechanism of inheritance might be different in different pedigrees (i.e., there is genetic heterogeneity).

The combination of the lack of a straightforward Mendelian inheritance pattern, the multifactorial nature of this disorder, and the impact of genetic heterogeneity means that large samples of subjects must be studied before any conclusions can be drawn. A recent meta-analysis concluded that few replicable findings would be likely to emerge in samples of fewer than 100 individuals (50 high-risk subjects and 50 carefully matched low-risk control subjects) (Pollock 1992). Thus, although few studies have samples this large, only investigations with a minimum of 20 individuals in a group (total of 40 subjects) will be relied on for this review, whenever possible.

Importance of Controls

As alluded to briefly above, investigations of individuals at high future risk for the development of alcoholism require a control group for optimal data interpretation. In the studies that incorporate an alcohol challenge, comparisons of individuals at higher and lower future risk for alcoholism can only be optimally interpreted when researchers control for other important factors that relate to the reaction to alcohol and the alcoholism risk (Schuckit 1992). Thus, the two subject groups must be comparable with respect to factors that impact on the distribution of alcohol in their bodies (e.g., the percentage of body fat approximated by the height-to-weight ratio) and factors that are likely to have an impact on the sensitivity to or the rate of metabolism of alcohol (e.g., recent smoking, drinking, drug use history, sex, age, and general physical status) (Schuckit and Klein 1991).

Parameters of the Alcohol Challenge

An additional methodological consideration is important in challenges carried out in individuals at higher and lower risk for alcoholism (Schuckit 1992). To establish optimal replications, the dose of alcohol or other drugs, the route of administration of the substance, and the time over which it is administered must be comparable across studies. Similarly, it is difficult to compare results from studies that only evaluated the reaction to alcohol with results from studies that exposed subjects to electric shock or deliberately contrived stressful situations as part of the challenge protocol.

Summary

Studies of trait markers of a predisposition toward alcoholism differ in their definition of alcoholism, the samples under study, and the methods used to evaluate those samples. The following section offers an overview of the most consistent results generated from the literature, trying whenever possible to place an emphasis on studies that used appropriate definitions of risk, relatively large samples, and appropriate research methodologies. With these thoughts in mind, it is possible to review some of the biological trait markers highlighted in the literature.

ENZYMES AND OTHER PROTEIN MARKERS OF RISK

The following potential markers consist of a disparate group of enzymes and other proteins that are fairly easy to measure, that have been shown to differ between alcoholic persons and control subjects, and for which some limited data are available regarding differences between groups at high and low risk for the future development of alcoholism.

Alcohol-Metabolizing Enzymes

The most convincing data relate to the importance of the multiple forms of the enzyme responsible for metabolizing acetaldehyde, the first breakdown product of ethanol. Although there are many aldehyde dehydrogenase (ALDH) isoenzyme forms, it is the variant known as the low K_m ALDH form that is present in the mitochondria of liver cells and that contributes most to the body's ability to break down the very low levels of acetaldehyde that develop soon after the consumption of low to modest doses of alcohol (Goedde et al. 1985). The relative or absolute absence of this mitochondrial form of ALDH results in high enough levels of acetaldehyde being released into the bloodstream after drinking to cause physiological effects. For individuals who are heterozygous for the absence of this ALDH form, the syndrome observed after drinking consists of facial flushing, palpitations, and some additional physical discomfort. Individuals who are homozygous, lacking any of this low K_m ALDH, are likely to become dramatically ill with nausea, vomiting, and wide fluctuations in blood pressure after less than one drink of alcohol (Goedde and Agarwal

1990; Harada et al. 1983; Suwaki and Ohara 1985). Full or partial absence of this enzyme characterizes one-half to one-third of Chinese, Japanese, Korean, and other related Asian groups. It appears as if individuals who are homozygous for the absence of this form of ALDH rarely, if ever, drink, whereas individuals who are heterozygous do tend to drink, but appear to consume less alcohol during evenings of drinking. There are data indicating that the lower levels of alcohol intake in heterozygous individuals are not solely a reflection of the adverse effects of the beverage, but occur at least in part because heterozygous individuals require less of the drug to achieve desired feelings of intoxication (Wall et al. 1992).

Thus, there are consistent and convincing data that the absence of a genetically controlled enzyme markedly lowers the risk for heavy drinking and subsequent alcoholism in Asian groups. There are no data documenting a similar intense flushing phenomenon among non-Asians, including Native American groups (Goedde et al. 1985).

Multiple isoenzyme forms of the primary enzyme responsible for the initial breakdown of alcohol, alcohol dehydrogenase, also exist. At least one "atypical" form has been identified, with speculations that it, too, might relate to the alcoholism risk, perhaps through affecting the rate of disappearance of alcohol from the blood (Meier-Tackmann et al. 1991; Yoshida 1992). However, few convincing data are available regarding differences between alcoholic persons and control subjects, and no supporting information has been generated from populations at high risk for the future development of alcoholism (Day et al. 1991; Yoshida 1992).

Other Enzymes and the Possible Impact of Neurochemical Systems

Many of the potential biological markers outlined in this section have a wide range of normal values. Others are affected by chronic heavy drinking, making it difficult to determine cause-and-effect relationships between them and the alcoholism risk. Thus, in contrast to the conclusions about ALDH, all of the additional potential markers described in this section must be considered to have at best a tentative relationship to alcoholism.

The first, and probably most widely studied, of these possible markers is the activity level of an enzyme important in the breakdown of a number of neurotransmitters, *monoamine oxidase* (MAO) (Schuckit et al. 1982; Sher 1983; Sullivan et al. 1990). Low activity levels of this enzyme in the brain, at least as implied by activity levels measured in blood platelets, are said to characterize a variety of psychiatric disorders ranging from schizophrenia to ASPD. The association with ASPD jeopardizes the ability to draw coherent conclusions from the literature, because of the possibility that lower MAO activity levels in alcohol-dependent individuals might reflect a subgroup of men and women with ASPD, rather than a phenomenon related specifically to alcohol dependence itself. An additional confounding variable is the finding that high levels of drinking can temporarily lower the MAO activities for weeks to months after abstention (Sullivan et al. 1978). Despite these caveats, several reports (rarely excluding relatives with ASPD from the sample) have demonstrated lower levels of MAO activity in children of alcoholic persons (Sher 1983; Tabakoff et al. 1988).

Additionally, an interesting marker for which at least preliminary data have been developed is *adenylate cyclase*. Compared with control subjects, alcoholic persons have decreased platelet activity of this enzyme (Tabakoff et al. 1988). Another finding relates to *cyclic adenosine monophosphate* levels; lymphocytes in alcoholic persons have been shown to have a 75% reduction in both basal and adenosine receptor–stimulated activity levels of this enzyme (Diamond et al. 1987). Of equal interest is the reduced ability of alcohol to stimulate this enzyme in white cells from alcohol-dependent individuals, even after several generations of cells are raised in tissue cultures.

With respect to specific, measurable genetic markers, perhaps the greatest interest in recent years has been focused on the possible relationship between the alcoholism risk and a specific allele of the dopamine 2 (D_2) receptor gene (Bolos et al. 1990; Noble et al. 1991; Turner et al. 1992). Although original reports of the possible association or linkage of this genetic material with alcoholism itself appeared promising, it has been difficult to replicate these findings. More recent reviews have questioned whether the original association was spurious, or they suggest that this marker might be tied to specific consequences associated with alcohol dependence, especially those that might predispose an individual toward an early or violent death (Conneally 1991; Smith et al. 1992). The latter observation is consistent with the possibility that additional markers might not relate directly to alcoholism but to the enhanced probability of being identified in studies as an "alcoholic case." These could include any genes that increase the risk for problems in alcoholic persons, such as alcohol-related liver disease, psychiatric sequelae, more severe withdrawal syndromes, and so forth (Hrubec and Omenn 1981). For example, there are data supporting the contention that only some alcoholic persons have a genetically controlled heightened predisposition toward developing severe neurological and psychiatric symptoms when their diet is relatively deficient in thiamine (one of the B vitamins). Thus, a genetically controlled deficiency in the thiamine-dependent enzyme transketolase might be used to identify individuals who carry a heightened risk for a specific consequence associated with alcoholism, Wernicke-Korsakoff syndrome (Mukherjee et al. 1987).

Finally, although it is of less immediate importance regarding biological markers of a predisposition toward alcoholism, future study of at least one neurochemical system is warranted. Data from both animal and human experiments indicate that manipulations of the level of the brain chemical serotonin affect levels of voluntary alcohol intake (Naranjo and Sellers 1985). Thus, drugs that either enhance or decrease serotonin activity can have an impact on drinking practices. In response to these studies, a number of laboratories are beginning to look at the possibility that children of alcoholic persons might differ from control subjects with respect to serotonin function. Some preliminary data from our own work has revealed that sons of alcoholic fathers exhibit a higher maximum velocity (V_{max}) for serotonin uptake, which might prevent this chemical from having easy access to other serotonin receptor systems (Rausch et al. 1991).

Summary

This overview of potential markers of alcoholism risk presented a heterogeneous group of proteins and chemicals that are attractive as markers because of the relative ease with which they can be measured. Impressive data are available regarding the relative or absolute absence of the low K_m form of ALDH as a marker of lowered alcoholism risk in Asian groups. However, with this exception, data relating to the other potential markers listed above all suffer from restrictions in sample sizes or the methodologies used, or both, problems that preclude any definitive conclusions regarding the relationship of the markers to future alcoholism risk. At the same time, this review highlights the interest in these potential markers and argues for the need for further research in these areas.

ELECTROPHYSIOLOGICAL MEASURES

Electroencephalographic procedures also carry the potential advantage of ease of measurement. The findings in this sphere grew out of comparisons between alcoholic persons and control subjects, which documented differences that apparently remained even after long periods of abstinence. The usefulness of these procedures is bolstered by the demonstration that many of the electrophysiological characteristics appear to operate under at least partial genetic control (Begleiter et al. 1984; Porjesz and Begleiter 1983).

The most extensively validated of these measures is the positive brain wave observed approximately 300 milliseconds after a rare and difficult-to-discriminate stimulus; that is, the P3 wave of the event-related potential (Begleiter and Porjesz 1988). The finding that, compared with control subjects, alcoholic persons have lower-amplitude P3 waves led to the observation that a similar phenomenon is true in at least one-third of the sons of alcoholic persons, even when they are tested fairly early in life (Begleiter et al. 1984). Although there is some evidence that the lower amplitude of this wave is most characteristic of individuals with relatives who have ASPD (Hesselbrock et al. 1992)—and although not all studies agree with the finding (Polich and Bloom 1988)—the diversity of studies that have documented this phenomenon makes it an important potential marker of risk, especially when testing of the event-related potential incorporates complex visual paradigms (Begleiter et al. 1984).

Another electrophysiological characteristic relates to the differences between alcoholic persons and control subjects with respect to patterns of power of the waveforms that are part of the usual background cortical electroencephalogram. Various reports have indicated that individuals at higher risk for the future development of alcoholism are likely to demonstrate relatively low levels of brain-wave activities in the alpha or lower voltage, faster frequency ranges, and a possible enhanced amount of beta activity (Ehlers 1993; Ehlers and Schuckit 1990; Gabrielli et al. 1982; Pollock et al. 1983). Although the ease of measurement of this factor is attractive, and although numerous studies have indicated the potential importance of the electroencephalogram pattern, the differences in these specific findings across investigations jeopardize any immediate impact that background cortical electroencephalogram studies might have as biological markers of the alcoholism risk.

MEASURES OF COGNITIVE IMPAIRMENT

The electrophysiological findings raise the possibility that alterations in brain waves reflect cognitive attributes of an individual that might relate to a predisposition toward alcoholism. Again, studies of cognitive attributes have the advantage of being noninvasive and relatively inexpensive. Unfortunately, however, impairments in cognition are likely to reflect a variety of influences not directly related to the alcoholism risk itself, including malnutrition, head trauma, severe stress, and fetal alcohol effects (Schuckit et al. 1987). Additional complicating factors can be seen in the relationship of cognitive measures to ASPD, conduct disorder, and attention-deficit disorder, all factors that are relatively independent of alcoholism but that increase the likelihood of secondary severe alcohol-related problems.

With these caveats in mind, comparisons of higher-risk and lower-risk sample groups by means of cognitive evaluations tend to report more similarities than differences. For example, children of alcoholic persons and children of control subjects have relatively similar findings regarding verbal and total intelligence scores, as well as cognitive styles, memory, and measures of school achievement (Schuckit et al. 1987). At the same time, some findings indicate a difference between children of alcoholic persons and children of control subjects, with the former being more likely to show relative impairments in logic and abstract reasoning, although not all studies agree (Drejer et al. 1985; Johnson 1987; Workman-Daniels and Hesselbrock 1987).

PERSONALITY CHARACTERISTICS

For decades it has been theorized that alcoholic individuals develop their problems as a result of a unique pattern of personality characteristics (Blane and Leonard 1987). If so, then these attributes would likely be enduring characteristics of an individual present from early in life and, thus, identifiable before the onset of alcohol dependence (American Psychiatric Association 1987). One genetically influenced and reliably diagnosed personality disorder, ASPD, is characterized by impulsivity and a disregard for rules beginning early in life and is a diagnosis closely associated with the future development of severe alcohol-related life problems (McGuffin and Thapar 1992). On the other hand, as discussed above, ASPD does appear to be an independent disorder with a different premorbid course, response to treatment, and posttreatment patterns of problems than are seen for the usual alcoholic patient (Hesselbrock 1991; Schuckit 1989).

Once the characteristics of the ASPD are set aside, comparisons of recently intoxicated alcoholic persons and control subjects are still likely to reveal a number of personality differences (Blane and Leonard 1987). However, these might be state markers associated with the recent effects of alcohol and associated life stresses, with little evidence that the majority of these attributes predated the alcohol dependence or remained after extended periods of abstinence (Kammeier et al. 1973; Vaillant 1982).

In the final analysis, there is attractive logic to the argument that personality characteristics might be used as markers of a predisposition toward the future development of alcoholism. Unfortunately, there are a host of confounding variables that must be controlled before such speculation can be validated. Once these characteristics are taken into account, there are few impressive findings indicating that a specific identifiable personality attribute can be reliably used in this context.

RESPONSE TO ALCOHOL AND DRUG CHALLENGES

This section describes a group of studies that have focused on variations in subjects' level of response to alcohol as potential predictors of future alcoholism risk.

Evidence of a Decreased Response to Alcohol

These studies grew out of anecdotal reports of some alcoholic persons who, from early in their drinking careers, were able to consume very large amounts of alcohol without obvious evidence of intoxication (Schuckit, in press [a], in press [b]). To evaluate the relationship of this phenomenon to the heightened risk for alcoholism, drinking but non-alcoholic sons of primary alcohol-dependent men (i.e., subjects at higher risk for future alcoholism) were matched with subjects with no known family history of alcoholism on drinking and drug use histories, age, education, smoking histories, height-to-weight ratio, and other relevant factors (Schuckit 1992). Higher-risk and lower-risk subjects were then tested under identical conditions, receiving acute doses of 0.75 ml/kg and 1.1 ml/kg of ethanol or placebo that were consumed over a 10-minute period. The subjects' reactions were then observed during the subsequent 3 to 4 hours (Schuckit, in press [b]; Schuckit and Gold 1988). After the alcohol challenges, the two groups had similar times to the development of peak blood alcohol levels, similar magnitudes of that peak, and (reflecting the care with which they were matched on their alcohol and drug use histories) virtually identical rates of disappearance of alcohol from the blood. However, in this sample, which eventually totaled 454 men (227 matched pairs), those at elevated risk for future alcoholism showed less intense responses to the alcohol challenges. These responses were measured through evaluations of their subjective feelings of intoxication, postdrinking levels of impairment in static ataxia or body sway, changes in electrophysiological measures, and alcohol-related alterations in prolactin, cortisol, and adrenocorticotropin hormone (Schuckit 1990, 1992).

Higher-risk and lower-risk young men originally tested at age 20 were subsequently followed up at approximately age 30 with personal interviews, reports about their behavior from a "significant other" such as a spouse, evaluations of blood markers of heavy drinking, and record searches. Data generated from the first 233 follow-ups, representing over 99% of the men eligible for follow-up by 1991, indicated that the decreased intensity of their reaction to alcohol at age 20 was a potent predictor of future severe alcohol-related life problems (Schuckit, in press [b]). Thus, almost 60% of the sons of alcoholic men who had demonstrated the lowest response to alcohol subsequently developed alcohol abuse or dependence, whereas the same was true for only 15% of the sons of alcoholic men in the higher response range. In other words, even after considering the impact of the family history of alcoholism, in this sample the diminished response to alcohol explained over 80% of the variance of the risk.

A meta-analysis of alcohol challenge studies using similar paradigms and focusing on the subjective responses to alcohol confirmed the conclusion that lower responses to this drug are more likely to characterize individuals at higher future risk for alcoholism than to characterize control subjects (Pollock 1992). At the same time, there are some studies that do not document the lower response to alcohol among individuals at risk for alcoholism. In general, these studies have used alternative testing procedures that involve administration of much lower doses of alcohol, or they have incorporated into the alcohol challenge paradigm manipulations of subjects aimed to evaluate either their response to psychological stress or their reactions to electric shock. Thus, the investigators indicate that the diminished response is not observed with all doses of alcohol or in stressful situations.

A phenomenon potentially related to the decreased reaction to alcohol has been described as the "antagonistic placebo response" (Newlin and Thomson 1991). In these experiments, sons of alcoholic persons demonstrated decreased heart rate, skin conductance, and pulse transit time when exposed to alcohol placebo, a response that was more intense among these men than it was among control subjects. This response has been hypothesized to be an attempt by an individual to maintain homeostasis, and it might contribute to the future alcoholism risk either as a potential mechanism related to the diminished response to alcohol or as a separate phenomenon. An additional group of investigators has reported that young men who have alcoholic relatives in multiple generations (but *not* those with only one generation of alcoholism) are more likely than control subjects to respond to an unavoidable shock with a greater change in heart rate and associated findings (Finn and Pihl 1988). Although more work needs to be done, the studies open up an additional parameter, pain or shock, that should be explored in additional studies. The exaggerated response to shock in these subjects appeared to be more likely to occur with moderate to low doses of alcohol than was true for control subjects. In a related finding, even after exposure to levels of alcohol as low as one to two drinks, individuals at higher future risk for alcoholism reported more dysphoric symptoms after both alcohol or placebo as part of a complex paradigm that required seven evening sessions and observations in a social context (de Wit and McCracken 1990). Another series of studies incorporating a stress-inducing paradigm showed evidence of higher baseline levels of heart rate in high-risk subjects than in control subjects (Hill et al. 1992).

In summary, the possible importance of characteristics incorporated in the reaction to alcohol varies with divergent types of subjects and research paradigms. There are data demonstrating that as a group, the sons of alcoholic men consistently show a diminished intensity of response to alcohol, with evidence from a large sample indicating that this diminished response is a powerful predictor of the future development of alcoholism. Additional research paradigms invoking different baseline measures (before alcohol) or stressful protocols indicate different results that, reflecting the divergent methodologies, are difficult to place into perspective.

Reactions to Other Drugs

The possibility that a diminished response to alcohol at age 20 is a potent predictor of the future development of alcohol abuse or dependence raises the question of whether individuals demonstrating this phenomenon might also exhibit a unique response to other substances. Although any substance of abuse might be incorporated into a challenge protocol, most studies to date have used brain depressants such as the benzodiazepines or barbiturates.

Our own acute challenge paradigm has been broadened to include two additional sessions with 0.12 and 0.20 mg/kg of diazepam infused intravenously over a 10-minute period. Data gathered from 126 men (63 matched high-risk and low-risk pairs) revealed that, with the possible exception of growth hormone, none of the subjective or objective measures of the response to diazepam differed between high-risk and low-risk subjects (Schuckit et al. 1991a, 1991b). However, using somewhat smaller samples and a paradigm with incremental increases in small doses of diazepam over a longer period, another group reported the possibility of a differential response to diazepam in sons of alcoholic persons (Cowley et al. 1992). Similar findings have been observed after challenges with a barbiturate (McCaul et al. 1990).

In summary, in contrast to the results of studies involving acute challenges with intoxicating doses of alcohol, the results from studies comparing high-risk and low-risk subjects on their responses to other brain depressants are contradictory. When one large sample of higher-risk and lower-risk men were given an acute challenge with intoxicating doses of diazepam, there was little consistent evidence of a diminished response to this agent among the men at higher risk. Others studies, using smaller samples and different challenge procedures, reported the possibility that an altered response to benzodiazepines or barbiturates might characterize individuals at high risk for future alcoholism. Additional studies will be required before any definitive answer can be generated.

REVIEW AND SYNTHESIS

Even after considering the important methodological issues that can affect the results, there are a number of possible biological markers of the alcoholism risk. These include a diminished response to an ethanol challenge, the absence of the low K_m form of ALDH, electrophysiological measures such as a diminished P3 amplitude, and several promising protein markers including MAO, adenylate cyclase, and cyclic adenosine monophosphate activity levels. It is important to note that even tentative conclusions can only be drawn from studies of moderately large samples focusing on individuals with primary alcohol-dependent relatives. On the other hand, by focusing on those studies that incorporated more appropriate methodologies, this review runs the risk of having overlooked other promising markers. Thus, a relatively comprehensive literature list has been included to allow the reader to go back to the original manuscripts and draw his or her own conclusions.

None of the potential markers discussed above is likely to constitute a necessary and sufficient condition for the development of alcoholism. In each case, there is likely to be an interaction between a level of vulnerability (e.g., a decreased intensity of reaction to alcohol) and social-psychological influences that affect the decision to drink, to imbibe with some level of regularity, or to expose oneself to high doses of alcohol (Schuckit, in press [a]). One overarching theme could be that each of the relevant factors might exert its influence by increasing the chances that in a heavy-drinking society an individual will drink heavily and regularly. For some men and women, this heavy drinking might occur as a consequence of their need to imbibe higher levels of alcohol to receive the same moderately intoxicating effects experienced by the usual drinker who does not share this diminished intensity of response to the beverage. This higher level of usual intake might then induce further levels of tolerance as both brain and liver enzymes adapt, with an increasing spiral of more and more alcohol required to have the desired effect. In this context, social and interpersonal factors might both reinforce the desirability of alcohol and increase the likelihood of a social support network that includes a disproportionate number of heavy-drinking friends, who might then also contribute to the likelihood of continued heavy drinking. Once psychological or physical dependence or both develop, it might be expected that the attributes of the dependence would themselves then contribute to a high likelihood of continuing to drink heavily.

It is possible that the decreased amplitude of the P3 wave, with its implied decreased ability to discriminate between subtle cues in the environment, might also be associated with the diminished alcohol response. However, genetic factors that affect P3 amplitude and the associated cognitive style might operate independently of the diminished response to alcohol through an increased level of impulsiveness, additional mechanisms that decrease a person's ability to learn from mistakes, or other types of influence.

Even if examples are limited to this small number of potential markers, a major point can be made. In addition to recognizing that no biological marker of alcoholism predisposition is likely to explain all of the variance in the risk for alcoholism among individuals, the findings reinforce the importance of searching for as many biological markers of risk as possible. These markers might represent the results of genetic heterogeneity or the probability that multiple genetic influences interact with the environment to explain the final alcoholism risk.

The intent of this chapter is to provide more than an overview of the current state of the art in the field of biological markers of vulnerability for alcoholism. Hopefully, readers will be able to use the methodological guidelines outlined herein in an effort to take these findings a step further. The more accurate and detailed our understanding of these biological markers becomes, the greater will be our ability to use this information to fashion general educational tools that will help increase the awareness among relatives of alcoholic persons of their heightened risk for this severe, incapacitating, and often fatal disorder. Although the very nature of the genetic influences operating in alcoholism precludes the identification of a 100% risk for any individual, as our levels of knowledge increase it is probable that those relatives of alcoholic persons with the highest (although not absolute) risk can be identified and become the focus for the most intensive prevention efforts. Similarly, further knowledge about the potential behavioral and psychological correlates of these biological factors might help clinicians and educators to develop specific psychological and behavioral techniques to decrease the risk for severe alcohol-related pathology among those individuals at risk who choose to drink.

REFERENCES

American Psychiatric Association: Diagnostic and Statistical Manual of Mental Disorders, 3rd Edition, Revised. Washington, DC, American Psychiatric Association, 1987

Begleiter H, Porjesz B: Potential biological markers in individuals at high risk for developing alcoholism. Alcohol Clin Exp Res 12:488–493, 1988

Begleiter H, Porjesz B, Bihari B, et al: Event-related brain potentials in boys at risk for alcoholism. Science 227:1493–1496, 1984

Blane H, Leonard K: Psychological Theories of Drinking and Alcoholism. New York, Guilford, 1987

Bolos AM, Dean M, Lucas-Derse S, et al: Population and pedigree studies reveal a lack of association between the dopamine D_2 receptor gene and alcoholism. JAMA 264:3156–3160, 1990

Booth BM, Cook CA, Blow FC: Comorbid mental disorders in patients with AMA discharges from alcoholism treatment. Hosp Community Psychiatry 43:730–731, 1992

Chakravarti A, Lander ES: Genetic approaches to the dissection of complex diseases. Banbury Report 33:307–315, 1990

Conneally PM: Association between the D_2 dopamine receptor gene and alcoholism. Arch Gen Psychiatry 48:664–666, 1991

Cowley DS, Roy-Byrne PP, Godon C, et al: Response to diazepam in sons of alcoholics. Alcohol Clin Exp Res 16:1057–1063, 1992

Day CP, Bashir R, James OF, et al: Investigation of the role of polymorphisms at the alcohol and aldehyde dehydrogenase loci in genetic predisposition to alcohol-related end-organ damage. Hepatology 14:798–801, 1991

de Wit H, McCracken SG: Ethanol self-administration in males with and without an alcoholic first-degree relative. Alcohol Clin Exp Res 14:63–70, 1990

Devor EJ, Cloninger CR: Genetics of alcoholism. Annu Rev Genet 23:19–36, 1989

Diamond I, Wrubel B, Estrin W, et al: Basal and adenosine receptor-stimulated levels of cAMP are reduced in lymphocytes from alcoholic patients. Proc Natl Acad Sci USA 84:1413–1416, 1987

Drejer K, Theilgaard A, Teasdale TW, et al: A prospective study of young men at high risk for alcoholism: neuropsychological assessment. Alcohol 9:498–502, 1985

Ehlers CL: EEG fast frequency activity and alcoholism risk in Native American men. Paper presented at the annual meeting of the Research Society for Alcoholism, San Antonio, TX, June 1993

Ehlers CL, Schuckit MA: EEG fast frequency activity in the sons of alcoholics. Biol Psychiatry 27:631–641, 1990

Finn PR, Pihl RO: Risk for alcoholism: a comparison between two different groups of sons of alcoholics on cardiovascular reactivity and sensitivity to alcohol. Alcohol Clin Exp Res 12:742–747, 1988

Gabrielli WF, Mednick SA, Volavka J, et al: Electroencephalograms in children of alcoholic fathers. Psychophysiology 19:404–407, 1982

Goedde HW, Agarwal DP: Pharmacogenetics of aldehyde dehydrogenase (ALDH). Pharmacol Ther 45:345–371, 1990

Goedde HW, Agarwal DP, Eckey R, et al: Population genetic and family studies on aldehyde dehydrogenase deficiency and alcohol sensitivity. Alcohol 2:383–390, 1985

Goodwin DW, Schulsinger F, Moller N, et al: Drinking problems in adopted and nonadopted sons of alcoholics. Arch Gen Psychiatry 31:164–169, 1974

Harada S, Agarwal DP, Goedde HW, et al: Aldehyde dehydrogenase isozyme variation and alcoholism in Japan. Pharmacol Biochem Behav 18:151–153, 1983

Hesselbrock MN: Gender comparison of antisocial personality disorder and depression in alcoholism. J Subst Abuse 3:205–219, 1991

Hesselbrock VM, Hesselbrock MN, Stabenau JR: Alcoholism in men patients subtyped by family history and antisocial personality. J Stud Alcohol 46:59–64, 1985

Hesselbrock VM, O'Connor S, Bauer L: P3 ERP amplitude, family history of alcoholism, antisocial personality disorder and the risk for alcoholism. Paper presented at the annual meeting of the International Society of Biomedical Research on Alcoholism, Bristol, England, June 1992

Hill SY, Steinhauer SR, Zubin J: Cardiac responsivity in individuals at high risk for alcoholism. J Stud Alcohol 53:378–388, 1992

Hrubec Z, Omenn GS: Evidence of genetic predisposition to alcohol cirrhosis and psychosis: twin concordances for alcoholism and its biological end points by zygosity among male veterans. Alcohol Clin Exp Res 5:207–212, 1981

Irwin M, Baird S, Smith T, et al: Use of laboratory tests to monitor heavy drinking by alcoholic men discharged from a treatment program. Am J Psychiatry 145:595–599, 1988

Johnson J: Cognitive performance patterns in school aged children from alcoholic and nonalcoholic families. Paper presented at the joint meeting of the Research Society on Alcoholism and the Committee on the Problems of Drug Dependence, Philadelphia, PA, June 1987

Kammeier M, Hoffman H, Loper R: Personality characteristics of alcoholics as college freshmen and at the time of treatment. J Stud Alcohol 34:390–399, 1973

Lie N: Follow-ups of children with attention deficit hyperactivity disorder (ADHD). Acta Psychiatr Scand 85 (suppl):5–40, 1992

McCaul ME, Turkkan JS, Svikis DS, et al: Alcohol and secobarbital effects as a function of familial alcoholism: acute psychophysiological effects. Alcohol Clin Exp Res 14:704–712, 1990

McGuffin P, Thapar A: The genetics of personality disorder. Br J Psychiatry 160:12–23, 1992

Meier-Tackmann D, Agarwal DP, Fritze G, et al: Distribution pattern of ADH_2 and $ALDH2$ genotypes: relationship to alcohol use and abuse. Paper presented at the joint meeting of European Society of Biomedical Research on Alcoholism and Biomedical Research on Alcoholism, Oslo, Norway, June 1991

Mukherjee AB, Svoronos S, Ghazanfari A, et al: Transketolase abnormality in cultured fibroblasts from familial chronic alcoholic men and their male offspring. J Clin Invest 79:1039–1043, 1987

Naranjo CA, Sellers EM (eds): Research Advances in New Psychopharmacological Treatments for Alcoholism. Amsterdam, Elsevier Science Publishers, 1985

Newlin DB, Thomson JB: Chronic tolerance and sensitization to alcohol in sons of alcoholics. Alcohol Clin Exp Res 15:399–405, 1991

Noble EP, Blum K, Ritchie T, et al: Allelic association of the D_2 dopamine receptor gene with receptor-binding characteristics in alcoholism. Arch Gen Psychiatry 48:648–654, 1991

Polich J, Bloom FE: Event-related brain potentials in individuals at high and low risk for developing alcoholism: failure to replicate. Alcohol Clin Exp Res 12:368–373, 1988

Pollock VE: Meta-analysis of subjective sensitivity to alcohol in sons of alcoholics. Am J Psychiatry 149:1534–1538, 1992

Pollock VE, Volavka J, Mednick SA, et al: The EEG after alcohol administration in men at risk for alcoholism. Arch Gen Psychiatry 40:857–881, 1983

Porjesz B, Begleiter H: Brain dysfunction and alcohol, in The Pathogenesis of Alcoholism. Edited by Kissin B, Begleiter H. New York, Plenum, 1983, pp 415–483

Rapaport MH, Tipp JE, Schuckit MA: A comparison of ICD-10 and DSM-III-R criteria for substance abuse and dependence. Am J Drug Alcohol Abuse 19:143–151, 1993

Rausch JL, Monteiro MG, Schuckit MA: Platelet serotonin uptake in men with family histories of alcoholism. Neuropsychopharmacology 4:83–86, 1991

Schuckit MA: Drug and Alcohol Abuse: A Clinical Guide to Diagnosis and Treatment, 3rd Edition. New York, Plenum, 1989

Schuckit MA: Populations genetically at high risk of developing alcohol abuse or dependence. Current Opinion in Psychiatry 3:375–379, 1990

Schuckit MA: Advances in understanding the vulnerability to alcoholism, in Advances in Understanding the Vulnerability to Alcoholism. Edited by O'Brien CP, Jaffe JH. New York, Raven, 1992, pp 93–108

Schuckit MA: A clinical model of genetic influences in alcohol dependence. J Stud Alcohol (in press [a])

Schuckit MA: Low level of response to alcohol as a predictor of future alcoholism. Am J Psychiatry (in press [b])

Schuckit MA, Gold EO: A simultaneous evaluation of multiple markers of ethanol/placebo challenges in sons of alcoholics and controls. Arch Gen Psychiatry 45:211–216, 1988

Schuckit MA, Klein JL: Correlations between drinking intensity and reactions to ethanol and diazepam in healthy young men. Neuropsychopharmacology 4:157–163, 1991

Schuckit MA, Goodwin DA, Winokur GA: A study of alcoholism in half-siblings. Am J Psychiatry 128:1132–1136, 1972

Schuckit MA, Shaskan E, Duby J: Platelet MAO activities in relatives of alcoholics and controls. Arch Gen Psychiatry 39:137–140, 1982

Schuckit MA, Butters N, Lyn L, et al: Neuropsychologic deficits and the risk for alcoholism. Neuropsychopharmacology 1:45–53, 1987

Schuckit MA, Hauger RL, Monteiro MG, et al: Response of three hormones to diazepam challenge in sons of alcoholics and controls. Alcohol Clin Exp Res 15:537–542, 1991a

Schuckit MA, Duthie LA, Mahler HIM, et al: Subjective feelings and changes in body sway following diazepam in sons of alcoholics and control subjects. J Stud Alcohol 52:601–608, 1991b

Sher KJ: Platelet monoamine oxidase activity in relatives of alcoholics (letter). Arch Gen Psychiatry 40:466, 1983

Sher KJ, Walitzer KS: Individual differences in the stress-response-dampening effect of alcohol: a dose-response study. J Abnorm Psychol 95:159–167, 1986

Smith S, O'Hara B, Persico A, et al: Genetic vulnerability to drug abuse. Arch Gen Psychiatry 49:723–727, 1992

Streissguth AP, Landesman-Dwyer S, Martin JC, et al: Teratogenic effects of alcohol in humans and laboratory animals. Science 209:353–361, 1980

Sullivan JL, Stanfield CN, Schanberg S, et al: Platelet monoamine oxidase and serum dopamine-B-hydroxylase activity in chronic alcoholics. Arch Gen Psychiatry 35:1209–1212, 1978

Sullivan JL, Baenziger JC, Wagner DL, et al: Platelet MAO in subtypes of alcoholism. Biol Psychiatry 27:911–922, 1990

Suwaki H, Ohara H: Alcohol-induced facial flushing and drinking behavior in Japanese men. J Stud Alcohol 46:196–198, 1985

Tabakoff B, Hoffman P, Lee J, et al: Differences in platelet enzyme activity between alcoholics and nonalcoholics. N Engl J Med 318:134–139, 1988

Turner E, Ewing J, Shilling P, et al: Lack of association between an RFLP near the D_2 dopamine receptor gene and severe alcoholism. Biol Psychiatry 31:285–290, 1992

Vaillant GE: Natural history of male alcoholism: is alcoholism the cart to sociopathy. Paper presented at the annual meeting of the American Psychiatric Association, Toronto, Ontario, May 1982

Wall TL, Thomasson HR, Schuckit MA: Subjective feelings of alcohol intoxication in Asians with genetic variations of ALDH2 alleles. Alcohol Clin Exp Res 16:991–995, 1992

Workman-Daniels KL, Hesselbrock V: Childhood problem behavior and neuropsychological functioning in persons at risk for alcoholism. J Stud Alcohol 48:187–193, 1987

Yoshida A: Genetics of alcohol metabolizing enzymes related to alcoholic problems. Paper presented at the annual meeting of the International Society for Biomedical Research on Alcoholism, Bristol, England, June 1992

Chapter 10

Eating Disorders

Denise M. Heebink, M.D., and Katherine A. Halmi, M.D.

The eating disorders are not diseases with a common cause, course, or pathology. They are best conceptualized as syndromes and classified by specific symptom constellations, which appear to result from a complex interplay of psychological, physiological, and environmental influences. The vast majority of persons who develop eating disorders are women.

Anorexia nervosa is a disorder characterized by an intense preoccupation with body weight and food, behavior directed at losing weight, peculiar patterns of handling food, intense fear of gaining weight, disturbance in body image, and amenorrhea. These patients lose weight by drastically reducing their food intake and disproportionately decreasing their intake of carbohydrates and fat. Some patients with anorexia nervosa adopt rigorous, compulsive exercise programs. Others attempt to lose weight by self-induced vomiting and laxative and diuretic abuse. They tend to determine their self-worth by distorted assessments of their body shape and weight. The intense fear of gaining weight continues to exist in the face of worsening cachexia and contributes to these patients' characteristic disinterest in and resistance to treatment. The failure of these anorexic patients to recognize the extent of their emaciation is potentially life threatening.

Bulimia nervosa was first described just over a decade ago and is a disorder in which the primary pathological behavior is binge eating, which is an episodic, uncontrolled, rapid ingestion of large quantities of food over a short period of time. The food consumed during a binge is usually high in calories and has a texture that facilitates rapid ingestion. Abdominal pain or discomfort, self-induced vomiting, sleep, or interruption by another person usually terminates the binge episode. Feelings of guilt, depression, and self-disgust follow. A purging episode aimed at preventing weight gain follows a binge and most often involves the use of cathartics such as self-induced vomiting, laxatives, diuretics, and enemas. A pattern of bingeing followed by severe food restriction or compulsive exercise is also common in this disorder. Bulimia most often develops after a diet. Depression, impulsive behaviors, substance abuse, and problems with interpersonal relationships are often seen in persons with bulimia nervosa.

NUTRITIONAL STATE VERSUS BIOLOGICAL TRAIT

The most potentially useful biological markers are those that are specific for the illness and have some predictive value for prognosis and treatment. In patients with eating disorders, there are disturbances in mood, eating behaviors, weight maintenance, and appetite modulation. How this symptom complex forms is unclear. Neuroendocrine and neurotransmitter disturbances are present in patients with eating disorders and have potential importance in the search for biological markers of this disorder. Most disturbances in these systems are thought to be primarily the result of malnutrition because they generally reverse with weight gain. Adding to the complexity of the search for biological markers in patients with eating disorders is that environmental stress, fluid and electrolyte imbalances, and a mood disorder can affect neurotransmitter and neuroendocrine functioning. Also, it is possible that the behaviors associated with these disorders are in some way an adaptation to a premorbid physiological disturbance.

Designing studies that would eliminate the effects of confounding variables (e.g., mood and nutritional state abnormalities seen in this patient group) is difficult, and prospective studies are impractical. To overcome this problem, investigators have studied patients with anorexia nervosa at various stages of their weight restoration and recovery. Also, patients with bulimia nervosa can be studied when they are actively bingeing and purging and after periods of abstinence from these behaviors.

No specific biological markers have been identified in patients with eating disorders, but much has been learned about potential markers and the pathophysiology of these disorders.

ENERGY REGULATION AND METABOLISM

Anorexia nervosa and bulimia nervosa both have high rates of relapse despite effective treatment. Psychological factors are thought to be the main contributors to relapse, but increasing evidence also supports a role for energy balance and metabolic abnormalities. These studies are reviewed, and potential biological markers are considered, in this section.

Energy Regulation Abnormalities

The subtype groupings of patients with eating disorders are important for meaningful comparisons in a discussion of energy balance and also highlight the heterogeneity within each diagnostic group.

Persons with anorexia nervosa usually demonstrate two types of eating and weight-control patterns. One type is the restricting anorexic patient who loses weight by food restriction (dieting). The other type is the bulimic anorexic patient who restricts food intake but has additional periods of bingeing and purging. Patients with bulimia nervosa are also classified into two subtype groupings: those with normal-weight bulimia with and without a history of antecedent anorexia nervosa.

Anorexia nervosa.   Beginning in the late 1970s, reports of energy balance differences in certain subgroups of patients with anorexia nervosa began to appear in the literature. Two groups reported that bulimic anorexic patients had a greater premorbid weight than nonbulimic anorexic patients (Beaumont et al. 1976). Others reported that anorexic patients who were previously obese gained weight more rapidly than those who were at normal weight before the onset of illness (Walker et al. 1979). Synthesis of these findings might suggest that patients with restricting anorexia require more calories than those with bulimic type to gain and maintain normal body weight.

More recently, other investigators have performed studies examining the caloric needs of different groups of patients with anorexia nervosa. Kaye et al. (1986a) found that restricting anorexic patients require 30%–50% more caloric intake than bulimic anorexic patients to maintain a stable weight. This difference was noted at weights as low as 75% of average body weight and at intervals of up to 1 year after weight restoration. Although it appears that compared with bulimic anorexic patients, restricting anorexic patients have a stable requirement for more calories to maintain their weight at various stages of illness and recovery, these investigators could not conclude that such differences were a trait and thus a potential biological marker rather than the consequence of years of bingeing and vomiting.

Work done by Weltzin et al. (1991) suggested that there was no difference in caloric requirements between subgroups of patients with anorexia nervosa, although this result may be an artifact of the units used to express caloric requirements in their study. Newman et al. (1987) investigated the caloric requirements for weight gain and maintenance in restricting and bulimic anorexic subgroups and in bulimic patients with and without a history of anorexia nervosa. As a group, anorexic patients with a history of bulimic symptoms required fewer calories to maintain weight than anorexic patients without a history of bulimia, although bulimic patients with a history of anorexia nervosa needed more calories to maintain their weight than bulimic patients without a history of anorexia.

In general, studies show that patients with anorexia nervosa have greater-than-normal caloric needs to maintain a stable weight during the first several weeks after weight restoration. However, at 6 months or longer after weight recovery, their caloric needs normalized (Kaye et al. 1986b). Later work by this same group suggested that this increased caloric need is partially the result of increased physical activity during refeeding (Kaye et al. 1988b). These findings support the hypothesis that increased metabolic needs in patients with anorexia nervosa are not a fixed trait and that treatment for weight maintenance in patients with anorexia must be continued vigilantly to prevent relapse when metabolic needs are high.

Bulimia nervosa. As described above, bulimic symptoms in anorexic patients are associated with a decreased caloric requirement for weight maintenance. To investigate this phenomenon further, Gwirtsman et al. (1989b) compared caloric requirements for weight maintenance in bulimic patients with those in a group of healthy control subjects. Bulimic patients ate significantly fewer calories per day to maintain their weight compared with control subjects—1,173 versus 1,694 kcal/day. A prior history of anorexia nervosa, differences in activity level, body weight, or laxative abuse did not seem to alter this caloric need. These results suggest an increased efficiency in caloric use and reductions in daily calorie expenditure in patients with bulimia nervosa.

Decreases in resting metabolic rate in normal-weight bulimic patients have been reported by several groups (Bennett et al. 1989; Devlin et al. 1990; Fernstrom et al. 1990). Altemus et al. (1991) found that in normal-weight bulimic women the resting metabolic rate was decreased significantly from baseline by a 7-week period of abstinence from bingeing and vomiting without weight loss. Another study of bulimic women who were abstinent from bingeing and vomiting for 2–3 weeks and whose weight was stable also showed decreased resting metabolic rate compared with that of healthy control subjects (Obarzanek et al. 1991).

Diet-induced thermogenesis reflects the energy cost of digesting, absorbing, and storing nutrients and is tied to functions of the sympathetic nervous system. Fernstrom et al. (1992) have shown that normal-weight bulimic patients have a profound blunting of diet-induced thermogenesis. Bulimic patients may be efficient at storing calories in their body tissues and gaining weight. An interesting aside is that one study showed that bulimic women did not differ from control subjects in body fat mass, fat cell size, or lipoprotein lipase activity (Devlin et al. 1990). The reduction in diet-induced thermogenesis is consistent with the reduction in resting metabolic rate that has been observed. Whether abnormalities of energy balance in patients with eating disorders result from abnormal eating patterns or from a metabolic predisposition merits further investigation.

Metabolic Abnormalities

In addition to energy intake and expenditure abnormalities, metabolic aberrations have been demonstrated in patients with anorexia nervosa and bulimia nervosa and may give further clues to the pathophysiological mechanisms that contribute to the onset and clinical course of eating disorders.

Anorexia nervosa. The metabolic and thyroid derangements found in anorexia nervosa are similar to those found in starvation, in certain chronic illnesses, and in some cases of depression. These derangements probably represent an adaptive response to inadequate caloric intake and physiological and psychological stress. In anorexia nervosa, thyroxine (T_4) levels are usually normal, triiodothyronine (T_3) levels are decreased (Miyai et al. 1975), and thyroid-stimulating hormone (TSH) levels are normal or slightly decreased (Kiyohara et al. 1989; Vigersky et al. 1976). Blunted or delayed TSH response to thyrotropin-releasing hormone (TRH) has been reported and suggests hypothalamic dysfunction (Casper and Frohman 1982). Kiyohara et al. (1989) reported that after weight recovery in a group of patients with anorexia, T_4 and TSH levels were unchanged and T_3 levels increased but still remained lower than those in control subjects. Earlier investigators reported lowered levels of T_4, T_3, TSH, and thyroxine-binding proteins and an abnormal TSH response to TRH; all showed a significant increase with refeeding (Tamai et al. 1986). Because of their potential reversibility with refeeding and their nonspecificity, thyroid abnormalities found in anorexia nervosa patients are unlikely candidates for biological markers.

Casper et al. (1988) studied menstruating, weight-recovered anorexic patients and nonrecovered, amenorrheic, underweight patients. Recovered patients showed glucose tolerance curves and insulin responses similar to those of healthy control subjects, whereas nonrecovered anorexic patients had persistently abnormal glucose tolerance curves and delayed insulin release. Unesterified free fatty acid levels were persistently higher in both groups of patients than in control subjects. This finding probably reflects the persistence of undereating in recovering anorexic patients. Abnormalities of glucose metabolism appeared to reverse with effective treatment in these patients.

Bulimia nervosa. Metabolic abnormalities associated with semistarvation have been reported with varying frequency in women with bulimia nervosa. Pirke et al. (1985) found elevated blood levels of β-hydroxybutyric acid, free fatty acids, and low T_3 levels—all metabolic signs of starvation—in a majority of anorexic and bulimic patients studied. Devlin et al. (1990) noted that TSH, but not T_3 and T_4, was significantly lower in bulimic patients compared with control subjects. Others have reported decreased T_3 levels in bulimic women (Fichter et al. 1990; Obarzanek et al. 1991). Blunted and delayed TSH responses to TRH stimulation have also been reported (Fichter et al. 1990). The effects of treatment on these metabolic indicators in bulimia nervosa are still to be determined.

Lower-than-normal fasting glucose levels have been found in bulimic women (Devlin et al. 1990; Pirke et al. 1985). Goldbloom et al. (1992) demonstrated that fasting glucose, alanine, pyruvate, fat-derived metabolites, insulin, and glucagon were similar in actively bingeing and purging bulimic women and healthy control subjects. They also measured plasma levels of C-peptide, which is secreted by the pancreas in equimolar amounts with insulin and whose hepatic extraction is fixed. The C-peptide level in bulimic patients was 50% of that in control subjects, indicating a decreased clearance of insulin in the patient group. Another group found that after an intravenous glucose challenge, the blood glucose level and the insulin-to-glucagon ratio remained lower in bulimic patients compared with control subjects for 45 minutes after injection. These observed physiological differences in the bulimic patients were also accompanied by an increased subjective craving for sweets, an enhanced urge to binge, and less subjective control over food intake compared with control subjects (Blouin et al. 1991). Insulin abnormalities might be a potential biological marker for these bulimic-type, subjective responses to increased blood glucose and merit further study.

HYPOTHALAMIC-PITUITARY-ADRENAL AXIS

Corticotropin-Releasing Hormone

Corticotropin-releasing hormone (CRH) is of theoretical interest in a discussion of potential biological markers in eating disorders because preclinical work has shown that exogenous CRH can produce hypothalamic hypogonadism (Rivier and Vale 1984), decreased sexual activity (Sirinathsinghji et al. 1983), decreased feeding (Britton et al. 1982), and hyperactivity (Sutton et al. 1982)—all physiological and behavioral changes associated with anorexia nervosa.

Anorexia nervosa. Hypercortisolism is well recognized in underweight anorexic patients (Walsh et al. 1978). Studies have supported a role for hypersecretion of endogenous CRH in producing this characteristic hypercortisolism (Gold et al. 1986; Hotta et al. 1986). Elevated levels of cerebrospinal fluid (CSF) CRH that normalize with weight restoration have also been reported in patients with anorexia nervosa (Hotta et al. 1986; Kaye et al. 1987a). This finding does suggest that CRH hypersecretion could be due to weight loss alone. On the other hand, the possibility that hypersecretion of CRH may antedate the weight loss in some anorexic patients—particularly those with depression—does exist, as Kaye et al. (1987a) did find a positive correlation between CSF CRH levels and depression in weight-restored but not in underweight patients.

CRH hypersecretion may have a role in maintaining anorexic behaviors and initiating a relapse and therefore may be a potentially useful biological marker.

Bulimia nervosa.   Normal-weight bulimic women have been shown to have normal (Walsh et al. 1987) and elevated (Mortola et al. 1989) 24-hour plasma cortisol levels. Nocturnal circadian patterns of cortisol production have been found to be both normal (Fichter et al. 1990) and elevated (Kennedy et al. 1989). Also, the response of cortisol and adrenocorticotropic hormone (ACTH) to CRH administration has been shown to be normal (Gold et al. 1986) and blunted (Mortola et al. 1989). Actively bingeing and vomiting bulimic patients have demonstrated normal levels of CSF ACTH, plasma ACTH, and cortisol, as well as decreased levels of CSF ACTH after a 30-day period of abstinence from bingeing and vomiting (Gwirtsman et al. 1989a). These conflicting CRH findings need to be clarified and simply may be related to dieting behavior.

Dexamethasone Suppression Test

The dexamethasone suppression test (DST) has been one of the most widely studied biological markers in psychiatry. Results of the DST have been found to be abnormal in some patients with depression, obsessive-compulsive disorder, weight loss and emaciation, Alzheimer's disease, and bulimia and anorexia nervosa. Studies are inconsistent in elucidating a relationship between failure to suppress cortisol production during a DST in patients with eating disorders and affective illness and the degree of weight loss (Fichter et al. 1990; Schweitzer et al. 1990). Inconsistently abnormal results on the DST, which is nonspecific and sensitive to weight fluctuations, are a shared feature of eating disorders and other psychiatric illnesses.

HYPOTHALAMIC-PITUITARY-OVARIAN AXIS

The hypothalamic-pituitary-ovarian axis has been widely investigated in patients with eating disorders because of these patients' concomitant menstrual abnormalities.

Anorexia nervosa.   Amenorrhea is an essential clinical feature in the diagnosis of anorexia nervosa and often precedes substantial weight loss (Halmi 1974). It is well established that basal levels of luteinizing hormone (LH), follicle-stimulating hormone, and estrogen are decreased and 24-hour LH secretion is abnormal in patients with anorexia nervosa. This pattern is similar to that found in cases of starvation but not in cases of affective illness. With weight restoration, the menstrual cycle usually returns and normal LH secretion patterns are reestablished in some but not all patients (reviewed by Weiner 1989). A diminished or absent response of LH to gonadotropin-releasing hormone (GnRH) has been a fairly consistent finding in patients with anorexia nervosa. However, regular injections of GnRH in underweight anorexic women have produced ovulation (Nillius and Wide 1975). This result suggests that pituitary cells manufacturing LH and follicle-stimulating hormone are understimulated in patients with anorexia nervosa because of hyposecretion of GnRH by the hypothalamus. A 10-year follow-up study of patients with a history of anorexia nervosa showed a robust response of LH and follicle-stimulating hormone to GnRH challenge independent of current eating disorder symptomatology (Halmi et al. 1991).

In general, available data do not strongly support a trait abnormality in the hypothalamic-pituitary-ovarian axis as causal or enduring in patients with anorexia nervosa, but certain biological vulnerabilities within this system could predispose an individual to the development of the illness. Aberrations are most likely present in the neurotransmitter systems that influence GnRH release.

Bulimia nervosa.   Amenorrhea and oligomenorrhea occur in the majority of women with bulimia. Intermittent dieting, purging behaviors, and psychological factors could contribute to neuroendocrine changes that produce menstrual abnormalities in bulimic patients.

Although not as exhaustively investigated as it has been in anorexia nervosa, the hypothalamic-pituitary-ovarian axis does appear to be abnormal in patients with bulimia nervosa. Levy et al. (1989) reported that bulimic patients have lower-than-normal basal LH and follicle-stimulating hormone levels and a greater-than-normal response to GnRH. Schweiger et al. (1992) found decreased pulsatile LH secretion in bulimic women with menstrual cycle irregularities but not in bulimic women with normal cycles. Although hypothalamic hypogonadism is one possible explanation for these findings, these investigators did find that elevated plasma cortisol, low T_3, and high β-hydroxybutyric acid levels were associated with abnormal gonadotropin secretion. Animal studies have shown decreased LH secretion after central application of exogenous CRH (Rivier et al. 1984). Increased serum cortisol may reflect increased CRH stimulation in bulimic patients with ovulatory abnormalities. Altogether, these results suggest that alterations in both endocrine and metabolic functions could contribute to menstrual irregularities in bulimia nervosa.

GROWTH HORMONE AND SOMATOMEDINS

Growth hormone (GH) levels have been investigated in both anorexia nervosa and bulimia nervosa as possible neuroendocrine markers. GH is secreted by the pituitary gland under the influence of hypothalamic growth hormone–releasing hormone (GHRH), various neurotransmitters, and peripheral feedback mechanisms. Somatomedin C is secreted from the liver in response to GH stimulation and promotes growth of target tissues.

Anorexia nervosa.   Evidence exists for an impaired regulation of GH in patients with anorexia nervosa, but the underlying mechanisms are unclear. Cabranes et al. (1988) reported increased GH levels in pubertal and postpubertal patients with anorexia nervosa and lower somatomedin C levels in pubertal but not in postpubertal anorexic patients. In studies of anorexic patients, the GH response to clonidine challenge was found to be similar to that of control subjects, but the GH response to GHRH was significantly higher in anorexic patients than in control subjects (Brambilla et al. 1989). This hyperresponsiveness to GHRH and the apparently normal response to clonidine in anorexic patients suggest decreased α-adrenergic sensitivity in these patients. Pirenzepine, a selective antagonist of muscarinic cholinergic receptors, is known to blunt the GH response to GHRH. In acutely ill anorexic patients, pirenzepine has been shown to block the GH response to GHRH only partially, whereas it completely suppressed the GH response in recovered anorexic patients (Rolla et al. 1991). The authors speculated that acutely ill anorexic patients may have increased cholinergic tone in the hypothalamus. Central cholinergic pathways appear to play a role in GH abnormalities seen patients with anorexia nervosa. Abnormalities in GH secretion appear to reverse with nutritional rehabilitation in patients with anorexia nervosa and are therefore not likely to be a useful biological marker.

An impaired GH response to challenges with L-dopa and insulin has been reported in emaciated and weight-restored anorexic patients (Brauman and Gregoire 1975; Halmi and Sherman 1979). Impaired prolactin response to chlorpromazine has been described in weight-restored anorexic patients (Owen et al. 1983). These findings suggest that an abnormality in the central dopamine system may not be related to nutritional factors alone in anorexic patients and deserves further attention as a potential biological marker.

Bulimia nervosa.   Normal-weight bulimic patients have been reported to have a significantly higher mean basal GH level and similar somatomedin C levels compared with control subjects (Levy and Malarkey 1988). These investigators also found that the GH response to TRH was greater in bulimic patients than in control subjects but that somatomedin C levels did not increase in response to GH hypersecretion in bulimic patients. These results suggest that somatomedin C is not affecting the GH hypersecretion in these patients. Other workers have found that in bulimic patients baseline GH levels after clonidine challenge are similar to those of healthy control subjects during the follicular phase, when estrogen status is less likely to affect receptor responsiveness (Kaplan et al. 1989). These results suggest that central abnormalities of noradrenergic receptor responsiveness and GH do exist in bulimic patients.

Another group found that bulimic patients and control subjects had a similar GH response to GHRH, clonidine, and insulin-induced hypoglycemia but that TRH increased GH secretion in bulimic patients but not in control subjects (Coiro et al. 1990). These results suggest that the GHRH-GH axis is intact in patients with bulimia but that GH secretion may be abnormally sensitive to TSH secretory systems.

Whether these GH abnormalities reverse with recovery from bulimia nervosa requires further investigation. Aberrations in GH secretion in both anorexic and bulimic patients may be related to disturbances in GH release or receptor dysfunction, influences of abnormalities in other neurotransmitter systems, or nutritional factors. It is possible that GH abnormalities are a response to fasting states in both bulimia and anorexia nervosa, rather than a response to weight loss alone.

NEUROTRANSMITTERS

Work in the past decade suggests that abnormalities in the neurotransmitter systems of persons with anorexia nervosa and bulimia nervosa may play an important role in the pathogenesis of those disorders. Dysfunction in a neurotransmitter system may be a biological marker that indicates a potential vulnerability for the development of an eating disorder.

Serotonin

Work with laboratory animals has shown that central serotonin (5-hydroxytryptamine; 5-HT) pathways modulate feeding. Administration of 5-HT antagonists results in increased food intake and a consequent weight gain; conversely, administration of 5-HT agonists decreases food intake. 5-HT appears to increase postprandial satiety rather than to decrease appetite (Blundell 1984).

The onset of an eating disorder is frequently marked by a weight-reducing diet—a common event in a weight-conscious culture. Recent work has shown that dieting alters brain 5-HT function more significantly in women than in men (Goodwin et al. 1987). Dieting also reduces the availability of circulating tryptophan, a precursor necessary for 5-HT synthesis, in women but not in men (Anderson et al. 1990). These findings suggest that biological factors along with psychosocial pressures on women to diet may account for the higher incidence of eating disorders in women.

Anorexia nervosa. Whether patients with anorexia nervosa have an abnormality in 5-HT activity that contributes to their abnormal feeding behaviors, relentless pursuit of thinness, and weight loss is an open question.

Low concentrations of CSF 5-hydroxyindoleacetic acid (5-HIAA), a major serotonin metabolite, have been found in low-weight anorexic women compared with themselves after weight restoration and with control subjects—a finding that suggests a starvation-dependent alteration in 5-HT functioning (Kaye et al. 1984a). In another study, Kaye et al. (1991a) found elevated CSF 5-HIAA levels in anorexic women compared with control subjects, suggesting that this trait contributes to pathological feeding behavior and weight loss.

One could speculate that the proclivity in anorexic patients to be rigid, inhibited, ritualistic, and perfectionist might also be associated with increased CSF 5-HIAA levels. Interestingly, these personality traits are also associated with obsessive-compulsive disorder, and 5-HT system abnormalities have been reported in patients with this disorder (Zohar et al. 1988). The association of low levels of CSF 5-HIAA with impulsive, suicidal, and aggressive behavior points to the opposite end of the spectrum (Asberg et al. 1976; Brown et al. 1979).

Peripheral studies of 5-HT activity are inconclusive. Blood platelets are believed to be similar to central monoaminergic neurons with respect to the uptake, storage, and release of 5-HT. Studies of platelet 5-HT uptake in patients with anorexia nervosa have shown no difference from control subjects (Weizman et al. 1986). Urinary excretion of 5-HIAA has been reported to be decreased in anorexic patients compared with control subjects, but it did return to normal with refeeding in a majority of patients (Riederer et al. 1982). Whole blood 5-HT levels in patients with anorexia were found to be higher than those in healthy control subjects, but a subgroup of anorexic patients with affective disorder had whole-blood 5-HT levels that were higher than all others (Hassanyeh and Marshall 1991).

Pharmacological challenge to the neuroendocrine system is recognized as a viable method of investigating brain 5-HT function. Compared with healthy control subjects, women with anorexia nervosa exhibit reduced prolactin responses to *m*-chlorophenylpiperazine (m-CPP), a direct 5-HT agonist, and L-tryptophan, a 5-HT precursor, in both the emaciated state and at normal weight (Brewerton et al. 1990). This work suggests that anorexic patients have reduced postsynaptic 5-HT receptor function in the hypothalamus.

Both 5-HT agonists and antagonists have been found useful in the treatment of anorexia nervosa. Cyproheptadine, a 5-HT antagonist, has been shown to facilitate weight gain in anorexic patients and probably acts on hypothalamic appetite centers to decrease satiety and increase food intake (Halmi et al. 1986). 5-HT reuptake inhibitors (e.g., clomipramine and fluoxetine) are effective in reducing obsessive-compulsive behaviors, which are also seen in relation to food and weight in anorexic patients. Both of these drugs also have been reported to be useful in the treatment of anorexia nervosa and may specifically target the characteristic obsessive-compulsive symptomatology (Kaye et al. 1991b; Lacey and Crisp 1980).

The studies reviewed suggest that alteration in the central 5-HT system could develop as a result of weight loss, persist long after weight restoration, and also contribute to the resistance to weight gain seen in patients with anorexia. Alternatively, it is possible that persons who develop anorexia nervosa have a preexisting dysfunction of the homeostatic mechanisms regulating the 5-HT system, which then becomes easily destabilized by food restriction and weight loss.

Bulimia nervosa.   The symptom patterns of bulimia nervosa and experimental work with animals suggest that an impaired serotonergic response may contribute to the blunted satiety and prolonged periods of rapid food ingestion seen in this illness (reviewed by Brewerton et al. 1990). In addition, disturbances in the 5-HT system have been reported in patients with impulsive behaviors (Asberg et al. 1976; Brown et al. 1979). The bingeing and purging behaviors of bulimic patients are suggestive of impulse-control and satiety-regulation problems and point to a possible role for 5-HT in their genesis.

Jimerson et al. (1992) reported that bulimic patients who binged more than twice a day had a lower CSF 5-HIAA level than control subjects and those who binged less often. This work does suggest that highly symptomatic, bulimic patients could have decreased presynaptic release of 5-HT, although earlier work suggested that as a group, patients with bulimia had normal levels of CSF 5-HIAA (Kaye et al. 1990b). Reduced CSF 5-HIAA levels were found in weight-restored, bulimic anorexic patients compared with restricting anorexic patients after probenecid administration (Kaye et al. 1984b). This finding also indicates that reduced 5-HT metabolism is associated with binge eating.

Peripheral studies of 5-HT regulation and activity are of interest in bulimia nervosa. Work by Kaye et al. (1988a) suggests that bingeing behavior by bulimic patients may be an attempt to increase 5-HT–mediated neurotransmitters and reduce hunger and dysphoria.This hypothesis is based on the fact that carbohydrate consumption can cause an insulin-mediated response that elevates the ratio of tryptophan to large neutral amino acids. This response in turn increases levels of tryptophan in the brain and promotes accelerated 5-HT synthesis and release. Platelet 5-HT uptake has been shown to be higher than normal in bulimic subjects, but no significant correlation among depression scores, body weight, or frequency of bingeing has been found (Goldbloom et al. 1990).

Neuroendocrine studies by Brewerton et al. (1990) demonstrated that bulimic patients given m-CPP had a blunted prolactin response compared with control subjects, suggesting an abnormality of postsynaptic serotonergic neurons. They also found that only bulimic patients with major depression had a blunted prolactin response to L-tryptophan, suggesting an involvement of both presynaptic and postsynaptic serotonergic neurons in this group. Work by McBride et al. (1991) has shown that these patients also have a reduced prolactin response to the 5-HT agonist fenfluramine—a finding that suggests abnormalities in central nervous system responses mediated by 5-HT.

Further evidence for the hypothesis that 5-HT neuropathways are involved comes from the beneficial effect seen when the serotonergic agent fluoxetine is used in patients with bulimia (Fluoxetine Bulimia Nervosa Collaborative Study Group 1992).

Altogether, there is enough evidence of serotonergic dysfunction in both anorexia nervosa and bulimia nervosa to justify a search for a biological marker within this neurotransmitter system.

Norepinephrine

Norepinephrine at near-physiological doses causes satiated animals to eat more and potentiates eating in hungry animals when administered into regions of the hypothalamus known to modulate feeding; this response is thought to occur through α_2-noradrenergic receptors (Leibowitz 1988). In addition, noradrenergic dysfunction can occur during starvation and altered nutritional states (Landsberg and Young 1978). An intrinsic abnormality in the noradrenergic system could contribute to the development and expression of symptoms in persons with eating disorders. Noradrenergic abnormalities are also found in affective illness, which is frequently present in these patients.

Anorexia nervosa. Norepinephrine metabolism appears to be reduced in patients with anorexia nervosa. This reduction at least partially represents a compensatory adaptation to the starvation state, as plasma norepinephrine and urinary 3-methoxy-4-hydroxyphenylglycol (MHPG) levels tend to increase as anorexic patients gain weight (Halmi et al. 1978) and undergo medical stabilization (Lesem et al. 1989). Blood pressure and pulse are dramatically reduced in the starvation state of this illness and normalize with refeeding. Isoproterenol challenge tests to evaluate postsynaptic cardiac β-adrenergic receptor responsiveness in patients with anorexia nervosa during refeeding have shown erratic secretion of plasma epinephrine in response to increasing doses of isoproterenol; a linear response was seen in healthy control subjects (Kaye et al. 1990d). Because presynaptic β-adrenergic receptors serve as a positive feedback loop for synaptic catecholamine secretion, these results may be explained by altered regulation of presynaptic adrenergic receptors during the refeeding of anorexic patients. Again, the nutritional state appears to influence adrenergic function in patients with anorexia nervosa.

Kaye et al. (1984a) found persistently low CSF norepinephrine levels in anorexic patients for almost 2 years after weight recovery. This finding does suggest that brain norepinephrine abnormalities may be an enduring finding in these patients and justifies a search for a biological marker for adrenergic dysfunction in anorexia nervosa.

Bulimia nervosa.   In extrapolating from animal work, one could consider bingeing behavior to be related to increased activity of α_2-noradrenergic systems in the hypothalamus (Leibowitz 1988). However, norepinephrine systems might also be affected by nutritional status, mood, neuroendocrine factors, physical activity, and fluid and electrolyte balance. This possibility, of course, makes it difficult to isolate a potential biological marker for bulimia nervosa.

Studies across a range of settings and methodologies have suggested that the activity of the sympathetic nervous system is decreased in bulimic patients. Plasma norepinephrine concentrations in patients with bulimia nervosa have been found to be lower than those in healthy control subjects (Kaye et al. 1990c), as have CSF norepinephrine concentrations (Kaye et al. 1990b, 1990c). Decreased release of norepinephrine probably contributes to an upregulation of peripheral adrenergic receptor sensitivity (Heufelder et al. 1985).

Various other factors, however, appear to affect noradrenergic activity and suggest a complex pathophysiology. Bingeing itself has been shown to increase plasma norepinephrine to a higher-than-normal level in bulimic patients, and abstinence from bingeing and vomiting appears to lower it—findings that suggest a state-dependent effect (Kaye et al. 1990c). It is also of note that in this study lower CSF levels of norepinephrine were associated with amenorrhea in bulimic women during periods of both bingeing and abstinence. In a another study of actively bingeing patients, CSF MHPG concentrations were normal (Jimerson et al. 1992). Also adding to the conundrum is work by Kaplan et al. (1989), who used the α_2 agonist clonidine in challenge tests in depressed and nondepressed bulimic patients. They found no evidence for adrenergic receptor abnormality at the hypothalamic level in either group. It is unlikely that a marker for noradrenergic activity in bulimia nervosa will be useful.

Dopamine

Animal studies have suggested a role for dopamine and its close links with the opiate system in modulating eating behavior and pleasure-reward responses to food (Morley and Blundell 1988).

No differences in the dopamine metabolite homovanillic acid were found in the CSF of bulimic and restricting anorexic patients after administration of probenecid (Kaye et al. 1984b). Earlier work by Halmi et al. (1983), which showed a reduced response of prolactin to chlorpromazine challenge and of GH to L-dopa challenge, suggested that patients with anorexia nervosa have a defect in the negative feedback system in dopamine synthesis, such as an impairment at the postsynaptic receptor site. Bulimic patients without a history of anorexia nervosa appear to have lower CSF levels of homovanillic acid and a less vigorous dopamine response to a clonidine challenge than bulimic patients with a history of anorexia nervosa (Kaplan et al. 1989; Jimerson et al. 1992). These findings suggest that abnormalities in the dopaminergic pathways could lead to decreased satisfaction after eating, which in turn may facilitate binge-eating behavior. The abnormal pleasure-reward response to food seen in both anorexia and bulimia nervosa patients could be related to dopamine and its role in addictive behaviors. A further search in this area for a marker is warranted.

NEUROPEPTIDES

The neuropeptides have received attention as potential biological markers. Because of their role in regulating satiety, appetite, mood, and neuroendocrine functions, they may contribute to the pathophysiology of eating disorders.

Opioids

Opioid agonists increase and opioid antagonists decrease food intake in animals and humans (Morley 1983).

Anorexia nervosa. In the CSF of severely underweight anorectic patients, higher-than-normal levels of opioid activity have been found;

that activity returns to normal when their weight is restored (Kaye et al. 1982). This is a curious finding because it is unclear whether elevation in opioid activity is a compensatory biological attempt to increase appetite during a time of low caloric intake or a protective response to help decrease the metabolic rate. An increase in opioid activity might partially explain the extreme preoccupation with food seen in these patients. CSF β-endorphin levels are lower than normal in underweight anorexic patients and after short-term restoration, but they return to normal after prolonged weight maintenance (Kaye et al. 1987b). β-Endorphin has been shown to stimulate feeding in animals, and a hypothesis that reduced levels of this peptide contribute to the food refusal observed in patients with anorexia nervosa is worth entertaining. Nevertheless, the reversibility of these changes with long-term weight maintenance suggests that CSF β-endorphin levels are related to state changes rather than to trait changes.

Brambilla et al. (1985) found that anorexic patients have elevated plasma β-endorphin levels, which did not correlate with the degree of weight loss but rather with depressive symptomatology. Later work by this same group showed an increased nocturnal secretion of β-endorphin and a loss of circadian rhythmicity (Brambilla et al. 1991). Plasma levels of β-endorphin reflect pituitary secretion of the peptide and may not necessarily reflect activity in the brain centers that regulate hunger and satiety. A peripheral action of this peptide on opiate receptors in the gastrointestinal tract might, however, exert some feedback influence on central nervous system centers and play a contributory role in the pathophysiology of anorexia nervosa, although this possibility seems remote.

Bulimia nervosa. Patients with bulimia most frequently report bingeing on sweet, high-fat foods—an eating pattern that could be related to findings that suggest that ingestion of sweets can increase endogenous opioid activity (reviewed by Fullerton et al. 1985).

CSF β-endorphin levels have been found to be lower than normal in normal-weight bulimic women and correlate inversely with the degree of depression (Brewerton et al. 1992). Plasma β-endorphin levels have been found to be decreased in bulimic patients and correlated with the severity of the eating disorder but not with the severity of depression in one study (Waller et al. 1986); however, these levels were increased in another study (Fullerton et al. 1986). Another interesting finding is that bulimic women who binged but had not purged by vomiting for 1 month before the study had normal plasma β-endorphin levels, whereas those who were actively bingeing and vomiting had elevated levels of plasma β-endorphin (Fullerton et al. 1988). In one brief trial, the opioid antagonist naloxone was found to decrease bingeing in bulimic patients (Mitchell et al. 1986). In another study, the opioid antagonist naltrexone decreased bingeing in bulimic patients only at doses high enough to produce hepatotoxicity (Mitchell et al. 1989).

An abnormality of the opioid system is present in bulimic patients, but whether it is the result of active bingeing and vomiting or starvation or is a trait feature that might predispose a person to bulimia is unclear from current data. Because the opioids are linked with pleasure-reward systems, it is also possible that the opioids may in some way contribute to the clinical impression that bulimic patients are addicted to their abnormal eating patterns, which at least seem to reduce anxiety if not to produce pleasure.

Cholecystokinin

Cholecystokinin (CCK) is secreted by the gastrointestinal system in response to food intake and is thought to signal the brain by way of the vagus nerve. CCK in both the central nervous system and the periphery has been shown in animals to promote satiety—a finding that has prompted investigation of its potential role in the etiology of eating disorders.

Anorexia nervosa.   Persons with anorexia nervosa have been found to experience more satiety and less-than-normal hunger while fasting and after eating; this condition reverses with short-term weight restoration (Halmi et al. 1989). In a study of fasting and postprandial plasma CCK concentrations in anorexic women, normal levels were found both when the women were underweight and after short-term weight restoration (Geracioti et al. 1992). These findings do not support a role for the hypersecretion of CCK in the etiology of anorexia nervosa.

Bulimia nervosa.   In theory, reduced CCK levels could be associated with bingeing behavior. Geracioti and Liddle (1988) found that after a meal bulimic women had a significantly impaired total plasma CCK response and abnormal postprandial satiety. Fasting CCK levels were normal. Interestingly, this group also found that a trial of tricyclic antidepressants tended to increase the postprandial CCK response and satiety. Abstinence from bingeing and vomiting alone might also account for this increase in postprandial CCK response.

Neuropeptide Y and Peptide YY

Neuropeptide Y (NPY) is abundantly found in the central nervous system. NPY has been shown in animals to be one of the most potent endogenous stimulants to feeding behavior and is selective for carbohydrate-rich foods (Stanley et al. 1985).

Peptide YY (PYY), even more potent than NPY in promoting feeding, is found in lower concentrations in the brain than NPY and is also selective for carbohydrate-rich foods (Morley et al. 1985). Because both peptides are found in the hypothalamus and powerfully modulate eating behavior, they could contribute to the pathophysiology of eating disorders and be hypothetical biological markers.

Anorexia nervosa. Underweight anorexic women have been found to have normal CSF PYY concentrations and elevated CSF NPY concentrations, which remained significantly elevated after short-term weight restoration (Kaye et al. 1990a). These investigators also found that CSF NPY levels normalized with long-term weight restoration in the women who regained regular menstruation but were elevated in those who remained amenorrheic or oligomenorrheic. This finding suggests that elevations in CSF NPY after weight gain may contribute to the persistent menstrual pathophysiology seen in some women with anorexia nervosa.

Elevations in NPY do not appear to stimulate eating in women with anorexia, who are notoriously reluctant to increase their food intake, but may play a role in their puzzling, obsessional interest in food and its preparation. This persistent elevation of NPY causes down-regulation of the NPY receptors that modulate feeding and so contributes to the food refusal and avoidance of sweets so characteristic of patients ill with anorexia nervosa.

Bulimia nervosa. CSF PYY concentrations have been found to be normal when bulimic patients are actively bingeing and vomiting and elevated after 30 days of abstinence. CSF NPY values remain normal before and after the abstinent period (Kaye et al. 1990a).

The cause of this reported elevation of PYY after abstinence from bingeing and vomiting in bulimic patients is unknown. The characteristic abnormal eating pattern could in some way alter the regulation of PYY secretion in the brain, and the sudden cessation of bingeing and vomiting could cause regulatory systems to dysfunction. Another intriguing interpretation of these data is that elevation of CSF PYY is a trait in persons vulnerable to the development of bulimia and that bingeing and vomiting are an attempt to normalize some intrinsic aberration. It is also possible that this PYY abnormality contributes to the uncontrollable drive to eat and the craving for sweets seen during binges.

Vasopressin and Oxytocin

Vasopressin is a neuropeptide of hypothalamic origin that is transported to the posterior pituitary for release into the systemic circulation. In the kidney, vasopressin controls free-water clearance. Oxytocin is structurally related to vasopressin and promotes uterine contraction during parturition and milk production during the postpartum period. Oxytocin appears to disrupt memory consolidation and retrieval, whereas vasopressin promotes the consolidation of learning. Oxytocin also inhibits vasopressin-induced release of ACTH from the anterior pituitary gland.

Anorexic patients have been shown to have an impaired ability to concentrate urine (Vigersky et al. 1976). Underweight anorexic patients have abnormally high levels of plasma and CSF vasopressin, which are gradually normalized with weight gain (Gold et al. 1983). Demitrack et al. (1990) have shown that underweight anorexic patients also have reduced CSF oxytocin levels, which return to normal with weight restoration. Although CSF vasopressin and oxytocin levels are unlikely markers for eating disorders, an interesting interaction between these neuropeptides might exist. Demitrack et al. hypothesized that a low level of oxytocin and a high level of vasopressin could work in concert to enhance the retention of distorted thinking and contribute to the anorexic patient's obsessional concerns about food.

Work by Nishita et al. (1989) showed that abnormalities in vasopressin secretion also occur during hypertonic saline infusion in underweight and weight-restored anorexic patients and in bulimic patients. Vasopressin abnormalities in the bulimic patients are probably epiphenomena of the electrolyte changes associated with self-induced vomiting.

NEUROIMAGING STUDIES

Neuroradiological abnormalities and postmortem morphological changes in the brains of patients with anorexia nervosa have been recognized. An increased brain ventricular size and sulcal widening on computed tomographic brain scans have been reported in a vast majority of underweight anorexic patients and about a third of bulimic patients. These abnormalities tend to reverse with improved nutrition and weight gain. Ventricular size has been inversely correlated with T_3 levels (Krieg et al. 1988, 1989). Magnetic resonance imaging has revealed that anorexic and bulimic patients have evidence of pituitary atrophy (Doraiswamy et al. 1990). Positron-emission tomography of underweight anorexic patients showed hypermetabolism in the caudate nucleus bilaterally that reversed with weight gain (Herholz et al. 1987). Brain structure and metabolic changes seen in these studies seem to reflect state changes only.

BONE MINERAL DENSITY

In patients with anorexia nervosa, decreased bone mineral density and an increased rate of osteoporosis are well established and may result in pathological bone fractures. Hypercortisolism, low nutrient intake, low body weight, early onset and enduring amenorrhea, low calcium intake, and reduced physical activity appear to play a role in the decreased bone density seen in patients with anorexia (reviewed by Salisbury and Mitchell 1991). Bulimic patients have been reported to have normal bone density (Newman and Halmi 1989).

CONCLUSION

Although specific biological markers that identify eating disorders and potentially predict prognosis and treatment outcome are still to be identified, this review does yield areas for further investigation. Pursuit of markers for energy balance and insulin abnormalities, CRH secretion aberrations, and serotonergic, noradrenergic, and dopaminergic neurotransmitter dysfunction appears most promising.

Alterations observed in neuroendocrine and neurotransmitter systems, energy regulation, and bone and brain structure in patients with eating disorders are embedded in a complex matrix of nutritional, psychological, and environmental factors that makes it difficult to discern what is cause and what is effect. It is probable in anorexia nervosa that intrinsic biological factors, dieting, and psychosocial influences are somehow catalytic; however, once weight loss and malnutrition occur, a downward spiral of physiological changes perpetuates the desire for more dieting and weight loss. In patients with bulimia nervosa, it is possible that extremes in food intake and purging set in motion neurochemical changes that somehow sustain the abnormal eating patterns, and a vicious cycle develops. Although the pathophysiology of eating disorders continues to be investigated and potential biological markers continue to be isolated, the precise etiology of both anorexia nervosa and bulimia nervosa remains unknown.

REFERENCES

Altemus M, Hetherington MM, Flood M, et al: Decrease in resting metabolic rate during abstinence from bulimic behavior. Am J Psychiatry 148:1071–1072, 1991

Anderson IM, Parry-Billings M, Newsholme EA, et al: Dieting reduces plasma tryptophan and alters brain 5-HT function in women. Psychol Med 20:785–791, 1990

Asberg M, Traskman L, Thoren P: 5-HIAA in the cerebrospinal fluid: a biochemical suicide predictor? Arch Gen Psychiatry 33:1193–1197, 1976

Beaumont PJV, George GCW, Smart DE: "Dieters" and "vomiters" in anorexia nervosa. Psychol Med 6:617–622, 1976

Bennett SM, Williamson DA, Powers SK: Bulimia nervosa and resting metabolic rate. International Journal of Eating Disorders 8:417–424, 1989

Blouin AG, Blouin JH, Braaten JT, et al: Physiological and psychological responses to a glucose challenge in bulimia. International Journal of Eating Disorders 10:285–296, 1991

Blundell JE: Serotonin and appetite. Neuropharmacology 23:1537–1551, 1984

Brambilla F, Cavagnini F, Invitti C, et al: Neuroendocrine and psychopathological measures in anorexia nervosa: resemblances to primary affective disorders. Psychiatry Res 16:165–176, 1985

Brambilla F, Massironi R, Ferrari E, et al: Alpha-2-adrenoceptor sensitivity in anorexia nervosa: GH response to clonidine or GHRH stimulation. Biol Psychiatry 25:256–264, 1989

Brambilla F, Ferrari E, Petraglia F, et al: Peripheral opioid secretory pattern in anorexia nervosa. Psychiatry Res 39:115–127, 1991

Brauman H, Gregoire F: The growth hormone response to insulin induced hypoglycemia in anorexia nervosa and control underweight normal subjects. J Clin Invest 5:289–295, 1975

Brewerton TD, Brandt HA, Lessem MD, et al: Serotonin in eating disorders, in Serotonin in Major Psychiatric Disorder. Edited by Coccaro EF, Murphy DL. Washington, DC, American Psychiatric Press, 1990, pp 153–184

Brewerton TD, Lydiard RB, Laraia MT, et al: CSF beta-endorphin and dynorphin in bulimia nervosa. Am J Psychiatry 149:1086–1090, 1992

Britton DR, Koob GR, Rivier J, et al: Intraventricular corticotropin-releasing factor enhances behavioral effects of novelty. Life Sci 31:363–367, 1982

Brown GL, Goodwin FK, Ballenger JC, et al: Aggression in humans correlates with cerebrospinal fluid amine metabolites. Psychiatry Res 1:131–139, 1979

Cabranes JA, Almoguera I, Santos JL, et al: Somatomedin-C and growth hormone levels in anorexia nervosa in relation to the pubertal or postpubertal stages. Prog Neuropsychopharmacol Biol Psychiatry 6:865–871, 1988

Casper RC, Frohman D: Delayed TSH response in anorexia nervosa following injection of thyrotropin-releasing hormone (TRH). Psychoneuroendocrinology 7:59–68, 1982

Casper RC, Pandey G, Jaspan JB, et al: Eating attitudes and glucose tolerance in anorexia nervosa patients at 8-year follow-up compared to control subjects. Psychiatry Res 25:283–299, 1988

Coiro V, Capretti L, d'Amato L, et al: Growth hormone responses to growth hormone-releasing hormone, clonidine and insulin-induced hypoglycemia in normal weight bulimic women. Neuropsychobiology 23:8–14, 1990

Demitrack MA, Lesem MD, Listwak SJ, et al: CSF oxytocin in anorexia nervosa and bulimia nervosa: clinical and pathophysiologic considerations. Am J Psychiatry 147:882–886, 1990

Devlin MJ, Walsh T, Kral JG, et al: Metabolic abnormalities in bulimia nervosa. Arch Gen Psychiatry 47:144–148, 1990

Doraiswamy PM, Krishnan KRR, Figiel GS, et al: A brain magnetic resonance imaging study of pituitary gland morphology in anorexia nervosa and bulimia. Biol Psychiatry 28:110–116, 1990

Fernstrom MH, Weltzin TE, McConaha C, et al: Resting metabolic rate and diet-induced thermogenesis are reduced in patients with normal weight bulimia, in Abstracts of European Winter Conference on Brain Research Annual Meeting, 1990

Fernstrom MH, Weltzin TE, Kaye WH: Metabolic changes, in Psychobiology and Treatment of Anorexia Nervosa and Bulimia Nervosa. Edited by Halmi KA. Washington, DC, American Psychiatric Press, 1992, pp 221–234

Fichter MM, Pirke KM, Pollinger J, et al: Disturbances in the hypothalamo-pituitary-adrenal and other neuroendocrine axes in bulimia. Biol Psychiatry 27:1021–1037, 1990

Fluoxetine Bulimia Nervosa Collaborative Study Group: Fluoxetine in the treatment of bulimia nervosa. Arch Gen Psychiatry 49:139–147, 1992

Fullerton DT, Getto CJ, Swift WJ, et al: Sugar, opioids and binge eating. Brain Res Bull 14:673–680, 1985

Fullerton DT, Swift WJ, Getto CJ, et al: Plasma immunoreactive beta-endorphin in bulimics. Psychol Med 16:59–63, 1986

Fullerton DT, Swift WJ, Getto CJ, et al: Differences in the plasma beta-endorphin levels of bulimics. International Journal of Eating Disorders 7:191–200, 1988

Geracioti TD, Liddle RA: Impaired cholecystokinin secretion in bulimia nervosa. N Engl J Med 319:683–688, 1988

Geracioti TD, Liddle RA, Altemus M, et al: Regulation of appetite and cholecystokinin secretion in anorexia nervosa. Am J Psychiatry 149:958–961, 1992

Gold PW, Kaye WH, Robertson GL, et al: Abnormalities in plasma and cerebrospinal-fluid arginine vasopressin in patients with anorexia nervosa. N Engl J Med 308:1117–1123, 1983

Gold PW, Gwirtsman H, Avgerinos TC, et al: Abnormal hypothalamic-pituitary-adrenal function in anorexia nervosa: pathophysiologic mechanisms in underweight and weight-corrected patients. N Engl J Med 314:1335–1342, 1986

Goldbloom DS, Hicks LK, Garfinkel PE: Platelet serotonin uptake in bulimia nervosa. Biol Psychiatry 28:644–647, 1990

Goldbloom DS, Zinman B, Hicks LK, et al: The baseline metabolic state in bulimia nervosa: abnormality and adaptation. International Journal of Eating Disorders 12:171–178, 1992

Goodwin GM, Fairburn CG, Cowen PJ: Dieting changes serotonergic function in women not men: implications for the aetiology of anorexia nervosa? Psychol Med 17:839–842, 1987

Gwirtsman HE, Kaye WH, George DT, et al: Central and peripheral ACTH and cortisol levels in anorexia nervosa and bulimia. Arch Gen Psychiatry 46:61–69, 1989a

Gwirtsman HE, Kaye WH, Obarzanek E, et al: Decreased caloric intake in normal-weight patients with bulimia: comparison with female volunteers. Am J Clin Nutr 49:86–92, 1989b

Halmi KA: Anorexia nervosa: demographic and clinical features in 94 cases. Psychosom Med 36:18–26, 1974

Halmi KA, Sherman BM: Prediction of treatment response in anorexia nervosa, in Biological Psychiatry Today. Edited by Obiols J, Ballus C, Monclus E, et al. New York, Elsevier/North Holland Biomedical, 1979, pp 609–614

Halmi KA, Dekirmenjian H, Davis JM, et al: Catecholamine metabolism in anorexia nervosa. Arch Gen Psychiatry 35:458–460, 1978

Halmi KA, Owen WP, Lasley E, et al: Dopaminergic regulation in anorexia nervosa. International Journal of Eating Disorders 2:129–133, 1983

Halmi KA, Eckert E, LaDu T, et al: Anorexia nervosa treatment efficacy of cyproheptadine and amitriptyline. Arch Gen Psychiatry 43:177–181, 1986

Halmi KA, Sunday S, Puglisi A, et al: Hunger and satiety in anorexia nervosa and bulimia nervosa. Ann N Y Acad Sci 575:431–444, 1989

Halmi KA, Stokes P, Eckert E, et al: FSH and LH responses to GnRH in anorexia nervosa patients and ten-year follow-up. Biol Psychiatry 2:305–307, 1991

Hassanyeh F, Marshall EF: Measures of serotonin metabolism in anorexia nervosa. Acta Psychiatr Scand 84:561–563, 1991

Herholz K, Krieg JC, Emrich HM, et al: Regional cerebral glucose metabolism in anorexia nervosa measured by positron emission tomography. Biol Psychiatry 22:43–51, 1987

Heufelder A, Warnoff, Pirke KM: Platelet alpha-2 adrenoceptor and adenylate cyclase in patients with anorexia nervosa and bulimia. J Clin Endocrinol Metab 61:1053–1060, 1985

Hotta M, Shibasaki T, Masuda A, et al: The responses of plasma adrenocorticotropin and cortisol to corticotropin-releasing hormone (CRH) and cerebrospinal fluid immunoreactive CRH in anorexia nervosa patients. J Clin Endocrinol Metab 62:319–324, 1986

Jimerson DC, Lesem MD, Kaye WH, et al: Low serotonin and dopamine metabolite concentrations in cerebrospinal fluid from bulimic patients with frequent binge episodes. Arch Gen Psychiatry 49:132–138, 1992

Kaplan AS, Garfinkel PE, Warsh JJ, et al: Clonidine challenge test in bulimia nervosa. International Journal of Eating Disorders 8:425–435, 1989

Kaye WH, Pickar D, Naber D, et al: Cerebrospinal fluid opioid activity in anorexia nervosa. Am J Psychiatry 139:643–645, 1982

Kaye WH, Ebert MH, Raleigh M, et al: Abnormalities in CNS monoamine metabolism in anorexia nervosa. Arch Gen Psychiatry 41:350–355, 1984a

Kaye WH, Ebert MH, Gwirtsman HE, et al: Differences in brain serotonergic metabolism between nonbulimic and bulimic patients with anorexia nervosa. Am J Psychiatry 141:1598–1601, 1984b

Kaye WH, Gwirtsman HE, Obarzanek E, et al: Caloric intake necessary for weight maintenance in anorexia nervosa: nonbulimics require greater caloric intake than bulimics. Am J Clin Nutr 44:435–443, 1986a

Kaye WH, Gwirtsman HE, George T, et al: Caloric consumption and activity levels in anorexia nervosa: a prolonged delay in normalization. International Journal of Eating Disorders 5:489–502, 1986b

Kaye WH, Gwirtsman HE, George DT, et al: Elevated cerebrospinal fluid levels of immunoreactive corticotropin-releasing hormone in anorexia nervosa: relation to state of nutrition, adrenal function, and intensity of depression. J Clin Endocrinol Metab 64:203–208, 1987a

Kaye WH, Berrettini W, Gwirtsman H, et al: Reduced cerebrospinal fluid levels of immunoreactive pro-opiomelanocortin related peptides (including beta-endorphin) in anorexia nervosa. Life Sci 41:2147–2155, 1987b

Kaye WH, Gwirtsman HE, Brewerton TD, et al: Bingeing behavior and plasma amino acids: a possible involvement of brain serotonin in bulimia nervosa. J Psychiatr Res 23:31–43, 1988a

Kaye WH, Gwirtsman HE, Obarzanek E, et al: Relative importance of caloric intake needed to gain weight and level of physical activity in anorexia nervosa. Am J Clin Nutr 47:987–994, 1988b

Kaye WH, Berrettini W, Gwirtsman H, et al: Altered cerebrospinal fluid neuropeptide Y and peptide YY immunoreactivity in anorexia and bulimia nervosa. Arch Gen Psychiatry 47:548–556, 1990a

Kaye WH, Ebert MH, Gwirtsman HE, et al: CSF monoamine levels in normal weight bulimia: evidence for abnormal noradrenergic activity. Am J Psychiatry 147:225–229, 1990b

Kaye WH, Gwirtsman HE, George DT, et al: Disturbances of noradrenergic systems in normal-weight bulimia: relationship to diet and menses. Biol Psychiatry 27:4–21, 1990c

Kaye WH, George DT, Gwirtsman HE, et al: Isoproterenol infusion test in anorexia nervosa: assessment of pre- and post-beta-noradrenergic receptor activity. Psychopharmacol Bull 26:355–359, 1990d

Kaye WH, Gwirtsman HE, George DT, et al: Altered serotonin activity in anorexia nervosa after long-term weight restoration. Arch Gen Psychiatry 48:556–562, 1991a

Kaye WH, Weltzin TE, Hsu LKG, et al: An open trial of fluoxetine in patients with anorexia nervosa. J Clin Psychiatry 52:464–471, 1991b

Kennedy SH, Garfinkel PE, Parienti V, et al: Changes in melatonin levels but not cortisol levels are associated with depression in patients with eating disorder. Arch Gen Psychiatry 46:73–78, 1989

Kiyohara K, Tamai H, Takaichi Y, et al: Decreased thyroidal triiodothyronine secretion in patients with anorexia nervosa: influence of weight recovery. Am J Clin Nutr 50:767–772, 1989

Krieg JC, Pirke KM, Lauer C, et al: Endocrine, metabolic and cranial computed tomographic findings in anorexia nervosa. Biol Psychiatry 23:377–387, 1988

Krieg JC, Lauer C, Pirke KM: Structural brain abnormalities in patients with bulimia nervosa. Psychiatry Res 27:39–48, 1989

Lacey JH, Crisp AH: Hunger, food intake and weight: the impact of clomipramine on a refeeding anorexia nervosa population. Postgrad Med J 56 (suppl 1):79–85, 1980

Landsberg L, Young JB: Fasting, feeding and the regulation of sympathetic activity. N Engl J Med 298:1295–1301, 1978

Leibowitz SF: Hypothalamic paraventricular nucleus: interaction between alpha-2-noradrenergic system and circulating hormones and nutrients in relation to energy balance. Neurosci Biobehav Rev 12:101–109, 1988

Lesem MD, George DT, Kaye WH, et al: State-related changes in norepinephrine regulation in anorexia nervosa. Biol Psychiatry 25:509–512, 1989

Levy AB, Malarkey WB: Growth hormone and somatomedin C in bulimia. Psychoneuroendocrinology 13:359–362, 1988

Levy AB, Dixon KN, Malarkey WIS, et al: Gonadotropin response to LRH in anorexia nervosa and bulimia. Biol Psychiatry 26:425–427, 1989

McBride PA, Anderson GM, Khait VD, et al: Serotonergic responsiveness in eating disorders. Psychopharmacol Bull 27:365–372, 1991

Mitchell JE, Laine DE, Morley JE, et al: Naloxone but not CCK-8 may attenuate binge-eating in patients with the bulimia syndrome. Biol Psychiatry 21:1399–1406, 1986

Mitchell JE, Christenson G, Jennings J, et al: A placebo-controlled, double-blind crossover study of naltrexone hydrochloride in outpatients with normal-weight bulimia. J Clin Pharmacol 9:94–97, 1989

Miyai K, Yamamoto T, Azukizawa M, et al: Serum thyroid hormones and thyrotropin in anorexia nervosa. J Clin Endocrinol Metab 40:334–338, 1975

Morley JE: Neuroendocrine effects of endogenous opioid peptides in human subjects: a review. Psychoneuroendocrinology 8:361–379, 1983

Morley JE, Blundell JE: The neurobiological basis of eating disorders. Biol Psychiatry 23:53–78, 1988

Morley JE, Levine AS, Grace M, et al: Peptide YY (PYY), a potent orexigenic agent. Brain Res 341:200–203, 1985

Mortola JF, Rasmussen DD, Yen SSC: Alterations of the adrenocorticotropin-cortisol axis in normal weight bulimic women: evidence for a central mechanism. J Clin Endocrinol Metab 68:517–522, 1989

Newman MM, Halmi KA: Relationship of bone density to estradiol and cortisol in anorexia nervosa and bulimia. Psychiatry Res 29:105–112, 1989

Newman MM, Halmi KA, Marchi P: Relationship of clinical factors to caloric requirements in subtypes of eating disorders. Biol Psychiatry 22:1253–1263, 1987

Nillius SJ, Wide L: Gonadotrophin-releasing hormone treatment for induction of follicular maturation and ovulation in amenorrhoeic women with anorexia nervosa. BMJ 3:405–408, 1975

Nishita JK, Ellinwood EH, Rockwell WJK, et al: Abnormalities in the response of plasma arginine vasopressin during hypertonic saline infusion in patients with eating disorders. Biol Psychiatry 26:73–86, 1989

Obarzanek E, Lesem MD, Goldstein DS, et al: Reduced resting metabolic rate in patients with bulimia nervosa. Arch Gen Psychiatry 48:456–462, 1991

Owen NP, Halmi KA, Lasley E, et al: Dopamine regulation in anorexia nervosa. Psychopharmacol Bull 19:4, 578, 1983

Pirke KM, Pahl J, Schweiger U, et al: Metabolic and endocrine indices of starvation in bulimia: a comparison with anorexia nervosa. Psychiatry Res 15:33–39, 1985

Riederer R, Toifl K, Kruzik P: Excretion of biogenic amine metabolites in anorexia nervosa. Clin Chim Acta 123:27–32, 1982

Rivier C, Vale W: Influence of corticotropin-releasing factor on reproductive functions in the rat. Endocrinology 114:914–921, 1984

Rolla M, Andreoni A, Belliti D, et al: Blockade of cholinergic muscarinic receptors by pirenzepine and GHRH-induced secretion in the acute and recover phase of anorexia nervosa and atypical eating disorders. Biol Psychiatry 29:1079–1091, 1991

Salisbury JJ, Mitchell JE: Bone mineral density and anorexia nervosa in women. Am J Psychiatry 148:768–774, 1991

Schweiger U, Pirke KM, Lasessle RG, et al: Gonadotropin secretion in bulimia nervosa. J Clin Endocrinol Metab 74:722–727, 1992

Schweitzer I, Szmukler GI, Maguire KP, et al: The dexamethasone suppression test in anorexia nervosa. The influence of weight, depression, adrenocorticotrophic hormone and dexamethasone. Journal of Psychiatry 157:713–717, 1990

Sirinathsinghji DJ, Rees LH, Rivier J, et al: Corticotropin-releasing factor is a potent inhibitor of sexual receptivity in the female rat. Nature 305:232–235, 1983

Stanley BC, Daniel DR, Chin AS, et al: Paraventricular nucleus injections of peptide YY and neuropeptide Y preferentially enhance carbohydrate ingestion. Peptides 6:1205–1211, 1985

Sutton RE, Koob GF, LeMoul M: Corticotropin-releasing factor produces behavioral activation in rats. Nature 297:331–333, 1982

Tamai H, Kobayashi N, Fukata S, et al: Paradoxical responses of plasma cortisol, adrenocorticotropic hormone and growth hormone to thyrotropin-releasing hormone and luteinizing hormone–releasing hormone in anorexia nervosa patients. Psychother Psychosom 46:147–151, 1986

Vigersky RA, Loriaux DL, Andersen AE, et al: Anorexia nervosa: behavioral and hypothalamic aspects. Clinical Endocrinology and Metabolism 5:517–535, 1976

Walker J, Roberts SI, Halmi KA, et al: Caloric requirements for weight gain in anorexia nervosa. Am J Clin Nutr 32:1396–1400, 1979

Waller DS, Kiser RS, Hardy BW et al: Eating behavior and plasma beta-endorphin in bulimia. Am J Clin Nutr 44:20–23, 1986

Walsh BT, Stewart JW, Levin J, et al: Adrenal activity in anorexia nervosa. Psychosom Med 40:499–506, 1978

Walsh BT, Roose SP, Katz JL, et al: Hypothalamic-pituitary-adrenal-cortical activity in anorexia nervosa and bulimia. Psychoneuroendocrinology 12:131–140, 1987

Weiner H: Psychoendocrinology of anorexia nervosa. Psychiatr Clin North Am 12(1):187–206, 1989

Weizman R, Carmi M, Tyano S, et al: High affinity [3H]imipramine binding and serotonin uptake to platelets of adolescent females suffering from anorexia nervosa. Life Sci 38:1235–1242, 1986

Weltzin TE, Fernstrom MH, Hansen D, et al: Abnormal caloric requirements for weight maintenance in patients with anorexia and bulimia nervosa. Am J Psychiatry 148:1675–1682, 1991

Zohar J, Insel TR, Zohar-Kadouch RC, et al: Serotonergic responsiveness in obsessive-compulsive disorder. Arch Gen Psychiatry 45:167–172, 1988

Chapter 11

Personality Disorders

Larry J. Siever, M.D., Bonnie J. Steinberg, M.D.,
Robert L. Trestman, Ph.D., M.D., and
Joanne Intrator, M.D.

Although personality disorders have traditionally been understood in the context of psychodynamic, psychosocial, or behavioral heuristic frameworks, emerging evidence implicates biological factors as important in the pathogenesis of these disorders. A greater appreciation of the underlying biology of personality disorders may provide an alternative or complementary perspective from which to understand these disorders, which are often refractory to treatment. Biological factors may represent the "building blocks" or "constitutional" factors from which personality is constructed. Although the nature of the personality construction or development depends on a variety of environmental factors, an increased awareness of the nature of these underlying biological substrates may help us to better understand how personality becomes disordered.

The impetus for new studies of the biology of personality disorder comes from several arenas. First, the advances of biological psychiatry through the application of neurobiological tools to the Axis I disorders invite their application to the Axis II disorders as well. Indeed, biological factors might more plausibly be implicated in the "trait" characteristics of the Axis II disorders than in the often state-related phenomena of the Axis I disorders. However, only recently has interest been generated in the biology of the personality disorders.

Second, the development of operationalized criteria and instruments for diagnosing personality disorders makes them a more attractive target for investigation. The DSM-III-R and DSM-IV (American Psychiatric Association 1987, 1994) categorization systems, although only having limited empirical underpinnings, provide a common, reliable vocabulary that may be utilized across research centers.

Third, an increasing appreciation of the role of heritability in the development of personality has an obvious corollary in the likelihood of

Our research was supported in part by a grant from the National Institutes of Health, National Center for Research Resources (RR00071), to the Mt. Sinai Medical Center and by grants from the National Institute of Mental Health (RO1-MH41131) and the Department of Veterans Affairs (Merit Award 7609004).

a stable biology of personality disorder (Goldsmith 1982). Studies of twins reared together and apart, as well as studies of monozygotic and dizygotic twins, provide strong support for genetic factors in the range of "normal" personality (Tellegen et al. 1988). Although definitive studies have yet to be performed with the personality disorders, adoptive studies (Cloninger et al. 1978) and twin studies (Torgersen 1984) support the heritability of underlying dimensions of personality disorder.

Finally, with the increasing awareness of the role of trauma in the pathogenesis of personality disorder (Herman et al. 1989), an emerging biology of posttraumatic stress disorder may yield another fruitful avenue from which to explore the biology of personality disorders. Thus, interest in the biology of personality, which had been largely confined to academic psychologists studying normal personality (Claridge 1985; Eysenck 1967), has become a focus for clinical psychiatrists interested in the biology of mental disorders.

Many of the studies of personality disorders have logically started with the investigation of biological variables implicated in the Axis I disorders. Original conceptualizations of the biology of personality disorder focused on personality disorders as representing variants of major Axis I disorders. For example, borderline personality disorder may be seen as a variant of affective disorder (Akiskal 1981). Accordingly, it was logical to apply biological tests implicated in the affective disorders to borderline personality disorders. Not surprisingly, state-related correlates such as the dexamethasone suppression test did not prove to be consistent correlates of personality disorder (L. J. Siever, J. Temple, H. Klar, R. Trestman, E. Coccaro: "DST and Depression in Personality Disorders," unpublished manuscript, July 1992), although more promising results were found with biological correlates of the affective disorders that were state independent, such as shortened rapid eye movement (REM) latency (Akiskal 1981; Siever and Davis 1991). Correlates of schizophrenia, which are generally more state invariant, generated promising results in the study of schizotypal personality disorder (Siever et al. 1993). Measures of the serotonin (5-hydroxytryptamine; 5-HT) system associated with suicide attempts (self-directed aggression) in depressed patients have been applied successfully to the investigation of impulsive aggression in personality disorders.

As our sophistication in the study of personality disorders has increased, investigators have relied more on biological measures that are stable over time (trait-related measures). These correlates have been linked not only to specific personality disorders, such as borderline or schizotypal personality disorders (diagnoses with extensive overlap in DSM-III-R), but are also being applied with promise to trait dimensions of the personality disorders.

In this chapter we discuss studies that use both specific personality disorder categories (primarily borderline and schizotypal personality disorder) and trait-dimensional clinical correlates (e.g., impulsivity or affective instability). Categorical comparisons offer the advantages of identifying associations with specific diagnoses used clinically. In contrast, dimensional studies rely on correlational analyses that may have greater power and more accurately reflect the distribution of these traits in the personality disorders but that do not precisely coincide with the DSM-III-R nomenclature. The DSM-III-R concept of "clusters" provides a heuristic starting point to organize both categorical and dimensional studies. Although there is some disagreement about the precise empirical validity of these clusters, which will be deemphasized in DSM-IV (American Psychiatric Association 1994), the groupings of the schizophrenia-related personality disorders ("odd" cluster), affective/impulsive personality disorders ("dramatic" cluster), and anxiety-related personality disorders ("anxious" cluster) provide a useful starting point from which to examine available data regarding the biology of personality disorder (Table 11–1).

At the end of each section, we give a clinical vignette based on patients who have participated in our investigative program of biological correlates of the personality disorders and describe these patients' laboratory findings.

SCHIZOPHRENIA-RELATED PERSONALITY DISORDERS

The schizophrenia-related personality disorders or odd cluster of DSM-III-R and DSM-IV personality disorders are composed of schizotypal, paranoid, and schizoid personality disorders. The hallmark of these disorders is a pervasive interpersonal and social isolation such that those persons affected are often perceived as "odd" and

Table 11–1. Proposed neurotransmitter systems in personality disorders

Personality disorder cluster	Dimensions	Neurotransmitter systems	Axis I related
Schizophrenia related	Cognitive/ perceptual	Dopaminergic	Schizophrenic disorders
Affective/ impulsive	Affect regulation; impulse control	Cholinergic; noradrenergic; serotonergic	Affective disorders; impulsive control disorders
Anxiety related	Anxiety	Noradrenergic; dopaminergic; serotonergic; GABAergic	Anxiety disorders

"loners." Although schizoid personality disorder emphasizes the preference for solitary activities and isolation without specific cognitive and perceptual distortions, paranoid personality disorder is characterized by a pervasive suspiciousness and sensitivity to potential malevolence of others. Schizotypal personality disorder, the prototype of these personality disorders, is the most severe; it includes eccentricities and specific cognitive and perceptual distortions among its criteria. An underlying dimension of impairment in these disorders is cognitive-perceptual organization, which may impair social relationships (Siever and Davis 1991). Although strong and specific data support a genetic relationship between schizophrenia and schizotypal personality disorder, only limited data support a relationship between schizophrenia and paranoid personality disorder. Newer concepts relating schizoid personality disorder to schizophrenia are as yet minimally defined. Thus, most biological studies have focused on the more severe prototypical disorder of this group—schizotypal personality disorder. These studies include psychophysiological testing, neuropsychological performance, neuroimaging, and neurotransmitter and neuroendocrine assessments (see Table 11–2).

Table 11–2. Proposed biological markers in schizophrenia-related personality disorders

Test	Finding
Information processing and psychophysiology	
Eye-movement impairment	Low gain; increased saccadic movements
Continuous Performance Task	Sustained attentional performance deficit
Backward Masking Task	Visual information-processing deficit
Evoked potential	Reduced amplitude; increased latency
Galvanic skin orienting response	Abnormal autonomic responsiveness to environmental stimuli
Visual reaction time	Increased
Computed tomography scan	Increased ventricle-to-brain ratio
Neuropsychological testing	Impaired performance on prefrontal tasks; possible impaired performance on frontal tasks
Neurochemistry	
Monoamine oxidase	Decreased
Plasma amine oxidase	Decreased
Homovanillic acid	Increased
Amphetamine challenge	Increased psychosis

Information Processing and Psychophysiological Tests

Eye-movement impairment. The majority of schizophrenic patients, at least half in most studies, evidence impaired eye movement when instructed to follow a continuously moving target (for a review, see Clementz and Sweeney 1990), as do approximately 50% of the relatives of schizophrenic patients (Holzman et al. 1984). Given the genetic relationship of schizotypal personality disorder to schizophrenia, subjects with the former would be expected to also demonstrate an increased prevalence of eye-movement dysfunction. Indeed, studies of volunteer populations selected by virtue of poor eye tracking (Siever et al. 1982a, 1984), as well as studies of volunteers selected by virtue of their schizotypic traits (Lencz et al. 1993; Simons and Katkin 1985), demonstrate an association between eye-movement dysfunction and schizotypal traits, or "schizotypy," specifically correlated with the interpersonal detachment or "deficit" traits of schizotypal personality disorder.

This association has been observed in clinical populations as well. Patients with schizotypal personality disorder demonstrated more eye-movement dysfunction than healthy control subjects, whereas patients with other personality disorders did not differ from control subjects (Moskowitz et al. 1992; Siever et al. 1990, 1993). Studies utilizing infrared detection of eye movements also suggest that there is eye-movement dysfunction in patients with schizotypal personality disorder, with global qualitative measures of tracking accuracy particularly associated with the deficit-like symptoms of schizotypal personality disorder (Moskowitz et al. 1992; Siever et al. 1990). Whether patients with paranoid or schizoid personality disorders exhibit eye-movement impairment is still open to investigation.

Continuous Performance Task. The Continuous Performance Task (CPT) is a test of sustained attentional performance that frequently has abnormal results in schizophrenic patients (Resvold et al. 1956). Abnormalities in the CPT have also been found in volunteers selected by virtue of their schizotypal characteristics (Neuchterlein 1987), in pilot studies of schizotypal patients (Wainberg et al. 1993), and in the offspring of schizophrenic patients (Cornblatt and Erlenmeyer-Kimling 1985; Neuchterlein 1983). An association between attentional deficits on the CPT and interpersonal deficits is suggested by the correlation between CPT abnormalities and social isolation in the offspring of schizophrenic patients (Cornblatt et al. 1992). In both schizotypal patients and their relatives, impairment on the CPT is related to the degree of schizotypal symptomatology (Siever et al. 1993). Studies utilizing the CPT provide further support for a relationship between attentional impairment and schizotypic traits, particularly traits reflecting interpersonal skill deficits.

Backward Masking Task. The Backward Masking Task is a visual information-processing task in which a stimulus is followed quickly by a "masking stimulus" that impairs the identification of the original target stimulus when the interval is very short. Compared with healthy control subjects, patients with schizotypal personality disorder and volunteers selected by virtue of schizotypal traits from a community sample require a longer interval between the presentation of the target stimulus and the onset of the mask to correctly identify the original target (Braff 1986; Merritt and Balogh 1989; Siever and Davis 1991).

Evoked potential studies. Electroencephalographic (EEG) responses to paradigms that require an individual to attend to an "oddball" or unexpected stimulus have been found to be abnormal in schizophrenic patients compared with control subjects (Pfefferbaum et al. 1984, 1989; Roth et al. 1980, 1981). Specifically, a positive wave at P300 is reduced in amplitude and increased in latency in schizophrenic patients compared with control subjects (Pfefferbaum et al. 1989). Similar abnormalities have been reported in patients with schizotypal personality disorder, but comparable abnormalities have been found in patients with borderline personality disorders (Kutcher et al. 1987). Alterations in P300 have also been found in college-student volunteers determined to be schizotypal by psychological screening inventories (Simons 1982). In one other study of personality disorder patients (Kalus et al. 1991), the N200 and P300 amplitudes observed in schizotypal personality disorder patients were intermediate between those observed in other personality disorder patients and healthy control subjects and those observed in schizophrenic patients.

Galvanic skin orienting response and visual reaction time. The galvanic skin orienting response, reflecting the autonomic responsiveness to environmental stimuli, has been reported to be abnormal in both schizophrenic subjects and schizotypal individuals selected from volunteer populations (Simons 1981). Schizotypal patients show an abnormal reaction time to visual stimuli similar to that observed in schizophrenic patients (Simons et al. 1982b).

Neuroimaging. An increased ratio of ventricle to brain has been one of the more robust biological findings in patients with chronic schizophrenia. Investigations to date of patients with schizotypal traits also suggest ventricular abnormalities. Adolescents with schizophrenia-spectrum diagnoses have been reported to have increased ventricular size (Schulz et al. 1983). Although some studies suggest decreased ventricular size in schizophrenic persons' offspring who have schizotypal traits (Cannon et al. 1990; Schulsinger et al. 1984), other studies of relatives of schizophrenic patients have shown tendencies toward increased ventricular size (Silverman et al. 1991, 1992).

Studies of clinically defined schizotypal patients also suggest that ventricular abnormalities may be present. Studies of patients with schizophrenia-related personality disorder reported increased ventricular size (Cazzullo et al. 1991). In another study, schizotypal patients demonstrated lateral ventricular enlargement, particularly on the left side, and a tendency toward left frontal horn enlargement (Siever et al. 1993) associated with impaired performance on the Wisconsin Card Sorting Test (WCST) (Grant and Berg 1948; Lucas et al. 1989; Siever et al. 1993). In exploratory analyses, increased ventricular size was associated with reduced concentrations of plasma homovanillic acid (HVA) and deficit-like symptoms and impairment on frontal neuropsychological task (Siever et al. 1993). Furthermore, increased ventricular size in schizotypal patients has been associated negatively with psychotic-like symptoms (Rotter et al. 1991). Preliminary findings of structural asymmetry parallel similar findings in severe chronic "Kraepelinian" schizophrenic patients. These exploratory results raise the possibility of a dimension of schizotypy grounded in structural impairment that is associated with neuropsychological and clinical deficits and hypodopaminergia.

Neuropsychological testing. Schizophrenic patients generally demonstrate impaired performance on tests sensitive to prefrontal dysfunction, such as the WCST. Because these performance decrements are associated with deficit symptoms, it has been hypothesized that schizotypal personality disorder patients with prominent deficit-like symptoms would show a similar association between frontal impairment and these deficit symptoms. Preliminary studies have suggested that schizotypal patients make more perseverative errors, make more perseverative responses, and complete fewer categories than patients with other personality disorders (deVegvar et al. 1993; Siever et al. 1993). Similar findings have been observed in symptomatic volunteers with schizotypy (Lyons et al. 1991; Raine et al. 1992). Schizotypal patients and relatives of schizophrenic patients also demonstrate abnormalities in other tests of prefrontal functions such as the Trails B Test (Reitan 1980); abnormalities on these prefrontal-related tasks correlate with deficit-related or nonpsychotic-like symptoms schizotypal personality disorder (deVegvar et al. 1993; Keefe et al. 1991; Siever et al. 1993).

Neurochemical Measures

Monoamine and plasma amine oxidase.   Both monoamine oxidase (MAO) and plasma amine oxidase have been reported to be decreased in "borderline schizophrenic" or schizotypal relatives of schizophrenic patients as well as in volunteers selected by virtue of schizotypal characteristics (Baron and Levitt 1980; Baron et al. 1980a, 1980b). Reduced MAO activity has been hypothesized to contribute to increased dopaminergic activity by decreasing its inactivation after reuptake from the synapse. However, data have been limited, and results of studies have been inconsistent.

Homovanillic acid.   HVA is the primary metabolite of dopamine in the brain. Its measurement affords an opportunity to assess dopaminergic activity and to test the hypothesis that increased dopamine contributes to the chronic psychosis of schizophrenia. Measurement of cerebrospinal fluid (CSF) HVA has not consistently differentiated schizophrenic patients from healthy control subjects (van Kammen et al. 1983), although there are suggestions of increases in patients with some paranoid subtypes (Rimon et al. 1971). However, numerous confounding artifacts make the interpretation of CSF HVA in schizophrenia problematic: chronic neuroleptic treatment, chronic institutionalization, and the theoretical considerations of cortical hypodopaminergia associated with subcortical dopamine excess (Davis et al., in press). In patients with schizotypal personality disorder, however, increases in CSF HVA have been found compared with levels observed in other personality disorder patients; mean CSF 5-hydroxyindoleacetic acid (5-HIAA) concentrations do not differ among groups. These CSF HVA concentrations correlated significantly with the number of "psychotic-like" or positive schizotypal personality disorder symptoms but not with the deficit-related criteria. Indeed, this association seemed to account for the group differences, because covariate analyses controlling for psychotic-like symptoms eliminate the statistical differences (Siever et al. 1993a). Consistent with these findings, CSF HVA also correlated positively with the Perceptual Aberration Scale of the Chapman Psychosis-Proneness Scale (Chapman et al. 1980b) but not with the Physical or Social Anhedonia Scales (Siever et al. 1993a).

Although plasma HVA is derived largely from the periphery, it may partially reflect central dopaminergic activity and has been found to be correlated with psychotic symptoms in drug-free schizophrenic patients (Davis et al. 1985; Pickar et al. 1986). Plasma HVA is also increased in patients with schizotypal personality disorder compared with control subjects and correlates significantly and positively with "positive" or psychotic-like symptoms (Siever et al. 1991b, 1993).

These findings suggest that increased dopaminergic activity is associated with the psychotic-like symptoms of schizotypal personality disorder.

Responses to amphetamine challenge. The psychotic-like symptoms of patients meeting criteria for both borderline personality disorder and schizotypal personality disorder—in contrast to those of "pure" borderline patients—worsened in response to an infusion of amphetamine (Schulz et al. 1988). Referential ideas and related psychotic-like symptoms were more prominent after the infusion. Further, preliminary study raises the possibility that schizotypal patients with prominent deficit-like symptoms may respond with enhancement of cognitive functioning after amphetamine infusion (Wainberg et al. 1993). These studies again suggest the potential dissociation of frontal cognitive function associated with relative hypodopaminergia from a subcortical-limbic psychosis associated with relative hyperdopaminergia in schizotypal patients.

Clinical Vignettes[1]

Mr. A is a 65-year-old, single, white man who lives alone and last worked 10 years ago as a clerk. Mr. A has long-standing difficulties with interpersonal relations, has no friends, and has never been in a significant relationship during his lifetime. He reports not having feelings, or a "lack of feeling, apathy" and is fearful of being rejected. He is often unkempt and frequently does not shower. He does report mild referential thinking, but he has never experienced delusions or hallucinations and has no magical thinking. He meets criteria for schizotypal personality disorder.

Mr. A is a good example of a patient who has schizotypal personality disorder with predominantly deficit-like symptoms. His serum HVA was in the low end of the normal range. His smooth pursuit eye movements were severely impaired (5.00; normal mean ± SD = 2.4 ± 0.7). He had a large number of perseverative errors in the WCST (37; normal mean ± SD = 14 ± 12), and he had marked improvement in WCST after amphetamine challenge. In addition, he went from three categories completed on the WCST to a perfect six categories completed after amphetamine challenge. His ventricle-to-brain ratio was greater than two SDs above the mean ratio (9.44; normal mean ± SD = 4.91 ± 1.82). Mr. A's deficit symptoms might be grounded in underlying alterations in brain structure that impair his information processing.

Mr. B is a 39-year-old, never married, unemployed white man who lives with his father. Mr. B has no close friends but reports having had them as

---

[1]The facts of each vignette have been modified to protect the identity of patients who have participated in our studies.

an adolescent. He has had romantic relationships with women; the longest was 14 months and he left abruptly. He feels uncomfortable around people, and feels it is better if people don't get to know him. He is suspicious, believing that other people usually have hidden motives for their actions. Mr. B reports having psychic experiences and using these to make predictions for bets on horse races. He also reports ideas of references. He has no hallucinations but at times does have perceptual disturbances such as hearing noises. He speech is vague and inappropriately abstract. His antisocial traits include substance abuse, fights, stealing, gambling, and sex with people he did not know well; he has been convicted on felony charges eight times. He meets criteria for schizoid, schizotypal, and antisocial personality disorder.

In his testing, Mr. B had a high number of nonperseverative errors but a normal number of perseverative errors. His serum HVA was high (14.7 ng/ml; normal mean $\pm$ SD = 7.7 $\pm$ 1.8), and his ventricle-to-brain ratio was normal. These findings would be consistent with Mr. B's positive or psychotic-like symptoms of schizotypal personality disorder.

Summary

Neurochemical studies of schizotypal personality disorder suggest that increases in dopaminergic activity may be associated with the psychotic-like symptoms of this disorder, whereas results of neuroimaging and neurochemical studies raise the possibility that some schizotypal individuals with prominent deficit symptoms are characterized by structural cortical dysfunction and possibly frontal hypodopaminergia. Increased dopaminergic activity in subcortical areas might contribute to the hypervigilance and stereotypical thinking implicated in psychotic distortions, whereas frontal hypodopaminergia may impair working memory and executive functions. These two pathophysiological dimensions of the schizophrenia spectrum may be more clearly differentiated in schizotypal personality disorder, whereas they are more likely to be too interactive in schizophrenia to be easily disentangled (Siever et al. 1993). Schizotypal individuals with prominent deficit symptoms and evidence of cognitive dysfunction and brain structure alterations, perhaps secondary to a neurodevelopmental abnormality, may be less susceptible to subcortical dopamine dysregulation than schizophrenic patients. Other schizotypal patients with prominent psychotic-like symptoms may evidence dysregulated dopamine activity without a prominent neurodevelopment impairment. Genetic data suggesting independent heritability of psychotic-like and negative symptoms (Kendler et al. 1991) suggest that these two underlying pathophysiological dimensions may be dissociated in the schizophrenia-spectrum personality disorder (Siever et al. 1993).

AFFECTIVE/IMPULSIVE
PERSONALITY DISORDERS

The affective/impulsive personality disorders (the dramatic cluster of DSM-III-R) include borderline, histrionic, narcissistic, and antisocial personality disorders. These disorders are each marked by an orientation to action and reactivity to the environment. Individuals with these personality disorders are often profoundly sensitive to changes in their interpersonal relationships and may respond with profound affective shifts, as is prototypical of borderline (and, to a lesser degree, of histrionic) personality disorders. Antisocial personality disorder may not be characterized by affective sensitivity and, indeed, may be marked by a relative insensitivity to emotional cues. However, antisocial individuals also display prominent impulsivity and aggression. Individuals with narcissistic personality disorder are sensitive to criticism and often respond to criticism with humiliation and rage. In general, these disorders are marked by a heightened engagement with the environment rather than the more fearful, inhibited behaviors of individuals with the anxious cluster of personality disorders.

Accordingly, biological studies investigating the dramatic cluster of disorders have been guided by theories emphasizing the affectively unstable features, the impulsivity, the psychopathy, and the behavioral dyscontrol of individuals meeting criteria for these personality disorders.

Affective instability describes rapidly shifting affective states that are exquisitely responsive to external stimuli. Individuals with affective instability may be extraordinarily sensitive to separation or frustration, stressors that might have only modest effects on others. At times these affective shifts may result in transient depressive episodes. In contrast to the often environmentally unresponsive and autonomous mood disorders of Axis I or the withdrawn, inhibited style of the anxious cluster, individuals with affective/impulsive personality disorders seek stimulation from the environment and, in turn, are very responsive to it. This trait has prompted the investigation of biological systems, such as the noradrenergic system, that mediate responsiveness to the environment.

Impulsivity is a central feature of borderline and antisocial personality disorders and to a lesser extent is expressed in histrionic and narcissistic personality disorders. A relative failure to suppress aggressive or otherwise risky behaviors with possible negative consequences may underlie the tendency toward fighting, irritability, drug abuse, promiscuity, and self-damaging acts characteristic of these disorders. Emerging evidence implicates biological abnormalities of behavior-inhibiting systems such as the 5-HT system in the expression of impulsivity.

The individual with antisocial personality disorder displays characteristics of impulsivity, usually without the affective instability typical of patients with borderline personality disorder. "Psychopathy" is another basic characteristic and is defined by glibness and disregard of others' feelings associated with manipulative and exploitative behaviors. In perhaps more subtle fashion, this same psychopathic pattern may be seen in individuals with narcissistic personality disorder. A growing body of work suggests that psychophysiological correlates of psychopathy include inadequate detection of emotional cues and reduced cortical arousal compared with that observed in psychiatrically healthy individuals.

Other studies have been driven by hypotheses of subcortical epileptiform activity underlying the behavioral dyscontrol observed in patients with affective/impulsive personality disorders, particularly younger patients with borderline personality disorder. The often concomitant finding of EEG abnormalities (Cowdry et al. 1985–1986), certain symptomatic similarities to temporal lobe epilepsy (Cowdry et al. 1985–1986), and partial clinical response to anticonvulsive agents (Gardner et al. 1987) have provided supporting evidence for this theoretical construct. A related avenue of investigation is based on possible subtle neurological dysfunction and structural abnormalities that may be related to "minimal" brain dysfunction and attentional disorders, such as adult attention-deficit hyperactivity disorder.

Twin studies provide some evidence for the heritability of these specific dimensions of the affective/impulsive personality disorders. Although there is an increased prevalence of borderline personality disorder in the relatives of borderline personality disorder patients (Zanarini et al. 1988), underlying traits such as impulsivity and affective instability may be independently heritable in the relatives of these patients and may interactively predispose individuals to borderline personality disorder (Torgersen 1992). Although monozygotic and dizygotic twin studies do not support the heritability of the categorical borderline personality disorder (Torgersen 1984), they do provide some support for genetic factors underlying dimensions of impulsivity and affective instability (Silverman et al. 1991). Subepileptiform disorders and attentional disturbances may potentially derive from early congenital damage and contribute to the psychopathology of these disorders. Furthermore, it is increasingly clear that early physical or sexual abuse, a common event in the background of many borderline personality disorder patients (Gallagher et al. 1992; Herman et al. 1989; Raczek 1992), may have long-lasting biological sequelae.

Thus, although these different theoretical frameworks may seem incompatible, there may be a parallel to the parable of the blind men examining an elephant. Some disturbances may apply more directly to some subpopulations with these personality disorders than to others, and for many individuals, interactions of these potentially separable psychobiological dimensions may contribute to the final personality disorder profile (see Table 11–3).

Information Processing and Psychophysiology

Neuropsychological tests.   Theories of subtle neurological dysfunction in patients with borderline personality disorder have been bolstered by neuropsychological testing studies that demonstrate that borderline personality disorder patients experience difficulties in separating essential from extraneous visual information. Subsequent recall of recently learned complex material is impaired and is partially correctable with auditory cues. These data support the possibility of limbic and temporal dyscontrol in patients with borderline personality disorder (O'Leary et al. 1991).

Neurological signs.   In support of subtle neurological deficit theories of some subpopulations of borderline patients, an increased incidence of neurological soft signs (including difficulty with complex movements and distinctions between right and left) have been found in borderline personality disorder individuals (Gardner et al. 1987).

Language processing.   Patients with psychopathy process both unemotional and emotional language differently than do psychiatrically healthy individuals. Unlike healthy individuals, individuals with antisocial personality disorder are unable to process emotionally charged words more quickly than neutral words, as tested by a lexical decision task (i.e., "Is this string of letters a word or is it not?") (Rubenstein et al. 1971). Although healthy individuals demonstrate differences in some components of the event-related potentials (ERPs) for emotional words compared with neutral words (Chapman et al. 1980a), this difference was not found in patients with psychopathy tested by a lexical decision task (Williamson et al. 1991). In verbal left/right dichotic listening tests (Hare and McPherson 1984; Raine and Venables 1987) and in studies of divided visual fields (Hare and Jutai 1988), patients with psychopathy may process both verbal and auditory language differently than healthy subjects, which may have implications for cerebral development of lateralization of language function. The inability to respond specifically to emotional stimuli may be related to the psychopathic patient's characteristic disregard both for others' feelings and for potential punishment.

EEG studies.   Excessive limbic neuronal discharge has been hypothesized to underlie many of the dyscontrol symptoms of borderline personality disorder and would predict the presence of EEG abnormalities.

Table 11–3. Proposed markers in affective/impulsive personality
disorders

Test or study	Finding
Information processing and psychophysiology	
Neuropsychological tests	Difficulties separating essential from extraneous visual information; impaired recall of recently learned complex material
Neurological signs	Increased neurological soft signs
Lexical decision task (language processing)	Abnormal
EEG studies	Abnormal EEG patterns, with limbic system correlation
Event-related potential	Prolonged latencies and decreased amplitudes in borderline personality disorder; prolonged early component and augmented middle component in antisocial personality disorder
EEG sleep studies	Decreased REM latency and increased REM density
Skin conductance	Decreased electrodermal response in anticipation of aversive stimuli in antisocial personality disorder
Computed tomography scan	No abnormalities noted
Neurochemistry	
Neuroendocrine studies	
TRH stimulation	No abnormalities noted
Dexamethasone suppression	No abnormalities noted
Platelet monoamine oxidase	Reduced
Neurotransmitter studies	
The cholinergic system	
Acetylcholinesterase challenge	Depressive syndrome
Muscarinic challenge	Depressive syndrome
Cholinomimetics and sleep	Increased REM sleep abnormalities
Cholinergic challenge	Increased mood response in affectively labile patients
The noradrenergic system	
Growth hormone response to clonidine	Elevated in irritable patients
Plasma NE	Possibly elevated
CSF MHPG	Possibly elevated
Plasma MHPG	Possibly elevated
Urinary VMA	Possibly elevated
Urinary NE + metabolites	Possibly elevated
The serotonergic system	
Basal metabolism	Decreased
Brain 5-HT and receptors	Decreased

Table 11–3. Proposed markers in affective/impulsive personality disorders *(continued)*

Test or study	Finding
CSF 5-HIAA	Decreased
Platelet 5-HT, IMI binding, and 5-HT$_2$ receptors	Decreased
Fenfluramine challenge	Decreased prolactin response
Buspirone challenge	Decreased prolactin response
m-CPP challenge	Decreased prolactin response
The endogenous opiate system	
Plasma β-endorphin	Elevated

Note. CSF = cerebrospinal fluid. EEG = electroencephalogram. 5-HIAA = 5-hydroxyindoleacetic acid. 5-HT = serotonin (5-hydroxytryptamine). IMI = imipramine. m-CPP = *m*-chlorophenylpiperazine. MHPG = 3-methoxy-4-hydroxyphenylglycol. NE = norepinephrine. REM = rapid eye movement. TRH = thyrotropin-releasing hormone. VMA = vanillylmandelic acid.

Indeed, increases in abnormal EEG patterns, coupled with behavioral symptoms similar to those commonly seen in patients with complex partial seizures, were found in borderline personality disorder patients compared with psychiatrically healthy control subjects (Cowdry et al. 1985–1986). However, other studies have shown that these EEG abnormalities correlate with transient psychotic symptoms (Cornelius et al. 1986) rather than with the traits of affective instability or impulsivity. Intravenous infusion of procaine, which stimulates limbic dyscontrol, produces dysphoria in borderline patients that is similar to their spontaneous dysphoric episodes, accompanied by simultaneous temporal-amygdala EEG abnormalities (Kling et al. 1987). Therefore, it is possible that behavioral dyscontrol and dysphoria have a behavioral correlate in limbic system abnormalities. These studies are consistent with the hypothesis that dyscontrol symptoms of borderline and other personality disorders of this cluster are related to dyscontrol of limbic system discharge. In contrast, other EEG studies (Hare and Craigen 1974) suggest that antisocial behavior may be associated with decreased cortical arousal as reflected by increased density of slow-wave cortical activity.

Event-related potentials. Auditory ERPs would also be expected to be sensitive to limbic and attentional dysfunction. Although studies of borderline patients have found abnormalities such as prolonged P3 latency and small P300 amplitude (Kutcher et al. 1987, 1989) and prolonged N100, P200, and N200 latency with attenuated amplitude (Drake et al. 1991), these differences are not specific to borderline personality disorder (Kutcher et al. 1987; Simons et al. 1982a). These abnormalities may reflect disturbances in a variety of processing domains.

A different profile of ERP abnormalities has been observed in patients with antisocial personality disorder. These patients have a longer latency in the early component of ERPs, possibly indicating an abnormality in lower brain stem regions (Josef et al. 1985). In the middle component of the ERP there is evidence for augmentation of response to several tasks (Raine 1989; Rohrbaugh and Gaillard 1983). The P300, which is part of the late component of the ERP, tends to be increased in patients with psychopathy, although this finding has been variable (Raine 1989; Raine and Venables 1987). This pattern is consistent with the model of psychopathic patients as sensation seekers or cortical augmenters who have increased perception of visual stimuli and are proficient at selectively attending to some stimuli and events and ignoring others (Quay 1965; Zuckerman et al. 1980).

EEG sleep studies. In patients with major depression, REM sleep latency is decreased and REM density is increased. Similarly, patients with borderline personality disorder have decreased and more variable REM sleep latency and increased REM density (Akiskal et al. 1985; McNamara et al. 1984). REM sleep latency may be further shortened and REM density may be further increased in borderline personality disorder patients with concurrent Axis I mood disorders (Lahmeyer et al. 1988; Reynolds et al. 1985). Family or personal past history of Axis I disorder may correlate with these sleep abnormalities as well (Lahmeyer et al. 1989). Thus, alterations in REM sleep may serve as a trait marker for several types of affective dysregulation.

Skin conductance. Psychophysiological studies have shown that psychopathic patients' electrodermal response to an aversive stimulus is normal, yet their electrodermal response in anticipation of this aversive stimulus is smaller than that in psychiatrically healthy control subjects (Hare and Craigen 1974). This result has been interpreted as evidence that psychopathic patients are deficient in fear conditioning (Lykken 1957). In addition, this small electrodermal response is accompanied by an increase in heart rate (Hare 1982; Oglaff and Wong 1990), a pattern that may reflect the operation of defensive coping mechanisms and the attenuation of anticipatory fear responses (Hare 1982; Venables 1987). If the skin conductance reflects the behavior inhibition system and the heart rate reflects the behavior activation system (Gray 1975), psychopathic patients have a weak behavior inhibition system and a normal behavior activation system or are more responsive to rewards than to punishments (Forth and Hare 1989). When there are competing goals of avoiding punishment while earning rewards, psychopathic patients are unable to inhibit an incorrect response even at the risk of punishment (Newman and Kossen 1980; Newman et al. 1985).

Neuroimaging. Findings of subtle neurological impairment in some borderline patients invited structural image studies of this disorder. However, studies to date using computed tomography (CT) to measure ventricular size or diffuse atrophy have been negative (Lucas et al. 1989). Future studies with magnetic resonance imaging (MRI) will allow for better resolution of relevant cortical and subcortical structures. This technique could reveal structural abnormalities in limbic structures and therefore provide more useful information than the present data from CT.

Neurochemistry

Neuroendocrine studies. Building on the success of studies of neuro-endocrine regulation and depression, early investigations of borderline and related personality disorder focused on hormone-stimulating or suppression tests. However, abnormal responses such as blunted response of thyroid-stimulating hormone to thyroid-releasing hormone and plasma cortisol escape from dexamethasone suppression have generally not been observed (for a review, see Lahmeyer et al. 1989), with only inconsistent findings of abnormalities in very early reports (Carroll et al. 1981; Sternbach et al. 1983; for a review, see Lahmeyer et al. 1989). This result may not be surprising because the affective instability of these disorders constitutes a persistent trait, whereas the hormonal abnormalities documented in major depressive disorder are for the most part state related.

Platelet monoamine oxidase. The findings of reduced platelet MAO in a variety of psychiatric disorders—including schizophrenia (Giller et al. 1980; Schildkraut et al. 1976), alcohol abuse (Major and Murphy 1978), and bipolar illness (Murphy and Weiss 1972)—have stimulated hypotheses that platelet MAO reductions are a vulnerability factor in psychiatric disorders (Buchsbaum et al. 1976). Reduced concentrations of MAO in platelets, if paralleled in brain, would imply that there is a greater availability of monoamines for release. This might contribute to increased affective lability. Platelet MAO has been found to be decreased in patients with borderline personality disorder (Lahmeyer et al. 1988; Yehuda et al. 1989) and decreased to a greater degree if the patients had concurrent antisocial personality disorder (Yehuda et al. 1989). The precise behavioral correlates of reduced platelet MAO in borderline personality disorder patients have yet to be defined but may include impulsivity (Schalling et al. 1987), suicidality (Buchsbaum et al. 1977), and psychopathy (Lidberg et al. 1985b).

Neurotransmitter Studies

The cholinergic system.   Increased cholinergic responsiveness has been implicated in major depressive disorder and is particularly associated with an increased susceptibility to dysphoric affects (Janowsky and Risch 1987; Janowsky et al. 1972). Acetylcholinesterase inhibitors and muscarinic agonists, which increase cholinergic availability in the brain, create a depression-like syndrome (Davis et al. 1978; Janowsky et al. 1974; Oppenheimer et al. 1979; Risch et al. 1981) and have antimanic properties (Davis et al. 1978; Janowsky et al. 1973). In healthy males, response to physostigmine correlates with the traits of irritability and emotional lability (Fritze et al. 1990). These observations invite the investigation of the cholinergic system in the affective/impulsive personality disorders (e.g., borderline disorder).

Similarly, studies of REM sleep latency (which is mediated by cholinergic activity) also raised the possibility of cholinergic abnormalities in patients with borderline personality disorder. Borderline patients, who have decreased and more variable REM sleep latency than psychiatrically healthy control subjects (Akiskal et al. 1985; McNamara et al. 1984), demonstrated an exaggerated reduction in REM sleep latency in response to cholinomimetics in preliminary studies (Bell et al. 1983). These results raise the possibility that supersensitivity to cholinomimetics may be associated with borderline personality disorder and perhaps more specifically with the trait of affective instability.

Stimulated by these suggestive leads, very preliminary studies from our laboratory do indeed indicate that personality disorder patients with the trait of affective instability have a differential depressive-like response to the acetylcholinesterase inhibitor physostigmine compared with other personality disorder patients who do not have affective instability (Steinberg et al., in press). Thus, increased responsiveness of cholinergic receptors might contribute to the affective instability in personality disorder patients.

The noradrenergic system.   Because the noradrenergic system modulates normal arousal and engagement with the environment, it is a logical candidate for investigation in patients who are excessively reactive to the environment. Patients with affective instability, particularly patients in the dramatic cluster (and to a lesser degree, those in the anxious cluster), are often excessively engaged with, and responsive to, the environment.

Preclinically, novel or threatening stimuli increase the activity in the locus coeruleus, the primary noradrenergic nucleus of the brain (Aston-Jones and Bloom 1981; Levine et al. 1990). Increased locus coeruleus activity is associated with irritable aggression in animal models (Lamprecht et al. 1972; Levine et al. 1990); decreased locus coeruleus firing is associated with vegetative activities such as eating, sleeping, and grooming (Aston-Jones and Bloom 1981) and is observed during withdrawal from the environment, for example, in infants in response to separation from the mother (McKinney et al. 1984). Thus, increased noradrenergic activity may be associated with heightened engagement with, and reactivity to, the environment, and decreased noradrenergic activity may similarly be associated with withdrawal from the environment.

A hyporesponsive noradrenergic system might be expected to decrease interaction with the environment, causing withdrawal, psychomotor retardation, and decreased concentration; these neurovegetative symptoms are classically associated with major depression (Siever and Davis 1985). Consistent with a hyporesponsive noradrenergic system, the growth hormone response to clonidine, an α_2-noradrenergic agonist, is decreased in major depression (Siever et al. 1982b). In addition, lipophilic β-blockers can induce depression as a side effect (Mann and Arango 1988). Thus, decreased activity of the noradrenergic system may be associated with decreased engagement with the environment.

In contrast, increased reactivity to environmental events might be expected to be associated with increased noradrenergic activity. Indeed, risk takers such as gamblers have increased measures of arousal (Eysenck 1967) and increased susceptibility to boredom and sensation seeking (Dickerson et al. 1987); their noradrenergic system also tends to be hyperactive (Roy et al. 1988). These individuals are impulsive and more physically active. Growth hormone responses to clonidine are increased in patients with attention-deficit hyperactivity disorder, a phenomenon that is reversible with methylphenidate treatment. Increased arousal and orientation to the environment in patients with increased noradrenergic indices may lead to a predisposition to direct their anger externally.

Hysteroid dysphoria, characterized by atypical depression and increased emotional responsiveness, especially to rejection, overlaps with borderline personality disorder. The symptoms of these patients respond best to MAO inhibitors, which stabilize noradrenergic transmission as well as that of other monoamines (Liebowitz and Klein 1981).

Increased responsiveness of the noradrenergic system in psychiatrically healthy control subjects and in personality disorder patients, as indicated by an increased or exaggerated growth hormone response to clonidine challenge, is correlated with irritability as defined by the Irritability Subscale of the Buss-Durkee Hostility Inventory (Buss and Durkee 1957; Coccaro et al. 1991). In an expanded cohort, personality disorder patients with increased irritability demonstrated increased indices of noradrenergic activity, both at baseline (plasma 3-methoxy-4-hydroxyphenylglycol [MHPG]) and after challenge with clonidine (Trestman et al. 1992).

It is thus possible that noradrenergic indices may in the future serve as biological markers, indicating increased engagement with and reactivity to the environment as a contributing factor to both affective instability and impulsivity.

The serotonergic system. The 5-HT system is a modulatory neurotransmitter that plays a primarily inhibitory or suppressive role in relation to aggression and punished behavior. Thus, it has been a useful starting point from which to investigate the biological basis of impulsivity and disinhibited aggression in the personality disorders. Preclinical studies link decreased serotonergic activity with aggression in animal models (Dichiara et al. 1971; for a review, see Winchel and Stanley 1991). The aggressive behavior can be reduced or blocked with the administration of a 5-HT precursor (Broderick and Lynch 1982) or 5-HT itself to animals in whom these neurons have been ablated (Dichiara et al. 1971; Stark et al. 1985). Further, serotonergic agents such as reuptake inhibitors tend to inhibit spontaneous (Molina et al. 1987) or induced (Kostowski et al. 1984; Stark et al. 1985) aggressive behavior. Consistent with these data, MAO inhibitors have been found to increase 5-HT more slowly in aggressive rats than in normal rats, suggesting a reduction in 5-HT capacity in aggressive rats (Valzelli 1967).

In general, aggressive behavior is associated with decreased indices of serotonergic activity in clinical studies as well. Studies of impulsivity and self-directed and other-directed aggression in humans include studies of individuals who have attempted suicide and completed suicide and of patients with parasuicidal or self-mutilating behavior. These studies help to delineate a generally consistent pattern of serotonergic disturbances in both forms of aggressive behavior.

Studies of basal metabolism. 5-HT and 5-HT receptors and metabolites are decreased in the brains of suicide victims, regardless of diagnosis (G. L. Brown et al. 1979; Ninan et al. 1984; Siever et al. 1991a; Van Praag 1983). Patients who have made suicide attempts, as well as some patients with parasuicidal behavior, have decreased CSF levels of 5-HIAA, the primary 5-HT metabolite. This observation holds true across a number of psychiatric diagnoses, including personality disorders, and suggests a correlation between self-directed aggression and decreased serotonergic activity (G. L. Brown et al. 1979; Siever et al. 1991a). Patients with self-mutilating behavior have significantly decreased platelet imipramine-binding sites, a measure of presynaptic 5-HT receptors, and increased indices of self-mutilation and impulsivity (Simeon et al. 1992). A decrease in platelet 5-HT$_2$ receptors has also been found in patients with suicidal ideation (Pandey et al. 1990). These studies collectively suggest that 5-HT contributes to the regulation of self-directed aggression.

Patients with personality disorders who are violent have fairly consistently demonstrated reduced indices of 5-HT. Decreased CSF 5-HIAA has been reported in patients who are physically aggressive (G. L. Brown et al. 1982), violent criminal offenders (Linnoila et al. 1983), murderers of sexual partners (Lidberg et al. 1985a) or of their own children (Lidberg et al. 1984), arsonists (Virkkunen et al. 1987), and aggressive children (Kruesi et al. 1990). Decreased platelet 5-HT in aggressive and impulsive patients has also been found (C. S. Brown et al. 1989). These findings taken together suggest decreased 5-HT release and increased up-regulation of postsynaptic receptors in patients with impulsivity or suicidality.

Challenge studies. Neuroendocrine challenge studies offer a means to assess dynamic functioning of central neurotransmitter functions. Central serotonergic activity may be assessed by measuring the change in plasma levels of prolactin in response to fenfluramine, a 5-HT–releasing and uptake-inhibiting agent. A blunted prolactin response to fenfluramine has been found in mood disorder and personality disorder patients with a history of at least one suicide attempt; further, in personality disorder patients, an inverse correlation has been noted between the prolactin response to fenfluramine and clinical indices of impulsivity and aggression (Coccaro et al. 1989b).

A number of other serotonergic agonists have been studied in these personality disorders with fairly consistent findings. The prolactin response to challenge with buspirone, a 5-HT_{1a} receptor agonist, has been found to correlate negatively with irritability in personality disorder patients (Coccaro et al. 1990). m-Chlorophenylpiperazine (m-CPP) is the active metabolite of trazodone and acts as a direct $5\text{-HT}_{1c,2,3}$ agonist. m-CPP challenge results in increased plasma levels of prolactin, cortisol, and growth hormone. Consistent with the findings regarding fenfluramine challenge, a negative correlation between prolactin response to m-CPP and measures of irritability and aggression in personality disorder patients has been observed in a preliminary study (Coccaro et al. 1989a). In contrast, challenge with clomipramine as a probe of central serotonergic functioning failed to discriminate between high suicidality and low suicidality in a population with mixed diagnosis (Golden et al. 1991). Decreased serotonergic activity may thus in the future serve as a marker for impulsivity and aggression in personality disorder patients.

Pharmacological studies. Emerging evidence supporting the effectiveness of selective 5-HT reuptake inhibitors in patients with impulsivity and aggression lends empirical support to the hypothesis that 5-HT is reduced in patients with disinhibited behavior. Patients with borderline personality disorder treated with fluoxetine demonstrate improvement in anger, affective lability, irritability, and impulsivity (Norden 1989); self-mutilation (Markovitz et al. 1991); and depression and impulsivity (Cornelius et al. 1990).

Impulsivity and impulsive aggression in the dramatic cluster of personality disorders have thus been associated with decreased transmission of 5-HT.

The endogenous opiate system. The endogenous opiate system may be involved in the modulation of impulsive aggressive behavior, particularly self-injurious behavior. For example, elevated plasma levels of β-endorphin have been found in patients with self-injurious behavior and personality disorder in preliminary studies (Konicki and Schulz 1981).

Clinical Vignette

Mr. C is a 39-year-old, twice-divorced Hispanic man who is currently unemployed but who has worked most of his life and run his own business at several points. Mr. C has a history of unstable interpersonal relationships, and he was violent toward both of his wives and his children. He describes impulsive rages and gets into frequent fights; on one occasion when a neighbor had spoken in a way he did not like, Mr. C got his shotgun and went to the neighbor's house to kill him (fortunately, the neighbor escaped). Mr. C has cut his wrists on two occasions. He complains of mood swings and feelings of emptiness and boredom. He is extremely sensitive to personal rejection and generally reacts with anger to rebuffs. He met criteria for borderline, histrionic, and paranoid personality disorders.

In his testing, Mr. C had abnormal smooth pursuit eye movements. He had a severely blunted prolactin response to fenfluramine (−0.2 ng/ml; threshold for blunting is ≤6 ng/ml) (Coccaro et al. 1989b), suggesting a hypoactive serotonergic system; it is interesting to hypothesize that this hypoactivity is related to Mr. C's impulsivity and aggression. He had a robust growth hormone response to clonidine (10.0 ng/ml; threshold for blunted response is ≤4 ng/ml). This response is consistent with findings of increased noradrenergic indices in patients who are irritable and hyperreactive to their environment.

Summary

A range of preclinical and clinical data is consistent with dimensions of affective instability and impulsive aggression in the dramatic cluster of personality disorders. Neuropsychological and psychophysiological testing has demonstrated abnormalities of information processing and response mediation, whereas electrophysiological findings are consistent with disinhibition models of behavior and limbic regulation. Neurotransmitter abnormalities in noradrenergic, cholinergic, and serotonergic systems are consistent with disturbed neuroregulatory mechanisms that modulate environmental engagement, affective arousal, and impulse inhibition. These psychobiological disturbances are generating a substantial body of research leading to more explicit hypotheses of the underlying pathophysiology of affective lability and impulse dyscontrol.

ANXIETY-RELATED PERSONALITY DISORDERS

The maladaptive patterns of behavior and cognition associated with the anxious cluster of personality disorders (avoidant, dependent, obsessive-compulsive, and passive-aggressive disorders) can be conceptualized as attempts to ward off anxiety. The biology and pathophysiology of this group of disorders have received less attention and are less well understood than the biology and pathophysiology of other personality disorders (see Table 11–4). One potentially useful association for characterizing the biology of these disorders is the significant comorbidity of avoidant personality disorder and social phobia, thought by some to be as high as 90% (Holt et al. 1992; Schneier et al. 1991; Turner et al. 1991, 1992; Widiger 1992). Obsessive-compulsive personality disorder may also be common in patients with social phobia; in one study, 61.8% of the patients with social phobia met all or nearly all of the criteria for obsessive-compulsive personality disorder. The biology of social phobia, which recently has been emerging (Potts and Davidson 1992), may thus shed light on the biology of some of the personality disorders in this cluster, and it will be discussed as it is relevant to our current understanding of these disorders.

There appears to be a relationship between other Axis I anxiety disorders (generalized anxiety disorder, panic disorder, and obsessive-compulsive disorder) and the anxious cluster of personality disorders,

Table 11–4.   Proposed markers in anxiety-related personality disorders

System	Finding
Hypothalamic-pituitary axis	No abnormalities noted
Noradrenergic system	Possibly increased indices
Serotonergic system	Possibly decreased indices
Dopaminergic system	Possibly decreased indices
GABAergic system	Possibly decreased indices

but the relationship does not have the same degree of specificity as social phobia and avoidant personality disorder. For example, obsessive-compulsive personality disorder may be associated with obsessive-compulsive disorder, but this association may be seen only in a minority of obsessive-compulsive disorder patients (Baer et al. 1990; Joffee et al. 1988) or not at all (Sciuto et al. 1991). It may be that markers of obsessive-compulsive disorder such as serotonergic (Rapoport 1991) or noradrenergic (Hollander et al. 1991) dysregulation play some part in obsessive-compulsive personality disorder as well. However, obsessive-compulsive disorder also has been associated with mixed personality disorder (Baer et al. 1990), dependent personality disorder (Steketee 1988, cited in Baer and Jenike 1992), avoidant personality disorder (Joffee et al. 1988), and histrionic personality disorder (Baer et al. 1990).

Panic disorder might be expected to be associated with some of the personality disorders in this spectrum. Although there is an overall increased incidence of anxiety-related personality disorders in patients with panic disorder, there is as yet no clear association between panic disorder and one or more of these personality disorders (Mellman et al. 1992; Reich and Troughton 1988). One group of researchers did find that phobic panic disorder patients were more likely to have dependent personality disorder (Reich et al. 1987); others found that patients with panic disorder had an increase in avoidant, histrionic, and dependent traits (Mavissakalian and Hamann 1988) or in avoidant and dependent traits (Pfohl et al. 1991). However, it is not clear whether the markers for panic disorder such as panic induction with lactate, yohimbine, or carbon dioxide are also markers for anxiety-related personality disorders.

Similarly, generalized anxiety disorder might be conceptualized as possibly related to avoidant or dependent personality disorders, but studies to date have not borne this relationship out (Gasperini et al. 1990). One study did find a relationship between generalized anxiety disorder and DSM-III compulsive personality disorder (Nestadt et al. 1992). It remains to be seen whether markers for generalized anxiety disorder such as decreased numbers of noradrenergic receptors (Cameron et al. 1990) are useful in identification of the anxiety-related personality disorders.

There is some evidence for heritability of anxious, excessive inhibition. Both "anxious" personality traits (Reich 1991a) and all personality disorders (Reich 1989, 1991b) are increased in family members of patients with these disorders. Monozygotic twins from the Norwegian twin registry had a significantly higher concordance for distress in social situations than did dizygotic twins (Torgerson and Kringlen 1978). The development of social phobia has been found to be related in part to genetic factors (Kendler et al. 1991).

Neurochemistry

Neuroendocrine studies.   There have been several studies of neuro-endocrine function in social phobia. No differences have been found between patients with social phobia and psychiatrically healthy control subjects in the hypothalamic-pituitary-adrenal axis (Uhde et al. 1991) or thyroid axis (Tancer et al. 1990b), other than one report of an exaggerated pressor response to thyrotropin-releasing hormone. (Tancer et al. 1990a). The absence of further studies of neuroendocrine abnormality reflects a parallel lack of hypotheses about pathophysiological disturbances in the neuroendocrine function of patients with the anxious cluster of disorders.

Pharmacological studies.   Symptomatic improvement in avoidant personality disorder has been observed with administration of irreversible MAO inhibitors (Deltito and Stam 1989; Liebowitz et al. 1990b) and reversible MAO inhibitors (Liebowitz et al. 1990b). MAO inhibitors increase the effective neurotransmission of monoamines. This suggests that monoamines may contribute to the pathology of the personality disorders in this cluster.

An important aspect of the anxious cluster of personality disorders is anxiety about interacting with the environment; indeed, β-blockers are effective in treating well-circumscribed forms of social phobia, especially performance anxiety (Liebowitz 1989). A blunted growth hormone response to clonidine has been noted in patients with social phobia compared with psychiatrically healthy subjects (Uhde et al. 1991). Although lactate infusion is known to produce panic attacks in patients with panic disorder, it does not regularly do so in patients with social phobia (Liebowitz et al. 1985). These studies collectively provide some evidence for the role of the noradrenergic system in social phobia and, by extension, in avoidant personality disorder.

The serotonergic reuptake inhibitor fluoxetine has been found to be useful for the treatment of core symptoms in patients with avoidant personality disorder (Deltito and Stam 1989), suggesting that decreased serotonergic availability may contribute to this disorder. Evidence for serotonergic involvement in social phobia comes primarily from treatment studies with serotonergic agents such as fluoxetine (Black and Uhde 1992; Liebowitz et al. 1991; Schneier et al. 1992; Sternbach 1990) and buspirone (Schneier et al. 1990).

One consistent finding in patients with social phobia has been a relationship between decreased dopamine and social phobia (Potts and Davidson 1992). Effectiveness of monoamine oxidase inhibitors and reversible monoamine oxidase inhibitors (Liebowitz 1992; van Vliet et al. 1992) in treating social phobia may imply a monoaminergic contribution to avoidant personality disorder as well.

Benzodiazepines have been found to be effective in treating social phobia in some (Davidson et al. 1991; Munjack et al. 1990; Ontiveros and Fontaine 1990) but not all (Liebowitz et al. 1990a) studies. Decreased GABAergic activity may thus correlate with social phobia and possibly with the anxious personality disorders.

Clinical Vignette

Ms. D is a 25-year-old, never-married, white woman who lives alone, has a master's degree in sculpture, and works in a clerical position. She has anxiety in social situations and seeks out individuals she perceives as less intimidating. She is also somewhat suspicious and believes friends have their own goals in mind. She describes her mood as "radically swinging" between periods of feeling "angry, scared, and content." She is sensitive to others' reactions to her, and she often fears that her boyfriend will leave her even though he is quite devoted. She is afraid to show her art or play her saxophone with her band in front of others. She meets criteria for avoidant personality disorder.

In her testing in our program, neuropsychophysiological correlates were normal. Ms. D's growth hormone response to clonidine was severely blunted, a finding demonstrated in patients with Axis I anxiety disorders (Uhde et al. 1991). The prolactin response to fenfluramine was robust in this inhibited, nonimpulsive patient. She showed a marked dysphoric response to physostigmine challenge, with a change of 10 points on the Depression Subscale of the Profile of Mood States (Lorr et al. 1971) on the drug day compared with the placebo day (normal mean $\pm$ SD = 1.8 $\pm$ 3.3). Her plasma HVA concentration was in the normal range.

Summary

These disorders are characterized by increased levels of anxiety in response to internal and external stimuli. Early investigations into the biology of these and related disorders suggest that possible increases in noradrenergic transmission and possible decreases in the dopaminergic, serotonergic, and GABAergic neurotransmitter systems may be potential markers for the anxious cluster of personality disorders.

NEW INVESTIGATIVE TOOLS

Exploration of tools such as functional neuroimagery and molecular biology will likely yield more information about the biology of personality disorders. Investigating and classifying personality disorders by gender, age, distribution of diagnosis, and nosological assessment may also further our understanding of the nature of the personality disorders.

Functional Neuroimagery

Functional neuroimagery allows the investigation of regional cerebral blood flow with single photon emission computed tomography (SPECT) or MRI with echo-planar technology; of regional metabolism with positron-emission tomography (PET); and of receptor binding with either SPECT or PET. These techniques allow for study of hypotheses involving potential regional cerebral disturbances, receptor function or distribution abnormalities, differential function in response to cognitive activation, and pretreatment and posttreatment differences.

To date, very few studies have been conducted with personality disorder patients. Two preliminary studies (Goyer et al. 1991; Raine et al. 1992) with PET report flow abnormalities, primarily in the frontal lobe, that correlate with aggressive behavior. These results are consistent with findings of similar correlations in a population of patients with closed head injuries who were examined with SPECT (Oder et al. 1992).

Molecular Biology

Recently, the chromosomal location of a polymorphic tryptophan hydroxylase site was identified in violent offenders and control subjects, and it was found to have significant relationships with 5-HT turnover as well as specific behavior associated with 5-HT function (Nielsen 1992). A normal personality trait was linked to the color-blindness gene (on the X chromosome). One of 16 personality factors was found to correlate with color blindness (Benjamin et al. 1992). As the genotypes for specific neurotransmitters and their regulation come to light in the future, further avenues of genetic investigation will open up for the pathophysiology of the personality disorders.

Methodological Considerations

Gender. Differences between female and male serotonergic systems have been noted. Females have increased imipramine-binding sites in animal (Ieni et al. 1985) and human (Arato et al. 1991) studies. Males and females respond differently to fenfluramine (McBride et al. 1990) and m-CPP (Charney et al. 1988).

Such considerations may apply to other neurotransmitter systems as well. Indeed, higher mean levels of monoamine metabolites were recently found in women compared with men, but these differences did not reach significance (Traskman-Bendz et al. 1992). Gender differences have been noted in platelet MAO, and indeed MAO varies with the menstrual cycle (Baron et al. 1980a). In contrast, in preliminary studies, no gender differences have been observed in associations of noradrenergic functioning (as measured by the growth hormone response to clonidine) with behavioral indices in personality disorder patients in our laboratory (Trestman et al. 1993).

Gender is also important in the epidemiology of the personality disorders. Several of these disorders, most notably in the affective/impulsive cluster, have an unequal gender distribution. To what extent this uneven distribution reflects underlying biological differences, learned methods of expression of emotions and drives, or cultural bias remains to be seen.

Age.   The effect of age (and the effect of its interaction with biology) on the diagnosis and the clinical progression of personality disorders has yet to be adequately studied. Geriatric patients who were clinically diagnosed with borderline personality disorder by a geropsychiatry team may not meet the full criteria by DSM-III-R or by the Diagnostic Interview for Borderlines (Gunderson et al. 1981; Rosowsky and Gurian 1991).

Nosological assessment.   Alternative methods of classifying personality disorders are a source of controversy. The DSM system of categorical classification uses familiar and clinically relevant personality disorder diagnoses. In contrast, a dimensional approach is more descriptive, and patients are classified according to specific traits that are more likely to have biological correlates (Siever and Davis 1991). This approach is consistent with a symptom-based method for pharmacological treatment. A number of dimensional systems have been proposed (Cloninger 1987; Costa and McRae 1990; Eysenck 1967), and their relative contribution to the understanding of the personality disorders has yet to be fully explored.

SUMMARY AND CONCLUSIONS

An increased appreciation of the biological underpinnings of personality disorders can have important psychopharmacological and psychotherapeutic implications. For example, selective 5-HT reuptake inhibitors are already proving useful in the treatment of impulsive personality disorders and, indeed, may have advantages over broader-spectrum antidepressants that enhance noradrenergic activity. Agents that decrease noradrenergic activity such as propranolol or clonidine may be useful in reducing the irritability associated with these disorders. Although largely untested, anticholinergic agents might conceivably prove of value in ameliorating the tendency toward dysphoric mood. Mood stabilizers and anticonvulsants may provide stability to irritable limbic foci.

From a psychotherapeutic vantage point, an increased understanding of the biological vulnerabilities of personality disorder patients may lead to more empathic understanding of their life experiences. The recognition of an underlying instability of affect, a subtle attention-deficit disorder, a tendency to disinhibited aggression, or a fearful and inhibited temperament may make more understandable the coping strategies the patient has chosen, usually on the basis of a less-than-optimal developmental experience. Such an empathic approach may permit the development of more adaptive coping strategies in the context of the patient experiencing the therapist's recognition of his or her underlying vulnerability.

Although the psychobiological study of personality disorders is still in its infancy, recent investigations have begun to define and explore potential biological mechanisms subserving basic personality disorder traits such as impulsivity or schizotypy. These investigations have been grounded in the approaches used to study the neurobiology of the Axis I disorders and suggest the applicability of new neurobiological tools to the study of the Axis II disorders as well. Promising leads include information processing, psychophysiological tests, and neurochemical measures such as subcortical hyperdopaminergia and frontal hypo-dopaminergia in the schizophrenia-related personality disorders; information processing and response mediation dysfunction, disinhibition of behavior and limbic regulation, and noradrenergic, cholinergic, and serotonergic dysregulation in the affective/impulsive personality disorders; and possibly increases in noradrenergic transmission and decreases in dopaminergic, serotonergic, and GABAergic neurotransmitter systems in the anxiety-related personality disorders. Although these tools are not yet applicable clinically for either Axis I or Axis II disorders, the investigative work in developing useful biological markers for the personality disorders continues.

REFERENCES

Akiskal HS: Subaffective disorders: dysthymic, cyclothymic and bipolar II disorders in the "borderline" realm. Psychiatric Clin North Am 4:25–46, 1981
Akiskal HS, Yerevarian BI, Davis GC, et al: The nosologic status of borderline personality: clinical and polysomnographic study. Am J Psychiatry 142:192–198, 1985
American Psychiatric Association: Diagnostic and Statistical Manual of Mental Disorders, 3rd Edition. Washington, DC, American Psychiatric Association, 1980
American Psychiatric Association: Diagnostic and Statistical Manual of Mental Disorders, 3rd Edition, Revised. Washington, DC, American Psychiatric Association, 1987
American Psychiatric Association: Diagnostic and Statistical Manual of Mental Disorders, 4th Edition. Washington, DC, American Psychiatric Association, 1994
Arato M, Frecska E, Tekes K, et al: Serotonergic interhemispheric asymmetry: gender differences in the orbital cortex. Acta Psychiatr Scand 84:110–111, 1991
Aston-Jones G, Bloom FE: Norepinephrine-containing locus coeruleus neurons in behaving rats exhibit pronounced responses to non-noxious environmental stimuli. J Neurosci 1:887–890, 1981

Baer L, Jenike MA: Personality disorders in obsessive compulsive disorder. Psychiatric Clin North Am 15:803–811, 1992

Baer L, Jenike MA, Ricciardi JN II, et al: Standardized assessment of personality disorders in obsessive-compulsive disorder. Arch Gen Psychiatry 47:826–832, 1990

Baron M, Levitt M: Platelet monoamine oxidase activity: relation to genetic load of schizophrenia. Psychiatry Res 3:69–74, 1980

Baron M, Levitt M, Perlman R: Human platelet monoamine oxidase and the menstrual cycle. Psychiatry Res 3:323–327, 1980a

Baron M, Levitt M, Perlman R: Low platelet monoamine oxidase activity: a possible biochemical correlate of borderline schizophrenia. Psychiatry Res 3:329–335, 1980b

Bell J, Lycaki H, Jones D, et al: Effect of preexisting borderline personality disorder on clinical and EEG sleep correlates of depression. Psychiatry Res 9:115–123, 1983

Benjamin J, Press J, Maoz B, et al: Linkage of a normal personality trait to the color-blindness gene, in Abstracts of the 31st Annual Meeting of the American College of Neuropsychopharmacology, American College of Neuropsychopharmacology, December 1992, p 161b

Black B, Uhde TW, Tancer ME: Fluoxetine for the treatment of social phobia (letter). J Clin Psychopharmacol 12:293–295, 1992

Braff DL: Impaired speed of information processing in non-medicated schizotypal patients. Schizophr Bull 7:499–508, 1986

Broderick P, Lynch V: Biochemical changes induced by lithium and L-tryptophan in muricidal rats. Neuropharmacology 21:671–679, 1982

Brown CS, Kent TA, Bryant SG, et al: Blood platelet uptake of serotonin in episodic aggression. Psychiatry Res 27:5–12, 1989

Brown GL, Goodwin FK, Ballenger JC, et al: Aggression in humans correlates with cerebrospinal fluid amine metabolites. Psychiatry Res 1:131–139, 1979

Brown GL, Ebert M, Goyer P, et al: Aggression, suicide and serotonin: relationship to CSF amine metabolites. Am J Psychiatry 139:741–746, 1982

Buchsbaum MS, Coursey RD, Murphy DL: The biochemical high risk paradigm: behavioral and familial correlates of low platelet MAO activity. Science 194:339–341, 1976

Buchsbaum MS, Haler RJ, Murphy DL: Suicide attempts, platelet monoamine oxidase and the average evoked response. Acta Psychiatr Scand 56:69–79, 1977

Buss AH, Durkee A: An inventory for assessing different kinds of hostility. Journal of Consulting Psychology 21:343–348, 1957

Cameron OG, Smith CB, Myung AL, et al: Adrenergic status in anxiety disorders: platelet alpha-2-adrenergic receptor binding, blood pressure, pulse, and plasma catecholamines in panic and generalized anxiety disorder patients and in normal subjects. Biol Psychiatry 28:3–20, 1990

Cannon TD, Sarnoff AM, Parnas J: Antecedents of predominantly negative- and predominantly positive-symptom schizophrenia in a high risk population. Arch Gen Psychiatry 47:622–632, 1990

Carroll BJ, Greden JF, Feinberg M, et al: Neuroendocrine evaluation of depression in borderline patients. Psychiatr Clin North Am 4:89–99, 1981

Cazzullo CL, Vita A, Giobbio GM, et al: Cerebral structural abnormalities in schizophreniform disorder and in schizophrenia spectrum personality disorders, in Advances in Neuropsychiatry and Psychopharmacology, Vol 1: Schizophrenia Research. Edited by Tamminga CA, Schulz SC. New York, Raven, 1991, pp 209–217

Chapman RM, McCrary JW, Chapman JA, et al: Behavioral and neutral analysis of connotative meaning: word classes and rating scales. Brain Lang 11:319–339, 1980a

Chapman SJ, Edell WS, Chapman JS: Physical anhedonia, perceptual aberration and psychosis proneness. Schizophr Bull 6:639–653, 1980b

Charney DS, Goodman WK, Price LH, et al: Serotonin function in obsessive-compulsive disorder. Arch Gen Psychiatry 45:177–185, 1988

Claridge G: Origins of Mental Illness. New York, Blackwell, 1985

Clementz BA, Sweeney JA: Is eye movement dysfunction a biological marker for schizophrenia? A methodological review. Psychol Bull 108:77–92, 1990

Cloninger CR: A systematic method for clinical description and classification of personality variants. Arch Gen Psychiatry 44:573–588, 1987

Cloninger CR, Christiansen KO, Reich T, et al: Implications of sex differences in the prevalence of antisocial personality, alcoholism, and criminality for familial transmission. Arch Gen Psychiatry 35:941–951, 1978

Coccaro EF, Siever LJ, Kavoussi R, et al: Postsynaptic function in aggression (NR183), in New Research Program and Abstracts: American Psychiatric Association 142nd Annual Meeting, San Francisco, CA, May 6–11, 1989a, p 112

Coccaro EF, Siever LJ, Klar H, et al: Serotonergic studies in affective and personality disorder patients: correlates with suicidal and impulsive aggression. Arch Gen Psychiatry 43:587–599, 1989b

Coccaro EF, Gabriel S, Siever LJ: Buspirone challenge: preliminary evidence for a role for central 5-HT$_{1a}$ receptor function in impulsive aggressive behavior in humans. Psychopharmacol Bull 26:393–405, 1990

Coccaro EF, Lawrence T, Trestman RL, et al: Growth hormone responses to intravenous clonidine challenge correlate with behavioral irritability in psychiatric patients and in healthy volunteers. Psychiatry Res 39:129–139, 1991

Cornblatt BA, Erlenmeyer-Kimling L: Global attentional deviance as a marker of risk for schizophrenia: specificity and predictive validity. J Abnorm Psychol 94:470–486, 1985

Cornblatt BA, Lenzenweger MF, Dworkin RH, et al: Childhood attentional dysfunctions predict social deficits in unaffected adults at risk for schizophrenia. Br J Psychiatry 161 (suppl 18):59–64, 1992

Cornelius JR, Brenner RP, Soloff PH, et al: EEG abnormalities in borderline personality disorder: specific or nonspecific. Biol Psychiatry 21:977–980, 1986

Cornelius JR, Soloff PH, Perel JM, et al: Fluoxetine trial in borderline personality disorder. Psychopharmacol Bull 26:151–154, 1990

Costa PT, McRae RR: Personality disorders and the five factor model of personality. Journal of Personality Disorders 4:362–371, 1990

Cowdry RW, Pickar D, Davies R: Symptoms and EEG findings in the borderline syndrome. Int J Psychiatry Med 15:201–211, 1985–1986

Davidson JRT, Ford SM, Smith RD, et al: Long-term treatment of social phobia with clonazepam. J Clin Psychiatry 52 (suppl 11):16–20, 1991

Davis KL, Berger PA, Hollister LE, et al: Physostigmine in mania. Arch Gen Psychiatry 35:119–122, 1978

Davis KL, Davidson M, Mohs RC, et al: Plasma homovanillic acid concentration and the severity of schizophrenic illness. Science 227:1601–1602, 1985

Davis KL, Kahn RS, Ko G, et al: Dopamine and schizophrenia: a reconceptualization. Am J Psychiatry (in press)

Deltito JA, Stam M: Psychopharmacological treatment of avoidant personality disorder. Compr Psychiatry 30:498–504, 1989

deVegvar ML, Keefe RSE, Moskowitz J, et al: Frontal lobe dysfunction and schizotypal personality disorder. Paper presented at the 146th annual meeting of the American Psychiatric Association, San Francisco, CA, May 1993

Dichiara G, Camba R, Spano PF: Evidence for inhibition by brain serotonin of mouse killing behavior in rats. Nature 233:272–273, 1971

Dickerson M, Hinchy J, Falve J: Chasing, arousal and sensation seeking in off-course gamblers. British Journal of Addiction 82:673–680, 1987

Drake ME Jr, Phillips BB, Pakalnis A: Auditory evoked potentials in borderline personality disorder. Clin Electroencephalogr 22:188–192, 1991

Eysenck H: The Biological Basis of Personality. Springfield, IL, Charles C Thomas, 1967

Forth AE, Hare RD: The contingent negative variation in psychopaths. Psychophysiology 26:676–682, 1989

Fritze J, Sofic E, Muller T, et al: Cholinergic-adrenergic balance, part II: relationship between drug sensitivity and personality. Psychiatry Res 34:271–279, 1990

Gallagher RE, Flye BL, Hurt SW, et al: Retrospective assessment of traumatic experiences (rate). Journal of Personality Disorders 6:99–108, 1992

Gardner DL, Cowdry RW: Pharmacotherapy of borderline personality disorder: a review. Psychopharmacol Bull 25:515–523, 1989

Gardner DL, Lucas PB, Cowdry RW: Soft sign neurological abnormalities in borderline personality disorder and normal control subjects. Journal of Nervous and Mental Disease 175:117–180, 1987

Gasperini M, Bataglia M, Diaferia G, et al: Personality features related to generalized anxiety disorder. Compr Psychiatry 31:363–368, 1990

Giller EL, Bierer L, Rubinow D, et al: Platelet MAO V_{max} and K_m in chronic schizophrenics. Am J Psychiatry 137:97–98, 1980

Golden RM, Gilmore JH, Corrigan MHN, et al: Serotonin, suicide and aggression: clinical studies. J Clin Psychiatry 52:61S–69S, 1991

Goldsmith HH: Genetic influences on personality from infancy to adulthood. Child Dev 54:331–355, 1982

Goyer PF, Andreason PJ, Semple WE, et al: Pet and personality disorders (abstract NR306), in New Research Program and Abstracts: American Psychiatric Association 144th Annual Meeting, New Orleans, LA, May 1991, p 121

Grant DA, Berg EWA: A behavioral analysis of degree of reinforcement and ease of shifting to new responses in a Weigl-type card sorting problem. J Exp Psychol 38:404–441, 1948

Gray JA: Elements of a Two-Process Theory of Learning. New York, Academic Press, 1975

Gunderson JG, Kolb JE, Austin V: The diagnostic interview for borderlines. Am J Psychiatry 138:869–903, 1981

Hare RD: Psychopathy and the personality dimensions of psychoticism, extraversion and neuroticism. Personality and Individual Differences 3:35–42, 1982

Hare RD, Craigen D: Psychopathy and physiological activity in mixed-motive game situations. Psychophysiology 11:197–206, 1974

Hare RD, Jutai JW: Psychopathy and cerebral asymmetry in semantic processing. Personality and Individual Differences 9:329–337, 1988

Hare RD, McPherson LOM: Psychopathy and perceptual asymmetry during verbal dichotic listening. J Abnorm Psychol 93:141–149, 1984

Herman JL, Perry JC, van der Kolk BA: Childhood trauma in borderline personality disorder. Am J Psychiatry 146:490–495, 1989

Hollander E, DeCaria C, Nitescu A, et al: Noradrenergic function in obsessive-compulsive disorder: behavioral and neuroendocrine responses to clonidine and comparison to healthy controls. Psychiatry Res 37:161–177, 1991

Holt CS, Heimberg RG, Hope DA: Avoidant personality disorder and the generalized subtype of social phobia. J Abnorm Psychol 101:318–325, 1992

Holzman PS, Solomon CM, Levin S, et al: Pursuit eye movement dysfunctions in schizophrenia: family evidence for specificity. Arch Gen Psychiatry 41:136–139, 1984

Ieni JR, Tobach E, Zukin SR, et al: Multiple 3H imipramine binding sites in brains of male and female Frawn-Hooded and Long-Evan rats. Eur J Pharmacol 112:261–264, 1985

Janowsky DS, Risch CS: Role of acetylcholine mechanisms in the affective disorders, in Psychopharmacology: The Third Generation of Progress. Edited by Meltzer HY. New York, Raven, 1987, pp 527–533

Janowsky DS, El-Yousef MK, Davis JM, et al: A cholinergic-adrenergic hypothesis of mania and depression. Lancet 2:632–635, 1972

Janowsky DS, El-Yousef MK, Davis JM, et al: Parasympathetic suppression of manic symptoms by physostigmine. Arch Gen Psychiatry 28:542–547, 1973

Janowsky DS, El-Yousef MK, Davis JM: Acetylcholine and depression. Psychosom Med 36:248–257, 1974

Joffee RT, Swinson RP, Regan JJ: Personality features of obsessive compulsive disorder. Am J Psychiatry 145:1127–1129, 1988

Josef NC, Lycaki H, Chayasirisobhon S: Brainstem auditory evoked potential in antisocial personality. Clin Electroencephalogr 16:91–93, 1985

Kalus O, Horvath TB, Peterson A, et al: Event related potentials in schizotypal personality disorder and schizophrenia (abstract 202). Biol Psychiatry 29:137A, 1991

Keefe RSE, Silverman JM, Amin F, et al: Frontal functioning and plasma HVA in the relatives of schizophrenic patients. Abstract presented at the annual meeting of the American College of Neuropsychopharmacology, San Juan, Puerto Rico, December 1991

Kendler KS, Ochs AL, Gorman AM, et al: The structure of schizotypy: a pilot multitrait twin study. Psychiatry Res 36:19–36, 1991

Kling MA, Kelner CH, Post RM, et al: Neuroendocrine effects of limbic activation by electrical, spontaneous, and pharmacological modes: relevance to the pathophysiology of affective dysregulation in psychiatric disorders. Prog Neuropsychopharmacol Biol Psychiatry 11:459–481, 1987

Konicki PE, Schulz CS: Rationale for clinical trials of opiate antagonists in treating patients with personality disorders and self-injurious behavior. Psychopharmacol Bull 25:556–563, 1981

Kostowski W, Valzelli L, Kozak W, et al: Activity of desipramine, fluoxetine and nomifensine on spontaneous and p-CPA–induced muricidal aggression. Pharmacological Research Communications 16:265–271, 1984

Kruesi MJ, Rapoport JL, Hamburger S, et al: Cerebrospinal fluid monoamine metabolites, aggression, and impulsivity in disruptive behavior disorders of children and adolescents. Arch Gen Psychiatry 47:419–426, 1990

Kutcher SP, Blackwood DHR, St. Clair D, et al: Auditory P300 in borderline personality disorder and schizophrenia. Arch Gen Psychiatry 44:645–650, 1987

Kutcher SP, Blackwood DHR, Gaskell DF, et al: Auditory P300 does not differentiate borderline personality disorder from schizotypal personality disorder. Biol Psychiatry 26:766–774, 1989

Lahmeyer HW, Val E, Gaviria FM, et al: EEG sleep, lithium transport, dexamethasone suppression and monoamine oxidase activity in borderline personality disorder. Psychiatry Res 25:19–30, 1988

Lahmeyer HW, Reynolds CF III, Kupfer DJ, et al: Biologic markers in borderline personality disorder: a review. J Clin Psychiatry 50:217–225, 1989

Lamprecht F, Eichelman B, Thoa NB, et al: Rat fighting behavior: serum dopamine-B-hydroxylase and hypothalamic tyrosine hydroxylase. Science 177:1214–1215, 1972

Lencz T, Raine A, Scerbo A, et al: Impaired eye tracking in undergraduates with schizotypal personality disorder. Am J Psychiatry 150:152–154, 1993

Levine ES, Litto WJ, Jacobs BL: Activity of cat locus coeruleus noradrenergic neurons during the defense reaction. Brain Res 531:189–195, 1990

Lidberg L, Asberg M, Sunquist-Stensman UB, et al: 5-Hydroxy-indoleacetic acid levels in attempted suicides who have killed their children (letter). Lancet 2:928, 1984

Lidberg L, Tuck JR, Asberg M, et al: Homicide, suicide and CSF 5-HIAA. Acta Psychiatr Scand 71:230–236, 1985a

Lidberg L, Modin I, Oreland L, et al: Platelet monoamine oxidase activity and psychopathy. Psychiatry Res 16:339–343, 1985b

Liebowitz MR: Phenelzine versus atenolol in social phobia: a placebo controlled study. J Clin Psychiatry 49:498–504, 1989

Liebowitz MR: Reversible MAO inhibitors in social phobia, bulimia and other disorders. Clin Neuropharmacol 15 (suppl 1):434A–435A, 1992

Liebowitz MR, Klein DF: Interrelationship of hysteroid dysphoria and borderline personality disorder. Psychiatr Clin North Am 4:67–87, 1981

Liebowitz MR, Fyer AJ, Gorman JM, et al: Specificity of lactate infusions in social phobia versus panic disorder. Am J Psychiatry 142:947–950, 1985

Liebowitz MR, Schneier F, Campeas R, et al: Phenelzine and atenolol in social phobia. Psychopharmacol Bull 26:123–125, 1990a

Liebowitz MR, Hollander E, Schneier F, et al: Reversible and irreversible monoamine oxidase inhibitors in other psychiatric disorders. Acta Psychiatr Scand Suppl 360:29–34, 1990b

Liebowitz MR, Schneier FR, Hollander E, et al: Treatment for social phobia with drugs other than benzodiazepines. J Clin Psychiatry 52 (suppl 11):10–15, 1991

Linnoila M, Virkkunen M, Scheinin M, et al: Low cerebrospinal fluid 5-hydroxy-indoleacetic acid concentration differentiates impulsive from nonimpulsive violent behavior. Life Sci 33:2609–2614, 1983

Lorr M, McNair DM, Droppleman LF: Manual—Profile of Mood States. San Diego, CA, Educational and Industrial Testing Service, 1971

Lucas PB, Gardner DL, Cowdry RW, et al: Cerebral structure in borderline personality disorder. Psychiatry Res 27:111–115, 1989

Lykken DT: A study of anxiety in the sociopathic personality. Journal of Abnormal and Social Psychology 55:6–10, 1957

Lyons MJ, Merla ME, Young L, et al: Impaired neuro-psychological functioning in symptomatic volunteers with schizotypy: preliminary findings. Biol Psychiatry 30:424–426, 1991

Major LF, Murphy DL: Platelet and plasma amine oxidase activity in alcoholic individuals. Br J Psychiatry 132:548–554, 1978

Mann JJ, Arango V: CNS adrenergic receptors and beta blockade. Postgraduate Medicine, A Special Report, February 29, 1988, pp 135–139

Markovitz PJ, Calabrese JR, Schulz SC, et al: Fluoxetine in the treatment of borderline and schizotypal personality disorders. Am J Psychiatry 148:1064–1067, 1991

Mavissakalian M, Hamann MS: Correlates of DSM-III personality disorder in panic disorder and agoraphobia. Compr Psychiatry 29:535–544, 1988

McBride PA, Tierney H, DeMeo M, et al: Effects of age and gender on CNS serotonergic responsivity in normal adults. Biol Psychiatry 27:1143–1155, 1990

McKinney WT, Moran EC, Kraemer GW: Separation in nonhuman primates as a model for human depression: neurobiological implications, in Neurobiology of Mood Disorders. Edited by Post RM, Ballenger JC. Baltimore, MD, Williams & Wilkins, 1984, pp 393–406

McNamara E, Reynolds CF III, Soloff PH, et al: EEG sleep evaluation of depression in borderline patients. Am J Psychiatry 141:182–186, 1984

Mellman TA, Leverich GS, Hauser P, et al: Axis II pathology in panic and affective disorders: relationship to diagnosis, course of illness, and treatment response. Journal of Personality Disorders 6:53–63, 1992

Merritt RD, Balogh DW: Backward masking spatial frequency effects among hypothetically schizotypal individuals. Schizophr Bull 15:573–583, 1989

Molina V, Ciesielski L, Gobaille S, et al: Inhibition of mouse killing behavior by serotonin-mimetic drugs: effects of partial alterations of serotonin neurotransmission. Pharmacol Biochem Behav 27:123–131, 1987

Moskowitz J, Lees S, Friedman L, et al: The relationship between eye tracking impairment and deficit symptoms (abstract 204). Biol Psychiatry 31:149A 1992

Munjack DT, Baltazar PL, Bohn PB, et al: Clonazepam in the treatment of social phobia: a pilot study. J Clin Psychiatry 51 (suppl 5):35–40, 1990

Murphy DL, Weiss R: Reduced monoamine oxidase activity in blood platelets from bipolar depressed patients. Am J Psychiatry 128:1351–1357, 1972

Nestadt G, Romanoski AJ, Samuels JF, et al: The relationship between personality and DSM-III Axis I disorders in the population: results from an epidemiological survey. Am J Psychiatry 149:1228–1233, 1992

Neuchterlein KH: Signal detection in vigilance tasks and behavioral attributes among offspring of schizophrenic mothers and among hyperactive children. J Abnorm Psychol 92:4–28, 1983

Neuchterlein KH: Converging evidence for vigilance deficit as a vulnerability indicator for schizophrenic disorders, in Controversies in Schizophrenia. Edited by Alpert M. New York, Guilford, 1987, pp 175–198

Newman JP, Kossen OS: Passive avoidance of learning in psychopathic and non-psychopathic offenders. J Abnorm Psychol 95:252–256, 1980

Newman JP, Widom CS, Nathan S: Passive avoidance in syndromes of disinhibition psychopathy and extraversion. J Pers Soc Psychol 48:1316–1327, 1985

Nielsen DA: CSF 5-HIAA, behavior and tryptophan hydroxylase genotype, in New Research Program and Abstracts: American Psychiatric Association 145th Annual Meeting, Washington, DC, May 1992, pp 112–113

Ninan PT, van Kammen DP, Scheinin M, et al: Cerebrospinal fluid 5-HIAA in suicidal schizophrenic patients. Am J Psychiatry 141:566–569, 1984

Norden MJ: Fluoxetine in borderline personality disorder. Prog Neuropsychopharmacol Biol Psychiatry 13:885–893, 1989

Oder W, Goldenberg G, Spatt J, et al: Behavioural and psychosocial sequelae of severe closed head injury and regional cerebral blood flow: a SPECT study. J Neurol Neurosurg Psychiatry 55:475–480, 1992

Oglaff JPR, Wong S: Electrodermal and cardiovascular evidence of a coping response in psychopaths. Criminal Justice and Behavior 17:231–245, 1990

O'Leary KM, Brouwers P, Gardner DL, et al: Neuropsychological testing of patients with borderline personality disorder. Am J Psychiatry 148:106–111, 1991

Ontiveros A, Fontaine R: Social phobia and clonazepam. Can J Psychiatry 35:439–441, 1990

Oppenheimer G, Ebstein R, Belmaker R: Effect of lithium on the physostigmine induced behavioral syndrome and plasma cyclic GMP. J Psychiatr Res 15:133–138, 1979

Pandey GN, Pandey SC, Janicak PG, et al: Platelet serotonin-2 receptor binding sites in depression and suicide. Biol Psychiatry 28:215–222, 1990

Pfefferbaum A, Wenegrat B, Ford J, et al: Clinical applications of P3 component of event-related potentials, II: dementia, depression and schizophrenia. Electroencephalogr Clin Neurophysiol 59:104–124, 1984

Pfefferbaum A, Ford JM, White PM, et al: P3 in schizophrenia is affected by stimulus modality, response requirements, medication status, and negative symptoms. Arch Gen Psychiatry 46:1035–1044, 1989

Pfohl B, Black DW, Noyes R, et al: Axis I and axis II comorbidity findings: implications for validity, in Personality Disorders: New Perspectives on Diagnostic Validity. Edited by Oldham JM. Washington DC, American Psychiatric Press, 1991, pp 145–161

Pickar D, Labarca R, Doran A, et al: Longitudinal measurement of plasma homovanillic acid levels in schizophrenic patients. Arch Gen Psychiatry 43:669–676, 1986

Potts NLS, Davidson JRT: Social phobia: biological aspects and pharmacotherapy. Prog Neuropsychopharmacol Biol Psychiatry 18:635–646, 1992

Quay HC: Psychopathic personality as pathological stimulation-seeking. Am J Psychiatry 122:180–183, 1965

Raczek SW: Childhood abuse and personality disorders. Journal of Personality Disorders 6:109–116, 1992

Raine A: Evoked potentials and psychopathy. Int J Psychophysiol 3:1–16, 1989

Raine A, Venables PH: Contingent negative variation, P3 evoked potentials and antisocial behavior. Psychophysiology 25:30–38, 1987

Raine A, Sheard C, Reynolds GP, et al: Pre-frontal structural and functional deficits associated with individual differences in schizotypal personality. Schizophr Res 7:237–247, 1992

Rapoport JL: Recent advances in obsessive-compulsive disorder. Neuropsychopharmacology 5:1–10, 1991

Reich JH: Familiality of DSM-III dramatic and anxious personality clusters. Journal of Nervous and Mental Disease 177:96–100, 1989

Reich J: Avoidant and dependent personality traits in relatives of patients with panic disorder, patients with dependent personality disorder, and normal controls. Psychiatry Res 39:89–98, 1991a

Reich J: Using the family history method to distinguish relatives of patients with dependent personality disorder from relatives of controls. Psychiatry Res 39:227–237, 1991b

Reich J, Troughton E: Frequency of DSM-III personality disorders in patients with panic disorder: comparison with psychiatric and normal control subjects. Psychiatry Res 26:89–100, 1988

Reich J, Noyes R Jr, Troughton E: Dependent personality disorder associated with phobic avoidance in patients with panic disorder. Am J Psychiatry 144:323–326, 1987

Reitan RM: Validity of the trail-making test as an indicator of organic brain damage. Percept Mot Skills 48:605–614, 1980

Resvold HE, Mirsky A, Sarason L, et al: A continuous performance test of brain damage. J Consult Psychol 20:343–350, 1956

Reynolds CF III, Soloff PH, Kupfer DJ, et al: Depression in borderline patients: a prospective EEG sleep study. Psychiatry Res 14:1–15, 1985

Rimon R, Roos BE, Rakkolainen V: The content of 5-HIAA and HVA in the CSF of patients with acute schizophrenia. J Psychosom Res 15:375–378, 1971

Risch SC, Cohen PM, Janowsky KS, et al: Physostigmine induction of depressive symptomatology in normal human subjects. Psychiatry Res 4:89–94, 1981

Rohrbaugh JW, Gaillard AWK: Sensory and motor aspects of the CNV, in Tutorials in ERP Research: Endogenous Components. Edited by Gaillard AWK, Ritter W. New York, North Holland, 1983

Rosowsky E, Gurian B: Borderline personality disorder in late life. Int Psychogeriatr 3:39–52, 1991

Roth WT, Pfefferbaum A, Horvath TB, et al: P3 reduction in auditory evoked potentials of schizophrenics. Electroencephalogr Clin Neurophysiol 49:497–505, 1980

Roth WT, Pfefferbaum A, Kelly AF, et al: Auditory event-related potentials in schizophrenia and depression. Psychiatry Res 4:497–505, 1981

Rotter M, Kalus O, Losonczy M, et al: Lateral ventricle enlargement in schizotypal personality disorder (abstract 287). Biol Psychiatry 29:173A, 1991

Roy A, Adinoff B, Linnoila M: Acting out hostility in normal volunteers: negative correlation with levels of 5-HIAA in cerebrospinal fluid. Psychiatry Res 24:187–194, 1988

Rubenstein H, Lewis SS, Rubenstein MA: Homographic entries in the internal lexicon: effects of systematicity and relative frequency of meanings. Journal of Verbal Learning and Verbal Behavior 10:57–62, 1971

Schalling D, Asberg M, Edman G, et al: Markers for vulnerability to psychopathology: temperament traits associated with platelet MAO activity. Acta Psychiatr Scand 76:172–182, 1987

Schildkraut JJ, Herzog JM, Orsulak PJ, et al: Reduced platelet monoamine oxidase activity in a subgroup of schizophrenic patients. Am J Psychiatry 133:438–440, 1976

Schneier FR, Campeas R, Fallon B, et al: Buspirone in social phobia, in Proceedings of the 17th Collegium Internationale of Neuro-Psychopharmacologium, Kyoto, Japan, September 14–18, 1990, p 141

Schneier FR, Spitzer RL, Gibbon M, et al: The relationship of social phobia subtypes and avoidant personality disorder. Compr Psychiatry 32:496–502, 1991

Schneier FR, Chin SJ, Hollander E, et al: Fluoxetine in social phobia. J Clin Psychopharmacol 12:62–64, 1992

Schulz SC, Koller MM, Kishore PR, et al: Ventricular enlargement in teenage patients with schizophrenia spectrum disorder. Am J Psychiatry 140:1592–1595, 1983

Schulz SC, Cornelius J, Schulz PM, et al: The amphetamine challenge test in patients with borderline disorder. Am J Psychiatry 145:809–814, 1988

Schulsinger F, Parnes J, Peterson E, et al: Cerebral ventricular size in the offspring of schizophrenic mothers. Arch Gen Psychiatry 41:602–606, 1984

Sciuto G, Diaferia G, Battaglia M, et al: DSM-III-R personality disorders in panic and obsessive-compulsive disorder: a comparison study. Compr Psychiatry 32:450–457, 1991

Siever LJ, Davis KL: Overview: Towards a dysregulation hypothesis of depression. Am J Psychiatry 142:1017–1031, 1985

Siever LJ, Davis KL: A psychobiological perspective on the personality disorders. Am J Psychiatry 148:1647–1658, 1991

Siever LJ, Haier, RJ, Coursey RD, et al: Smooth pursuit eye tracking impairment: relation to other "markers" of schizophrenia and psychobiologic correlates. Arch Gen Psychiatry 39:1001–1005, 1982a

Siever LJ, Uhde TW, Silberman E, et al: The growth hormone response to clonidine as a probe of noradrenergic reception responsiveness in affective disorder patients and controls. Psychiatry Res 6:293–302, 1982b

Siever LJ, Coursey RD, Alterman IS, et al: Impaired smooth-pursuit eye movement: vulnerability marker for schizotypal personality disorder in a normal volunteer population. Am J Psychiatry 141:1560–1566, 1984

Siever LJ, Keefe R, Bernstein DP, et al: Eye tracking impairment in clinically identified schizotypal personality disorder patients. Am J Psychiatry 147:740–745, 1990

Siever LJ, Kahn RS, Lawlor BA, et al: Critical issues in defining the role of serotonin in psychiatric disorders. Pharmacol Rev 43:509–525, 1991a

Siever LJ, Amin F, Coccaro EF, et al: Plasma homovanillic acid in schizotypal personality disorder patients and controls. Am J Psychiatry 148:1246–1248, 1991b

Siever LJ, Amin F, Coccaro EF, et al: Cerebrospinal fluid homovanillic acid in schizotypal personality disorder. Am J Psychiatry 150:149–151, 1993a

Siever LJ, Kalus O, Keefe R: The boundaries of schizophrenia. Psychiatric Clin North Am 16:217–244, 1993b

Silverman JM, Pinkham L, Horvath TB, et al: Affective and impulsive personality disorder traits in the relatives of patients with borderline personality disorder. Am J Psychiatry 148:1378–1385, 1991

Silverman JM, Keefe RSE, Losonczy MF, et al: Schizotypal and neuro-imaging factors in relatives of schizophrenic probands. Paper presented at the Society of Biological Psychiatry Annual Meeting, April 1992

Simeon D, Stanley B, Frances A, et al: Self-mutilation in personality disorders: psychological and biological correlates. Am J Psychiatry 149:221–226, 1992

Simons RF: Electrodermal and cardiac orienting in psychometrically high risk subjects. Psychiatry Res 4:347–356, 1981

Simons RF: Physical anhedonia and future psychopathology: a possible electrocortical continuity. Psychophysiology 19:433–441, 1982

Simons RF, Katkin W: Smooth pursuit eye movements in subjects reporting physical anhedonia and perceptual aberrations. Psychiatry Res 14:275–289, 1985

Simons RF, MacMillan FW, Ireland FB: Anticipatory pleasure deficit in subjects reporting physical anhedonia: slow cortical evidence. Biol Psychology 14:297–310, 1982a

Simons RF, MacMillan FW, Ireland FB: Reaction-time cross over in preselected schizotype subjects. J Abnorm Psychology 91:414–419, 1982b

Stark P, Fuller RW, Wong DT: The pharmacologic profile of fluoxetine. J Clin Psychiatry 46:1647–1658, 1985

Steinberg BJ, Trestman RL, Siever LJ: The cholinergic and noradrenergic neurotransmitter systems and affective instability in borderline personality disorder, in Biological and Neurobehavioral Studies in Borderline Personality Disorder. Edited by Silk KR. Washington, DC, American Psychiatric Press (in press)

Steketee G: Personality traits and diagnoses in obsessive compulsive disorder. Paper presented at the annual meeting of The Association for the Advancement of Behavior Therapy, November 1988

Sternbach HA: Fluoxetine treatment of social phobia. J Clin Psychopharmacol 10:230–231, 1990

Sternbach HA, Fleming J, Extein I, et al: The dexamethasone suppression and thyrotropin releasing hormone tests in depressed borderline patients. Psychoneuroendocrinology 8:459–462, 1983

Tancer ME, Stein MB, Uhde TW: Effects of thyrotropin-releasing hormone on blood pressure and heart rate in social phobia patients, panic disorder patients, and normal controls: results of a pilot study. Biological Psychiatry 27:781–783, 1990a

Tancer ME, Stein MB, Gelernter CS, et al: The hypothalamic-pituitary-thyroid axis in social phobia. Am J Psychiatry 147:929–933, 1990b

Tellegen A, Lykken DT, Bouchard TJ Jr, et al: Personality similarity in twins reared apart and together. J Pers Soc Psychol 54:1031–1039, 1988

Torgersen S: Genetic and nosologic aspects of schizotypal and borderline personality disorders. Arch Gen Psychiatry 41:546–554, 1984

Torgersen S: The genetic transmission of borderline personality features displays multidimensionality, in Abstracts of the American College of Neuropsychopharmacology Annual Meeting, 1992, p 23

Torgerson AM, Kringlen E: Genetic aspects of temperamental differences in infants: a study of same-sexed twins. Journal of the American Academy of Child Psychiatry 17:438–444, 1978

Traskman-Bendz L, Alling C, Oreland L, et al: Prediction of suicidal behavior from biologic tests. J Clin Psychopharmacol 12:21S–26S, 1992

Trestman RL, Coccaro EF, Mitropoulou V, et al: Differential biology of impulsivity, suicide and depression in the personality disorders, in Proceedings of the XXIII Congress of the International Society of Psychoneuroendocrinology, Madison, WI, 1992, p 92

Trestman RL, deVegvar M, Coccaro EF, et al: The differential biology of impulsivity, suicide, and aggression in depression and in personality disorders. Biol Psychiatry 33:46A–47A, 1993

Turner SM, Beidel DC, Borden JW, et al: Social phobia: Axis I and II correlates. J Abnorm Psychol 100:102–106, 1991

Turner SM, Beidel DC, Townsley RM: Social phobia: a comparison of specific and generalized subtypes and avoidant personality disorder. J Abnorm Psychol 101:326–331, 1992

Uhde TW, Tancer ME, Black B, et al: Phenomenology and neurobiology of social phobia: comparison with panic disorder. J Clin Psychiatry 52 (suppl 11):31–40, 1991

Valzelli L: Drugs and aggressiveness. Adv Pharmacol 5:79–108, 1967

van Kammen DP, Mann LP, Sternberg DE, et al: Dopamine beta-hydroxylase activity and homovanillic acid in spinal fluid in schizophrenics with brain atrophy. Science 220:974–976, 1983

Van Praag HM: CSF-5HIAA and suicide in nondepressed schizophrenics. Lancet 2:977–978, 1983

van Vliet IM, den Boer JA, Westenberg HG: Psychopharmacological treatment of social phobia: clinical and biochemical effects of brofaromine, a selective MAO-A inhibitor. Eur Neuropsychopharmacol 2:21–29, 1992

Venables PH: Psychophysiology and crime: theory and data, in Biological Contributors to Crime Causation. Edited by Maffitt TE, Medrick SA. Dordrecht, Netherlands, Martinus Nijhoff, 1987, pp 3–13

Virkkunen M, Nuutila A, Goodwin FK, et al: Cerebrospinal fluid metabolite levels in male arsonists. Arch Gen Psychiatry 44:241–247, 1987

Wainberg ML, Trestman RL, Keefe RS, et al: CPT in schizotypal personality disorder. Paper presented at the 146th annual meeting of the American Psychiatric Association, San Francisco, CA, May 1993

Widiger TA: Generalized social phobia versus avoidant personality disorder: a commentary on three studies. J Abnorm Psychol 101:340–343, 1992

Williamson S, Harpur T, Hare R: Abnormal processing of affective words by psychopaths. Psychophysiology 28:260–273, 1991

Winchel RM, Stanley M: Self-injurious behavior: a review of the behavior and biology of self-mutilation. Am J Psychiatry 148:306–317, 1991

Yehuda R, Southwick SM, Edell WS, et al: Low platelet monoamine oxidase activity in borderline personality disorder. Psychiatry Res 30:265–273, 1989

Zanarini MC, Gunderson JG, Marino MF, et al: DSM-III disorders in the families of borderline outpatients. Journal of Personality Disorders 2:292–302, 1988

Zuckerman M, Buchsbaum MS, Murphy DL: Sensation seeking and its biological correlates. Psychol Bull 88:187–214, 1980

Chapter 12

Childhood Psychiatric Disorders

Dorothy E. Grice, M.D., Ann M. Rasmusson, M.D., and James F. Leckman, M.D.

Over the past 30 years, the field of psychiatry and our understanding of psychiatric illness have undergone profound changes. Psychodynamic theories have been joined by the products of neuroscience and psychopharmacology. Advances in neurobiology and genetics have added dimensions to psychiatric research that now allow us to consider the pathophysiology of psychiatric illness at the molecular level. With technological advances in the neurosciences, research in biological psychiatry, once confined exclusively to adult psychiatric illnesses, has extended into child psychiatry. Perhaps the most compelling aspect of the empirical and theoretical research in child and adult psychiatry is the potential for more accurate diagnosis and treatment of many of the disabling and often chronic disorders that afflict psychiatric patients.

Neurobiological and molecular research in child psychiatry has followed an approach that has guided much of medical research. As Goodwin and Roy-Byrne (1987, p. 1693) discussed, the "medical model" employed in biological psychiatry emerged from infectious disease and "inborn error of metabolism" models. These models contain the theoretical assumption that the presence (or lack) of a single agent determines a disease state and that elimination (or replacement) of that agent is corrective.

Phenylketonuria (PKU) was the first inherited mental retardation syndrome linked to a biochemical disorder. PKU is characterized by elevated serum phenylalanine due to a deficiency in phenylalanine hydroxylase, the hepatic enzyme that converts phenylalanine to tyrosine. In PKU, fetal central nervous system (CNS) development is normal because of maternal metabolism of phenylalanine. However, in the neonatal period, phenylalanine levels rise and CNS maldevelopment results.

Supported in part by National Institute of Mental Health Grants MH49351 and MH18268. We thank Drs. George M. Anderson, Donald J. Cohen, and Mark A. Riddle for their thoughtful comments.

The elucidation of the molecular pathophysiology in PKU led to the development of routine PKU screening for all neonates and prenatal diagnostic techniques for some high-risk families. Once vulnerable individuals are detected, phenylalanine levels can be controlled through dietary measures, allowing for normal cerebral development.

PKU exemplifies the reductionistic disease model common in medical research. Once the primary pathological locus was identified, the range of molecular abnormalities (mutations) at that locus was determined and biological markers were defined. As a result, an accurate and cost-effective screening test was developed, and novel treatment strategies were designed. Other research continues in the areas of increased prenatal identification and gene attenuation.

The need for biological markers in childhood psychiatry is apparent because researchers in other fields have made great strides in developing treatments for various illnesses based on their discovery of biological markers using the reductionistic model of disease. In child psychiatry, research efforts are capitalizing on the explosion of knowledge in the areas of molecular genetics and developmental neurosciences.

However, in child psychiatry, attempts to determine the primary pathological loci of disease have been largely unsuccessful. However, there are notable exceptions, such as in fragile X syndrome and possibly some forms of attention-deficit hyperactivity disorder (ADHD; see Attention-Deficit Hyperactivity Disorder section).

In this chapter, we examine current definitions and examples of biological markers (e.g., genetic, neurochemical, neuroanatomical) and explore the general utility of putative biological markers in child psychiatry with regard to selected childhood psychiatric disorders.

DEFINITION OF BIOLOGICAL MARKERS

A biological marker can be defined as a measurable biological characteristic that signifies the presence of a particular disease or disease state (either before or after clinical symptoms are manifested), distinguishes one disease process from others that are otherwise clinically indistinguishable, or permits clinicians to monitor the course of an illness. In medicine, biological markers have been employed successfully and dramatically, allowing physicians to determine vulnerability to disease (PKU), detect new-onset pathological processes before they become clinically evident (glucose tolerance test during pregnancy), predict relapse before it is clinically detectable (prostate-specific antigen assay), confirm specific diagnoses and monitor clinical course (cardiac isoenzymes), and even direct specific treatments (tumor markers). Medical uses of such markers provide models of their potential use in child psychiatric illness.

Restated, there are two primary ways in which biological markers are useful in the management of clinical disorders: as trait markers and as state markers. As a general rule, trait markers allow the identification of a specific pathological process independent of the clinical expression of the disorder. A trait marker does not fluctuate with disease manifestations and can be assayed at any point in an illness, whether during the prodromal, the active, or the remitted phase. As a result, trait markers may be used to identify quiescent disease or determine the presence of vulnerability to disease in an otherwise asymptomatic individual.

The other use of biological markers is in monitoring the course of a disorder. Utilized in this way, biological markers are state dependent. The state marker may be a hallmark of illness manifestation or recrudescence and is often employed to assist the clinician in monitoring the course of disease. State markers reflect the pathophysiology of a disorder, and changes in the measure indicate important clinical change. State markers can direct therapeutic choices and aid in the determination of appropriate treatment interventions.

DEVELOPMENT OF BIOLOGICAL MARKERS

In psychiatry, the determination of pathophysiological mechanisms of disease has been hampered by the fact that the CNS is one of the most complex and least accessible anatomic structures in the body. Although in the past researchers had to rely on postmortem tissue and animal models to determine even the fundamentals of brain organization and function, technological advancements in neurochemistry, molecular biology, and in vivo imaging techniques have opened new avenues of research. For example, researchers now are able to directly measure concentrations of relevant substances in living brain tissue with magnetic resonance spectroscopy. However, the potential use of many of these techniques has not yet been fully realized in patients with psychiatric disease.

In child psychiatry, research can be even more complex for two reasons: 1) there is a relative lack of postmortem tissue available for study, and 2) it may be difficult to differentiate between normal developmental changes and pathophysiological changes indicative of specific disease processes.

A significant problem in the design of diagnostic biological-marker studies is bias in recruitment, evaluation, and follow-up of study subjects, such that the spectrum of disease examined may be inadequate. It is ethically problematic to ask children (and adults) to serve as healthy matched or comorbid control subjects in invasive studies of disease from which they do not suffer. It is likewise untenable to involve those with disease unless the potential benefits of the study clearly outweigh the risks. Therefore, such studies tend to be done only on patients manifesting the most extreme forms of the disorder. As discussed by Goldberg (1987), such selective scrutiny of the Gaussian extremes of disease distorts the statistical significance of findings and the value of biological markers thus derived.

A broad range of measures could be employed as putative biological markers. In child psychiatric research, investigators have focused on CNS neuroanatomy, characterization of cerebral spinal fluid (CSF) neurotransmitters and metabolites, peripheral models of CNS activity (e.g., platelet function), and neuropharmacological challenge studies.

MARKERS IN SPECIFIC CHILDHOOD DISORDERS

A selected survey of child psychiatric disorders follows. Although biological research has been undertaken in virtually every childhood psychiatric disorder (e.g., developmental disorders, depression, eating disorders, obsessive-compulsive disorder, and disruptive behavior disorders), very few markers that satisfy the above criteria have been identified in child psychiatry. In addition to the problems discussed above, many studies have been hampered by small samples sizes, ascertainment biases, variable phenotypical classifications, specificity of findings, and reproducibility of results.

In this chapter, we discuss four childhood psychiatric disorders—fragile X syndrome, autism, Tourette's syndrome, and ADHD—and the status of biological markers in each syndrome. Fragile X syndrome is a rare example of a childhood disorder with a well-determined biological marker. Recent advances in research on autism, Tourette's syndrome, and ADHD also have shown promise. Autism is a disorder in which putative biological markers (neurochemical and neuroanatomical) have been identified in subsets of patients with the disorder, although the underlying pathophysiological explanations for these traits are unknown at this time. The vertical transmission of Tourette's syndrome within families is known to be genetically determined, although nongenetic factors also contribute to the phenotypical expression of this disorder. If a single vulnerability gene can be isolated, robust trait markers for Tourette's syndrome should become readily available. Last, researchers in ADHD recently identified a genetic marker for a small ADHD subgroup.

Fragile X Syndrome

Multiple factors have been implicated in producing mental retardation syndromes, including prenatal (chromosomal abnormalities, inborn errors of metabolism, complications of pregnancy), perinatal (prematurity, kernicterus), postnatal (infections, toxins, trauma), and sociocultural (emotional, social, or environmental deprivation) factors (Wong and Ciaranello 1987). X-linked mental retardation syndromes generally were grouped together until the discovery in the late 1960s of a specific cytogenetic defect, later termed fragile X, that was associated with a substantial subgroup of individuals with X-linked mental retardation (Lubs 1969).

The typical presentation of males affected with fragile X syndrome includes mental retardation, macroorchidism, and prominent ears. Other clinical features include characteristic faces, connective tissue abnormalities, and increased head circumference during childhood (Turner et al. 1980).

The true prevalence of fragile X syndrome is not known. It has been estimated that between 30% and 50% of families with X-linked mental retardation have the fragile X syndrome (Turner et al. 1980).

The genetic defect that causes fragile X syndrome is located near the end of the long arm of the X chromosome at the Xq27.3 band (Yunis et al. 1978). Transmission patterns of fragile X syndrome are known to be X linked, although it is an unusual dominant disorder because of a number of features (Sherman et al. 1984, 1985). Of the carrier females, 30% demonstrate some degree of mental retardation. Although the majority of males with the fragile X chromosome are mentally retarded, approximately 20% of males who have an early form of the genetic defect are phenotypically normal and are not mentally impaired (see below). Daughters of these nonpenetrant males are also mentally normal. However, the grandsons and granddaughters of nonpenetrant males are often affected with the syndrome.

Analysis of mental impairment patterns in pedigrees shows that the risk of mental impairment depends on the position of individuals in the pedigree and that the severity of the syndrome increases through progressive generations. This pattern of transmission is known as *anticipation* (Sherman et al. 1984, 1985).

Recent molecular studies have revealed the mechanisms behind the variable transmission and expression of fragile X syndrome. In 1991, Verkerk et al. isolated a gene *(FMR-1)* that is expressed in the brain and testes. The mutation site at the *FMR-1* gene is of variable length and contains an unusual repetitive sequence of cytosine-guanine-guanine, $(CGG)_n$, and a CpG island with specific methylation patterns (Oberle et al. 1991; Pieretti et al. 1991).

The variation of DNA length at the *FMR-1* mutation site has been ascribed to differences in the $(CGG)_n$ sequences (Kremer et al. 1991). Normal X chromosomes have a range of 6–54 base-pair amplifications of the CGG sequence, with 29 being the most common number of repeats. Nonpenetrant males and carrier females have inserts from 52 to 600 base pairs, called premutations. Males with the full mutation (who exhibit full clinical features of fragile X syndrome) have amplifications from 600 to 3,000 base pairs (Fu et al. 1991; Pergolizzi et al. 1992). All alleles with more than 52 repeats (i.e., those found in fragile X families) are meiotically unstable. In carrier females, the risk of expansion from a premutation to a full mutation during meiosis correlates with the size of the premutation allele (Fu et al. 1991). When meiotic induction occurs, male offspring of the carrier female will have the full mutation and express fragile X syndrome.

The genetic and cytogenetic findings in fragile X syndrome offer a basis for the variable phenotypical expression in families with the fragile X site and resolve questions about the mechanisms of anticipation in this syndrome. The *FMR-1* gene has been identified, and although its gene product has not yet been determined, it is of note that the *FMR-1* gene is highly expressed in the brain and testes, the two organs most specifically affected in fragile X syndrome. Additionally, the molecular premutations associated with phenotypical severity are beginning to be explored (Freund et al. 1993; Reiss et al. 1993).

To assess the status of the fragile X trait markers as a model for a biological marker in child psychiatry, it is useful to compare the features of current fragile X markers with the criteria for a well-defined genetic marker set forth by Goldin et al. (1986).

The first criterion is that the marker—the *FMR-1* gene—be associated with a specific condition (i.e., fragile X syndrome). Although other genetic neurological disorders (e.g., Huntington's disease and myotonic dystrophy [Redman et al. 1993] and Kennedy's disease [Amato et al. 1993]) have a similar molecular configuration of repetitive base-pair sequences at the aberrant locus, research indicates that the *FMR-1* gene and its associated features are specifically associated with fragile X syndrome.

The second criterion is that the trait marker be heritable. Fragile X syndrome is of definite genetic origin, transmitted vertically through generations. The *FMR-1* gene is the heritable marker. Questions remain about factors that determine both the range and variation of phenotypes in fragile X families. For example, little research has been done on subgroups that carry premutations (variable repeats of less than 600 base pairs).

The third feature of a robust genetic trait marker is that it is state independent. The advances in fragile X syndrome research exemplify how identification of an accurate state-independent (i.e., trait) marker leads to the development of valuable clinical interventions. Preclinical diagnosis of fragile X syndrome is now possible, as are early psychological, social-emotional, and academic interventions for affected individuals.

The fourth criterion for a genetic marker set forth by Goldin et al. (1986) is that the marker be associated with increased risk of the disorder in relatives of the affected individual. Again, data on the fragile X syndrome illustrate the power of an accurately determined genetic marker. Because the molecular basis of anticipation (increasing severity of a condition as it passes through subsequent generations) in fragile X syndrome has become understood, researchers can examine the molecular aspects of a range of clinical phenotypes and inform families regarding their genotype and potential risk status.

Research on fragile X syndrome exemplifies how careful clinical and phenotypical study (i.e., delineation of fragile X syndrome from other X-linked mental retardation syndromes) advances biological and genetic research and can yield important biological trait markers of disease. Lubs's discovery of the fragile X site was the product of serendipity, clinical acumen, and careful development of scientific methodology. Molecular genetic breakthroughs in fragile X syndrome have resulted in model biological trait markers. Clinicians now are able to offer family and genetic counseling regarding vulnerability to fragile X syndrome, ameliorative or prophylactic intervention strategies for affected individuals, and early, even prenatal, diagnosis of fragile X syndrome.

Autism

In our current understanding of autism and pervasive developmental disorders, etiological heterogeneity is assumed. Genetic defects and maternal-fetal complications such as exposure to infectious agents during gestation, dysmaturity, gestational bleeding, and medication ingestion during pregnancy have all been proposed as causative. The presence of minor physical anomalies in autistic children has led to a hypothesis that the etiology is a first-trimester insult.

Thus, although the fundamental origins of autism remain controversial, many researchers propose interactional models in which genetic and nongenetic factors (particularly in the maternal-fetal environment) serve as incremental insults to the developing fetus, neonate, and infant, ultimately leading to the clinical expression of autistic disorders in childhood.

Although there is considerable phenotypical heterogeneity in the clinical presentation of autism, the description by Kanner (1943) remains integral to current understanding of the disorder. He emphasized the extreme aloneness and self-isolation of these individuals, as well as their obsessive desire for sameness. DSM-III-R criteria (American Psychiatric Association 1987) emphasize three major aspects of autism. Children with autism have impaired social interactions, such as poor performance in social play, inadequate peer relationships, and an inability to seek comfort from others. Communication difficulties are prominent, including limitations in verbal, nonverbal, and imaginative activities. Autistic individuals also manifest a restricted repertoire of interests and activities (e.g., attachment to unusual objects, stereotypic body movements, or preoccupation with one narrow field of interest).

In the general population, autism is thought to affect 2–5 individuals per 10,000, although these numbers vary depending on the clinical criteria used in various studies (Zahner and Pauls 1987). Autism affects boys more commonly than girls, with ratios ranging from 2:1 to 5:1 (Tsai and Beisler 1983; Tsai et al. 1987; Wing 1981). Closer examination of the gender distribution within this disorder has shown that although girls are underrepresented as a whole, they tend to be more severely impaired when they are affected (Tsai et al. 1987; Young et al. 1990) and have poorer outcomes compared with autistic boys (Lotter 1974). Biological explanations of this disparity remain undetermined.

In the past, autism was seen as a disorder of developmental arrest, with loss of skills and age-appropriate mastery typically occurring at 2–3 years of age. More recent studies, including retrospective examination of home movies (Adrien et al. 1991; Rutter 1985), indicate that autistic prodromal behaviors can be detected in early infant life. These findings offer further evidence of the early biological grounding of this disorder.

Because autism is currently seen as a final functional expression of multiple pathological genetic and developmental events, it does not fit the reductionistic model of disease causality. The search for biological markers in autism has been difficult, presumably because of the complex genesis of this disorder.

Although genetic studies have been able to identify select subgroups of autistic individuals, they have not demonstrated the presence of uniform anomalies—either in the particular type of mutation (e.g., trisomy, deletion, translocation) or the chromosomal site—that are consistent across the clinical spectrum of autism. In efforts to integrate these findings, a stress diathesis model has been invoked. Some researchers hypothesize that genetic factors result in a predisposition to developmental difficulties. The genetic potential for maldevelopment is subsequently expressed after interactions with pathological environments (Rutter 1985).

These models suggest that autism itself is not inherited, but rather a genetic defect in social function, language, or communication. Specific environmental agents and cues would then affect the exact nature, severity, and timing of the clinical manifestations of autism (Folstein and Rutter 1988). If this disorder is heritable, an increased incidence of autism—and perhaps a range of cognitive disorders—should be found in siblings of autistic children. Research in this area has been contradictory.

An examination of the biological studies of autism allows us to look at two biological markers that have been reported: hyperserotonemia and hypotrophy of the cerebellar vermis. A number of studies of autism have measured serotonin concentrations in whole blood and in platelets, the main repository for serotonin in the peripheral system. Elevated levels of serotonin in autistic individuals have been a relatively consistent research finding (for a review, see G. M. Anderson et al. 1990). Up to 30%–40% of autistic individuals are hyperserotonemic. Neurochemically, there are a number of potential explanations for elevated platelet serotonin: increased synthesis of serotonin, altered tryptophan metabolism, abnormal degradation of serotonin by monoamine oxidase, and enhanced uptake or storage of serotonin (G. M. Anderson et al. 1990).

Hyperserotonemia may be a selective marker for an as-yet poorly defined subpopulation of autistic patients rather than for all phenotypes of autism. Although many research groups have reported elevated blood serotonin levels in autistic individuals, this finding has been difficult to interpret with respect to both its clinical relevance and its neurochemical basis. Hyperserotonemia has been found to be familial within autistic families (Levanthal et al. 1990). However, autistic individuals who have elevated serotonin tend to be those with severe mental retardation. Because some nonautistic mentally retarded individuals demonstrate hyperserotonemia, doubts have been raised about the specificity of this finding (Oikawa et al. 1978).

The question of the heritability of autism remains open. For instance, it is not clear whether elevated serotonin is state or trait dependent. In addition to potential genetic influences, platelet serotonin levels are also known to vary with age and in response to certain medications. The dynamics of normal platelet uptake, storage, and release of serotonin are not well defined. How these processes are altered in autism and the relationship between this peripheral metabolic defect and CNS function remain to be determined. CSF studies of serotonin and its metabolites have not correlated with the peripheral platelet findings.

Hyperserotonemia, the most reliable and reproducible finding in autism, may be heuristically important. Some data indicate that serotonin influences nerve growth through effects on growth cone motility and synapse formation (Haydon et al. 1987). It is possible, for example, to imagine that an early dysregulation in serotonin metabolism could potentially yield pervasive, global changes in neuronal organization and cell migration, either directly or through second-messenger systems. Manifestation of these changes, most likely under developmental regulation, would occur during childhood development, with clinical evidence for the disorder emerging only as critical developmental periods are reached. If, for example, the aberration of serotonin function were environmentally cued (meaning that it could occur at different stages of neuronal organization), the timing and severity of the environmental insult would ultimately influence the clinical features of the disorder. This model also allows for the wide spectrum of symptoms and features in autism.

Neuroanatomic research has offered potential trait markers for autism. Specifically, a convergence of neuropathological findings and the results of in vivo neuroimaging studies indicates that some autistic subjects have a hypoplastic cerebellar vermis as well as hypoplasia of the cerebellar hemispheres (Arin et al. 1991; Courchesne et al. 1988; Ritvo et al. 1986). Although this finding has been widely replicated, the question of the specificity of the finding to autism remains in doubt, as many control and comparison subjects show similar defects (Piven et al. 1992).

At this stage in the delineation of the pathophysiology of autism, serotonin measurements seem to hold promise as prototypes of future biological markers in this disorder. It is possible to imagine that once the exact nature of the alteration of platelet serotonin metabolism in autism is determined, CNS studies of serotonin metabolism will be directed in accordance with these findings, with the ultimate goal being to understand the neurochemical and biological pathways that are affected in autism. Similarly, it may be possible to identify discrete neuropathological findings associated with some forms of autism.

Tourette's Syndrome

Tourette's syndrome is a chronic neuropsychiatric disorder of childhood onset. Expression of Tourette's syndrome is under the influence of genetic factors; the developmental epoch of the individual; gender; and environmental factors; including in utero and hormonal microenvironments. Tourette's syndrome serves as an exemplary model for the complexity of genetic, biological, and environmental interactions. In part because of these properties, identification of reliable biological markers in Tourette's syndrome has been, thus far, unsuccessful.

Although proposed over a century ago, Georges Gilles de la Tourette's description of this syndrome has largely withstood the test of time. In 1885, clinical features described by Tourette included the presence of motor and phonic tics, obsessive thoughts, compulsive behaviors, and a hereditary pattern of transmission. Although coprolalia and echolalia were featured as core symptoms in Tourette's original description, it is now appreciated that fewer than 50% of individuals with Tourette's syndrome manifest these symptoms. In our current understanding, Tourette's syndrome is characterized by an array of motor and phonic tics as well as by a variety of associated symptoms, including behavioral problems such as the aforementioned obsessive-compulsive symptoms, attentional and neurocognitive problems, increased impulsivity, and social difficulties. Up to 50% of individuals with Tourette's syndrome have concurrent diagnoses of ADHD.

Tourette's syndrome usually presents when individuals are between ages 2 and 16 years, with the mean age at onset being 7 years (Bruun 1988). Typically motor tics are seen first, with involvement of the head and neck being common. Tics vary in body location and can be simple (e.g., eye blinking or sniffing) or complex (e.g., shoulder jerk in concert with a facial grimace and a brief phonic utterance). Over time, tics are often joined by sensorimotor phenomena, ritualistic behaviors, and obsessional thoughts (Leckman et al. 1992). Sensorimotor phenomena include a premonitory urge to execute a tic. A premonitory urge is often likened to an itch that needs to be scratched (Leckman et al. 1993). It precedes the tic and is relieved with the performance of the tic.

Although the transmission of Tourette's syndrome is highly penetrant, there is a significant disparity in the rates of occurrence between sexes. Boys are more commonly affected than girls, with ratios ranging from 2:1 to 4:1 depending on the population under study. The prevalence of Tourette's syndrome is estimated to be 9.3 per 10,000 for boys and 1 per 10,000 for girls (King and Noshpitz 1991). Recent genetic findings offer a partial explanation for this disparity. Family studies show that Tourette's syndrome and some forms of obsessive-compulsive disorder are alternative phenotypical expressions representing the same genetic anomaly. Further analysis reveals that females are more likely to display obsessive-compulsive symptoms, whereas males more commonly manifest tics and have a higher incidence of disruptive behaviors (Pauls and Leckman 1986; Pauls et al. 1986). The natural history studies of Tourette's syndrome show that the most severe symptoms typically remit by young adulthood (Bruun 1988; Burd et al. 1986).

The familial nature of Tourette's syndrome and tic disorders has led investigators to search for patterns of inheritance and genetic markers of Tourette's syndrome. Family and twin studies (and, more recently, genetic linkage studies) have yielded evidence that Tourette's syndrome, chronic tics, and obsessive-compulsive disorder are related and represent a spectrum of clinical phenotypes that are transmitted vertically through families as an autosomal dominant trait (Pauls and Leckman 1986, 1988; Pauls et al. 1991). Genetic linkage studies continue, and although over 80% of the genome has been excluded, the gene has yet to be identified (Pakstis et al. 1991). Another approach that may yield biological markers for Tourette's syndrome is the search for genes that, when present in conjunction with the Tourette's syndrome gene, influence an individual's phenotypical expression of Tourette's syndrome (Comings et al. 1991). Candidate genes include those coding for dopamine receptors and dopamine transporters (Gelernter et al. 1990).

Although the exact pathophysiology of Tourette's syndrome remains unclear, a number of studies have implicated the basal ganglia and related cortical and thalamic structures as the primary affected anatomic sites (for a review, see Chappell et al. 1990). Magnetic resonance imaging studies show significant differences in the volumetric measurements of the basal ganglia and the corpus callosum of Tourette's syndrome individuals compared with control subjects (Peterson et al. 1993, in press). Altered glucose metabolism (Stoetter et al. 1992) and regional cerebral blood flow (Riddle et al. 1992) in the basal ganglia and the frontal lobes have been demonstrated through positron-emission tomography and single photon emission computed tomography, respectively. The questions of whether brain imaging ultimately will be clinically useful to discern an anatomic biological marker for Tourette's syndrome and whether brain images are genetically influenced or are state markers require further investigation.

Concurrent with anatomical studies, research in the area of neurotransmitters and neurochemistry has implicated involvement of the central monoaminergic systems (dopaminergic, serotonergic, and noradrenergic) represented in the basal ganglia. Pharmacological challenge studies and clinical trials have indicated that disruptions in the dopaminergic system (Shapiro et al. 1989) and the noradrenergic system (Leckman et al. 1986) occur in patients with Tourette's syndrome. CSF studies have indicated that there may be alterations in the opioid system (Haber et al. 1986) and the dopamine system (Butler et al. 1979; Cohen et al. 1978; Singer et al. 1982). A postmortem study of Tourette's syndrome patients demonstrated diffuse decreases in serotonin, tryptophan, and 5-hydroxyindoleacetic acid (5-HIAA) levels in cortical and subcortical brain sites (G. M. Anderson et al. 1992).

Although it is difficult to comment assuredly that the neuroanatomical and neurochemical findings noted above will ultimately be found to be specifically associated with Tourette's syndrome, many of these studies demonstrated robust and significant changes in brain areas or brain neurochemistry in Tourette's syndrome patients when they were compared with control groups. Research on Tourette's syndrome has repeatedly implicated the involvement of the basal ganglia and associated corticothalamic and limbic structures that contain the central monoamine systems. These findings are supported by a previously determined understanding of brain structure and function. For example, the basal ganglia are functionally involved in movement, and dopamine plays an integral role in the regulation of movement.

In Tourette's syndrome and tic disorders, heritability, the second criterion, is well established through family studies and genetic linkage studies. Although the actual genetic factor(s) has not been isolated, research thus far reminds us of the importance of well-described phenotypes. For example, astute clinical assessment and sophisticated genetic analysis were used to identify tic-related obsessive-compulsive disorder as an alternative expression of the typical Tourette's syndrome phenotype. It is also important to recall that not every presentation of a disorder with known genetic etiology is necessarily genetic in origin. Instead, it may be a sporadic case or a phenocopy.

In sum, the heterogeneous biological, biochemical, and neurochemical findings in Tourette's syndrome are provocative, as is the evidence for the complex and interacting pathophysiology that underlies the expression of Tourette's syndrome. Given the strength of the evidence that a single locus plays a major role in the transmission of Tourette's syndrome, perhaps the most propitious direction in the pursuit of a biological marker for Tourette's syndrome is to continue the search for the Tourette's syndrome gene. Identification of a genetic marker would lead to more accurate and timely diagnosis of Tourette's syndrome and would promote the development of early intervention strategies, genetic counseling, or even techniques of genetic prevention.

Attention-Deficit Hyperactivity Disorder

ADHD is a clinical syndrome in which symptoms of motor restlessness, impulsivity, inattention, and distractibility result in suboptimal social and academic function. This disorder is more prevalent in boys, by a ratio of approximately 8:1, and affects between 1% and 5% of the population (J. C. Anderson et al. 1987). Family studies also have shown that relatives of children with ADHD have a substantially higher risk of ADHD, antisocial personality, and depression (Biederman et al. 1986, 1987).

Previous studies directed toward establishing the etiology of ADHD have invoked the neurotransmitter hypothesis (Zametkin and Rapoport 1987)—in part because of the observed therapeutic effects of stimulant medications in ADHD. The dopamine system was first implicated. For instance, administration of amphetamine led to a decline in CSF homovanillic acid (HVA) (the major metabolite of central dopamine) levels in subjects with ADHD, whereas baseline CSF HVA levels were normal (Shetty and Chase 1976). In another study, the ratio of HVA to probenecid was found to be lower in 6 boys with the disorder than in 26 control subjects undergoing evaluation for other disorders (B. A. Shaywitz et al. 1977). These clinical findings were supported by basic research revealing that selective lesion of the dopamine system in rats caused hyperactivity and later learning deficits (S. E. Shaywitz and B. A. Shaywitz 1982).

Hypotheses regarding the etiology of ADHD also invoke malfunction of the noradrenergic system (Zametkin and Rapoport 1987). Dextroamphetamine, monoamine oxidase inhibitors, and desipramine are among the most effective agents in the treatment of ADHD; all these medications reproducibly suppress 3-methoxy-4-hydroxyphenylglycol (MHPG) levels in plasma and urine (MHPG is the major metabolite of CNS norepinephrine in humans). In addition, children with ADHD were observed to have greater vascular pressor responses on standing compared with control subjects (despite equal increases in plasma norepinephrine), suggesting that postsynaptic α-adrenergic receptors may be supersensitive in children with ADHD (Mikkelsen et al. 1981).

However, these neurophysiological abnormalities have not been found to be sensitive or specific for ADHD, and no diagnostically predictive markers for ADHD have been developed as a result of this line of inquiry. Central neurotransmitter system function is dynamic, interactive, and reflective of a number of factors, including the impact of comorbid psychopathology and stress. Indices of central neurotransmitter system function are thus difficult to interpret neurophysiologically (for a review, see Rasmusson et al. 1990).

Brain imaging studies have also been undertaken with the hope of defining either metabolic or neuroanatomic abnormalities in ADHD. For instance, Zametkin et al. (1990) found that adults with ADHD that had persisted since childhood (and who had at least one child with the disorder) had significantly reduced glucose metabolism in 30 of 60 regions of the brain. However, the degree to which such a profile predicts ADHD has not been established.

Most recently, the clinical profile of ADHD has been predictively linked in a subset of patients to the presence of a mutation in the human thyroid receptor-β gene. Hauser et al. (1993) studied 104 subjects from 18 families with generalized resistance to thyroid hormone. The latter is a syndrome in which elevations in triiodothyronine (T_3) and thyroxine (T_4) are accompanied by inappropriately high levels of thyrotropin-releasing hormone. To varying degrees, peripheral and central tissues are believed to be resistant to the metabolic impact of thyroid hormone because of structural abnormalities of the cellular thyroid receptor deriving from specific mutations in exons 9 and 10 of the $hTR\beta$ gene. Such mutations were found in 13 of the 18 families studied. In addition, the likelihood of having ADHD was found to be 10 times higher in children with generalized resistance to thyroid hormone and 15 times higher in affected adults.

Thus, even though ADHD is the common clinical phenotype of heterogeneous pathophysiological and environmental processes (Weiss 1990), in the subgroup of ADHD patients described by Hauser et al. (1993), either the clinical syndrome of generalized resistance to thyroid hormone or its underlying genetic abnormality may be considered a predictive marker for ADHD. This finding may guide future inquiries into processes by which specific genetic abnormalities lead to particular phenotypical presentations. For instance, molecular links between the thyroid receptor and genes involved in the homeostasis of catecholamine neurotransmitter systems have been postulated. Also, it is not difficult to imagine how thyroid hormone resistance in the brain might lead to decreased brain glucose metabolism, decreased available energy, and difficulty in maintaining an actively focused state.

Locating the genetic abnormality underlying ADHD in this subset of affected patients may allow early presumptive diagnosis of this disorder. Ameliorative behavioral, academic, and pharmacological treatments could then be initiated before significant functional decline occurs. Curative genetic therapy for this particular subtype of ADHD may also be developed.

CONCLUSION

Research involving biological markers has generated a substantial amount of neurobiological, neurochemical, and neuroanatomical data about childhood psychiatric disorders. As seen in the above examples, biological markers may be found in subpopulations of patients with a specific disorder, but may not be present in all individuals with that disorder. Conversely, genetic biological markers may be present in individuals who manifest no obvious signs of a disorder. Because biological markers measure one facet of a syndrome, they may fall short of representing the full dimensions of the disease etiology and potential.

In conclusion, research into the phenomenology and causation of childhood psychiatric disease makes some implicit but often necessary assumptions regarding current psychiatric nosology. Because diagnosis in child psychiatry is still largely grounded in clinical presentation, current classification systems categorize groups based on clinical similarities and, in doing so, often presume underlying etiological homogeneity. Although some presentations of disease may be derived from similar pathophysiological mechanisms, clinical similarity does not necessarily reflect common causation (Leckman et al. 1987). Additionally, it would be improvident not to recall that many symptoms cross diagnostic categories and may represent other etiologically homogeneous mechanisms that are not yet recognized by current diagnostic schema.

Because they are derived from underlying pathophysiological processes, biological markers can serve as both confirmation of and challenge to nosological systems. In this way, biological markers encourage critical reexamination of disease classifications while demonstrating direct clinical utility through more accurate diagnosis, delineation of pathophysiological mechanisms, and determination of appropriate treatment strategies.

REFERENCES

Adrien JL, Faure M, Perrot A, et al: Autism and family home movies: preliminary findings. J Autism Dev Disord 21:43–49, 1991

Amato AA, Prior TW, Barohn RJ, et al: Kennedy's disease: a clinicopathologic correlation with mutations in the androgen receptor gene. Neurology 43:791–794, 1993

American Psychiatric Association: Diagnostic and Statistical Manual of Mental Disorders, 3rd Edition, Revised. Washington, DC, American Psychiatric Association, 1987

Anderson GM, Horne WC, Chatterjee D, et al: The hyperserotonemia of autism. Ann N Y Acad Sci 600:331–340, 1990

Anderson GM, Pollack ES, Chatterjee D, et al: Postmortem analysis of subcortical monoamines and amino acids in Tourette's syndrome, in Advances in Neurology, Vol 58. Edited by Chase TN, Friedhoff AJ, Cohen DJ. New York, Raven, 1992, pp 123–133

Anderson JC, Williams S, McGee R, et al: DSM-III disorders in pre-adolescent children: prevalence in a large sample from the general population. Arch Gen Psychiatry 44:69–76, 1987

Arin DM, Bauman ML, Kemper TL: The distribution of Purkinje cell loss in the cerebellum in autism (abstract). Neurology (suppl 1)41:307, 1991

Biederman J, Munir K, Knee D, et al: A family study of patients with attention deficit disorder and normal controls. Psychiatry Res 20:263–274, 1986

Biederman J, Munir K, Knee D, et al: High rate of affective disorders in probands with attention deficit disorder and in their relatives: a controlled family study. Am J Psychiatry 144:330–333, 1987

Bruun RD: The natural history of Tourette's syndrome, in Tourette's Syndrome and Tic Disorders: Clinical Understanding and Treatment. Edited by Cohen DJ, Bruun RD, Leckman JF. New York, Wiley, 1988, pp 21–40

Burd L, Kerbeshian J, Wilkenheiser M, et al: Prevalence of de la Tourette syndrome in North Dakota adults. Am J Psychiatry 143:787–788, 1986

Butler IJ, Koslow SH, Seifert WE Jr, et al: Biogenic amine metabolism in Tourette's syndrome. Ann Neurol 6(1):37–39, 1979

Chappell PB, Leckman JF, Pauls D, et al: Biochemical and genetic studies in Tourette's syndrome: implications for treatment and future research, in Application of Basic Neuroscience to Child Psychiatry. Edited by Deutsch SI, Weizman A, Weizman R. New York, Plenum, 1990, pp 241–255

Cohen DJ, Shaywitz, BA, Caparulo B, et al: Chronic, multiple tics of Gilles de la Tourette's disease. CSF acid monoamine metabolites after probenecid administration. Arch Gen Psychiatry 35:245–250, 1978

Comings DE, Comings BG, Muhleman D, et al: The dopamine D2 receptor locus as a modifying gene in neuropsychiatric disorders. JAMA 266:1793–1800, 1991

Courchesne E, Yeung-Courchesne R, Press GA, et al: Hypoplasia of cerebellar vermal lobules VI and VII in autism. N Engl J Med 318:1349–1354, 1988

Folstein SE, Rutter ML: Autism: familial aggregation and genetic implications. J Autism Dev Disord 18:3–30, 1988

Freund LS, Reiss AL, Abrams MT: Psychiatric disorders associated with fragile X syndrome in the young female. Pediatrics 91:321–329, 1993

Fu YH, Kuhl BP, Pizzuti A, et al: Variation in the CGG repeat at the fragile X site results in genetic instability: resolution of the Sherman paradox. Cell 67:1047–1058, 1991

Gelernter J, Pakstis AJ, Pauls DL, et al: Gilles de la Tourette syndrome is not linked to D2-dopamine receptor. Arch Gen Psychiatry 47:1073–1077, 1990

Goldberg SC: Persistent flaws in the design and analysis of psychopharmacology research, in Psychopharmacology: The Third Generation of Progress. Edited by Meltzer HY. New York, Raven, 1987, pp 1005–1012

Goldin LR, Nurnberger JI Jr, Gershon ES: Clinical methods in psychiatric genetics, II: the high risk approach. Acta Psychiatr Scand 74:119–128, 1986

Goodwin FK, Roy-Byrne PP: Future directions in biological psychiatry, in Psychopharmacology: The Third Generation of Progress. Edited by Meltzer HY. New York, Raven, 1987

Haber SN, Kowall NW, Vonsattell JP, et al: Gilles de la Tourette syndrome: a postmortem and neurohistochemical study. J Neurosci 75:225–241, 1986

Hauser P, Zametkin AJ, Martinez P, et al: Attention deficit hyperactivity disorder in people with generalized resistance to thyroid hormone. N Engl J Med 328:997–1001, 1993

Haydon PG, McCobb DP, Kater SB: The regulation of neurite outgrowth, growth cone motility, and electrical synaptogenesis by serotonin. J Neurobiol 18:197–215, 1987

Kanner L: Autistic disturbances of affective content. Nervous Child 2:217–250, 1943

King RA, Noshpitz JD: Tic disorders, in Pathways of Growth: Essentials of Child Psychiatry, Vol 2. New York, Wiley, 1991, pp 299–314

Kremer EJ, Pritchard M, Lynch M, et al: Mapping of DNA instability at the fragile X to a trinucleotide repeat sequence p(CGG)n. Science 252:1711–1714, 1991

Leckman JF, Ort S, Anderson GM, et al: Rebound phenomenon in Tourette's syndrome after abrupt withdrawal of clonidine: behavioral, cardiovascular, and neurochemical effects. Arch Gen Psychiatry 43:1168–1176, 1986

Leckman JF, Weissman MM, Pauls DL, et al: Family genetic studies and identification of valid diagnostic categories in adult and child psychiatry. Br J Psychiatry 151:39–44, 1987

Leckman JF, Pauls DL, Peterson BS, et al: Pathogenesis of Tourette's syndrome: clues from the clinical phenotypes and natural history, in Advances in Neurology, Vol 58. Edited by Chase TN, Friedhoff AJ, Cohen DJ. New York, Raven, 1992, pp 15–24

Leckman JF, Walker DE, Cohen DJ: Premonitory urges in Tourette's syndrome. Am J Psychiatry 150:98–102, 1993

Levanthal BL, Cook EH Jr, Morford M, et al: Relationship of whole-blood serotonin and plasma norepinephrine with autistic families. J Autism Dev Disord 20:499–511, 1990

Lotter V: Factors related to outcome in autistic children. Journal of Autism and Childhood Schizophrenia 4:263–277, 1974

Lubs HA: A marker X chromosome. Am J Hum Genet 21:231–244, 1969

Mikkelsen E, Lake CR, Brown GL, et al: The hyperactive child syndrome: peripheral sympathetic nervous system function and the effect of D-amphetamine. Psychiatry Res 4:157–69, 1981

Oberle I, Rousseau F, Heitz D, et al: Instability of a 550-base pair DNA segment and abnormal methylation in fragile X syndrome. Science 252:1097–1102, 1991

Oikawa K, Deonauth J, Breidbart S: Mental retardation and elevated serotonin levels in adults. Life Sci 23(1):45–47, 1978

Pakstis AJ, Heutinik P, Pauls DL, et al: Progress in the search of genetic linkage of Tourette's syndrome: an exclusion map covering more than 50% of the autosomal genome. Am J Hum Genet 48:281–294, 1991

Pauls DL, Leckman JF: The inheritance of Gilles de la Tourette syndrome and associated behaviors: evidence for autosomal dominant transmission. N Engl J Med 315:993–997, 1986

Pauls DL, Leckman JF: The genetics of Tourette's syndrome, in Tourette's Syndrome and Tic Disorders: Clinical Understanding and Treatment. Edited by Cohen DJ, Bruun RD, Leckman JF. New York, Wiley, 1988, pp 91–101

Pauls DL, Towbin KE, Leckman JF, et al: Gilles de la Tourette syndrome and obsessive compulsive disorder. Arch Gen Psychiatry 43:1180–1182, 1986

Pauls DL, Cohen DJ, Heimbuch R, et al: Familial pattern and transmission of Gilles de la Tourette syndrome and multiple tics. Arch Gen Psychiatry 38:1091–1093, 1991

Pergolizzi RG, Erster SH, Goonewardena P, et al: Detection of full fragile X mutation. Lancet 339:271–272, 1992

Peterson B, Riddle MA, Cohen DJ, et al: Reduced basal ganglia volumes in Tourette's syndrome using 3-dimensional reconstruction techniques from magnetic resonance images. Neurology 43:941–949, 1993

Peterson B, Leckman JF, Duncan, J et al: Corpus callosum morphology from MR images in Tourette's syndrome. Psychiatry Res (in press)

Pieretti A, Zhang F, Ying-Hui F, et al: Absence of expression of the FMR-1 gene in fragile X syndrome. Cell 66:817–822, 1991

Piven J, Nehme E, Simon J, et al: Magnetic resonance imaging in autism: measurement of the cerebellum, pons, and fourth ventricle. Biol Psychiatry 31:491–504, 1992

Rasmusson AM, Riddle MA, Leckman JF, et al: Neurotransmitter assessment in neuropsychiatric disorders of childhood, in Application of Basic Neuroscience to Child Psychiatry. Edited by Deutsch SI, Weizman A, Weizman R. New York, Plenum, 1990, pp 33–59

Redman JB, Fenwick RG, Fu YH, Pizzuti A: Relationship between parental trinucleotide GCT repeat length and severity of myotonic dystrophy in offspring. JAMA 269:1960–1965, 1993

Reiss AL, Freund L, Abrams MT, et al: Neurobiological effects of the fragile X premutation in adult women—a controlled study. Am J Hum Genet 52:884–894, 1993

Riddle MA, Rasmusson AM, Woods SW, et al: SPECT imaging of cerebral blood flow in Tourette's syndrome, in Advances in Neurology, Vol 58. Edited by Chase TN, Friedhoff AJ, Cohen DJ. New York, Raven, 1992, pp 207–211

Ritvo ER, Freeman BJ, Scheibel AB, et al: Lower Purkinje cell counts in the cerebella of four autistic subjects: initial findings of the UCLA-NSAC autopsy research report. Am J Psychiatry 143:862–866, 1986

Rutter M: Infantile autism and other pervasive developmental disorders, in Child and Adolescent Psychiatry: Modern Approaches. Edited by Rutter M, Hersuv L. Oxford, England, Blackwell, 1985, pp 545–566

Shapiro ES, Shapiro AK, Fulop G, et al: Controlled study of haloperidol, pimozide, and placebo for the treatment of Gilles de la Tourette syndrome. Arch Gen Psychiatry 46:722–730, 1989

Shaywitz BA, Cohen DJ, Bower WB: CSF monoamine metabolites in children with minimal brain dysfunction: evidence for alteration of brain dopamine. J Pediatr 90:67–71, 1977

Shaywitz SE, Shaywitz BA: Biological influences in attentional disorders, in Developmental Behavioral Pediatrics. Edited by Levine MD, Carey WB, Crocker AC, et al. Philadelphia, PA, WB Saunders, 1982, pp 746–755

Sherman SL, Morton NE, Jacobs PA, et al: The marker X syndrome: a cytogenetic and genetic analysis. Ann Hum Genet 48:21–37, 1984

Sherman SL, Jacobs PA, Morton NE, et al: Further segregation analysis of the fragile X syndrome with special reference to transmitting males. Hum Genet 69:3289–3299, 1985

Shetty T, Chase TN: Central monoamines and hyperkinesis of childhood. Neurology 26:1000–1006, 1976

Singer HS, Butler IJ, Tune LE, et al: Dopaminergic dysfunction in Tourette's syndrome. Ann Neurol 2:361–366, 1982

Stoetter B, Braun AR, Randolph C, et al: Functional neuroanatomy of TS: limbic-motor interactions studies with FDG PET, in Advances in Neurology, Vol 58. Edited by Chase TN, Friedhoff AJ, Cohen DJ. New York, Raven, 1992, pp 213–226

Tsai L, Beisler JM: The development of sex differences in infantile autism. Br J Psychiatry 142:373–378, 1983

Tsai L, Steward MA, August G: Implication of sex differences in the familial transmission of infantile autism. J Autism Dev Disord 11:165–173, 1987

Turner G, Daniel A, Frost M: X-linked mental retardation, macro-orchidism, and the Xq27 fragile site. J Pediatr 96:837–841, 1980

Verkerk AJ, Pieretti M, Sutcliffe JS, et al: Identification of a gene (FMR-1) containing a CGG repeat coincident with a breakpoint cluster region exhibiting length variation in fragile X syndrome. Cell 65:905–914, 1991

Weiss G: Hyperactivity in childhood. N Engl J Med 323:1413–1415, 1990

Wing L: Sex ratios in early childhood autism and related conditions. Psychiatry Res 5:129–137, 1981

Wong DL, Ciaranello RD: Molecular biological approaches to mental retardation, in Psychopharmacology: The Third Generation of Progress. Edited by Meltzer HY. New York, Raven, 1987

Young JG, Brasie JR, Leven L: Genetic causes of autism and the pervasive developmental disorders, in Applications of Basic Neuroscience to Child Psychiatry. Edited by Deutsch SI, Weizman A, Weizman R. New York, Plenum, 1990, pp 1183–1216

Yunis JJ, Sawyer JR, Ball DW: The characterization of high resolution G-banded chromosomes of man. Chromosoma 67:293–307, 1978

Zahner GEP, Pauls DL: Epidemiological surveys of infantile autism, in Handbook of Autism and Pervasive Developmental Disorders. Edited by Cohen DJ, Donnellan AM. New York, Wiley, 1987, pp 199–207

Zametkin AJ, Rapoport JL: Neurobiology of attention deficit disorder with hyperactivity: where have we come in 50 years? J Am Acad Child Adolesc Psychiatry 26:676–686, 1987

Zametkin AJ, Nordahl TE, Gross M, et al: Cerebral glucose metabolism in adults with hyperactivity of childhood onset. N Engl J Med 323:1361–1366, 1990

Afterword to Section II

Jack M. Gorman, M.D., and Laszlo A. Papp, M.D.,
Section Editors

The first solid evidence that mental disorders are substantially determined by biological factors originated from successful medication treatment trials. In fact, the most obvious—but frequently overlooked—biological marker of a psychiatric illness or symptom is its response to the acute and chronic administration of specific medications. The finding that medications can control specific mental phenomena revolutionized the field; a series of symptom-specific psychotropic medications were developed, with subsequent research into their mechanisms of action. The "pharmacologic dissection" strategy of psychiatric research began to cut through traditional diagnostic categories, established new directions for research, and restructured the entire practice of psychiatry.

The growing success of biological treatments in psychiatry significantly expedited the search for other biological markers. The ideal biological marker is specific, sensitive, and readily observable. If a procedure is required for using the marker, it should be harmless, quick, and readily reproducible. A state marker is present only during symptomatic episodes, whereas a trait marker should persist regardless of the manifest symptoms. In general, a trait marker is considered to be more stable—unaffected by treatment status and capable of identifying asymptomatic carriers.

The research strategies most frequently used in the search for the ideal marker start with monitoring a series of biophysiological and biochemical measures in untreated patients, challenging the patients with specific pharmacological agents, and evaluating the direct and indirect signs of central neurotransmitter abnormalities. Investigators follow the same parameters throughout the course of the illness, rechallenge the symptom-free patients pharmacologically, and use various comparison groups to establish specificity. The application of epidemiology, sophisticated genetic techniques, and the latest advances in biotechnology supplements these strategies. The testimony of success is the rich and diverse data base documented by these chapters.

The traditional strongholds of biological research in schizophrenia, anxiety, mood disorders, and substance use disorders have been joined in this section by three relative newcomers: personality, childhood, and eating disorders. The tremendous theoretical and clinical impact of the successful biological treatment of a disorder that was thought to be medication resistant is amply documented in the chapter on personality disorders. The availability of safe, noninvasive biological procedures and tests finally allowed the evaluation of biological abnormalities in younger patients: children with psychiatric illness and adolescents with eating disorders. New methodologies will also open up the possibility of testing the children of adult psychiatric patients for biological predictors. The model for this type of research is presented in the chapter on alcoholism. The assessment of multiple risk factors in the children of alcoholic patients is our best hope to prevent the illness.

The benefits of biological markers in psychiatry are manifold. Biological markers could objectively identify patients with a manifest illness, predict the illness in carriers, and provide a rationale for early prevention. Some markers may give guidelines for the duration of treatment, whereas others may serve as screening devices in the general population.

"Biopsychiatry" and the promise of control of psychiatric symptoms had enormous social and political consequences. Mental illness started to look more like any other medical condition, and thus began the movement to "remedicalize" psychiatry, destigmatize mental illness, and provide insurance coverage for psychiatric treatment on par with that provided for other medical therapies. The unfortunate side effect of this process—the artificial split between "biological" versus "psychological" theories and treatments—continues to damage the profession and confuse the patient. Reiterating our "Foreword" to this section, we would like to emphasize again the need to incorporate all valid findings—psychological and biological—into an ideologically unbiased understanding of mental illness. The information presented in the preceding chapters is an attempt to stimulate and broaden psychiatric thinking.

III

Ethics

III

Ethics

Section III

Ethics

Foreword

Jeremy A. Lazarus, M.D., Section Editor

It has been a pleasure to serve as a section editor for the *Review of Psychiatry* series. Some 20 years of working with the issue of ethics in the American Psychiatric Association (APA) has provided me with a pragmatic base to address highly controversial ethical dilemmas. The opportunity to bring together a group of authors to elucidate these issues in a more comprehensive way has been both stimulating and rewarding for me.

We psychiatrists, as members of the medical profession, subscribe to the oldest set of ethical guidelines of any profession. The Hippocratic oath has been the cornerstone of medical ethics, along with additions from Maimonides and the monastic tradition. In the last 20 years, however, there has been a substantial shift away from these principles. Today, patients' rights, informed consent, and social justice are the pressing issues in medical ethics. New life-sustaining technologies have expanded the envelope of ethical thinking, and marginally beneficial care has contributed to skyrocketing medical costs. The APA, recognizing the unique nature of the psychiatrist-patient relationship, broadened the American Medical Association's (AMA's) *Principles of Medical Ethics* by adding the "Annotations Especially Applicable to Psychiatry." Along with the APA's "Opinions of the Ethics Committee," these stand as the official positions of organized psychiatry.

Psychiatry has confronted ethical problems related to confidentiality, informed consent, sexual misconduct, and the fundamental nature of the doctor-patient relationship. The AMA has provided broad assistance in promulgating ethical opinions that have been integrated as positions of the APA in areas such as conflicts of interest, managed care, self-referral, and gifts from industry. The APA Ethics Committee has developed ethical positions based on the ethical dilemmas brought to its attention.

Ethical problems usually involve conflicts between various ethical principles. Although there may be clear-cut answers for some problems, most require a careful examination and balancing of the underlying principles. In addition, one's value system, exclusive of medical ethics, may play a significant role in the process of ethical decision making. While reading this section, please keep in mind the fundamental ethical principles of autonomy, beneficence, justice, and honesty. These will most often be the principles in conflict.

This section is not a comprehensive review of every ethical problem for psychiatry; rather, it contains chapters relevant to common ethical dilemmas facing each of us. Although it could be used as an end point for the topics presented, it will hopefully serve as a starting point for ongoing ethical exploration.

In Chapter 13, Jay E. Kantor, Ph.D., carefully delineates several very sensitive areas of ethics in research, training, and experimental therapies. The very nature of the illnesses that psychiatrists treat pushes the questions about informed consent and honesty to the center of our attention. Our awareness of the power of the doctor-patient relationship and the attendant risk of exploitation makes these issues especially relevant.

Robert M. Wettstein, M.D., in Chapter 14, then focuses on confidentiality, the bedrock of the psychiatrist-patient relationship. The basic honesty required by both the patient and the psychiatrist is supported by the confidential relationship; however, third-party review has strained the ability to maintain confidentiality. In addition, the alteration of the therapeutic process by external review can have a detrimental influence on the development of a therapeutic alliance. Dr. Wettstein has focused on some confidentiality concerns not covered as broadly in previous literature, such as child abuse and treatment of patients who have been victimized by sexual misconduct.

We have expanded the scope of psychiatric practice to include specialized training in forensic psychiatry. This expansion has brought up new dilemmas of an ethical nature that are discussed in Chapter 15 by Robert Weinstock, M.D., Gregory B. Leong, M.D., and J. Arturo Silva, M.D. Organized forensic psychiatry, through the American Academy of Psychiatry and the Law, has taken an active role in delineating the special ethical problems encountered in forensic work. Although the academy has followed the ethical principles of the APA, there has also been a push to clarify certain dilemmas about which the APA's "Annotations Especially Applicable to Psychiatry" are silent. Collaboration among the American Academy of Psychiatry and the Law, the APA Ethics Committee, and the APA Council on Psychiatry and Law has served an important function in elaborating these special problems.

The next subject, discussed in Chapter 16 by Jeremy A. Lazarus, M.D., and Steven S. Sharfstein, M.D., is the impact of managed care on the fundamental values of psychiatry. The unique influence of economics on ethics will need ongoing exploration. With the impact of both health care reform and our society's diminishing patience with the explosion in health care costs, psychiatrists face dilemmas every day involving changing paradigms of treatment and financial pressures.

Conflicts about undertreatment and overtreatment, and the inherent ethical problems arising in managed care, are illustrated by case vignettes.

In Chapter 17, on nonsexual exploitation and boundary violations, Donna Elliott Frick, M.D., summarizes this complex ethical and therapeutic subject. The theoretical and actual experience of what level of boundary violation causes harm or is exploitative is given close scrutiny. Dr. Frick guides us in assessing the risks associated with boundary violations.

In Chapter 18, Glen O. Gabbard, M.D., discusses the multifaceted and destructive effects of doctor-patient sexual relationships. A review of doctor and patient vulnerabilities, evaluation of the types of physicians involved in sexual misconduct, and the traumatic effects on the patient are all considered. Dr. Gabbard's rich experience in the theoretical and practical aspects of this problem is greatly appreciated.

Although covering several major areas in ethics, this section does not include discussions about forced treatment, certain conflicts of interest, suicide, euthanasia, abortion, or disagreements between psychiatry and religion. These should be areas for future review.

Chapter 13

Ethical Issues in Psychiatric Research and Training

Jay E. Kantor, Ph.D.

RESEARCH ISSUES

Psychiatric research seems to have an ethically suspect public image. To some extent, that negative image reflects reality. However, often the image is unrealistically tinted by the eye of the beholder. On the justifiable side of the public's negative bias is the behavioral sciences' long history of complicity in what would currently be considered abuse of research subjects' rights to informed consent and to refuse to serve as research subjects. Perhaps the most generally known examples of these abuses include instances relating to the use of psychosurgery (Breggin 1982; *Kaimowitz v. Department of Health* 1973) and the experimental use of psychoactive agents such as lysergic acid diethylamide (LSD) (Macklin 1982) on unknowing subjects.

Psychiatric and related "scientific" findings about human behavior have also been used to justify horrendous governmental actions. The Nazis' program of "racial hygiene" included some concern about heritable undesirable physical characteristics. However, the program mainly seized on behavioral scientists' claims and recommendations about heritable and immutable undesirable behavioral characteristics to justify the extermination and sterilization of races and individuals who supposedly carried those characteristics in their genes. Psychiatrists were heavily involved in the theory and implementation of these policies (Lifton 1986; Proctor 1988).

Even without its research aspects, psychiatric treatment presents an ambivalent picture to the public. Part of the negative public view derives from fears and misconceptions about mental illness. Psychiatry has no infectious germs to demonstrate to the public as the causes of mental illness. Not only are the causes complex, but there is often disagreement within the profession about etiologies and about appropriate treatments. Those uncertainties are reflected in laypersons' anxiety when they try to comprehend diseases that can neither be demystified by showing slides of bacteria nor are foreseeably curable by some new antibiotic or preventable with a vaccination. Indications of genetic causes may produce more apprehension than hope, and indications of sources within family dynamics may be threatening enough to induce public resentment and defensive derision. The public's qualms about psychiatric experimentation partially reflect its underlying horror and fear of mental illness itself. Those fears are probably exacerbated by the high visibility of some unhospitalized mentally ill persons, the public's inability to differentiate among types and degrees of mental illness, and the concomitant widespread tendency to see all mentally ill persons as potentially dangerous.

Putting aside history and public misconceptions, there are a number of areas of research and training that still present true ethical dilemmas. True ethical dilemmas differ from instances of intentional unethical actions by self-interested researchers. Ethical dilemmas reside in domains in which the researcher intends to act ethically, but either the ethically appropriate course of action is not self-evident or the researcher is not aware that an ethical issue exists. In these times of competition for scarce research funds and other incentives to be first in the race for funding, fame, and glory, there are always dangers of intentional breaches of ethical behavior in science. There are well-publicized instances of fudged data and of thefts of ideas and research results. The increasing reliance on drug company funding for ongoing research and support may serve as an incentive to skew results in order to gain the continued favor of the sponsor (DePalma 1993).

Intentional misconduct by self-interested scientists who believe they are acting unethically but think they can get away with it is assumed to be self-evidently wrong, and such misconduct is not discussed here (Frommer et al. 1990; Pellegrino 1992). However, subtle instances of unethical actions (in which researchers rationalize justifications for practices that they really believe are unethical) are worth noting. For example, a researcher-clinician may dredge up inappropriate clinical reasons for keeping a psychiatric patient in the hospital in order to complete a drug study, while really believing that the patient is ready for discharge. A more complex example is the practice of avoiding United States' consent regulations by doing research in countries that have less stringent requirements. Some such researchers may adopt a legal positivist approach for the sake of convenience rather than for the sake of real moral conviction, arguing that the practices cannot be construed as unethical if those countries have no laws barring them. Or they may rationalize a justification, arguing that the regulations in this country are unfairly stringent. Although those arguments may have some real philosophical basis, they are often offered without any underlying moral conviction. In general, such conduct does not demand ethical analysis so much as it does self-examination of motivation by the researchers and careful independent monitoring of the ethical underpinnings of research projects by institutional review boards, peer reviewers, and journals (Chop and Silva 1991).

Despite the general attention now being paid to ethical issues in research, there is some indication that attention to the ethical aspects of studies is still lacking in the formulation, approval, and monitoring of research protocols in published studies (Fletcher 1990; Lane et al. 1990). Journals should establish clear policies in regard to publishing data obtained in unethical ways. Perhaps journals should reject papers that are wanting in ethical validity with the same rigor that they use to reject papers that are scientifically invalid. It has been argued that the consequences of adopting such exclusionary policies would be to lose findings important to society and cause the needless repetition of research (Levine 1988). However, it is quite possible that the existence of widespread exclusionary policies by journals would very quickly bring research studies up to ethical snuff.

Many of the ethical issues in clinical research and in health care delivery in general fall into the same overall categories. These include problems related to obtaining informed consent, problems about telling the truth, the limits of confidentiality, and issues about the just and fair resolution of conflicts between the rights or interests of individual persons and the interests of society in general.

In fact, although the present emphasis on ethics in clinical medicine has many sources, among the most important of these sources was the worldwide focus on ethical issues in research that resulted from the disclosures at the Nuremberg Trials about Nazi research. That focus led to the Nuremberg Code (Trials of War Criminals Before the Nuremberg Military Tribunals 1949) and the Helsinki Declaration (World Medical Association 1964, 1975), which—although concentrating on protecting the rights of research subjects—were each influential on subsequent thinking about the ethics of clinical care. Moreover, in the United States, interest in the rights of patients in "pure" clinical treatment situations was heightened after disclosure of ethically suspect research projects like the Tuskegee syphilis studies (Brandt 1978) and the Willowbrook hepatitis research (Goldby et al. 1971; Ramsey 1970).

The overlap of interest in research ethics and clinical care ethics is itself indicative of a major source of ethical dilemmas for researchers. Commonly, the medical researcher is also a medical clinician, and the research itself often has immediate clinical implications. The professional obligations of the person taking on the role of researcher may be at odds with the professional obligations of the person who takes on the role of clinician. The conflicting goals of each profession may raise particularly difficult dilemmas for the professional who is both clinician and researcher and is working with research subjects who are also potential patients because they are ill.

Although the ethical issues relating to clinical research and those relating to clinical education of physicians may seem to be unrelated, there are some fundamental connections between them. Unlike the goal of individual patient care, which is to treat the individual patient, in pure clinical research and much of clinical training the primary goals are usually external to the interests and benefit of the individual patient or research subject (President's Commission for the Study of Ethical Problems 1983). That is not to say that the individual patient or research subject may not benefit by the intervention of the trainee or by the process or results of the research project. It is to say that such possible benefits would be secondary to the intent of the research or training. In both instances, researchers sometimes seem to be guided by utilitarian, rather than autonomy-based, approaches to ethics. Utilitarian ethics are concerned with producing good results for society, even if good consequences must be achieved at the expense of individuals' autonomy. In some levels of training, the primary intention is to provide the trainee with the expertise to help future patients without requiring immediate supervision or constant guidance. In the case of nontherapeutic research, the primary goal is to gain information that, once collected and put through the digestive system of scientific analysis, eventually will meet the utilitarian goal of benefiting society at large.

To see the ethical issues in psychiatric research and training more clearly, it is useful to begin by briefly discussing present views of the ethical underpinnings of the physician-patient relationship in the context of "pure" patient care. Then, those views will be used to examine the general medical research and training relationship. Finally, the focus will be narrowed to the special ethical problems that arise in psychiatric research and training relationships.

Clinical Care Ethics

Under present views of the clinical care physician-patient relationship, the physician has a prima facie obligation to respect the patient's autonomy (New York State Task Force on Life and the Law 1992; *Schloendorff v. Society of New York Hospital* 1914). That obligation places limits on the terms that may be set in creating a physician-patient treatment contract. The normal adult patient is presumed to have the right to self-determination in regard to decisions about treatments. In the autonomy view, the traditional medical ethical principle of nonmaleficence ("Do no harm") still persists as an absolute obligation of the physician, and the patient cannot demand that the physician perform harmful acts. That places some limits on the patient's right to self-determination. The physician also retains a strong affirmative obligation to work for the benefit of the patient. However, the physician's affirmative duty to do good (the duty of beneficence) for a patient is constrained not only by the patient's right to reject the physician's subjective opinion of what would be good for him or her, but also by the patient's right to reject treatment that could objectively be determined to be for his or her good or in his or her interests. In Kant's words, persons are to be treated and respected as "rational wills" and as "ends in themselves and never solely as means to an end" (Kant 1785/1959). That means that the unconsenting person cannot be used merely as a means or tool that is useful to achieve some desirable goal, even if that goal is the good of the person himself or herself.

A number of subsidiary or derivative rights are found under the broadly autonomous right to self-determination. First among these, and really a restatement of the right to self-determination, is the patient's right to consent or refuse to consent to treatment. Added to that, perhaps somewhat paternalistically, are demands made on the physician to give the patient sufficient understandable information to use to make an informed, voluntary decision about whether to undergo complex (or invasive and risky) suggested or possible therapies that are appropriate to treat his or her condition (Simon 1992). Requirements to voluntarily provide information about commonly known or less risk-laden procedures, therapies, or medications are less stringent. However, the physician has an obligation to explain these options and provide information about them if asked by the patient, and the patient retains the right to refuse to consent even to these procedures. Under this right of informed consent, the patient must be told his or her diagnosis and be informed of the possible options for treatment, the probable risks and benefits of each option, and the likely consequences of rejecting treatment altogether (Council on Ethical and Judicial Affairs 1992).

Clearly, the process of fully informed consent would require that patients be told the truth about their condition, as well as the truth about the probable outcomes of possible choices and about what is intended to be done to or for them. To lie or even withhold the truth would be to infantilize patients rather than treat them as self-governing, responsible adults. It is generally accepted that patients may waive the exercise of their rights and may consent to allow the physician to make all decisions for them. Nevertheless, even under that caveat, it is also generally agreed that patients alone have that right to decide to withdraw from active participation in their care. Moreover, they always retain the right to become reinvolved.

Autonomy approaches also demand that patients have the right to make voluntary choices about treatment. Unraveling the meaning of "voluntary choice" is problematic and raises issues that, as we shall see, are quite relevant to the ways in which consent is obtained from subjects to join and continue to participate in research and training programs. A voluntary choice would be one made free of coercion, duress, or deceit.

The overriding difficulty regarding voluntary uncoerced choices about psychiatric treatment is that patients are in treatment precisely because their ability to make rational, autonomous decisions is compromised. In fact, some define a psychiatric illness as a condition that constrains autonomy in some way (Edwards 1981; Moore 1984). There are many other problems in determining whether a consent is voluntary and uncoerced. For example, it is clear that a decision to accept a therapy cannot be called fully voluntary if the physician had withheld information about commonly available and accepted effective alternatives to that therapy. On the other hand, it is not clear that an uninsured or poor patient who is "forced" to choose a minimally effective but acceptable inexpensive treatment alternative can be said to have made a voluntary choice. Similarly, it is not clear that a choice to choose or forgo a therapy could be said to be voluntary if obtaining an alternative therapy would require the expenditure of great effort. Consider, for example, the issue of voluntariness in regard to abortion choices in states in which a woman must travel hundreds of miles to find a physician willing to perform an abortion.

Research Ethics

Research projects present wide and varying ranges of invasiveness and risks to the research subject. Projects may run the gamut of invasiveness from studies involving only the observation of the subject with no physical intervention on the subject or his or her environment to experimental projects that hold the possibility of irreversible physiological or psychological damage or death to the subject.

Observational studies.   Even seemingly noninvasive, purely observational studies present ethical dilemmas. These studies may raise issues about the violation of rights to privacy and thus, in turn, about consent. It could be argued that in some settings, such as public streets, persons have no right to demand that their consent be obtained before purely observational studies of their behavior are done, as long as their anonymity is guarded in published studies. Here it would be asserted that to impose restrictions on the observers would be a violation of their First Amendment freedoms. As well, it could be argued that persons in public places must expect that they might be observed by others who may have any number of reasons for doing so. However, even in such seemingly innocuous cases, a strict Kantian might argue that to observe unconsenting persons as if they were mere objects raises issues about respect for the dignity of those persons. It might be said that such studies conducted without consent may not be forbidden by law, but still may be morally suspect.

There are other instances in which observational studies raise deeper issues about privacy and consent. Consider, for example, observational or epidemiological studies done in psychiatric treatment facilities. A person entering a psychiatric facility for the purpose of treatment may have to expect that his or her consent for treatment encompasses not only agreeing to formal therapeutic meetings with psychiatrists, but also acquiescing to observation by ward staff that is intended to help in his or her treatment. However, it is doubtful whether a person entering the facility solely for treatment can be said to have also implicitly consented to be observed by researchers interested only in collecting data about the behavior of patients in psychiatric wards. Unlike the public streets, the hospital, publicly funded or not, is a setting that has a primary presumptive mission of providing treatment to those who come there.

A typical patient's bill of rights (New York City Health and Hospitals Corporation 1988) is ambiguous about the obligation to obtain consent for noninvasive research, stating that patients have the right to "refuse to participate in research and any human experimentation affecting care and treatment. Such care and treatment shall be performed only with your effective informed consent," and defining experimentation as "the physician's departure from standard medical practice of treatment for the purpose of obtaining new knowledge or testing of an hypothesis" (pp. 6–7).

It might be argued that patients who agree to receive treatment at teaching or research hospitals must assume that in doing so they are implicitly agreeing to be the subjects of noninvasive research studies, including observational studies, or to serve as "practice pieces" for training. However, that argument assumes that patients always have the choice to go to another hospital if they do not wish to serve as research or training subjects. The ability to choose another hospital may be an unreal option for patients who are indigent or involuntarily hospitalized. One of the objections to the Willowbrook hepatitis research involved such an issue about the opportunity to choose alternative care. In the Willowbrook research, parents' consent was requested to enroll their retarded children as subjects in a project intended to develop a vaccine against hepatitis. The children were to be infected with hepatitis as part of the project. Although parents were not forced to consent to have their retarded children put into the hepatitis study, agreeing to consent resulted in immediate placement of the child in the institution, whereas a refusal to consent meant waiting years for placement in Willowbrook with no other institutions available. Faced with the option of caring for a profoundly retarded child at home for years, many parents consented in order to get the placement (Goldby et al. 1971).

These arguments raising ethical questions about unconsenting observational studies might also be raised in regard to beliefs that there is no need to obtain consent before doing studies on discarded human tissue, fluids, or other products (Pellegrino 1992).

Strictly observational studies using ill persons as subjects also raise ethical issues when clinician-researchers do not intervene to treat a disease when treatment is available. In this regard, we could mention the Tuskegee syphilis research project (Brandt 1978). Physician-researchers studying the long-term effects of untreated syphilis on infected black males were criticized on a number of ethical grounds. Among the criticisms was that the clinician-researchers did not offer treatment to the diseased subjects even when they knew that effective treatment was available. Part of that criticism is based on the argument that a formal physician-patient treatment contract was violated. The clinician-researchers told the subjects that they were to be taken on as patients and medicated, even though they were actually given only placebo. However, there might have been ground for criticism even if the clinician-researchers had not entered a formal treatment relationship with the subjects but had just stood by and observed persons suffering from a treatable illness without either offering to treat them or informing them that treatment was available. The medical profession's contract with society gives clinicians a licensed privilege to practice medicine, but also implies the imposition of some degree of Good Samaritan obligation to help those who need medical care (Moseley 1985; Ratzan 1985).

Related issues have to do with the obligations of a researcher who has reason to believe that an ill research subject has not been receiving adequate care from clinicians (Brennen 1992; Lind 1992) and with the obligations toward a subject's family members when research appears to establish a genetic etiology for a disorder. Genetic studies also raise issues about confidentiality if the subject is unwilling to divulge information to family members (Alexander et al. 1992; Rosenfeld 1984).

Many of these ethical difficulties in strictly observational studies could be avoided if the subjects either are already receiving the best available care for their condition or are informed of the available alternatives for care and referred to those care options if they so choose. In fact, that is also an argument for running randomized trials of experimental therapies against the best available therapies rather than against inactive placebos. One response to the problem has been more willingness to take patients off placebos and put them on the experimental therapy before the completion of a study when there is a strong early indication that the therapy under investigation is effective.

The short-term consequences of adopting these approaches might be to limit subject pools or even to make many research protocols unfulfillable or incomplete (Marquis 1983). With that difficulty in mind, there are attempts to defend research practices that include unconsenting deceit of subjects; rigid adherence to completing a randomized clinical trial, even in the face of strong early evidence of the efficacy or inefficacy of the therapy being evaluated; and failure to treat an existing illness for the sake of completing a study. These attempts are based on utilitarian arguments that the long-term benefits to society provide sufficient justification to override the duties to individual subjects (Marquis 1983). However, those who argue along those consequentialist lines also must take into account the possibility that the general societal distrust of all research will be furthered if the details of such studies become public. That increasing distrust may result in the public's reluctance to permit almost any sort of research.

If there is an indication that a project will raise issues about confidentiality, such as studies involving genetic linkage or dangerousness, a policy delineating the limits of confidentiality should be created before the onset of the study and incorporated into the informed consent process.

Distinction between therapeutic and nontherapeutic research. Primarily because of ethical considerations, there has been an attempt to make a distinction between "therapeutic" research, which is innovative therapy performed primarily for the benefit of the "subject," and nontherapeutic research, which is performed for other purposes. The American Medical Association distinguishes between "clinical investigation primarily for treatment" and "clinical investigation primarily for the accumulation of scientific knowledge" (Council on Ethical and Judicial Affairs 1992). Distinctions between the categories are not hard and fast, although there are clear instances of each.

Therapeutic research. Therapeutic research—also called "experimental therapy," "innovative therapy," or "investigational therapy" (Levine 1988; President's Commission for the Study of Ethical Problems 1983)—is usually performed with therapies that appear to show promise of efficacy but have not yet been approved for the intended application through the full clinical trial process demanded by federal regulations. With innovative therapy, the intention to benefit the recipient is considered more important than any coexistent intentions to gain pure knowledge or to help patients in the future. Stringent experimental protocols required for nontherapeutic research are put aside in order to benefit the individual recipient, and the recipient of the therapy is more properly described as a "patient" than as a "subject."

The use of experimental therapies, although intended primarily for the benefit of the patient, is not free of ethical difficulties. Both researchers and patients should be constantly aware of the danger of being overly enthusiastic and hopeful about the benefits of unproven therapies (Rutstein 1970). Also present are issues about reimbursement for the use of such therapies. Very often, patients are asked to pay for at least part of the costs of innovative therapies. These costs may or may not be covered by third-party payers. It might be argued that as long as a therapy has not gone through the entire clinical trial proof process and therefore is not yet an "accepted remedy," requiring payment by recipients should be considered unethical (Pellegrino 1992).

There are also conceptual problems having to do with the distinction between "therapeutic" and "nontherapeutic" research. For example, randomized clinical trials that test a new therapy against inactive placebos rather than available standard therapies are probably better categorized as nontherapeutic research, even though they may give some persons their only chance to receive a possibly effective therapy. The fact that the subject has only a possibility of receiving the trial therapy (and no chance of receiving a standard therapy) means that his or her interests are taken as secondary to the researchers' interest in doing a stringent statistical study. Randomized clinical trials that use best available therapies as controls are more justifiably categorized as therapeutic. That is especially true if provisions are made to move a subject from a group if there are strong early indications that the subject would greatly benefit from a move.

Nontherapeutic research. As a clear example of nontherapeutic research, we could think of toxicity trials of a drug intended for schizophrenia that use rats as subjects. The testing is done solely with the intent to test the toxic effects of the drug. The rats cannot suffer from schizophrenia and thus could not benefit from the results of the testing. Other clear examples of nontherapeutic research might include attempts to induce psychoses or psychological stresses in mentally healthy human subjects (Zimbardo 1981). Conceptually problematic examples might include testing of methods to control dangerous behavior exhibited by mentally ill persons. In instances in which the dangerous behavior is directed toward others and is not clearly a product of the subject's mental illness, it would take convoluted reasoning to argue that such research is performed directly for the benefit of the subject (Capron 1973; Simon 1992). For example, experimental measures used to lower the sex drives of sexual offenders may lead to shortened prison terms and lessened chances of suffering repeat arrests and so may be claimed to be "for the good" of the offender. However, when the primary intent of using experimental measures is to benefit or protect society, those gains for the subjects are more properly categorized as incentives to take part in the research rather than as direct benefits to the health of the subject (Macklin 1982).

In nontherapeutic research, as far as the research methodology and results are concerned, the individual subject or candidate for being a research subject may be quite expendable. The confounding factors due to the complexities or seriousness of study candidates' medical needs may, in fact, make them inappropriate subjects for the particular research study even if they might have benefited medically from taking part in the study. Wholly nontherapeutic invasive research is probably the exception when speaking of psychiatric research. Psychiatric research usually studies a pathology and, aside from toxicity tests, uses a subject population that suffers from the pathology and may benefit directly from the research.

However, in instances in which psychiatric disorders are characterized by complex cognitive and affective dysfunctions, there are limits to the ability to find or induce such disorders in nonhuman subjects. There are concomitant difficulties in using animals to test the effectiveness of therapies targeted at correcting complex cognitive and affective deficits. Thus, even putting aside the many ethical issues about the use of nonhuman animals in research (Regan 1983), some experimental drugs and procedures may raise consent issues because they must be brought very quickly to the level of testing on humans.

Informed Consent in Psychiatric Research

As is true of obtaining consent for psychiatric treatment, the most common problems with enlisting subjects for psychiatric research have to do with questions about the putative subjects' capacity to give voluntary consent.

Psychiatric patients have certain vulnerabilities that may interfere with their capacity to give fully voluntary informed consent for research. Medical patients may be said to lack autonomy because their physical illness, or its symptoms, interfere with their ability to live their lives in the ways they would wish to. Although the seriousness of the symptoms or prognosis may place enormous mental pressures on medical patients presented with the option to try experimental therapies, somatic illness does not inherently cast doubt on the patient's ability to make rational decisions. On the other hand, the psychiatric patient's illness has directly to do with his or her ability to make reasonable, rational decisions. Despite that, much of the current thinking in regard to the adult psychiatric patient's right to refuse treatment in clinical care places a burden of proof on providers to show that a patient lacks the capacity to make decisions about treatment (Hermann 1990; New York State Task Force on Life and the Law 1992). That presumption of capacity to make treatment decisions should imply a comparable presumption of capacity to give consent for participation as a research subject.

Consent by patients with decisional capacity.   Decisional capacity would be indicated by the putative subject's ability to comprehend all that is included in the informed consent for the research. That would include a capacity to understand the study, the purpose of the study, and the foreseeable risks and benefits for the subject. There is no prima facie ethical reason to prohibit psychiatric patients or any other persons from agreeing to take part in studies that involve deceit of the subjects or use of placebo, as long as those aspects of the study are explained to the candidate as part of the consent process.

There are factors that complicate determinations of decisional capacity in mentally impaired patients. For example, present criteria for determining capacity emphasize cognitive ability and de-emphasize the role of affective determinants that may interfere with decision making. A depressed patient may have the cognitive capacity to understand what is at stake in health care decisions and may be considered decisionally capable even though there may be doubts about his or her affective capacity to appreciate the consequences of his or her decisions. This unresolved problem has particular importance when a decision may have serious and irreversible consequences (Bursztajn 1993; Drane 1984; Ganzini et al. 1993; Spielman 1992). A second important factor is that mentally impaired patients may go in and out of decisional capacity. The possibility of shifting capacity in volunteer subjects who agreed to participate while they had the capacity to do so may raise doubts about their ability to later exercise their right to withdraw their consent.

There are other pressures that might interfere with the decisionally capable patient's ability to give voluntary consent to participate in research.

Psychiatric inpatients' chances of discharge are often tied to the image they present to staff of cooperativeness, compliance, and good behavior. Compliance is sometimes measured by criteria that have only vague connections to the patient's mental health or illness. Whether or not a patient is issued or denied a pass may depend more on whether his or her behavior in the ward or on pass is judged socially acceptable to hospital staff than on the behavior's connection to the state of the patient's illness. Patients become aware of these factors or may believe that they are operant even if they are not. Patients may fear that a refusal to participate as a research subject may adversely affect the quality of the clinical care they will receive.

On the other hand, a patient's trust that a medical professional would never place a patient in harm's way, as well as the presence of transferential factors that induce cooperation, might cause the patient to consent too easily to participation. Very likely it was these trust factors that enabled physician-researchers to enlist subjects in the Tuskegee research and in the Jewish Chronic Disease Hospital cancer research, where elderly patients were inoculated with living cancer cells without their fully informed consent (Levine 1992). To prevent this abuse of trust, it has been suggested that physicians should never be involved in nontherapeutic research with patients they are treating (Beecher 1970). Although that approach may be desirable because it avoids an appearance of conflict of interest, it may be unnecessary if steps are taken to ensure the initial and continued voluntariness of participation. In the consent process, it should be truthfully emphasized that refusal to consent, or a decision to withdraw from the study, will neither interfere with the quality of clinical treatment the patient will receive nor affect decisions about discharge. Researchers should also be vigilant for signs that a candidate's willingness to participate or to continue to participate comes from less than rational motives (Pellegrino 1992).

The diminished decisional capacity of some mentally ill persons may also raise issues about the underrecruitment of persons who could benefit from therapeutic studies. For example, many homeless, uninstitutionalized mentally ill persons may lack the social or mental wherewithal to find out about research of potential benefit to them. Those same social and mental factors may also cause problems in monitoring the compliance of these persons with study protocols. Although the latter may be a factor that influences neglect in attempts at recruitment, there may still be an ethical obligation to actively recruit members of underserved populations for therapeutic studies that show promise of benefit to them.

Once unconsented deceit and outright duress are removed from the picture, problems still remain with respect to determining what types of incentives are reasonable, noncoercive inducements for becoming a research subject. Classically, this issue has been raised in regard to prisoners; some have argued that influences such as the possibilities of early release and of a break from the prison routine cast doubt on prisoners' ability to freely volunteer to participate as subjects (Capron 1973). The more general argument has been offered that any pay for participation in research other than minimal reimbursement for expenses is unduly seductive to persons in need of money (Freund 1969). However, in our economic system, persons are allowed to choose to work at risky occupations for gain. Thus, it could be argued that, as long as putative subjects are truthfully informed of the purposes, methods, and foreseeable risks of a project, they have a right to be "hired" as participants in nontherapeutic research.

A more straightforward example of an unfair incentive is promising to give standard, or even the best available, treatment to ill participants who could not otherwise afford such treatment. The analogy to being "employed" as a subject in nontherapeutic research fails here. The Willowbrook project was one instance of this practice. With persons suffering from serious illness, a choice to participate under such circumstances could be seen as less than voluntary because it is reasonable to assume that the "choice" was made out of desperation. It might be argued that these practices are simply examples of the free-market system in medical care affording indigent persons access to care they could not ordinarily obtain. However, encouraging these practices with that justification might very well lead to a situation in society in which indigent persons will be forced to "volunteer" to participate as subjects in order to get anything more than basic medical care.

Participation by subjects lacking decisional capacity. In clinical care, the adoption of autonomy-based approaches has affected the ways in which decisions are made for patients who lack decisional capacity. Past approaches were based on a presumption for treatment and, at times, a "best interests" approach to decision making. The trend now is to attempt to recognize a patient's right to self-determination even after the patient has lost the capacity to make decisions (*Cruzan v. Director, Missouri Department of Health* 1990; New York State Task Force on Life and the Law 1992). Patients may express their wishes about future treatment before losing capacity by means of advance directives such as living wills, or they may designate persons to make decisions regarding care. A designated surrogate, familiar with the patient's life values, may make decisions for the patient who lacks capacity by projecting decisions that the patient would have made if he or she still had decisional capacity ("substituted judgment"). If a projection of wishes is not possible, the surrogate decides using a best interests standard that weighs the benefits and burdens of interventions to the patient.

By the same reasoning, we could say that a subject who was fully informed of the foreseeable risks and benefits of becoming a research subject while he or she had decisional capacity and who agreed to continued participation even in the event of losing that capacity should remain a subject after that capacity is lost. The subject should be withdrawn from the study if previously agreed-on conditions for withdrawal are satisfied or if unpredicted harmful events should occur in the course of the project (Winston et al. 1993).

Surrogate consent for research. Surrogate consent for participation on behalf of persons who lack decisional capacity raises other issues. (Although the problem of research involving children has not been specifically addressed in this chapter, the following discussion is applicable to that issue.) Traditionally, surrogates are empowered only to make decisions in regard to treatment. It is reasonable to assume that a surrogate designated by the patient could either project the patient's wishes in regard to treatment or could act in the best interests of the patient. It is also reasonable to assume that a surrogate designated by the courts, a patient's next of kin, or even a hospital ethics committee would be able to use an "average reasonable person" standard to decide what therapies are in a patient's best interests. Thus, there would appear to be strong arguments to support permitting surrogate consent for therapeutic research that held the promise of benefit to the patient.

Although at least a rough consensus may exist about the treatment therapies an average reasonable patient would consent to, there is no consensus about the average person's actual willingness to volunteer to participate in nontherapeutic research. Thus, the American Medical Association's opinion is that "a legally authorized representative of the [minor or mentally incompetent] subject" may give proxy consent for nontherapeutic studies "under circumstances in which informed and prudent adults would reasonably be expected to volunteer themselves or their children as subjects" (Council on Ethical and Judicial Affairs 1992, p. 38).

Doubtless, the major reason for the use of "captive" populations like decisionally incapable institutionalized persons and elderly nursing home residents (Ratzan 1980) as major sources of nontherapeutic research subjects is that these are the populations that suffer the pathologies under investigation. However, when we factor in the past use of prisoners and military personnel and the continuing widespread use of undergraduate and graduate students (each of which are groups prey to various forms of duress), we seem to get an indication that the scientific community cannot depend on the "average prudent person in the street" to step forward to volunteer as a subject. Considering the fact that use of unconsenting persons as subjects in nontherapeutic research treats them solely as means to an end and violates their autonomy rights, it is doubtful whether surrogate consent for participation should be permitted unless strong evidence exists that the putative subject would have volunteered to participate or unless the research is totally risk free.

PSYCHIATRIC TRAINING ISSUES

It is probable that most commonly occurring ethical issues tied directly to the training of clinical psychiatrists fit into one of two categories. One category of problems derives from a pervasive unclarity about the nature of the trainee-patient relationship. The second category consists of problems that arise when there is conflict between trainee and supervisor.

Trainee-Patient Relationship

It would be an exaggeration to insist that all levels of trainee-patient interactions in psychiatric clinical training are primarily intended to achieve goals external to the welfare of the individual patient. Clearly, there is a difference between the nature and purpose of the contact made with patients by a second-year medical student and those made by a third-year psychiatric resident.

When speaking of the preclinical and early clinical training period, it is difficult to dispute the claim that the primary intent of the student-patient interaction is to benefit the student rather than the patient. The student at that stage is still paying tuition for the right to learn medicine rather than being paid by the patient or third-party payer for treatment services rendered. Undeniably, undergraduate medical students do help in the care of patients. For instance, students in early clinical years may gather histories and may have a secure competence to perform necessary diagnostic procedures. Those tasks directly help in the care of the patient and also ease the burden of senior staff, who then may have more time to work with patients. Medical students may even help in the care of psychiatric patients simply by providing personal interaction with them.

The interaction of medical students with patients may result in a number of negative effects. The majority of medical students do not choose psychiatry as a specialty, and some students look on the required psychiatry rotation as a vacation or necessary burden that they must endure in between what they believe are more important and difficult clinical rotations. Those negative attitudes or lack of commitment may have effects on patients. Successful psychiatric treatment often still depends on rapport between provider and patient. The typical psychiatric patient seen by medical students in teaching hospitals is likely to be socially, educationally, and culturally different from the typical medical student. Many of these patients are chronically mentally ill (Nadelson and Robinowitz 1987).

Even the dedicated inexperienced medical student may have fears about interacting with such patients, especially if there is a suspicion that the patient is dangerous. Supervising residents who have negative feelings toward patients may encourage medical students to have the same negative feelings. That is most likely to happen when the patient presents with diagnoses that are still thought of as having a voluntary component and are tied to socially undesirable behaviors. These behaviors usually include substance abuse, abusive language, and bad hygiene. Some medical students may lack sufficient life experience or confidence to enable them to take on attitudes of dispassionate empathy rather than of blame. Constant exposure to chronically mentally ill persons or to elderly patients may lead to a sense of futility about the efficacy of psychiatric treatment

Trainee-Supervisor Relationship

Pressures to stay in the good graces of a supervising resident who has negative attitudes toward the institution or toward patients—or a medical student's lack of self-confidence when assigned a load of undersupervised tasks—may cause a student's initial humane feelings toward patients to be replaced with negative attitudes and behavior.

Compounding or causing such problems is the belief still held by some supervising physicians that the best way to teach medical students is to toss them in with patients and let them try to fend for themselves. That is a greater problem in understaffed institutions with large patient loads. It is not uncommon for students to be asked to perform tasks that are beyond their competence. Under such circumstances, even the best-intentioned and humane inexperienced medical student may make mistakes that could have long-term negative consequences for fragile mentally ill patients.

Pressures to obtain clinical experience and fears that the patient will reject contact with medical students sometimes encourage continuation of the long-discredited practice of medical students introducing themselves to patients as "Doctor." The practice is commonly encouraged or condoned by supervising residents. Sometimes attempts are made to mitigate the deception by encouraging use of the term "student doctor." The practice is sometimes rationalized with the claim that patients know the difference between students and experienced physicians. However, even entering medical students are unaware of the distinctions, for example, between students, interns, and year one postgraduate students. There is no reason to believe that the typical patient has any better knowledge of the distinctions. The fact that the term "student doctor" is used to give the impression that the student is a physician belies the claim that patients are believed to know the difference.

Although hospital patients may have a theoretical right to refuse contact with medical students, many of the obstacles to the exercise of that right already mentioned in regard to the refusal to participate in research are operant here. For instance, there is the limited decisional capacity of many of the patients. In this respect, it is a rare teaching hospital that has a mechanism that truly empowers the decisionally incapable patient to reject contact with medical students. Patients who do have decisional capacity may be subject to the fears already mentioned in regard to rejecting participation in research. These include apprehension that they will be labeled as noncompliant. That apprehension has more force if the patient believes that the student with whom he or she would prefer not to interact is a physician. As is the case with research, the claim that patients can choose to seek treatment elsewhere if they prefer not to be "practice pieces" for training is usually unrealistic, particularly when applied to the indigent, severely mentally disabled patients so frequently seen in teaching hospitals.

As psychiatrists-in-training achieve more years of training and experience, it becomes more reasonable to defend the position that their primary function is to provide care to the patients with whom they interact. Nonetheless, it would appear to be an obligation of the institution or individual resident to fully inform patients about the credentials of the caregivers treating them. That obligation is not mitigated by the claim that disclosure is unnecessary because all residents are supervised by attending psychiatrists. There is even less mitigation when, as is common, such supervision is perfunctory.

Professional Conflict

Ethical issues having to do with conflict between professionals and those in charge of them are not peculiar to the medical student–resident or resident–attending physician relationships. The old conception of professionals as having autonomy in their occupations has become increasingly irrelevant when applied to the medical profession. More and more physicians are employees of institutions or managed health care arrangements. These organizations have administrative bureaucracies that put limits on the physician's autonomy, and they may themselves be subject to the control of private or public third-party payers.

Despite what has been written here about the presumption that medical students lack expertise in the early stages of training, there are occasions when their professional disagreements with supervisory staff may be justified and worthy of a hearing. It is probable that programs that enable students and residents to air and discuss conflict without fear of repercussions will produce better doctors. Perhaps the data indicating that abused children become abusive parents (Smith and Adler 1991) should be applied to the trainee-mentor relationship in medicine.

CONCLUSION

Ethically acceptable methods of performing psychiatric research and doing training differ little from the methods of doing pure clinical work in an ethical way. Primarily, one must avoid the temptation to unthinkingly follow the well-trodden paths of least resistance when confronted with ethical quandaries. These paths typically include rigid adherence to existing law and policies, dependence without reflection on rules set by internal unit mechanisms, and acceptance of the presumption that the good will of the involved individuals will suffice to produce ethically correct actions.

True ethical practice requires constant reflection and reexamination of underlying assumptions. The worn paths are often inadequate for the goals of recognizing and resolving old as well as newly emerging ethical issues. At the least, fully functioning institutional mechanisms (e.g., well-trained and active institutional review boards, hospital ethics committees) are necessary. These should be kept in open liaison with the ethics mechanisms in professional associations, which in turn should be open to constant reevaluation of existing codes of ethics. Constant self-examination by the individual is necessary. However, regulatory mechanisms are also needed to provide the carrots of guidance and, sometimes, the sticks of sanctions for violation of ethical principles.

REFERENCES

Alexander JR, Lerer B, Biron M: Ethical issues in linkage studies of psychiatric disorders. Br J Psychiatry 160:98–102, 1992

Beecher HK: Research and the Individual: Human Studies. Boston, MA, Little, Brown, 1970

Brandt AM: Racism and research: the case of the Tuskegee syphilis study. Hastings Cent Rep 8(6):21–29, 1978

Breggin PR: The return of lobotomy and psychosurgery (reprinted with author's note), in Psychiatry and Ethics. Edited by Edwards RB. Buffalo, NY, Prometheus, 1982, pp 350–388

Brennen TA: Researcher as witness (editorial). J Clin Ethics 3(4):308–309, 1992

Bursztajn HJ: From PSDA to PTSD: the Patient Self-Determination Act and post-traumatic stress disorder. J Clin Ethics 4(1):71–73, 1993

Capron AM: Medical research in prisons: should a moratorium be called? Hastings Cent Rep 3(3):4–6, 1973

Chop RM, Silva MC: Scientific fraud: definitions, policies, and implications for nursing research. J Prof Nurs 7(3):166–171, 1991

Council on Ethical and Judicial Affairs: Code of Medical Ethics. Chicago, IL, American Medical Association, 1992

Cruzan v Director, Missouri Department of Health, 110 S Ct 2841 (1990)

DePalma A: Universities' reliance on companies raising vexing questions on research. The New York Times, March 17, 1993, p B9

Drane JF: Competency to give an informed consent: a model for making clinical decisions. JAMA 252:925–927 1984

Edwards RB: Mental health as rational autonomy. J Med Philos 6:309–322, 1981

Fletcher JC: Ethical aspect of research involving elderly subjects. J Clin Ethics 1:285–286, 1990

Freund PA: Some reflections on consent. Daedalus 98:314, 1969

Frommer PL, Ross J Jr, Benson JA Jr, et al: 21st Bethesda conference: ethics in cardiovascular medicine, Task Force IV: scientific responsibility and integrity in medical research. J Am Coll Cardiol 16(1):24–29, 1990

Ganzini L, Lee AL, Heintz RT, et al: Is the Patient Self-Determination Act appropriate for elderly persons hospitalized for depression? J Clin Ethics 4(1):46–50, 1993

Goldby S, Krugman S, Edsall G, et al: The Willowbrook letters. Lancet 1:749, 966–967, 1078–1079, 1971; 2:95, 1971

Hermann DHJ: Autonomy, self-determination, the right of involuntarily committed persons to refuse treatment, and the use of substituted judgment in medication decisions involving incompetent persons. Int J Law Psychiatry 13:361–385, 1990

Kaimowitz v Department of Health, No 73-19434-AW (Cir Ct of Wayne County, Michigan, 1973)

Kant I: Foundations of the Metaphysics of Morals (1785). Translated by Beck LW. Indianapolis, IN, Bobbs-Merrill, 1959

Lane WL, Casel CK, Bennet W: Ethical aspects of research involving elderly subjects: are we doing more than we say? J Clin Ethics 1:278–284, 1990

Levine RJ: Ethics and Regulation of Clinical Research, 2nd Edition. New Haven, CT, Yale University Press, 1988

Levine RJ: Clinical trials and physicians as double agents. Yale J Biol Med 65(2):65–74, 1992

Lifton RJ: The Nazi Doctors: Medical Killing and the Psychology of Genocide. New York, Basic Books, 1986, pp 110–114

Lind SE: The institutional review board: an evolving ethics committee. J Clin Ethics 3:278–282, 1992

Macklin R: Man, Mind and Morality: The Ethics of Behavior Control. Englewood Cliffs, NJ, Prentice-Hall, 1982, pp 116–117

Marquis D: Leaving therapy to chance. Hastings Cent Rep 13(4):40–47, 1983

Moore MS: The concept of mental illness, in Law and Psychiatry: Rethinking the Relationship. Cambridge, England, Cambridge University Press, 1984, pp 182–216

Moseley R: Excuse me, but you have a melanoma on your neck! Unsolicited medical opinions. J Med Philos 10(2):163–170, 1985

Nadelson CC, Robinowitz CB: Medical academics and economics: continued conflict or resolution? in Training Psychiatrists for the '90s: Issues and Recommendations. Edited by Nadelson CC, Robinowitz CB. Washington, DC, American Psychiatric Press, 1987, pp 11–22

New York City Health and Hospitals Corporation: Patient's Bill of Rights. New York, New York City Health and Hospitals Corporation, Office of Patient Relations, 1988, pp 6–7

New York State Task Force on Life and the Law: When Others Must Choose: Deciding for Patients Without Capacity. Albany, NY, Health Research, 1992

Pellegrino ED: Beneficence, scientific autonomy and self-interest:ethical dilemmas in clinical research. Cambridge Quarterly of Healthcare Ethics 4:361–369, 1992

President's Commission for the Study of Ethical Problems in Medicine and Biomedical and Behavioral Research: Implementing Human Research Regulations. Washington, DC, U.S. Government Printing Office, 1983

Proctor RN: The destruction of "lives not worth living," in Racial Hygiene: Medicine Under the Nazis. Cambridge, MA, Harvard University Press, 1988, pp 177–222

Ramsey P: The Patient as Person. New Haven, CT, Yale University Press, 1970

Ratzan RM: Being old makes you different: the ethics of research with elderly subjects. Hastings Cent Rep 10(5):32–42, 1980

Ratzan RM: Unsolicited medical opinion. J Med Philos 10(2):147–162, 1985

Regan T: Implication of the rights view, in The Case for Animal Rights. Berkeley, CA, University of California Press, 1983, pp 382–393

Rosenfeld A: At risk for Huntington's Disease: who should know what and when? Hastings Cent Rep 14(3):5–8, 1984

Rutstein DD: The ethical design of human experiments, in Experimentation With Human Subjects. Edited by Freund PA. New York, George Braziller, 1970, pp 383–401

Schloendorff v Society of New York Hospital, 211 NY 125, 129–30, 105 NE 92 (1914)

Simon RI: Concise Guide to Psychiatry and Law for Clinicians. Washington, DC, American Psychiatric Press, 1992

Smith JA, Adler RG: Children hospitalized with child abuse and neglect: a case-control study. Child Abuse Negl 15:437–445, 1991

Spielman B: Patient decisions and psychiatric hospitals: quandaries of the Patient Self Determination Act. Developments in Mental Health Law 12(1):1–3, 15–19, 1992

Trials of War Criminals Before the Nuremberg Military Tribunals Under Control Council Law No 10, Vol 2. Washington, DC, U.S. Government Printing Office, 1949, pp 181–182

Winston ME, Winston SM, Appelbaum PS, et al: Can a subject consent to a "Ulysses contract"? in Cases in Bioethics, 2nd Edition. Edited by Crigger B. New York, St. Martin's Press, 1993, pp 151–157

World Medical Association: Declaration of Helsinki: Recommendations Guiding Medical Doctors in Biomedical Research Involving Human Subjects. Adopted at the 18th World Medical Assembly, Helsinki, Finland, 1964. Revised at the 29th World Assembly, Tokyo, Japan, 1975

Zimbardo PG: The ethics of introducing paranoia in an experimental setting. A Review of Human Subjects Research 3(10):276–283, 1981

Chapter 14

Confidentiality

Robert M. Wettstein, M.D.

Confidentiality is often considered the sine qua non of psychiatric treatment. Absent confidentiality, it is argued, the patient would refuse to enter psychiatric care, would fail to develop the trust in the therapist, and would fail to share the information needed to accomplish treatment. The importance of preserving confidentiality is evident through its proclamation in the Hippocratic oath 2,500 years ago (Beauchamp and Childress 1989).

With the increasing complexity of contemporary society, confidentiality has come into conflict with other interests, some belonging to the patient and others to society. The patient-centered Hippocratic tradition has become less useful to today's practitioner. Thus, confidentiality has perhaps become the most prevalent type of ethically troubling incident for mental health professionals (Pope and Vetter 1992). Confidentiality was found to be the most frequent ethical principle intentionally violated by psychologists (Pope and Bajt 1988). Formal charges of breach of confidentiality against American Psychiatric Association members and processed through the American Psychiatric Association have increased in frequency over recent decades, according to the most recently published data (Moore 1985). Increasing incursions into the privacy of the psychiatrist-patient relationship from largely nonclinical interests make confidentiality of enduring if not increasing importance, although some physicians in exasperation have abandoned the notion in practice as a mythical fiction (Siegler 1982).

In this chapter, I review several aspects of confidentiality, primarily from the perspective of ethics rather than law. The chapter will bring to light empirical findings relevant to confidentiality. Although empirical findings do not themselves resolve fundamental ethical dilemmas, they may help guide the decision maker to the appropriate decision. Empirical work also reveals how clinicians actually, or might, manage ethical conflicts.

First, I will review and discuss some concepts relevant to confidentiality, including definitions and justifications. Then, I will present

I am grateful to Joel E. Frader, M.D., who reviewed the manuscript, and William J. Winslade Ph.D., J.D., who critiqued some of the chapter's conceptualizations. Any errors are mine.

some of the empirical data on confidentiality. The next sections cover child abuse reporting and the duty to protect third parties from patients. These situations are taken to be paradigm cases that illustrate the psychiatrist's conflicting ethical obligations to the patient and society. Only a few of the specific problem areas of confidentiality can be considered in any detail here.

DEFINITIONS

At the outset, it is important to distinguish among privacy, confidentiality, and testimonial privilege. *Privacy* is a complex concept that is largely self-regarding, in other words, focused on itself as the subject (Winslade and Ross 1985). It expresses a zone or area of private life free from government intrusion and has been recently recognized constitutionally as well. Thus, the state and others have limited access to the person, whether the body or the mind. The latter, informational privacy, is the principal concern here.

Confidentiality, as distinct from privacy, is an ethical duty of nondisclosure. The recipient of confidential information must protect that information from access by others and resist disclosing it. In contrast to privacy, confidentiality necessarily involves another party with whom private information is shared on the basis of trust. Thus, privacy applies to individuals, whereas confidentiality is applicable to relationships (Dyer 1988). A patient can suffer a loss of privacy, but not necessarily sacrifice confidentiality; when confidentiality is breached, however, both occur (Beauchamp and Childress 1989).

Confidentiality is typically addressed as a concern of professional ethics rather than law, although there are many statutes and regulations that prescribe and proscribe the release of confidential information either orally or from medical records. Furthermore, ethical standards, which are established by professional organizations, are often incorporated into legal standards of practice by medical licensure boards, giving them additional influence. Legal obligations about releasing records as opposed to patient communications may differ, but the ethical considerations are identical.

The notion that psychiatrist-patient confidentiality always supersedes all other interests has been abandoned by the organized profession, most psychiatrists, and the public. The patient-centered view of confidentiality has given way to the recognition that the psychiatrist has ethical and moral responsibilities to others as well. Thus, there are both ethical and legal exceptions to confidentiality, the most important of which is patient waiver of confidentiality. These exceptions either permit or require (i.e., mandatory reporting statutes) otherwise confidential information to be released by the therapist.

The term *breach of confidentiality* is often used loosely and improperly. Some therapists have claimed that every loss of confidentiality, no matter what the reason or mechanism, constitutes a breach of confidentiality. However, in this chapter, *breach of confidentiality* is defined as the unconsented release of patient information in the absence of a legal compulsion or authorization to release it. A loss of confidentiality through the patient's voluntary waiver is not a breach of confidentiality or infringement on his or her moral claim to informational privacy. It does not violate the patient's autonomy, since that is his or hers to allocate. Similarly, a therapist who reports a child abuse victim to a child protective services agency under a mandatory reporting statute is not breaching the patient's confidentiality. And a therapist who warns an endangered third party, contrary to the patient's wishes, in a jurisdiction where the therapist has a legal responsibility to protect a third party is not breaching that patient's confidentiality.

By this definition, a breach of confidentiality always violates the profession's ethics with regard to confidentiality; a therapist is not ethically permitted to breach confidentiality, and there are no permitted breaches. Legal exceptions to confidentiality thereby become ethical exceptions as well. By contrast, those psychiatrists who retain the view that confidentiality may never be sacrificed for other interests are saying that even a patient-initiated release of information is a breach of that psychiatrist's personal ethics or morality (Suarez and Balcanoff 1966); by the present account, such a disclosure is not a violation of the profession's ethics.

The relationship between ethical and legal standards of professional conduct is complex. A breach of confidentiality from an ethical viewpoint often, but not always, corresponds to a breach of confidentiality from a legal viewpoint. Ethical and legal breaches of confidentiality are not always coincident. Ethical standards of professional conduct may be more stringent than legal standards. Ethically, the psychiatrist is charged with the responsibility to "safeguard patient confidences within the constraints of law" (American Psychiatric Association 1993, Section 4). In effect, the profession's ethics have accommodated the society's interests in obtaining otherwise private information.

Having subordinated the ethical code to the law, the profession and the psychiatrist may not properly claim that the psychiatrist is only obligated to the patient's interests. If the law requires a release of confidential information, then the psychiatrist is ethically required to do so, although there may be competing ethical obligations. Further, once the psychiatrist obeys the law, his or her conduct would not be unethical, at least from the standpoint that a profession's ethics determine standards of professional conduct. Nevertheless, the presence of a law, and the ethical obligation of the psychiatrist to obey it, does not resolve the ethical and moral conflicts, but it does complicate them (Beauchamp and Childress 1989). Psychiatrists may perceive their conduct to be unethical when it is contrary to the best interests of the patient or others. By definition, the code creates dilemmas for the therapist when the law requires or allows the therapist to act in a manner contrary to the best interests of the patient or others.

A violation of confidentiality law constitutes a legally actionable tort, which, standing alone, would be considered an ethical breach. Conversely, releasing private information, though legally permissible, may in some circumstances constitute an ethical breach. An example of such an ethical breach is when a psychiatrist knows that the executor of an estate will use the requested information about the deceased patient for purposes of defaming the patient; the executor may have legal access to the information, but it may be unethical for the psychiatrist to reveal it. Other examples include the psychiatrist's failing to inform the patient of the consequences of consenting to information disclosure or the psychiatrist's disclosing more information than is necessary for a given purpose. In some cases, the law about releasing confidential information may be ambiguous or nonexistent.

Privilege, on the other hand, is strictly a legal concept, although it too has its origins in principles of ethics. Privilege refers to a statutory rule of evidence that makes that information admissible or not in court during litigation (Weiner and Wettstein 1993). Privilege is a rule of nondisclosure in court. As such, testimonial privilege encompasses just a small portion of the confidentiality concerns faced by clinicians. Exceptions to the testimonial privilege often, but not always, correspond to the exceptions to confidentiality as defined by the profession's ethics.

The type and extent of information subject to confidentiality and privilege are not always clearly identified. Most respected are the patient's communications, along with the fact of treatment. Beyond that, the therapist's observations, interpretations, diagnosis, treatment recommendations, and test or laboratory data and information provided by family members are not necessarily as readily protected, although the claim can be made that they should be. The distinction made here is the privacy of the patient versus that of the therapist or family (Winslade and Ross 1985).

BASIS OF CONFIDENTIALITY

Two fundamental ethical traditions form the basis for confidentiality of health care information: deontology and utilitarianism.

From the deontological perspective, confidentiality honors an individual's autonomy and respects his or her human dignity. Though not a moral principle itself, confidentiality respects the person's privacy interests. By corollary, some states have granted confidentiality legal constitutional status. Utilitarians, in contrast, emphasize the instrumental value of confidentiality. In this regard, confidentiality is seen as necessary to protect and preserve the psychiatrist-patient relationship. In short, confidentiality is necessary for health care, whether for this patient or any other. The consequentialist sees confidentiality as protecting an intimate or trusting relationship, whereas the deontologist keeps information confidential out of respect for the patient's privacy.

Under either ethical theory, the competent patient retains the right to control confidential information whether or not its release would be harmful. This right helps to promote the patient's autonomy and self-determination. Similarly, the incompetent patient may not autonomously release confidential information. The patient, rather than the therapist, is the source for this control and its waiver. Further, the expectation of control should rest with the patient, not the therapist (Winslade and Ross 1985), although that may conflict with the unequal power noted in many fiduciary relationships. Thus, when a therapist urges a position of absolute or strict confidentiality and refuses to release information (in court or otherwise) even though this release is requested by the patient, the autonomy interests of the patient are offended, as they are by paternalism generally. Therapist-centered informational control is not the predominant view of ethics codes, society, or most practitioners, and it is easy to neglect the patient's autonomy in this regard.

EMPIRICAL ASPECTS OF CONFIDENTIALITY

Research regarding confidentiality has focused on nonpatient community samples, patients (outpatients and inpatients), and health care professionals. Researchers have investigated a variety of aspects of confidentiality, including attitudes, preferences, expectations, behavior, past experiences, and knowledge of the relevant ethical principles and law. Empirical work on child abuse reporting has also been done, but this work will be reviewed separately (see "Mandatory Child Abuse Reporting"). Research has often been directed toward confirming or rejecting the utilitarian hypothesis of confidentiality: in other words, that confidentiality is essential to mental health treatment and that in the absence of confidentiality, individuals will avoid or delay seeking treatment, terminate it prematurely, or fail to disclose important information to the therapist, thus impairing treatment.

Community Samples

In a public opinion poll of 2,131 people (Harris 1979), respondents were concerned about their privacy, especially governmental intrusion. However, they were less critical of physicians' management of their confidentiality than they were of that by 17 other professions. Just 17% of the sample believed that physicians should better manage the confidentiality of their medical records.

A telephone survey of another group revealed that the respondents expected psychotherapists to maintain patient confidentiality, except when the patient consented to release information (Rubanowitz 1987). When presented with specific case vignettes about future violence or suicide and asked whether the therapist should breach confidentiality, respondents were usually in accord with professional ethics codes. Respondents, however, were also inclined to believe that therapists should report the use of illegal drugs, the confession of a past crime, or the occurrence of child abuse.

Two other groups of nonpatients, when asked to assume the role of a psychiatrist or psychologist, also were more likely than the professionals themselves to breach confidentiality when presented with complex case vignettes involving criminal behavior or substance use (Lindenthal and Thomas 1982, 1984). Persons in both sample groups expressed concern that therapists might breach their confidence if they were in treatment, and one-third of each sample claimed that this concern kept them from entering treatment.

Of a sample of high school and college students, 71% thought that psychologists consider "everything" in treatment to be confidential (D. J. Miller and Thelen 1986). Persons in an adult education sample said they would be less willing to discuss past criminal behavior with a therapist if no statutory evidentiary privilege existed; only 26% of the sample knew that one in fact existed (Shuman and Weiner 1982).

Patient Samples

Confidentiality attitudes, values, and expectations. Studies of clinical populations have concluded that most patients value, expect (anticipate), and prefer that their treatment will be held in confidence (McGuire et al. 1985). In one study, 68% of former outpatients stated that "everything" in mental health treatment was confidential (D. J. Miller and Thelen 1986). A study of family practice outpatients revealed that patients expected far more confidentiality from their physicians than the physicians in fact said they provided (Weiss 1982). For example, although 17% of patients thought that their physicians would discuss their case with a spouse or significant other, 51% of house staff physicians said they would do so. Contrary to expectations, patients who received treatment in a private office and those who received treatment in a clinic had similar perceptions of confidentiality (Weiss et al. 1986).

Using differing methods, several studies have examined whether, and to what degree, patient knowledge of the limits to confidentiality affects participation in treatment. Using an analog therapy interview situation with undergraduates, Woods and McNamara (1980) found that the assurance of confidentiality increased self-disclosure. In two other studies, to varying degrees depending on the recipient, patients said they would react negatively if confidential information were released without their consent (Appelbaum et al. 1984; Schmid et al. 1983). More than half of the patients in an outpatient psychiatric sample stated that an unconsented release of information "would adversely affect the therapeutic relationship" (Appelbaum et al. 1984, p. 114). These patients reacted more negatively to the unconsented release of records than to oral disclosure. In an outpatient study that, at intake, manipulated information about the limits of confidentiality in treatment, those patients who had received more information about the limits of confidentiality acknowledged "fewer socially unacceptable sexual thoughts and behaviors" (Taube and Elwork 1990). Similarly, self-reports of parolees' past sex crimes increased as perceived confidentiality of the interview increased (Kaplan et al. 1990).

Some research findings on patients have tended to reject the utilitarian hypothesis. One study found that the inhibitory effect on willingness to disclose information in treatment produced by increasing knowledge about the limits of confidentiality in treatment could be overcome by emphasizing the importance of self-disclosure in therapy (Muehleman et al. 1985). Another study found that self-disclosures did not decrease after confidentiality limits were detailed (Haut and Muehleman 1986). Finally, patients still incriminated themselves in civil commitment evaluations even after they were given a right to remain silent (R. D. Miller et al. 1985).

Patients often say they want to be informed of the limits of confidentiality (D. J. Miller and Thelen 1986). They state that discussions about confidentiality should occur before treatment begins rather than at any other time (D. J. Miller and Thelen 1986). If, however, patients are informed about the limits of confidentiality, many say they would react adversely by deciding to be less forthcoming (D. J. Miller and Thelen 1986).

As might be expected, patients' reactions to breach of confidentiality may depend on their attitudes about release of information (Vande-Creek et al. 1987), the nature and seriousness of their problems (Merluzzi and Brischetto 1983), the type of information being released (Simmons 1968), and the identity of the recipient (Appelbaum et al. 1984).

Past experiences.   In one outpatient group, 28% said they had asked their therapists about confidentiality, and 47% admitted to having withheld information in therapy, mostly about sexual thoughts and behavior (Shuman and Weiner 1982).

On the other hand, 9% of psychiatric outpatients (Lindenthal and Thomas 1982) and 15% of psychological outpatients (Lindenthal and Thomas 1984) claimed they had evidence that their therapist had breached their confidentiality. More than half of a current outpatient sample perceived a confidentiality violation by their therapists; those who stated their confidentiality had been violated in therapy placed a lower value on confidentiality and privacy (McGuire et al. 1985).

Knowledge base.   Studies indicate that patients are not that knowledgeable about confidentiality law and ethical codes. Only one-third of high school students knew they could obtain treatment for drug abuse or sexually transmitted diseases without parental knowledge (Cheng et al. 1993). Just 28% of psychiatric outpatients (Appelbaum et al. 1984) and 17% of psychiatric inpatients (Schmid et al. 1983) knew of legal rules regarding release of confidential information. Of another psychiatric outpatient sample, 27% knew that there was a statutory evidentiary privilege in their state (Shuman and Weiner 1982). Finally, outpatients in two other samples had general knowledge about confidentiality but not its limitations and exceptions (Hillerbrand and Claiborn 1988).

Clinician Samples

Confidentiality attitudes and values.   Research supports the clinical lore that therapists believe that patients value confidentiality. Nearly all (96%) of surveyed Florida mental health professionals reported they discuss confidentiality with their patients (Otto et al. 1991). One-third of psychologists reported they discuss confidentiality with a patient at the initial contact (Baird and Rupert 1987). Three-quarters of psychology doctoral training clinics have a written confidentiality policy (Bernard and O'Laughlin 1990). But some therapists contend that they, rather than the patient, know best when to reveal confidential information; one-third of Massachusetts psychiatrists surveyed rejected patient waiver as an exception to psychiatrist-patient privilege (Suarez and Balcanoff 1966).

Among surveyed California psychotherapists, 79% responded that patients would be less self-disclosing if they knew the limits of confidentiality (Wise 1978). Thus, only 11% of that group typically discussed these limits with patients; most did so only when an issue arose during treatment. Similarly, 87% of group psychotherapists reported that they discussed confidentiality with prospective group members, but only 32% explained that there were limits to confidentiality (Roback et al. 1992). In contrast, a recent study revealed that 98% of doctoral psychologists said they informed patients of the limits of confidentiality; 60% of patients were informed *prior to the beginning of therapy*, and 83% were informed by the third session (Somberg et al. 1993).

Past experiences.   Some studies have documented that in the past therapists disclosed confidential information to third parties, especially when confronted with potential violence to third parties (Givelber et al. 1984; Pope et al. 1987; Wise 1978) or child abuse (see "Mandatory Child Abuse Reporting"). Even psychoanalysts providing individual therapy or analysis in office practices admitted that they shared information with colleagues treating spouses of their patients in 84% of the cases (Szasz and Nemiroff 1963). Given that all such data are retrospective, it is not possible to reliably determine the frequency of these occurrences. Similarly, clinicians responding to other studies that presented hypothetical case vignettes indicated that they *would* breach a patient's confidentiality under specified conditions (Baird and Rupert 1987; Lindenthal and Thomas 1980, 1982, 1984; Otto et al. 1991; Weiss 1982).

Therapists reported a variety of adverse consequences resulting from confidentiality breaches. Texas psychiatrists reported that some patients prematurely terminated treatment after unconsented release of information to third parties or court testimony (Shuman and Weiner 1982). Roback et al. (1992) reported that when a group psychotherapy member breached another group member's confidentiality, there was decreased group cohesiveness, anger at the violator, and reduced self-disclosure, as well as withdrawals from the group.

Knowledge base.   To varying degrees, clinicians are knowledgeable about the applicable confidentiality principles of ethics and law. Therapists' responses vary widely as to whether a given behavior by a therapist is ethical (Pope et al. 1987). To some extent, this variability can be taken to represent lack of familiarity with codes of professional ethics.

Half of the Texas psychiatrists surveyed knew there was a statutory testimonial privilege in their state (Shuman and Weiner 1982), and three-quarters of the Massachusetts psychiatrists surveyed knew there was none (Suarez and Balcanoff 1966). Two-thirds of surveyed Florida psychiatrists were aware of that state's privilege that applied to them, whereas 81% of Florida psychologists knew of it (Otto et al. 1991). Florida social workers and counselors were much less well informed, however. Mental health professionals were poorly informed about the extent of confidentiality and privilege and thus misinformed their patients about the limits of confidentiality in treatment (Otto et al. 1991).

Summary and Discussion

Although there are conflicting data and many methodological problems, available research generally supports the utilitarian hypothesis of confidentiality, at least for some patients. However, not every patient is concerned about confidentiality and not to the degree that clinicians might imagine. Not every patient would be deterred from entering or fully participating in treatment if the limits to confidentiality were fully explained. Patients generally value confidentiality and expect and trust that their therapists will preserve it, although they may not be familiar with the specific rules of law or ethics regarding confidentiality. Patient trust appears to be more predicated on clinicians' professional ethics than on legal rules, given how ignorant most patients are about the latter.

From the available research data (which are largely self-report), there appear to be several, rather than one, empirically derived standards of practice with regard to informing patients about confidentiality and its limits. To various degrees and at various times, patients in fact are informed about these issues. Practice standards may change for psychologists, because the current American Psychological Association's *Ethical Principles of Psychologists and Code of Conduct* (1992) newly requires that discussions of confidentiality, including its limitations, occur "at the outset of the relationship and thereafter as new circumstances may warrant" (Section 5.01), unless contraindicated. This process has been called "forewarning" or "prewarning" (Faustman and Miller 1987), but it has often been rejected because of the likelihood that the patient will have forgotten the warnings by the time that the potential confidentiality breach arises in treatment or because patients may be deterred from fully participating in treatment.

In contrast, the American Psychiatric Association (1993, Section 4) does not require warnings of the limits of confidentiality at any time during treatment, but only specifies that confidentiality should be discussed when particular situations arise in which information is requested by, or should be released to, third parties. However, clinicians have been encouraged to review the specific limits of confidentiality before discussing human immunodeficiency virus infection with a patient (American Psychiatric Association 1988/1992).

Because patients vary so widely in the importance they place on confidentiality, it becomes more important for the clinician to discuss confidentiality and its limits with the patient sooner rather than later in treatment. Many clinicians need to improve their detailing of the limits of confidentiality. In many clinics and institutions, the limits of confidentiality are increasingly set forth in written contracts or information brochures, usually as part of the process of obtaining informed consent to treatment (Somberg et al. 1993).

MANDATORY CHILD ABUSE REPORTING

Mandatory child abuse reporting statutes have been extant in the United States for the last quarter century. Child abuse reports are among the most common intrusion on the confidentiality of health care information. In 1989, more than 2.4 million reports of suspected child abuse were officially filed, a number that has increased over the years (Daro and Mitchel 1990). We do not know how many reports were filed without the knowledge or consent of the victim and perpetrator. Only half of the cases reported by professionals and 15% of the cases reported anonymously are ever substantiated (Zuravin et al. 1987).

Mandatory child abuse reporting is primarily designed to identify, protect, and treat the child victim, but it has also been used to treat and punish the perpetrator (Smith and Meyer 1984). Child abuse reporting statutes generally require that mental health professionals and others formally report suspected child abuse or neglect without regard for whether the individual or family is currently in treatment for the problem at hand. The child need not be at risk of life-threatening or imminent harm before reporting is mandated, which is the basis for the emergency exception to confidentiality. In fact, reporting is usually made on the basis of recent past abuse rather than future abuse. The clinician is not responsible for investigating the complaint, nor should that be done. By law, the mandated reporter also is not to consider the likely outcomes of reporting; in other words, reporting remains mandatory even if it does more harm than good to the treatment or to the people involved. Although the statutes provide immunity from civil suits for good-faith reporting, they also prescribe civil and possibly criminal penalties for failure to report (Watson and Levine 1989). The statutes, however, vary as to the definitions of abuse and neglect, reportable circumstances, and who is a mandated reporter; for example, some do not require reports when the perpetrator discloses the abuse (Smith and Meyer 1984).

Empirical Findings

Studies of actual or hypothetical child abuse reporting by mental health professionals consistently reveal a significant amount of nonreporting. As many as 75% of clinicians reported that they did not in the past or would not, given a specific case vignette, report a case of suspected child abuse, with an average failure-to-report rate of 40% (Brosig and Kalichman 1992). Factors relevant to a failure to report include characteristics of the clinician (e.g., attitudes, training, experience) or of the case (e.g., type, severity, and evidence of abuse), legal considerations, and organizational influences. Clinicians appear to fall into patterns as to whether they are consistent reporters, inconsistent ("discretionary") reporters, or nonreporters (Zellman 1990). Compared with nonpsychiatric physicians and school principals, psychologists and psychiatrists were more likely to be discretionary rather than consistent reporters (Zellman 1990).

Nonreporters of child abuse provide a variety of rationales for their failure to report. These include the belief that there was insufficient evidence of abuse or neglect, unwillingness to breach confidentiality, anticipated disruption in treatment or the family unit itself, poor quality of child protective services, and the claim that the clinician could better help the child or family (Zellman 1990).

Treating a population of sex offenders, Berlin and colleagues (1991) provided some cogent data to support the utilitarian hypothesis with regard to child abuse reporting. After the Maryland reporting statute was broadened to mandate child abuse reporting when this abuse was disclosed by sex offenders in treatment (in addition to mandating this reporting when the abuse was disclosed by their victims), self-referrals for treatment and self-reported relapses by those already in treatment abruptly ended (Berlin et al. 1991). Anecdotal information has also revealed harmful results of reporting distant-past abuse, whether this abuse is reported by adults who were victimized as children or by offenders who later enter treatment (Weinstock and Weinstock 1988).

Although many clinicians assume (consonant with the utilitarian hypothesis) that reporting suspected child abuse will necessarily interfere with treatment, that has not been demonstrated. Watson and Levine (1989) examined clinical records after child abuse was in fact reported or was discussed with the patient but not reported. Negative outcomes, usually termination, occurred in 31% of the cases in which the perpetrator was in treatment and in 17% of the cases involving third-party perpetrators (e.g., mother's boyfriend, not in treatment). A positive outcome occurred in 7% of the former and 33% of the latter cases. Positive results of reporting were thought to occur by virtue of strengthening the therapeutic alliance via reporting to an outside agency (i.e., the therapist becomes a "protector" against the perpetrator). The authors concluded that reporting abuse is "not always detrimental . . . and may even be helpful" and that "trust, not absolute confidentiality . . . is essential for the psychotherapeutic relationship" (Watson and Levine 1989, p. 255). Even more positive effects of mandatory reporting were obtained by Harper and Irvin (1985), who studied cases on a child psychiatry inpatient unit. Mandatory reporting strengthened the therapeutic alliance with the parents through external limit setting and enhanced the child's well-being with almost no negative results.

Ethical Issues and Conflicts

Mandatory child abuse reporting laws pose a sharp conflict between two pairs of responsibilities: 1) promoting the best interests of the patient and maintaining the confidentiality of an evaluation or course of treatment and 2) protecting the child (whether or not the child is the reporter's patient) and obeying the law (American Psychiatric Association 1993, Section 3; American Psychological Association 1992, Principle F). Whether they report or not, clinicians are also obligated to "do no harm." Clinicians are faced with choosing between complying with the law, a social (control) responsibility, and pursuing what they may believe to be the child's best interests. Reporting statutes present conflicts between law and professional ethics and between competing professional ethical duties. They often pit the interests of the child against those of the perpetrator and the self-interests of the therapists against the interests of their patients. Of course, it is often unclear what constitutes the best interests of the adult patient or the allegedly abused child. Further, the consequences of the clinician's intervention or lack thereof for the adult patient and abused child may also be uncertain.

The proponents of mandatory child abuse reporting statutes assert that social interests such as protecting children easily outweigh confidentiality because the risk of physical or emotional (i.e., developmental) injury to the child exceeds the risk of emotional harm to the patient from disclosure (Weisberg and Wald 1984). Its detractors contend that mandatory reporting, due to underreporting and overreporting, offers uncertain benefits to children and society, undermines confidentiality, "usurps" professional judgment, and is ultimately "counterproductive" (Agatstein 1989).

The ethical conflicts are especially troublesome when the child is not the patient, when the offender (whether incestuous or extrafamilial) is in treatment for the child abuse, when the offender is already incarcerated (in a sexual offender treatment program in prison), when past abuse rather than ongoing abuse is at issue, or when the perpetrator can be prosecuted because of and with the psychiatrist's mandated report. (In the last case, the psychiatrist in effect acts as an informant and is compelled to testify at the criminal trial against the patient, which is permitted by some evidentiary privilege laws.) In any one or a combination of these situations, there are increased risks that reporting will be antitherapeutic, will fail to protect the specified child victim or future potential victims at large, or will be punitive.

Some mental health clinicians defensively avoid the ethical conflict by colluding with the patient to surreptitiously deny or minimize this and all future abuse allegations ("I won't ask and you shouldn't tell"), by overscrupulously complying with the reporting law to avoid personal liability, by defying the law by never reporting, by refusing to work with sexual offenders or abused children, or by remaining ignorant of the technicalities of the reporting statute. Some "discretionary" reporters, though violating the law, search for a solution to the ethical conflict by improperly assuming responsibilities such as investigation of the abuse allegations.

When the clinician resolves the conflict in favor of reporting, the potential harmfulness of the report, and perhaps even the conflict itself, can be mitigated with several interventions. The clinician honors the beneficence duty by informing the family that suspected child abuse will be reported and exploring the reaction to that information (Racusin and Felsman 1986). The mandatory reporting statutes do not require that the family be informed, but it may help maintain the therapeutic alliance, especially if the perpetrator is not in treatment and external limits are needed. It may even be possible to obtain the family's consent to filing the report. The clinician may also explain to the family that the report is required as a matter of law and is not designed to punish or deprive. Having (pre)warned the patient or family as to the limits of confidentiality is also ethically useful here.

Beyond the use of some clinical devices to mitigate the ethical conflict or the harm that ensues from reporting, psychiatrists are charged by the American Psychiatric Association (1993) with "contributing to an improved community" (Section 7). In this regard, reforms of the child abuse reporting statutes have been proposed. These reforms include making reporting elective rather than mandatory; excluding mandatory reporting when the perpetrator is already in treatment and compliant with it or when the reports would be based on the perpetrator-patient's disclosures to the therapist; excluding reports of distant-past child abuse that has ceased; prohibiting criminal prosecutions based on or using the patient's disclosures to the therapist, including the reporter's testimony "against" the patient; permitting clinicians to use professional discretion in deciding whether or not to file; eliminating criminal sanctions for failure to report; and sharpening the definition of abuse and neglect so it is less ambiguous (Agatstein 1989; Coleman 1986; R. D. Miller and Weinstock 1987; Smith and Meyer 1984; Weinstock and Weinstock 1988). Enactment of these proposals, at least for perpetrators in treatment, may help shift the balance of interests back toward respecting confidentiality, as opposed to the trend toward criminal prosecution of child abusers that has been evident in recent years (Wettstein 1992). The reemphasis on promoting therapeutic considerations in the long term would be welcome, given that so many who are abused become abusers themselves (Berlin et al. 1991).

DUTY TO PROTECT THIRD PARTIES

The therapist's duty to protect the public from a potentially violent patient was created two decades ago after the two California Supreme Court decisions in *Tarasoff* (1974, 1976). Even before this case arose, however, the American Psychiatric Association's first annotated principles indicated, as they still do today, that "psychiatrists at times may find it necessary, in order to protect the patient or the community from imminent danger, to reveal confidential information disclosed by the patient" (American Psychiatric Association 1973, Section 9). The danger in many duty-to-protect third-party situations, however, is not "imminent," so the duty can well exceed the reach of this ethical principle.

The contemporary legal duty to protect is based on both case law and, more recently, statutory law. These statutes, present in nearly half the states, immunize the therapist from third-party liability once the therapist complies with the law by taking some prescribed action such as warning the victim, notifying the police, or civilly committing the patient (Weiner and Wettstein 1993). The statutes have been designed to limit the therapist's liability unleashed through case law in that state or other states and to allow for a variable amount of professional discretion in the discharge of therapists' obligations (Appelbaum et al. 1989).

The duty to protect resembles child abuse reporting in several respects. Both are legally derived mandates imposed on health care professionals that create legal standards of care, and both are relatively recent phenomena. Both immunize the therapist from personal liability for releasing otherwise confidential information. Both involve the therapist as social control agent and triangulate the interests of the patient, the clinician, and the potential victim.

Empirical Findings

Frequency of warning and reporting. The prevalence of breaching confidentiality to protect third parties has not been well studied. Wise (1978) found that 38% of psychotherapists had warned someone of a patient's violent threats in the prior year and 50% had done so in their practice lifetimes. Givelber and colleagues (1984) found that 14% of psychiatrists nationally warned third-party victims in the previous year. Of these, 45% thought that doing so was contrary to their best clinical judgment—a greater percentage than that reported when information was disclosed to third parties for other purposes. Since *Tarasoff*, therapists claimed they were increasingly inclined to warn potential third-party victims of their patients (Wise 1978).

On a related issue involving a study of therapists' opinions about mandatory reporting, group therapists favored mandatory reporting laws when patients threatened physical harm to identified others (89%), more so than to nonidentified others (29%) (Roback et al. 1992).

Outcomes of warning and reporting. Few studies provide any quantitative data about the outcomes when therapists notify potential victims or call the police about violent patients. In a small study of institutional psychiatrists, warnings that were not discussed with the patient ahead of time—or warnings that the investigator believed post hoc were not warranted—were associated with negative results such as subsequent violence, suicide, and feelings of betrayal and rage (Beck 1982). However, most warnings had no apparent impact on the patient or the treatment, and a few were said to have reduced the likelihood of violence. In another study, premature terminations of inpatient and out-patient treatment were reported after the psychiatrist notified the threatened victim (Beck 1985). In summary, the available research does not permit a conclusion as to the respective frequencies of possible outcomes of trying to protect third parties.

Therapists also appear to misunderstand the duty to protect as involving a duty to warn rather than to protect the intended victim (Beck 1985; Givelber et al. 1984). Some mistake it for a duty to prevent suicide (Wise 1978).

Ethical Issues and Conflicts

As noted, the duty to protect third parties extends the available ethical and legal exceptions to confidentiality in emergency situations. Disclosing otherwise confidential information in psychiatric (i.e., life-and-death) emergencies has been ethically well justified, but many *Tarasoff*-like clinical situations cannot be so characterized. Although the interest in preventing physical harm to another person readily trumps the patient's privacy interests in principle, violating confidentiality in a given case is justifiable only when it in fact promotes the victim's safety.

Frequently, however, clinicians have erroneously believed that non-clinical warning of the victim rather than therapeutic intervention is required to discharge their responsibilities under the law. Some duty-to-protect statutes have contributed to this problem by emphasizing the need for notifying the police and victims, while minimizing the usefulness of clinical judgment and discretion in managing potentially violent patients. Further, the immunity provisions for reporting provide an incentive to automatically report any patient's violent threats, even when there is no violent intent or means to accomplish the act or when a clinical resolution such as hospitalization would have been satisfactory. The coercive influence of the law then substitutes for professional judgment. If asked, clinicians may then acknowledge that their warnings were counterproductive in reducing the risk of violence and were contrary to their clinical judgment and the therapeutic interests of the patient.

In effect, too often the duty to protect can function as a mandatory reporting statute. Perhaps without noticing, clinicians have grown to accept the clinical duty to protect with its attendant costs to clinical care. The risk is that clinicians may have resolved the conflict among the interests of the patient, victim, and themselves in their own favor, contrary to the responsibility of a professional. In contrast, a professional is obligated to honor the interests of the patient above his or her own.

Unlike child abuse reporting, no criminal sanctions apply for failing to protect an injured third party, but therapists nevertheless face a variety of ethical perils. Although the therapist who warns an intended victim based on an empty threat of violence might still enjoy statutory immunity, that disclosure might not be ethical if there is no reasonable basis for revealing confidential information. Ethical problems might also occur if the warning were predicated on the therapist's best interests, if the extent of the disclosure far exceeded that which was needed to protect the victim, if the patient were already in custody, or if the therapist knew that the warning would precipitate violence by the victim. There might be similar ethical reservations when a therapist warns a victim knowing that the patient deliberately confabulated the threat to harass the purported victim via the therapist. More uncertain still would be the therapist's warning, in a nonemergency situation, if the law in the jurisdiction in question did not provide for a duty to protect in the first place.

As is the case in child abuse reporting, several clinical-ethical techniques may be useful in maximizing the therapeutic potential for third-party warnings while minimizing their harm. Assuming that the therapist decides to warn the specified victim rather than clinically manage the potential violence, the therapist can involve the patient in the reporting, obtain the patient's consent to warn, have the patient make the telephone warning while he or she is still in the therapist's office, invite victims who are significant others into the treatment with the patient, and at least inform the patient as soon as possible about the need to warn (Roth and Meisel 1977; Wulsin et al. 1983). In this way, the patient's treatment interests need not be sacrificed for the protection of an unknown person, and the relationship with the patient may be less adversarial. At times, it may be desirable from an ethics perspective for the therapist to incur some personal risk of third-party liability when the likelihood of patient violence is small but the risk of violating confidentiality is substantial (Weinstock 1988).

Prosecution use of third-party warnings. Recent legal developments in California raise the ethical stakes of the duty to protect in a manner unforeseen by most. Case law involving homicides committed after third-party warnings has held that the warnings, in addition to the patient's statements that gave rise to them, are admissible in the subsequent criminal prosecutions of the patient, including death penalty determinations (*People v. Wharton* 1991). Thus, the therapist becomes a prosecution witness against the patient (usually by then he or she is a former patient). When the patient is familiar with this law of privilege, whether through the therapist's prior discussions or independently, the therapist could become a target for the patient's violence (Leong et al. 1992; *Menendez v. Superior Court* 1992). Of course, in these criminal prosecutions, as in many prosecutions involving mandatory child abuse reports, the risk of further harm to the victim has long ago ceased.

This turn of events increases concerns about still another potential misuse of psychiatry—one that increases the risks of violence against the therapist. Many will doubt whether violent patients will be as willing to seek care and whether therapists will be as available to care for them. Many will wonder more about the value of third-party warnings versus the increasing sacrifice of confidentiality through loss of a testimonial privilege in criminal trials. But some will claim that patient knowledge of the possibility of compelled psychiatric testimony about possible statements and behavior will deter patients from becoming violent (Klotz 1991). Whatever the outcomes, these developments will certainly complicate how therapists resolve their legal obligations to protect others, treat the patient, and secure their own personal and professional livelihoods.

CONCLUSION

With changes in society come changes in the practice of medicine. The role, identity, and function of psychiatrists have already changed and will continue to change in the future. Along with these changes come increasing incursions into the physician-patient relationship and confidentiality and the growth of legal exceptions to confidentiality. There have been many such incursions, and there will always be more. Confidentiality is a dynamic concept, and the ethics and law regarding confidentiality continue to evolve. As a profession, psychiatry has had to abandon its stance that the psychiatrist owes a duty just to the patient, although some may still cling to this notion. No longer do psychiatrists own complete control over information generated clinically, if they ever did. Confidentiality is no longer of overriding importance, overcoming all other interests. Treatment relationships are no longer simply, and forever, dyadic. Thus, confidentiality is better viewed as a spectrum concept than a categorical one; absolute confidentiality no longer exists, and degrees or levels of confidentiality fit the clinical realities. Yet psychiatry as a profession is ambivalent about this state of affairs (Gillon 1985). Although the psychiatric profession recognizes that psychiatric treatment and privacy no longer trump all other interests, we still tend to think and act as if they do.

Even without the claim that confidentiality supersedes all other interests, many therapists assert that treatment cannot proceed in the absence of absolute confidentiality. Review of the available data, however, provides some—but not universal—support for the consequentialist hypothesis. This hypothesis may be more or less correct for certain patients, categories of patients (e.g., sex offenders and repeatedly violent patients in treatment), or treatment situations (involuntary treatment). This issue awaits further study.

Although we may understand something about the value of confidentiality in psychiatry, the heart of the ethical dilemmas regarding violation of confidentiality lies elsewhere. Decisions about whether to violate confidentiality in a particular case are often predicated on the "best interests" of the patient or a third party. Regrettably, ascertaining what constitutes the best interests of the parties is complex, and the impact of any potential clinical intervention or lack thereof is fraught with uncertainty. Rarely can we say with confidence that warning an endangered third party or reporting suspected child abuse, in contrast to the available alternatives, will clearly promote that party's best interests. Equally problematic are attempts to total the benefits and burdens to the respective parties, along with any duty to respect persons.

Especially because confidentiality can no longer be guaranteed, we need to facilitate patient trust in the psychiatrist. There is much that psychiatry can do here. Psychiatry can work to ensure that confidentiality exceptions remain limited in scope, that information is released only to the extent and the persons necessary to accomplish that purpose, and that records are securely protected. Psychiatrists must educate patients about the boundaries of confidentiality and about who has access to their records and communications. Psychiatrists need to give patients more responsibility for this information, improve patient access to records, involve patients in decision making about release of information, and reaffirm that the patient, and no one else, retains the locus of control of information. Through this work, psychiatrists demonstrate their honesty and commitment to the treatment, reassure the patient, and increase the patient's trust and confidence in their work together.

REFERENCES

Agatstein DJ: Child abuse reporting in New York State: the dilemma of the mental health professional. New York Law School Law Review 34:117–168, 1989

American Psychiatric Association: The principles of medical ethics with annotations especially applicable to psychiatry. Am J Psychiatry 130:1058–1064, 1973

American Psychiatric Association: AIDS policy: confidentiality and disclosure (Am J Psychiatry 145:541, 1988), superseded by Position Statement on Confidentiality, Disclosure, and Protection of Others, 1992

American Psychiatric Association: The Principles of Medical Ethics With Annotations Especially Applicable to Psychiatry. Washington, DC, American Psychiatric Association, 1993

American Psychological Association: Ethical Principles of Psychologists and Code of Conduct. Washington, DC, American Psychological Association, 1992

Appelbaum PS, Kapen G, Walters B, et al: Confidentiality: an empirical test of the utilitarian perspective. Bull Am Acad Psychiatry Law 12:109–116, 1984

Appelbaum PS, Zonana H, Bonnie R, et al: Statutory approaches to limiting psychiatrists' liability for their patients' violent acts. Am J Psychiatry 146:821–828, 1989

Baird KA, Rupert PA: Clinical management of confidentiality: a survey of psychologists in seven states. Professional Psychology: Research and Practice 18:347–352, 1987

Beauchamp TL, Childress JF: Principles of Biomedical Ethics, 3rd Edition. New York, Oxford University Press, 1989

Beck JC: When the patient threatens violence: an empirical study of clinical practice after *Tarasoff*. Bull Am Acad Psychiatry Law 10:189–201, 1982

Beck JC: Violent patients and the *Tarasoff* duty in private psychiatric practice. Journal of Psychiatry and Law 13:361–376, 1985

Berlin FS, Malin HM, Dean S: Effects of statutes requiring psychiatrists to report suspected sexual abuse of children. Am J Psychiatry 148:449–453, 1991

Bernard JL, O'Laughlin DL: Confidentiality: Do training clinics take it seriously? Law and Psychology Review 14:59–69, 1990

Brosig CL, Kalichman SC: Clinicians' reporting of suspected child abuse: a review of the empirical literature. Clinical Psychology Review 12:155–168, 1992

Cheng TL, Savageau JA, Sattler AL, et al: Confidentiality in health care. JAMA 269:1404–1407, 1993

Coleman P: Creating therapist-incest offender exception to mandatory child abuse reporting statutes—when psychiatrists know best. University of Cincinnati Law Review 54:1113–1152, 1986

Daro D, Mitchel L: Current Trends in Child Abuse Reporting and Fatalities: The Results of the 1989 Annual Fifty State Survey. Washington, DC, National Committee for the Prevention of Child Abuse, 1990

Dyer AR: Ethics and Psychiatry: Toward Professional Definition. Washington, DC, American Psychiatric Press, 1988

Faustman WO, Miller DJ: Considerations in prewarning clients of the limitations of confidentiality. Psychol Rep 60:195–198, 1987

Gillon R: Confidentiality. Br Med J 291:1634–1636, 1985

Givelber DJ, Bowers WJ, Blitch CL: *Tarasoff*, myth and reality: an empirical study of private law in action. Wisconsin Law Review 1984:443–497, 1984

Harper G, Irvin E: Alliance formation with parents: limit-setting and the effect of mandated reporting. Am J Orthopsychiatry 55:550–560, 1985

Harris L: Most people think doctors do a good job of protecting the privacy of their records. Hosp Community Psychiatry 30:860–861, 1979

Haut MW, Muehleman T: Informed consent: the effects of clarity and specificity on disclosure in a clinical interview. Psychotherapy 23:93–101, 1986

Hillerbrand ET, Claiborn CD: Ethical knowledge exhibited by clients and nonclients. Professional Psychology: Research and Practice 19:527–531, 1988

Kaplan MS, Abel GG, Cunningham-Rathner J, et al: The impact of parolees' perception of confidentiality of their self-reported sex crimes. Annals of Sex Research 3:293–303, 1990

Klotz JA: Limiting the psychotherapist-patient privilege: the therapeutic potential. Criminal Law Bulletin 27:416–433, 1991

Leong GB, Eth S, Silva JA: The psychotherapist as witness for the prosecution: the criminalization of *Tarasoff*. Am J Psychiatry 149:1011–1015, 1992

Lindenthal JJ, Thomas CS: A comparative study of the handling of confidentiality. J Nerv Ment Dis 168:361–369, 1980

Lindenthal JJ, Thomas CS: Psychiatrists, the public, and confidentiality. J Nerv Ment Dis 170:319–323, 1982

Lindenthal JJ, Thomas CS: Attitudes toward confidentiality. Administration in Mental Health 11:151–160, 1984

McGuire JM, Toal P, Blau B: The adult client's conception of confidentiality in the therapeutic relationship. Professional Psychology: Research and Practice 16:375–384, 1985

Menendez v Superior Court, 834 P2d 786 (Cal Sup Ct 1992)

Merluzzi TV, Brischetto CS: Breach of confidentiality and perceived trustworthiness of counselors. Journal of Counseling Psychology 30:245–251, 1983

Miller DJ, Thelen MH: Knowledge and beliefs about confidentiality in psychotherapy. Professional Psychology: Research and Practice 17:15–19, 1986

Miller RD, Weinstock R: Conflict of interest between therapist-patient confidentiality and the duty to report sexual abuse of children. Behavioral Sciences and the Law 5:161–174, 1987

Miller RD, Maier GJ, Kaye K: *Miranda* comes to the hospital: the right to remain silent in civil commitment. Am J Psychiatry 142:1074–1077, 1985

Moore RA: Ethics in the practice of psychiatry: update on the results of enforcement of the code. Am J Psychiatry 142:1043–1046, 1985

Muehleman T, Pickens BK, Robinson F: Informing clients about the limits to confidentiality, risks, and their rights: is self-disclosure inhibited? Professional Psychology: Research and Practice 16:385–397, 1985

Otto RK, Ogloff JRP, Small MA: Confidentiality and informed consent in psychotherapy: clinicians' knowledge and practices in Florida and Nebraska. Forensic Reports 4:379–389, 1991

People v Wharton, 280 Cal Rptr 631 (Cal Sup Ct 1991)

Pope KS, Bajt TR: When laws and values conflict: a dilemma for psychologists. Am Psychol 43:828–829, 1988

Pope KS, Vetter VA: Ethical dilemmas encountered by members of the American Psychological Association. Am Psychol 47:397–411, 1992

Pope KS, Tabachnick BG, Keith-Spiegel P: Ethics of practice: the beliefs and behaviors of psychologists as therapists. Am Psychol 42:993–1006, 1987

Racusin RJ, Felsman JK: Reporting child abuse: the ethical obligation to inform parents. Journal of the American Academy of Child Psychiatry 25:485–489, 1986

Roback HB, Ochoa E, Block F, et al: Guarding confidentiality in clinical groups: the therapist's dilemma. Int J Group Psychother 42:81–103, 1992

Roth LH, Meisel A: Dangerousness, confidentiality, and the duty to warn. Am J Psychiatry 134:508–511, 1977

Rubanowitz DE: Public attitudes toward psychotherapist-client confidentiality. Professional Psychology: Research and Practice 18:613–618, 1987

Schmid D, Appelbaum PS, Roth LH, et al: Confidentiality in psychiatry: a study of the patient's view. Hosp Community Psychiatry 34:353–355, 1983

Shuman DW, Weiner MS: The privilege study: an empirical examination of the psychotherapist-patient privilege. North Carolina Law Review 60:893–942, 1982

Siegler M: Confidentiality in medicine—a decrepit concept. N Engl J Med 307:1518–1521, 1982

Simmons DD: Client attitudes toward release of confidential information without consent. J Clin Psychol 24:364–365, 1968

Smith SR, Meyer RG: Child abuse reporting laws and psychotherapy: a time for reconsideration. Int J Law Psychiatry 7:351–366, 1984

Somberg DR, Stone GL, Claiborn CD: Informed consent: therapists' beliefs and practices. Professional Psychology: Research and Practice 24:153–159, 1993

Suarez JM, Balcanoff EJ: Massachusetts psychiatry and privileged communication. Arch Gen Psychiatry 15:619–623, 1966

Szasz TS, Nemiroff RA: A questionnaire study of psychoanalytic practices and opinions. J Nerv Ment Dis 137:209–221, 1963

Tarasoff v Regents of the University of California, 529 P2d 553 (Cal Sup Ct 1974), vacated; 551 P2d 334 (Cal Sup Ct 1976)

Taube DO, Elwork A: Researching the effects of confidentiality law on patients' self-disclosures. Professional Psychology: Research and Practice 21:72–75, 1990

VandeCreek L, Miars RD, Herzog CE: Client anticipations and preferences for confidentiality of records. Journal of Counseling Psychology 34:62–67, 1987

Watson H, Levine M: Psychotherapy and mandated reporting of child abuse. Am J Orthopsychiatry 59:246–256, 1989

Weiner BA, Wettstein RM: Legal Issues in Mental Health Care. New York, Plenum, 1993

Weinstock R: Confidentiality and the new duty to protect: the therapist's dilemma. Hosp Community Psychiatry 39:607–609, 1988

Weinstock R, Weinstock D: Child abuse reporting trends: an unprecedented threat to confidentiality. J Forensic Sci 33:418–431, 1988

Weisberg R, Wald M: Confidentiality laws and state efforts to protect abused or neglected children: the need for statutory reform. Family Law Quarterly 18:143–212, 1984

Weiss BD: Confidentiality expectations of patients, physicians, and medical students. JAMA 247:2695–2697, 1982

Weiss BD, Senf JH, Carter JZ, et al: Confidentiality expectations of patients in teaching hospital clinics versus private practice offices. Soc Sci Med 23:387–391, 1986

Wettstein RM: A psychiatric perspective on Washington's sexually violent predators statute. University of Puget Sound Law Review 15:597–633, 1992

Winslade WJ, Ross JW: Privacy, confidentiality, and autonomy in psychotherapy. Nebraska Law Review 64:578–636, 1985

Wise TP: When the public peril begins: a survey of psychotherapists to determine the effects of *Tarasoff*. Stanford Law Review 31:165–190, 1978

Woods KM, McNamara JR: Confidentiality: its effect on interviewee behavior. Professional Psychology 11:714–721, 1980

Wulsin LR, Bursztajn H, Gutheil TG: Unexpected clinical features of the *Tarasoff* decision: the therapeutic alliance and the "duty to warn." Am J Psychiatry 140:601–603, 1983

Zellman GL: Child abuse reporting and failure to report among mandated reporters. Journal of Interpersonal Violence 5:3–22, 1990

Zuravin SJ, Watson B, Ehrenschaft M: Anonymous reports of child physical abuse: are they as serious as reports from other sources? Child Abuse Negl 11:521–529, 1987

Chapter 15

Ethics and Forensic Psychiatry

Robert Weinstock, M.D., Gregory B. Leong, M.D.,
and J. Arturo Silva, M.D.

The American Academy of Psychiatry and the Law (AAPL), generally acknowledged as the principal forensic psychiatric organization in the United States, defines forensic psychiatry as "a sub-specialty of psychiatry in which scientific and clinical expertise is applied to legal issues in legal contexts embracing civil, criminal, correctional or legislative matters; forensic psychiatry should be practiced in accordance with guidelines and ethical principles enunciated by the profession of psychiatry" (American Academy of Psychiatry and the Law 1991). An important part of this definition is that it clarifies that the psychiatric profession—not the law—determines forensic psychiatric ethics. Forensic psychiatrists provide invaluable data to the legal system. Although in many cases the ethics of psychiatry and of law can coincide, the interaction of the two systems with differing goals and ethics can present an ethical challenge.

Forensic psychiatry recently received official recognition by the American Board of Medical Specialties. In October 1994, the American Board of Psychiatry and Neurology is scheduled to administer its first test for added qualifications in forensic psychiatry, and the current certifying American Board of Forensic Psychiatry will cease operation this year. The practice of forensic psychiatry, however, is not solely confined to forensic psychiatrists. Many psychiatrists commonly perform forensic tasks in their clinical work and need some familiarity with psychiatric ethics in the legal context. For example, psychiatrists can be asked to testify in malpractice cases as to the standard of care or in civil commitment hearings regarding their patients. If a psychiatrist is asked to testify on a legal issue about which he or she has no knowledge, the very minimum competent service would necessitate that the psychiatrist attempt to familiarize himself or herself with the legal issue—or claim an inability to give an opinion.

In addition to the legal areas specified above, "forensic psychiatry" frequently is used to specify all areas in which psychiatry and law interrelate, such as the legal regulation of psychiatry or the treatment of criminal offenders. It has become virtually impossible for all psychiatrists to avoid some encounters with the law and with the broader definition of forensic psychiatry. Some knowledge of forensic psychiatry and its ethics, therefore, is crucial for all psychiatrists.

As physicians, psychiatrists are held to the principles of medical ethics as promulgated by the American Medical Association (AMA) (American Psychiatric Association 1993). The American Psychiatric Association (APA) has elaborated on the AMA's ethical principles to conform to psychiatric practice in *The Principles of Medical Ethics With Annotations Especially Applicable to Psychiatry* (hereafter *Annotations*; American Psychiatric Association 1993). In 1987, AAPL adopted ethical guidelines for the practice of forensic psychiatry—last revised in 1991 (American Academy of Psychiatry and the Law 1991)—that are supplemental to the APA *Annotations.*

Ethical guidelines for the practice of forensic psychiatry adopted by AAPL have been an important development. However, they still do not address many controversial issues in forensic psychiatry. In this chapter, we discuss the forensic psychiatrist's role, some of the philosophical debates relevant to forensic psychiatric practice that underlie continuing ethical controversies, the pertinent APA *Annotations* and AAPL guidelines, and some continuing dilemmas and subjects of debate.

PSYCHIATRY AND THE ADVERSARY SYSTEM

The law often seeks out opinions of experts, including psychiatrists. Frequently, though, perhaps because of highly publicized unpopular decisions, forensic psychiatry receives unwarranted blame for the functioning and problems inherent in the legal adversary system. Because differences of opinion in psychiatry are common, attorneys on either side often can find experts with honest, legitimate viewpoints conforming to their side. Moreover, because forensic psychiatrists apply psychiatry to legal issues, disagreement can exist not only about diagnoses but also over the interpretation of the legal issue or the application of psychiatry to the legal issue. Legitimate disagreement, however, differs from the relatively rare, dishonest "hired gun"—a professional embarrassment who will make a case for whoever does the hiring.

Differences in the role of the attorney and that of the forensic psychiatrist also can cause confusion. Attorneys clearly and appropriately are agents for one side in our legal system and make the best one-sided argument they can, regardless of their true beliefs. Forensic psychiatrists, in contrast, as witnesses take an oath "to tell the truth, the whole truth, and nothing but the truth." Appelbaum (1990) has claimed that *truth* is the forensic psychiatrist's main duty. However, the legal system often obscures truth by rules of evidence. The goal of each attorney is to present a biased favorable version of the case. In the polemics of the legal proceeding, truth can be distorted or obscured, often intentionally by one or both attorneys, or even by the legal rules of evidence themselves. Controversy exists as to whether the forensic psychiatrist has an affirmative obligation at least to try to bring out the whole truth, including limitations of knowledge and uncertainty (Katz 1984), or whether that should be left to the adversary process and the expectation of efficacious cross-examination that in reality may never occur.

Attorneys may try to influence the forensic psychiatrist to alter some aspects of an opinion or change the emphasis. Altering language to present a point of view more effectively presents no problem, but a substantive change does. However, the dividing line between the two may be difficult to draw. Many forensic psychiatrists participating in the adversary process see no problem with putting a "spin" on the facts or cooperating with an attorney to put a favorable face on a case by emphasizing favorable aspects and de-emphasizing or even omitting others. At the extreme, hired guns will be dishonest and distort data or psychiatric opinions to favor "their" side or to favor their own personal agenda (Diamond 1990). A survey of forensic psychiatrists showed that the "hired gun" issue was considered to be the most serious ethical problem (Weinstock 1986). There is the opposite danger, however, that forensic psychiatrists who honestly believe themselves to be right will conclude that any psychiatrist on the other side must be a hired gun. In reality, the opposing expert may have only an honest difference of opinion.

Sometimes psychiatrists rationalize their distortion of data as compensating for legal system deficiencies. For example, they may help commit a "dangerous" person with no active mental disorder or automatically equate a mental disorder with incompetency in a death row inmate to forestall an imminent execution. Even though the outcome might be desirable in a particular case, both the individual expert's credibility and that of the entire psychiatric profession may be undermined, and such practices cannot be condoned. Nevertheless, any psychiatrist retains the right to refuse to participate in any forensic case when he or she believes participation to be ethically inappropriate for either personal or professional reasons. A treating psychiatrist may not always have such a luxury if ordered to testify in court despite any objections he or she may raise.

THE ABSENCE OF A TRADITIONAL PHYSICIAN-PATIENT RELATIONSHIP: ETHICS AND LIABILITY

Some forensic psychiatrists see no problem in doing essentially whatever the legal system wishes, believing that the absence of a physician-patient relationship justifies this role. Rappeport (1991) is of the opinion that ethical practice can be achieved primarily through the formalities of informed consent—for example, through the forensic psychiatrist's making the nature, purpose, and consequences of the examination clear. However, caution is necessary because interviewing skills may engender rapport and consequent slippage of any previously given warnings. The medical tradition of physician as healer and helper could lead some individuals to trust a psychiatrist to help them even if the forensic role was properly disclosed.

Many forensic psychiatrists believe no doctor-patient relationship at all exists when the psychiatrist is functioning in a forensic capacity. Although the law generally recognizes the absence of a physician-patient relationship as precluding malpractice, the law itself acknowledges role complexities and that forensic psychiatrists are hired specifically for their professional expertise. They could be found liable for certain acts as a result of their retaining some medical responsibility despite the absence of the traditional physician-patient context. In the New York case *Twitchell v. McKay* (1980), the court found a physician doing a quasi-judicial evaluation for an insurance company liable for damage done while manipulating a knee during the evaluation, even if not for the expert's opinion. Because the physician "represented his skill to be such as ordinarily possessed by physicians in the community," the court found the treatment test for the presence of malpractice liability to be too narrow. However, in the later New York case *Ferguson v. Wilson* (1986), the court limited liability to the duty undertaken (such as the evaluation itself) and not for any opinion regarding disability.

The AMA Council on Ethical and Judicial Affairs states that "the physician's responsibilities to his patient are not limited to the actual practice of medicine" (American Medical Association 1986, p. 24). In a situation analogous to a forensic examination, a preemployment examination by a physician, the AMA states that "the physician should release only that information which is reasonably relevant to the employer's decision regarding that individual's ability to perform the work required by the job" (American Medical Association 1986, p. 24). Thus, medical ethics apply in the analogous preemployment physical examination situation in which the purpose is an evaluation for an employer and not treatment as it is traditionally understood. Ethical sanctions also are possible even in the absence of legal liability.

Forensic psychiatrists generally also have the legal protection of judicial immunity, provided to all witnesses when they testify in court. Similarly, they usually have quasi-judicial immunity for forensic evaluations that are not court ordered. However, in a recent case that the California Supreme Court declined to review (*Susan A. v. County of Sonoma* [1991]), liability for defamation was held to be possible if the expert is hired by one of the adversaries and not by the court and if the defamation happened outside of court testimony. It is not clear whether immunity would still be found for the forensic psychiatrist's quasi-judicial opinion itself if the forensic psychiatrist was hired by an adversary. Liability for defamation or even ordinary negligence may not be protected by malpractice insurance. It therefore could be financially disadvantageous, at least in California, to ignore those aspects of a doctor-patient relationship that would make malpractice and its insurance relevant.

Forensic psychiatrists also have some ethical responsibility to an evaluee, no matter who hired them. For example, being unnecessarily abusive to an evaluee in a forensic examination could lead to ethical—if not legal—sanctions. However, unlike a therapeutic evaluation, a forensic examination appropriately might be more confrontational and might likely involve exploration of upsetting conflictual issues more rapidly than should be done in a therapeutic interview. Even a therapeutic evaluation, however, might explore upsetting issues for diagnostic purposes. Controversy still exists regarding the extent of such sometimes-competing responsibilities, in the absence of a full-blown fiduciary physician-patient relationship, and the physician's primary duty to look after a patient's welfare and interests (Weinstock et al. 1990). Ethical sanctions by the APA and other professional organizations are not contingent on legal liability.

Moreover, professional licensing boards can remove licenses for gross negligence or unethical behavior. However, in *Missouri Board of Registration for the Healing Arts v. Levine* (1991), court testimony was not considered to be medical practice, so even false court testimony was considered irrelevant to removal of a medical license. In this case, the absence of a traditional physician-patient relationship was protective. It therefore remains significant that there are many legal protections from liability for forensic psychiatrists that are not available to general psychiatrists.

CONFLICTING RESPONSIBILITIES IN FORENSIC PSYCHIATRY

Appelbaum (1990) claimed that the forensic psychiatrist retains the principles of beneficence and nonmaleficence (central to medical ethics), but in court these principles lose their primacy to justice and do not govern the relationship. Appelbaum further stated that the possible harm from the evaluation is what endows it with value. He did emphasize, however, that it is possible and desirable to aid the evaluee in ways compatible with the primary purpose of the evaluation, such as recommending treatment and avoiding gratuitous harm like the disclosure of irrelevant, embarrassing, or harmful information—even if the psychiatrist was hired by the side opposing the evaluee.

Some others still maintain that they owe a duty only to the person retaining their services. However, it is unclear why a forensic psychiatrist should uniquely be considered as having only a single, uncomplicated duty and not as a "double" or multiple agent. In some states, such as California, therapists not only have duties to a patient but also can have duties to others who may be harmed by the patient. Therapists can also be used to help convict their patients after a child abuse report (*People v. Stritzinger* 1983), without the added requirement that such a conviction be helpful to a child. They also can be used to prove premeditation and deliberation for first-degree murder and to help obtain a death penalty sentence for their former patients (*People v. Wharton* 1991), regardless of whether there is any ongoing danger. Thus, the need to balance conflicting duties has become a necessity for all practitioners. Therapists can be forced into situations in which the government may try to utilize them as "undercover detectives" by encouraging patients to trust them and reveal self-incriminating statements that could later be used against them in a criminal trial. Despite the serious conflicts involved in deciding how to act, guidelines for balancing conflicting duties and responsibilities generally are nonexistent.

Hundert (1987, 1990) proposed a method for resolving ethical dilemmas in which either choice produces internal distress because some ethical value is compromised. He recommends trying to balance the competing values by placing them on opposite sides of a scale and weighing their importance. Brody (1988) similarly described a method of resolving conflicting appeals. However, both of these methods do not give any higher-order rules on how to prioritize conflicting values. When decision making involves conflicting values, the problems, after other clarifications are made, eventually will be found to exist at some higher level. Philosophy itself gives no way to resolve competing ethical justifications (Rosner 1990). Because forensic psychiatry functions at the interface between law and medicine, ethical conflicts frequently arise.

PHILOSOPHICAL UNDERPINNINGS OF FORENSIC PSYCHIATRIC ETHICS

Two major ethical schools exist in philosophy—the deontological (duty) school and the utilitarian (consequentialist) school. Either, if taken to its extreme, produces problems. For example, the ultimate deontological commitment to truth would entail telling an assassin where to find a victim or telling a Nazi court about a person's Jewish heritage. Other deontological arguments (such as preservation of life or doing to others what you would have them do to you) or consequentialist arguments (such as achieving the most good for the most people) are needed to provide justifications for not telling the truth to an assassin or to a Nazi court. Similarly, if it could be demonstrated that swiftly and publicly executing someone for every murder would lower the murder rate, a purely utilitarian rationale could be made for swiftly executing people arbitrarily designated as the murderer in order to lower the crime rate. It takes other utilitarian arguments (such as the value of the security of knowing that the government will not execute you arbitrarily) or deontological values of justice and fairness to provide contrary reasons.

Weinstock et al. (1990) proposed retaining traditional Hippocratic medical values as one factor in the balancing process when an individual functions as a forensic psychiatrist. *Primum non nocere* ("first, do no harm") is a fundamental precept of medical ethics dating back to Hippocratic medical tradition in ancient Greece. Although not specifically stated in the current AMA Principles of Medical Ethics, which emphasize a contractual theory of medical practice, this precept appears in the opinions of the AMA Council on Ethical and Judicial Affairs (American Medical Association 1986, p. 38) statement that "in the ethical tradition expressed by Hippocrates and continually affirmed thereafter, the role of the physician has been a healer." Moreover, according to the AMA, "A physician's responsibilities to his patient are not limited to the actual practice of medicine" (1986, p. 24).

When a physician testifies in court, Hippocratic medical values may be less important and lose their primacy to truth and justice, but probably still should remain a consideration (Weinstock et al. 1991) because forensic psychiatrists still introduce themselves as physicians with the title "Doctor," despite any subsequent disclaimers about their current role. Hippocratic medical values could necessitate refusing to perform certain roles when the harm done by truthful participation would be too great. In such circumstances, it could be most ethical to refuse to participate at all or to follow Diamond (1990) and participate only on behalf of one side (such as the defense)—but only if the truth justifies that side's position. Although others assert that the profession has an obligation to be available to both sides, that may not be true if the legal system is trying to do things seriously contrary to medical ethics, which may be true in capital cases in either some or all roles. The AMA and APA have taken the position that it is unethical to participate in a legally authorized execution, but to date such restrictions have been limited to participating in the actual killing itself (e.g., giving a lethal injection, pronouncing but not certifying death, or serving as witnesses in a medical role) (Skolnick 1993). In a survey, forensic psychiatrists were found to be divided regarding the ethics of contributing in any way to a death penalty verdict (Weinstock 1986), so the ethics on indirect death penalty participation remain unresolved and controversial. Because forensic psychiatrists routinely are asked to participate in various aspects of the process, this question remains relevant for the profession (Foot 1990) and is not solely a personal ethical or moral issue, despite some assertions to the contrary.

STONE'S CHALLENGES TO FORENSIC PSYCHIATRY

In a luncheon address to AAPL in October 1982, Stone (1984) called forensic psychiatry a "moral minefield" and set out an important intellectual challenge to forensic psychiatry to clarify its ethics that has only partially been answered. Although Stone himself decided that the ethical problems were so serious that he would not participate in court, his concerns can be seen as an intellectual challenge rather than precluding involvement. At the time, the forensic psychiatric profession had not developed any ethical guidelines other than those formulated by the APA (American Psychiatric Association 1993).

In his important challenge, Stone expressed concern about the ambiguity of the intellectual and ethical boundaries of forensic psychiatry. He considered the boundary problems to be 1) whether psychiatry can say anything clearly true to which the courts should listen; 2) the risk that the forensic psychiatrist will go too far and twist the rules of justice and fairness to help the patient; 3) the opposite risk that the forensic psychiatrist will deceive the patient to serve justice and fairness; and 4) the possibility that forensic psychiatrists will alternatively be seduced and assaulted by the power of the adversarial system, thereby hurting the profession's image and integrity. He asserted that the APA *Annotations* were irrelevant as guidelines for forensic psychiatrists. However, many of the *Annotations* do address issues that are applicable to forensic practice, despite Stone's criticism.

According to Stone (1984), philosophical problems add to the difficulties. The problem of free will and determinism is crucial when considering whether deterministic, psychodynamic causal factors preclude responsibility or leave a sphere of free will somehow untouched (as Kant believed). The unity of self is relevant to questions of multiple personality, dissociative reactions, and unconscious forces generally. With respect to the mind-brain problem, if mind states are reducible to brain states, then neurobiological explanations could provide a full account of human psychology. However, these explanations are irrelevant if mind and brain are totally distinct. If mind-brain interaction occurs, the nature of the interaction is crucial (Stone 1984). Unresolved philosophical conflicts, therefore, have more than academic intellectual interest, but it is probably unreasonable to place the burden of resolving them on psychiatry. In these situations the forensic psychiatrist probably should present the relevant scientific data and distinguish those data from his or her opinion on the moral or legal issue, ultimately to be decided by the trier of fact (the judge or jury), and about which the psychiatrist may not have any special knowledge or expertise.

The chasm between science and morality, according to Stone (1984), is important. Science tries to discover causal explanation of behavior, but morality presupposes the absence of such implications. Forensic psychiatry tries to bridge the chasm between science and morality, but has not reached a consensus. Nevertheless, according to Stone (1984), forensic psychiatrists often present their values as if they were facts.

Appelbaum's standard of truth is claimed by Stone (1992) to be more appealing in the abstract than as a useful guide to conduct. He claims that Appelbaum's standard is closer to honesty. This approach, therefore, appears to be essentially the same as forensic psychiatrist Diamond's honesty standard (Diamond 1990). David Bazelon, a justice on the District of Columbia Circuit Court of Appeals who authored the short-lived "product rule" insanity standard (*Durham v. United States* 1954), tried to increase the role of psychiatrists and their testimony in the courtroom, along with wanting psychiatrists to recognize and accede in court to the higher ethical framework of the adversarial system's search for justice. However, according to Stone, Bazelon failed to consider how psychiatrists could reconcile the ethical imperative of the healing profession with the adversarial goals of criminal prosecution. Stone thinks that medicine has not yet solved the problem of how to balance the particular good of the identified patient against the general good of the unidentified masses. He claims that we lose our practical ethical guidelines when we try to serve such a greater good in the courtroom, as opposed to fulfilling our ethical responsibilities to a patient in treatment (Stone 1984, 1992).

According to Stone (1992), Tancredi's solution of justice as a beneficence pertains to a society of unidentified persons but does not address the physician's ethical duty to ease the suffering of particular identified patients. However, because even treating psychiatrists have been given increased legal and ethical duties to society that may conflict with their responsibilities to a patient (e.g., reporting of suspected child abuse), Stone's distinction may have lost some of its relevance. According to Stone, Appelbaum's standard of truth fails because psychiatrists such as the psychiatrist in Texas who routinely predicts in death penalty cases with 100% certainty that defendants will continue to be dangerous (the so-called "Dr. Death") may honestly believe that everyone they examine is dangerous—just as those who always testify for the defense in capital cases believe in their position (Stone 1984). However, "Doctor Death" may be in violation of the AMA and APA guidelines to perform competent service because an assertion of 100% confidence in a patient's future dangerousness lacks a scientific basis. He also may be violating AAPL's current ethical guideline of "striving for objectivity."

Stone considers the Hippocratic maxims to first do no harm and to do whatever you can to help your patient as the ethical dialectic of medical practice. As clinicians, we struggle within this contradiction. We have not found the synthesis, but we know the boundaries of the ethical debate. When we give social justice, the needs of the state, advancement of science, or the American system of justice greater weight than helping patients and doing no harm, the ethical compass wanders and we lose our ethical boundaries (Stone 1984).

Stone proposes an adversarial standard in which forensic psychiatrists would openly accept that they were selected in a biased fashion to be partisan expert witnesses with the responsibility of putting forth the best possible case for their side, much like lawyers. Like lawyers, they would probably no longer need to take an oath to tell the truth. Unlike lawyers, forensic psychiatrists take an oath to tell the truth, the whole truth—not the partisan truth. They do not reveal that they have been selected to make the best case possible for the hiring side. Stone considers total candor about what in his opinion usually really occurs in court as one possible and probably desirable solution. Otherwise, he considers it impossible to sweep the ethical problems of forensic psychiatry under the rug of intelligible adversarial ethics (Stone 1984). This proposal, although it has some significant virtues, would require a change in how all expert testimony is utilized, not just the testimony of forensic psychiatrists, so it is not really fair to suggest that forensic psychiatrists alone are responsible for the problems of the legal adversary system, or that they alone could change the legal system. However, Stone's proposal would prevent some attorneys and witnesses from having it both ways—for example, the expert taking an oath to tell the whole truth but then presenting a one-sided, biased version of the truth. His proposal also implies pessimism about the possibility of getting experts to try to reveal the whole truth.

Stone (1992) recently discussed Appelbaum's proposal that forensic psychiatry have its own ethics based on truth and based on its own ethical principles divorced from medicine. Stone believes that this proposal does not solve forensic psychiatry's ethical problems because it still does not deal with the seductive power of the forensic psychiatrist, who can instill inappropriate trust in an evaluee. Stone believes that ethical problems arise any time a psychiatrist leaves the clinical situation. For example, he considers psychiatrists in managed care situations as behaving more like business people. Similarly, he believes forensic psychiatrists begin to act like attorneys and start to advocate for their side by making a one-sided case that may even distort the facts to help the case. Only the revelation of dishonesty by the other side, with its resultant destruction of credibility—not truth itself—becomes a limiting factor. Outside of the treatment situation, Stone believes we lose the forces that reinforce our ethics. Tancredi and Weisstub (1986) criticized Stone for not having solutions, but that is not necessarily the job of a critic. Nevertheless, Stone's challenge to forensic psychiatry does not in our opinion necessitate nonparticipation. The challenge can be seen as highlighting the need for caution and for awareness of ethical complexities, as well as for increased training in ethics.

ETHICAL SURVEYS OF FORENSIC PSYCHIATRISTS

A survey of AAPL forensic psychiatrists suggested that a very large percentage of forensic psychiatrists believe that medical and psychiatric ethics should be a consideration for forensic psychiatrists (Weinstock et al. 1991). A large number also believed that they had a responsibility both to an evaluee and to society, regardless of who hired them. An earlier survey of forensic psychiatrists indicated a belief that the death penalty, because of its special seriousness, should be handled differently (Weinstock 1988). Another survey showed a clear difference of opinion regarding the ethics of a forensic psychiatrist contributing in any way to a death penalty verdict (Weinstock 1986).

Even though a majority vote clearly should not itself determine ethics, the results of these surveys seem most consistent with a need to balance ethical values, retaining traditional medical ethics as one factor in the balancing process (Weinstock et al. 1990). Of course, this method does not give guidance regarding how to make a specific ethical decision. Higher-order decision rules could be useful; however, at some level no clear guidance could be given and individual decision making would still become inevitable. Guidelines and decision rules at some point are insufficient, and the psychiatrist must do his or her own balancing. In controversial situations, consultation should be obtained from ethics committees or those with expertise in professional ethics. When actions are debatable, sanctions should not be applied; however, that does not relieve the practitioner from the need to try to reach the most ethical solution.

CONFLICTS BETWEEN VALUES OF MEDICINE AND LAW

Forensic psychiatry entails the application of psychiatry and medicine with their core values of beneficence and nonmaleficence to the law with its emphasis on resolution of disputes, justice, retribution, deterrence, and sometimes rehabilitation. A valid ethical question exists as to whether psychiatrists as consultants to the legal system should bring medical values to the law and attempt to influence the law with those medical values. Alternatively, should they carry out the legal system's requests even when legal ends conflict with medical ends and values? For example, should efforts be made only in the direction of making the law more humanitarian? Should all efforts to obtain a death sentence be avoided? Should the forensic psychiatrist merely answer any question the legal system asks for which an answer can be provided, without questioning the legal system's goals? No consensus exists.

The two major approaches to forensic psychiatry are probably best enunciated by two prominent late California forensic psychiatrists, Pollack and Diamond. Pollack (1974) thought forensic psychiatric consultation was concerned primarily with the ends of the legal system—justice—as opposed to the therapeutic objectives of the medical system. In contrast, Diamond (1992) thought that the forensic psychiatrist brought psychiatric expertise and ethics to the legal system and should endeavor to participate in a fiducial manner only in ways consistent with medical ethics. Diamond would participate only if he agreed with the goals of the legal system, or he would endeavor to change its goals through participation in complex controversial cases, the appellate process, or legislative testimony. The psychiatrist in his view was no mere technician to be used however the law saw fit. Just as a treating psychiatrist probably would not treat a patient so that the patient could achieve goals contrary to those of the psychiatrist in any significant way (e.g., a goal to be a more effective embezzler of company funds or a more efficient drug dealer), forensic psychiatrists should agree to participate only if they basically agree with the ways in which their testimony will be used. Diamond would only testify for the defense in criminal cases because that was most consistent with his personal view of medical ethics. However, truth in court was an even higher value, so he refused most cases, participating in only about 10% of the cases in which he was asked to consult. He would not agree to participate in any case in which the defense attorney planned to use legal technicalities to obscure or withhold part of the truth, despite the attorney's legal right to do so.

When there was ambiguity, Pollack would try to determine what the legal system really wanted, much as a judge might do. In contrast, Diamond interpreted ambiguities in ways consistent with his own values and those of the medical profession but did so in a totally open and honest manner. Sometimes he would even try to change legal criteria he believed were wrong and would present his reasons for doing so. An example of their different approaches would be their interpretations of the *M'Naghten* insanity defense, which was interpreted in a more restrictive way by Pollack than by Diamond. However, even Pollack interpreted this defense much more broadly than some prosecution-oriented forensic psychiatrists, who interpret it so narrowly that almost no defendants would qualify, no matter how psychotic they might be, if they had even the slightest idea of the nature and wrongfulness of their offense.

Pollack and Diamond both agreed that before testifying in court about a legal issue, psychiatrists have a responsibility to become familiar with the legal criteria, after which they could express an opinion on the issue. That is part of the expertise of forensic psychiatry, despite the fact that some jurisdictions limit the giving of "ultimate-issue" opinions. Other psychiatrists, however, have advised not expressing an opinion on the ultimate legal issue but only on the psychiatric issues, thereby leaving the ultimate-issue decision to the trier of fact (Katz 1992). Because knowledge of the legal issue is important for knowing how to focus the psychiatric evaluation, some special forensic expertise or training remains relevant. Undoubtedly, however, if a psychiatrist is unable to ascertain the existing criteria for a legal issue, an opinion about it should not be given, especially if the psychiatrist fails to state the specific criteria he or she is utilizing.

IMPARTIALITY, HONESTY, AND OBJECTIVITY

It is often stated that impartiality is demonstrated by being willing to testify for either side in a case, dependent on the facts. However, such a record does not necessarily demonstrate honesty because a true "hired gun" will testify for whatever side pays the fee. Diamond (1959) claimed that true impartiality is impossible because we all have biases. He recommended that "impartiality" be replaced in guidelines by "honesty" (Diamond 1990). This change was implemented by AAPL in 1989. Even if experts were initially impartial, Diamond thought the adversary process would cause them to become biased toward their opinions. He considered impartiality to be rare—even at the outset—because of the forensic psychiatrist's ideological views, a desire to please the attorney, or a desire to be hired for the case. Diamond also thought that objectivity was unrealistic. Katz (1992) recommends replacing objectivity with "disciplined subjectivity." In addition to AAPL removing "impartiality" from its original ethical guidelines and replacing it with "honesty," it also has changed "objectivity" to a need to "strive for objectivity." This change recognized the need not to accept a subjective opinion too readily but to look for other discrepant evidence and to try to reach an opinion all could accept. Perhaps that is close to Katz's disciplined subjectivity. Nevertheless, some expert witnesses still claim impartiality or see it as an ideal.

Although few forensic psychiatrists probably would agree with Diamond about never participating for the prosecution, many more have problems in participating for the prosecution in capital cases. Testimony solely for the defense should be considered a valid option (Weinstock et al. 1992). It is not necessary to be equally ready to testify for either side. However, it is important to demonstrate honesty because some experts who testify for only one side may do so dishonestly or by exaggerating the case. In the civil arena, such problems arise in some jurisdictions in which some experts in personal injury or workers' compensation cases testify only for plaintiff or defense sides and may tend to exaggerate the case to please the hiring side. Such behavior, even if done for ideological reasons, does not meet the standard of total honesty required by Diamond; rather, it falls into Diamond's categorization of a "hired gun" (Diamond 1990).

IS IT NECESSARY FOR FORENSIC PSYCHIATRY TO HAVE ITS OWN ETHICS?

Appelbaum (1992) correctly stated that courts and legislatures have not addressed the problems with forensic psychiatric testimony and that it is very easy to qualify as an expert without expertise in a specific area. Prosecution for perjury is rare. As proposed by Appelbaum, voluntary peer review of testimony can be educational but will not affect the least-ethical, unconcerned practitioner. Appelbaum proposed that forensic psychiatry elaborate a code of ethics based on a fundamental set of principles rather than utilize the APA method of ad hoc responses to problems. He believes such ethical principles should be formulated de novo and not as an offshoot of the APA *Annotations* (American Psychiatric Association 1993).

Although a more systematic formulation of forensic psychiatric ethics based on principles may be desirable and forensic psychiatry might do well to enforce the ethics of its own subspecialty, it is unclear why these ethics should not be derived from the APA *Annotations* (American Psychiatric Association 1993). It is also unclear why forensic psychiatry is inherently different from psychiatric consultation to other systems in which medical ethics clearly continue to apply. With the development of managed care and cost controls, interactions between varying systems have become common, even if they are problematic (Stone 1992). Ethics also serve many functions. In addition to a punitive role, some ethical guidelines provide an inspirational aid for the ethical psychiatrist trying to resolve a dilemma in the best way possible in situations where conflicting responsibilities are present or a lack of consensus exists (Dyer 1988). Ethical concerns are necessary to combat the temptation of high fees, offered by some trial lawyers, to make the best case possible for that attorney regardless of the truth—although such behavior by attorneys may be considered ethical.

The recognition of forensic psychiatry as a subspecialty of psychiatry and the decision by AAPL to have ethics enforced by the APA is most consistent with the position that medical ethics is one consideration in the ethical balancing process and that certain aspects of a physician-patient relationship still are applicable. The APA enforces the AMA ethical principles, as elaborated in the *Annotations* (American Psychiatric Association 1993). AAPL has devised ethical guidelines that are supplemental to those of the APA and can be used as advisory by them. The strong relevance of medical and psychiatric ethics indicated in surveys of forensic psychiatrists shows that most forensic practitioners do not believe forensic psychiatry has unique ethical principles totally separate from those in medicine. The recent greater cooperation by the APA with organized forensic psychiatry and its official recognition as a subspecialty also speaks to the practicality of this procedure. Nevertheless, if practical, it could be advantageous for AAPL also to hold ethics hearings (Halpern 1990). Perhaps, to limit liability, only reprimands and warnings could be given, thereby also avoiding the necessity of reporting to the National Data Bank.

APA ETHICAL ANNOTATIONS AND OPINIONS: THEIR RELEVANCE FOR FORENSIC PSYCHIATRY

The *Annotations* (American Psychiatric Association 1993) address many aspects of forensic psychiatry, even if not in any systematic way (see Table 15–1 for the relevant AMA ethical principles). Some examples relevant to forensic psychiatry include Section 1, Annotation 1, which requires psychiatrists to preclude gratifying their own needs by exploiting a patient and to be vigilant about the impact of conduct on the boundaries of the doctor-patient relationship and thus upon the patient's well-being. Section 1, Annotation 4, prohibits physician participation in a legally authorized execution. This injunction has been narrowly interpreted by AMA and APA to proscribe giving lethal injections, determining (but not certifying) death, or serving as a witness in a professional capacity. Section 2, Annotation 1, has been revised to find sexual activity with a current or former patient unethical. The reasons for that are general exploitation of emotions arising from treatment and the inherent inequality in the psychiatrist-patient relationship. Section 3, Annotation 1, recognizes that although it would be unethical to engage in illegal activities if they bear directly on practice, it might not be unethical to engage in illegal activities such as those

Table 15–1. American Medical Association principles of medical ethics relevant to forensic psychiatry

Principle 1: A physician shall be dedicated to providing competent medical service with compassion and respect for human dignity.

Principle 2: A physician shall deal honestly with patients and colleagues, and strive to expose those physicians deficient in character or competence, or who engage in fraud or deception.

Principle 3: A physician shall respect the law and also recognize a responsibility to seek changes in those requirements which are contrary to the best interests of the patient.

Principle 4: A physician shall respect the rights of patients, of colleagues, and of other health professionals, and shall safeguard patient confidences within the constraints of the law.

Principle 7: A physician shall recognize a responsibility to participate in activities contributing to an improved community.

involved in protesting social injustice if such activities do not bear on the image of the psychiatrist or on his or her ability to treat patients ethically. However, no such prior assurance could be given. Section 4, Annotation 6, refers to the need to express the nature, purpose, and lack of confidentiality at the beginning of an evaluation for security purposes, a job, or determining legal competence. Section 4, Annotation 9, refers to the need, if doubt exists, to try to preserve patient confidences and to question the need for court disclosure. Section 4, Annotation 13, refers to the need not to perform a psychiatric evaluation before a person has access to or availability of legal counsel unless the care is for the sole purpose of treatment. Section 7, Annotation 3, states that it is unethical to offer opinions about public figures without an examination. Section 7, Annotation 4, states that a personal examination is required before certifying a patient for civil commitment.

Many of the Opinions of the APA Ethics Committee (American Psychiatric Association 1992) also are relevant. The number of a particular opinion refers to the enumerated ethical principle listed in Table 15–1.

Opinion 1C makes it clear that giving a lethal dose of a sedative to a prisoner is unethical because a physician is a healer, not a killer. Opinion 2U clarifies that it is unethical for a forensic psychiatrist to split a fee with attorneys. Opinion 2Z states that it is unethical to submit to pressure to give a dishonest expected opinion as a forensic examiner for a state. Opinion 2BB states that because of overriding confidentiality responsibilities, a defense forensic psychiatrist should not report to the Ethics Committee a psychiatrist who had sex with a patient unless there is imminent public danger or legal compulsion.

Opinion 4E states that developing a speculative psychological pro-file of a mass murderer for the police is not unethical. Opinion 4J states that it can be ethical not to disclose to state authorities that a child was abused if the therapist is working effectively on the problem. However, in some states reporting still may be legally required. Ethics here may conflict with state law. It would also be ethical, however, to decide to obey the state law. Opinion 4K states that confidences survive death, and that it is unethical for confidential information about, for example, a deceased mother to be released to her daughter, even though some jurisdictions give the daughter a legal right to the information, espe-cially if the daughter is the estate's executor. In such instances, confi-dentiality should be maintained. However, the information could be released if there is a specific court order to do so. Opinion 4L states that it is ethical to offer a diagnosis based solely on record review to deter-mine whether a suicide was a result of illness. Opinion 4P clarifies that exceptions to confidentiality after death can be made to protect others from imminent harm. Opinion 4R clarifies that if a psychiatrist is asked or subpoenaed to testify in a child custody dispute after having seen the couple in therapy and one party wants the psychiatrist to testify and the other does not, a confidentiality objection should be raised by the psychiatrist. The court may find proper legal compulsion and con-sider the best interests of the child paramount. Opinion 4U states that a psychiatrist who treated a member of a murdered family and then testified in court could agree to be a consultant to a television company producing a program about the case only if nothing new and no new insights other than those made public at trial were revealed. There is a danger, however, of creating a bad image of the profession. The opinion clarifies that the issue of the nontreating forensic psychiatrist is not ad-dressed in this analysis. Opinion 4Z reiterates that an abusing father of a patient who committed suicide has no ethical right to the records even if he is executor of the estate. If he has a legal right, it is suggested that the court be petitioned regarding the need for disclosure or to limit disclosure to what is relevant to a legally proper question. Courts can be asked to examine the records privately *in camera.*

Opinion 7A states that it is ethical to testify for the state in a criminal case about a defendant's competency based on medical records, with-out examining the defendant. The opinion does not clarify whether—as is the case with AAPL's guidelines—there is a necessity to try to exam-ine the defendant and whether there is an affirmative obligation to in-dicate a lack of an examination as a limitation to an opinion in any reports or testimony. Opinion 7B states that it is ethical to consult to a Catholic Diocese regarding marriage annulments on the basis of re-ports and other information, without a personal examination, because to rule otherwise would deprive many agencies of the benefit of psy-chiatric consultation.

AAPL ETHICAL GUIDELINES

AAPL developed ethical guidelines in 1987, last revised in 1991, that were designed to be supplemental to those of APA. AAPL has no enforcement mechanism, so its guidelines are advisory to APA, which enforces the *Annotations* (American Psychiatric Association 1993) through hearings held by the local district branches. AAPL's *Ethical Guidelines for the Practice of Forensic Psychiatry* (American Academy of Psychiatry and the Law 1991) consist of sections on confidentiality, consent, honesty and striving for objectivity, qualifications, and procedures for handling complaints of unethical conduct. They clarify some issues not directly addressed by the APA, as well as emphasizing some other issues already included by the APA.

Confidentiality is of concern because respect for the individual's right to privacy and the maintenance of confidentiality are major concerns of the psychiatrist performing forensic evaluations. The psychiatrist maintains confidentiality to the extent possible given the legal context. Special attention is paid to any limitations on the usual precepts of medical confidentiality. An evaluation for forensic purposes begins with notice to the evaluee of any limitations on confidentiality. Information or reports derived from the forensic evaluation are subject to the rules of confidentiality as they apply to the evaluation. Any disclosure is restricted accordingly.

The consent section clarifies that the informed consent of the subject of a forensic evaluation is obtained when possible. When consent is not required, notice is given to the evaluee of the nature of the evaluation. If the evaluee is not competent to give consent, substituted consent is obtained in accordance with the laws of the jurisdiction.

The section on honesty and striving for objectivity states that although the forensic psychiatrist may be retained by one party to a dispute, he or she adheres to the principles of honesty and striving for objectivity and performs his or her clinical evaluation and the application of the data obtained to the legal criteria in that spirit.

The qualifications section states that "expertise in the practice of forensic psychiatry is claimed only in areas of actual knowledge and skills, training and experience." The last section clarifies that the chairperson of AAPL's Committee on Ethics will consult in confidence with members and others. Because AAPL does not hold ethics hearings, ethics complaints are referred to APA or other relevant organizations.

Under each section, AAPL has a commentary section that expounds on the guidelines. Under confidentiality, it clarifies that an evaluee should be informed that although the examiner is a psychiatrist, he or she is not the evaluee's doctor. It also states that "there is a continuing obligation to be sensitive to the fact that although a warning has been given, there may be slippage and a treatment relationship may develop in the mind of the examinee." The psychiatrist should ensure that confidential information he or she has received does not fall into the hands of unauthorized persons. The psychiatrist should clarify with a potential retaining attorney whether an initial screening conversation before a formal agreement will interdict consultation to the opposite side if the psychiatrist turns down the case. Also, the psychiatrist in a treatment situation (whether inpatient, outpatient, parole, probation, or conditional release) should be clear about any limitations on the usual principles of confidentiality and communicate these to the patient. The psychiatrist should become aware of institutional confidentiality policies and clarify them if no policy exists.

Regarding consent, the commentary section (like Section 4, Annotation 13, of APA's *Annotations*) states that forensic evaluations of a person should not be done before access to, or availability of, legal counsel, except for emergency medical care and treatment.

The commentary under the section about honesty and striving for objectivity states that a forensic psychiatrist should enhance the honesty and objectivity of his or her work by basing his or her forensic opinions, reports, and testimony on all the data available to him or her. The forensic psychiatrist should distinguish between verified and unverified information, as well as among clinical "facts," "inferences," and "impressions." "The impression that a psychiatrist in a forensic setting might distort his/her opinion in the service of the party which retained him/her is especially detrimental to the profession and must be assiduously avoided."

Honesty, objectivity, and the adequacy of an examination may be called into question when an evaluation is offered without a personal examination. If after earnest effort it is not possible to conduct a personal examination, it is possible to render an opinion on the basis of other information. However, under such circumstances the forensic psychiatrist has a responsibility to ensure that any statement of his or her opinion, reports, and testimony based on that opinion clearly indicate that there was no personal examination and the opinion expressed is thereby limited. In child custody cases, it may be inappropriate to comment on a parent's fitness if that parent has not been seen.

Contingency fees, in which payment is made after the case is settled and is dependent on a favorable outcome, should not be accepted, but retainers are acceptable because they do not interfere with honesty or striving for objectivity. Contingency fees also are prohibited by the AMA Council on Ethical and Judicial Affairs (American Medical Association 1986, p. 25). However, the AMA does permit use of a lien to collect payment as long as the amount of the fee and its payment are not contingent on the outcome or amount of any settlement (American Medical Association 1986, p. 33). Also, a treating psychiatrist generally should avoid agreeing to be an expert witness or to perform an evaluation of his or her patient for legal purposes because a forensic evaluation usually requires that other people be interviewed, and testifying may adversely affect the treatment situation. However, AAPL recognizes that in some instances this double agentry is unavoidable, so there is no absolute prohibition against being both treater and evaluator (Miller 1990). It is also stated in AAPL's commentary that although AAPL's Committee on Ethics does not express an opinion about an actual case, it is available to consult regarding specific issues or hypothetical cases. Its chairperson is also prepared to consult with the chairs of APA district branch ethics committees, the APA Ethics Committee, or similar committees in other countries.

CONTINUING ETHICAL CONTROVERSIES

AAPL's Committee on Ethics (Weinstock 1992) has expressed written opinions that deliberate distortion of data by omitting relevant information is unethical because of the AAPL requirements for honesty and the APA requirement for competent medical service. The case considered was one in which a defendant's forensic psychiatrist, who considered an evaluee's diagnosis to be paranoid schizophrenia, omitted from his report any mention of illicit drug use on the night of a crime. Also, the committee considered it unethical for a prosecution forensic psychiatrist to give an explanation of the nature and purpose of an examination to a defendant but then say nothing when the defendant stated that he knew the psychiatrist was trying to help him and then proceeded to reveal detrimental information, such as the defendant's attorney's defense strategy, privileged information about other crimes, or irrelevant information about sexual orientation. Such information could unfairly benefit the prosecution or be admitted into the trial under the expert witness exception to the hearsay rule, or be used to foster bias and discrimination against the defendant. The committee considered the AAPL requirement of sensitivity to slippage to have been violated. Slippage refers to the tendency of an evaluee to begin to believe that a fiduciary therapeutic physician-patient relationship exists despite an explanation of the nature and purpose of the evaluation before the start of the interview. APA confidentiality requirements might also be violated, although this issue has not yet been addressed by the APA. A recent survey of AAPL members (Weinstock et al. 1991) showed support, in decreasing order, for the following guidelines, which are not currently part of the ethical guidelines:

1. Medical and psychiatric ethics remain a consideration when performing a forensic evaluation.

---

2. The forensic psychiatrist should not distort data.
3. Sex between a forensic psychiatrist and an evaluee is unethical as long as the case remains in litigation.
4. Because of the seriousness of the matter, an opinion should not be given in a death penalty case without a personal examination, regardless of whether court decisions hold such testimony permissible.
5. As a physician, a forensic psychiatrist owes some responsibility both to an evaluee and society, regardless of who pays the fee.

There is currently debate within AAPL as to whether sex between a forensic psychiatrist and an evaluee is adequately covered in the current APA *Annotations*. The problem is that the APA *Annotations* refer to a physician-patient relationship. It could be claimed that a forensic evaluation does not involve this traditional relationship. However, the recent modification in 1993 to the APA *Annotations* clarifies that in addition to transference problems the power imbalance is one reason that sex is unethical. The latter reason would appear most applicable to forensic psychiatry.

ETHICAL COMPLEXITIES AND GUIDELINES

There are many other ethical dilemmas in which ethical requirements and the legal regulation of psychiatry can produce conflicts. One example is the legal requirement in some states to report past child abuse even if the future risk has been resolved therapeutically. We will not review these areas except to emphasize the difference between the ethical and the legal requirements. Ethical requirements are not identical to legal ones and can be more stringent. It can be ethical, but not legal, to break the law under circumstances of conflict, but it is not ethically required to break the law and go to jail for contempt of court in forensic psychiatry. It is ethical to follow the law after raising appropriate objections. Such problems are likely to arise with more frequency in states, such as California, in which therapists now can be ordered in capital cases to testify against their patients solely to achieve a death sentence.

Forensic psychiatry is a complex ethical enterprise, but ethical complexity does not detract from its legitimacy. Occasional dishonest "hired guns" should not detract from the profession. Instead, ethical guidelines should be enforced in cases in which dishonesty could be proven. On the other hand, honest differences of opinion need no apology. In all fields, a "battle of the experts" can occur in court as long as any difference of opinion is possible. Ethical dilemmas indicate that some ethics training should be a required fundamental part of forensic psychiatric training and should not be minimized. Some familiarity with ethics is needed for any psychiatrist participating in forensic evaluations. Ethical dilemmas often require ethical forensic psychiatrists to make their own balancing efforts in conjunction with consultation with experts in the profession. Simple rules and guidelines cannot always provide the answer. A recent survey showed that 93.8% of the forensic psychiatrists surveyed had encountered ethical problems in their work, demonstrating an important sensitivity to ethical problems (Weinstock 1986), although it is unclear whether they saw ethical problems in their own work or that of others.

Ethical guidelines provide a start in resolving ethical problems, but they do not help when there is a conflict between principles. Moreover, the fundamental principles are not made explicit in existing guidelines, nor are rules given on how to prioritize principles. Perhaps truth should be predominant, but many questions still remain. Are there circumstances in which traditional medical values preclude participation? How much weight should be given to traditional Hippocratic medical ethics? Do forensic psychiatrists have an ethical responsibility primarily to the attorney who does the hiring or to try to tell the whole truth? The lack of consensus leaves much room for variability in the resolution of ethical dilemmas. In our opinion, sanctions should not be applied when significant legitimate differences of opinion occur, but only when there is general consensus. However, the lack of a consensus does not mean the absence of an important and real ethical dilemma. It should not be assumed that participation necessarily is ethical just because there lacks a consensus about what not to do in a particular set of circumstances.

The recognition of forensic psychiatry as a subspecialty, the enforcement of ethics by the APA, and the belief of most forensic psychiatrists that medical and psychiatric ethics are relevant in their work provide a rationale for current ethics procedures. Many residual differences of opinion remain, which is not surprising considering the interaction of two systems with very different goals and ethics. Unless decided arbitrarily, simple answers do not always exist, necessitating continued vigilant examination and debate. Complexity, however, does not detract from the significance or legitimacy of an endeavor. Psychiatrists without special expertise and training should obtain consultation from subspecialists in complex cases. Ethics in forensic psychiatry present an important, exciting challenge for any psychiatrist entering the forensic arena, but psychiatrists with proper knowledge, training, and familiarity with the relevant legal issues and criteria should not avoid confronting this challenge.

REFERENCES

American Academy of Psychiatry and the Law: Ethical Guidelines for the Practice of Forensic Psychiatry. Bloomfield, CT, American Academy of Psychiatry and the Law, 1991

American Medical Association: Current Opinions of the Council on Ethical and Judicial Affairs. Chicago, IL, American Medical Association, 1986

American Psychiatric Association: Opinions of the Ethics Committee on the Principles of Medical Ethics With Annotations Especially Applicable to Psychiatry. Washington, DC, American Psychiatric Association, 1992

American Psychiatric Association: The Principles of Medical Ethics With Annotations Especially Applicable to Psychiatry. Washington, DC, American Psychiatric Association, 1993

Appelbaum PS: The parable of the forensic psychiatrist: ethics and the problem of doing harm. Int J Law Psychiatry 13:249–259, 1990

Appelbaum PS: Forensic psychiatry: the need for self-regulation. Bull Am Acad Psychiatry Law 20:153–162, 1992

Brody BA: Life and Death Decision Making. New York, Oxford University Press, 1988

Diamond BL: The fallacy of the impartial expert. Archives of Criminal Psychodynamics 3:221–236, 1959

Diamond BL: The psychiatric expert witness: honest advocate or hired gun, in Ethical Practice in Psychiatry and the Law. Edited by Rosner R, Weinstock R. New York, Plenum, 1990, pp 75–84

Diamond BL: The forensic psychiatrist: consultant versus activist in legal doctrine. Bull Am Acad Psychiatry Law 20:119–132, 1992

Durham v United States, 214 F2d 862 (1954)

Dyer AR: Ethics and Psychiatry. Washington, DC, American Psychiatric Press, 1988

Ferguson v Wilson, 499 NYS 2d 356 (1986)

Foot P: Ethics and the death penalty: participation by forensic psychiatrists in capital trials, in Ethical Practice in Psychiatry and the Law. Edited by Rosner R, Weinstock R. New York, Plenum, 1990, pp 207–217

Halpern AL: Adjudication of AAPL ethical complaints: a proposal, in Ethical Practice in Psychiatry and the Law. Edited by Rosner R, Weinstock R. New York, Plenum, 1990, pp 171–174

Hundert EM: A model for ethical problem solving in medicine with practical applications. Am J Psychiatry 144:839–846, 1987

Hundert EM: Competing medical and legal ethical values: balancing problems of the forensic psychiatrist, in Ethical Practice in Psychiatry and the Law. Edited by Rosner R, Weinstock R. New York, Plenum, 1990, pp 53–74

Katz J: The Silent World of Doctor and Patient. New York, The Free Press, 1984

Katz J: "The fallacy of the impartial expert" revisited. Bull Am Acad Psychiatry Law 20:141–152, 1992

Miller RD: Ethical issues involved in the dual role of treater and evaluator, in Ethical Practice in Psychiatry and the Law. Edited by Rosner R, Weinstock R. New York, Plenum, 1990, pp 129–150

Missouri Board of Registration for the Healing Arts v Levine, 808 JW 2d 440 (Mo App 1991)

People v Stritzinger, 34 Cal 3d 505, 668 P2d 738 (1983)

People v Wharton, 53 Cal 3d 523, 609 P2d 290 (1991)

Pollack S: Forensic Psychiatry in Criminal Law. Los Angeles, University of Southern California, 1974

Rappeport J: Ethics and forensic psychiatry, in Psychiatric Ethics, 2nd Edition. Edited by Block S, Chodoff P. New York, Oxford University Press, 1991, pp 391–413

Rosner R: Forensic psychiatry: a subspecialty, in Ethical Practice in Psychiatry and the Law. Edited by Rosner R, Weinstock R. New York, Plenum, 1990, pp 19–29

Skolnick AA: Health professionals oppose rules mandating participation in executions. JAMA 269:721–723, 1993

Stone AA: The ethical boundaries of forensic psychiatry: a view from the ivory tower. Bull Am Acad Psychiatry Law 12:209–219, 1984

Stone AA: Paper presented as part of panel on controversial ethical issues in forensic psychiatry at the 23rd Annual Meeting of the American Academy of Psychiatry and the Law, Boston, MA, October 15–18, 1992

Susan A. v County of Sonoma, 2 Cal App 4th 88, 3 Cal Rptr 2d 27 (1991)

Tancredi LR, Weisstub DN: Law, psychiatry, and morality: unpacking the muddled prologomenon. Int J Law Psychiatry 9:1–38, 1986

Twitchell v McKay, 434 NYS 2d 516 (1980)

Weinstock R: Ethical concerns expressed by forensic psychiatrists. J Forensic Sci 31:176–186, 1986

Weinstock R: Controversial ethical issues in forensic psychiatry: a survey. J Forensic Sci 33:176–178, 1988

Weinstock R: Opinion by AAPL's Committee on Ethics. AAPL Newsletter 17:5–6, 1992

Weinstock R, Leong GB, Silva JA: The role of traditional medical ethics in forensic psychiatry, in Ethical Practice in Psychiatry and the Law. Edited by Rosner R, Weinstock R. New York, Plenum, 1990, pp 31–51

Weinstock R, Leong GB, Silva JA: Opinion by AAPL forensic psychiatrists on controversial ethical guidelines: a survey. Bull Am Acad Psychiatry Law 19:237–248, 1991; erratum 19:393, 1991

Weinstock R, Leong GB, Silva JA: The death penalty and Bernard Diamond's approach to forensic psychiatry. Bull Am Acad Psychiatry Law 20:197–210, 1992

Chapter 16

Changes in the Economics and Ethics of Health and Mental Health Care

Jeremy A. Lazarus, M.D., and Steven S. Sharfstein, M.D.

The high costs of medical care have created a crisis in access and quality of services for many in the United States and have led to rapid changes in the structure and financing of health services. "Managed care" and "managed competition" are terms and techniques that have been invented in an effort to get a handle on the escalating cost of care. As a percentage of the gross national product and in actual dollars, health care expenditures have risen significantly. In 1980, the national health expenditure represented 9.1% of the gross national product. By 1985, this percentage had risen to 10.5% and by 1993 to 14%, or just over $900 billion dollars.

The rising costs of health care and other benefits have left little room for real growth in wages and salaries. According to data in a 1990 report, the average total compensation for full-time workers—including wages, health care, pension benefits, and other contributions—rose to $29,712 in 1989 from an inflation-adjusted $28,117 in 1973. But only $273 of the $1,591 gain went to wages and salaries, whereas $878 of the increase went to health insurance and $440 dollars went to other forms of benefits. In 1973, group health benefits accounted for 2.3% of workers' total compensation; by 1989, that had risen to 5.1% of total compensation (U.S. Department of Commerce 1990).

The pressures of health bills on corporation and household budgets have forced many of the changes that we are experiencing in the new market for health and mental health care. There is now a broad consensus among all payers, including the government and the private sector, that health care costs must be constrained and reined in.

THE NEW MARKET FOR MENTAL HEALTH CARE—PROSPECTIVE PAYMENT AND MANAGED CARE

For the past decade, we have witnessed a change in many of the rules of reimbursement, with a movement away from traditional fee-for-service payment toward the direction of prospective payment—that is, fixed prices and incentives for increased competition within these contained costs. This effort is designed to create a market structure for the delivery of health care and to change the utilization of care in the direction of efficiency and effectiveness (Stoline et al. 1988).

An example of this approach is the Medicare diagnosis-related group (DRG) system. Introduced in 1983, this system was designed to control hospitalization costs by imposing a system of preset fees for hospital stays. DRGs are a "per-case" payment system that pays the hospital a standard fee per hospital stay for a specific diagnosis, modified by age, comorbid conditions, or the performance of a procedure. The average payment per hospital stay was adjusted for each of approximately 470 DRGs to reflect expected differences in the cost of care for patients with different clinical conditions. From the beginning, it was recognized that DRGs for psychiatry were less accurate than those for surgical and most nonsurgical care and that there might be untoward consequences of bringing psychiatric care into the system. Because of that, specialty hospitals and specialized units in general hospitals were exempted from this prospective payment system.

In addition, alternative delivery systems modifying the fee-for-service system have proliferated. These include the growth of health maintenance organizations (HMOs) and preferred provider organizations (PPOs). Both methods are an effort to create financial risk sharing for providers of care to contain costs. In addition, utilization management of traditional insurance-based benefits has now led to the virtual ubiquity of managed care in the new medical marketplace. This shift from fee-for-service medicine to managed care presents a number of challenges to professional values and ethics.

Fee-for-service reimbursement has its pros and cons from a societal and ethical perspective. It offers flexible choice of providers and a system of accountability whereby patients can hire and fire their physicians, and there is no incentive to skimp on care provided. The disadvantages of fee for service include the incentive to provide more services with higher costs. That has been cited as one of the major culprits in the escalating cost of health care. The inability to predict costs is caused in part by the seemingly insatiable demand of consumers, whose requests for care are highly influenced by professional judgment. Approaches with 100% insurance coverage are rapidly becoming systems of the past.

One modification in the fee-for-service arrangement is the PPO, in which a group of providers agrees to accept a discounted fee as reimbursement for a group of employees. This payment is accepted as payment in full, and there is an agreement not to bill patients for additional services. In addition, the PPO system has been the basis for the development of "networks" of providers who are considered to be efficient and effective. The "carving out" of mental health benefits and the movement to selected providers in a PPO have been one change brought about by managed care. If the patient decides to seek treatment outside of the PPO network, it can become quite expensive.

Capitation is the purest form of prospective payment, and the largest growing segment of managed care is the HMO. In return for a prospective payment, a provider organization agrees to provide all necessary care to a group for a predetermined period of time, typically 1 year. The total payment is independent of the amount of services eventually given and, as such, clearly is an incentive to provide less, not more, care. This payment arrangement also protects the enrollees against further financial loss from illness, unless the patients need treatment for a condition not covered by the HMO and must seek care outside of the HMO. That often happens with treatment for serious mental illness, which may have minimum coverage within the HMO. One issue is whether patients are aware in advance of some of these inside limits or restrictions on HMOs, and whether they would have joined that HMO with the knowledge that mental illness treatment is not adequately covered. Managed care, as exemplified by PPO "carve outs" and HMOs, creates many ethical dilemmas for psychiatrists.

THE CHANGING ROLE OF PSYCHIATRISTS IN THE CONTEXT OF MANAGED CARE

In the effort to contain costs, a particular focus is on the most expensive provider of mental health services—the psychiatrist. How can this expensive and scarce resource be used most effectively in the diagnosis and treatment of mental disorders and substance abuse? At present, as we move from a fee-for-service to a prospective payment system, this area of discussion is evolving rapidly. Psychiatrists are trained in the medical diagnosis and treatment of mental disorders. They also receive training in psychotherapy and in the management of long-term care. Managed care, with its focus on short-term treatment, medication management, and efficiency, is pushing the practice of psychiatry in the direction of acute medical and biological interventions. Longer-term psychotherapy or other psychosocial interventions either are not covered or are diverted to lower-cost mental health professionals.

Many psychiatrists treat individual patients in solo office practice with traditional fee-for-service arrangements, and many utilize extended psychotherapy for these patients. Increasingly, unless patients can pay for this care out-of-pocket, these treatments are being denied or not covered by third-party insurance, either public or private. In prepaid settings, a growing part of the health economy, psychiatrists are employed to be part of the diagnostic evaluation process, to supervise other mental health professionals who may provide short-term psychotherapeutic treatment, and to manage medications of fairly large panels of patients. They also may be called on to consult with their medical colleagues about patients with comorbid medical and psychiatric conditions. Moving into salaried situations and away from private practice represents a challenge to many in our profession. It also represents a challenge to the ethics of psychiatric practice, to the quality of care for our patients, and to the future for our profession and its identity.

The new economic terrain creates unprecedented ethical dilemmas for psychiatrists, other physicians, and mental health professionals generally. The process of utilization review, the expectations of the organizations that pay for care (with their understandable focus on cost containment), and the demands of outside regulatory bodies all pose possible conflict-of-interest problems for the professions. How one goes about accommodating these conflict-of-interest situations, making these conflicts overt to the ultimate consumer of care—the patient—as well as to others with stakes in health care economics, is a major challenge. These ethical issues are the focus of the rest of this chapter.

Psychiatrists, like other physicians, have been trained in ethics with a historical and traditional focus on the Hippocratic oath. The doctor as patient advocate has received the broadest attention (Abrams 1986; Furrow 1988; May 1986). This focus has been predominantly on both doing the best for the individual patient and doing no harm. Over the last two decades, however, there has been a significant change in physician and patient values, with more of an emphasis on patient autonomy and informed consent. In this value system, as opposed to "doctor knows best," the patient has at least as much choice in choosing or refusing treatment as the physician does (Pellegrino et al. 1991). In addition, the definition of "patient" is now being broadened in some insurance plans to mean groups of patients. Thus, in certain systems, the psychiatrist may need to do what is best or do no harm to groups of patients served. Groups of patients may choose systems of care that ration, allocate, capitate, or in some other manner divide resources among a whole group. In the public sector, rationing or allocation plans are ready to be implemented (e.g., the Oregon plan). Many other states are proposing similar plans. If health care reform includes global budgets or budget targets, these plans may increase.

The increased emphasis by health care philosophers and those involved in health care reform on the incorporation of the ethical principle of justice may alter the traditional one doctor–one patient paradigm. Many prominent health care philosophers emphasize this principle (Gillon 1985; Rawls 1971). Others provide models that incorporate the justice principle of equal, fair opportunity as a premise underlying the fair distribution of health care resources (Daniels 1985). In his discussion, Daniels described a model in which a society's health care resources are divided based on what an individual would benefit from in order to attain opportunities that would be available to him or her if there were no health problem. Other ethical principles will always need to be balanced with the justice principle. Thus, autonomy, beneficence, nonmaleficence, and honesty will need integration with justice. In ethical decision making, when conflicts arise among these principles, one needs to consider whether there is an overriding principle or, if not, to choose one basic principle over another (Dyer 1988).

Other authors provide different models applicable to hospital ethics committees and to the teaching of medical ethics (Hundert 1987). Pellegrino (1993) questions whether any ethical principles will survive to see medical ethics go through this period of crisis whose outcome is uncertain. The enormous pressure exerted by economic considerations puts the purity of the philosophical discussion in a titanic clash with societal and global financial concerns (Veatch 1990). Any society needs to determine at some point how much of its resources will go toward health, education, transportation, and other equally important societal necessities. Because of the skyrocketing costs of health care, those involved in it must take a responsible view of the limits any society will ultimately place on these costs.

American social values already seem to be undergoing some underlying shifts. Value systems concerning health care reform have changed from the egalitarianism of the 1960s to a model incorporating social and distributive justice as the dominant value (Goldfield 1992). Although there may be strong opposition in libertarian or egalitarian camps, there appears to be more widespread support for justice considerations in governmental bodies. Indeed, justice considerations appear to help strike a balance between societal value systems. Thus, there may be a basic package of health care benefits as opposed to unlimited and equal health care. There could also be the opportunity to purchase additional health care benefits beyond the basic package. In addition, individuals would have the right to choose their provider or provider groups.

The manner in which an individual psychiatrist or groups of psychiatrists view current ethical dilemmas will be strongly influenced by both their predominant societal values and their professional values. To fairly judge these emerging ethical dilemmas, one must be willing to put oneself into a value system that may not exactly reflect one's own deeply held beliefs. Indeed, several parallel systems of health care delivery may result in different ethical value systems existing side by side. Fee-for-service practice most likely will continue along the libertarian and autonomy model, the utilitarian model will function in certain allocation scenarios, and the justice model will function in prepaid and capitated health plans. Unless the society and its professionals develop a uniform value system, it may be impossible to do otherwise.

The crossroads between ethics and economics have been addressed in the recent literature. Conflicts of interest are addressed by several authors (Lomasky 1987; Lynn 1988; Relman 1985; Tancredi and Edlund 1983; Todd 1991). Other authors address how economic dilemmas precipitate ethical questions (Dougherty 1988; Schiedermayer et al. 1989). Ethical changes associated with new systems of care are also addressed (Engelhardt and Rie 1988; Povar and Moreno 1988). Some health care philosophers, however, appear to approach all of the bioethical issues with some caution, noting how changing times (Pellegrino 1993) and bioethical methods and models (Clouser 1990) are suspect. The use of institutional ethics committees in decisions to limit care is addressed by several authors (Brennan 1988; Fleetwood et al. 1989; Perkins and Saathoff 1988). The fundamental question about whether psychiatrists can be ethical in an unethical world is addressed by Fink (1989) and Webb (1990).

The ethical positions of the American Psychiatric Association (APA) are derived from the American Medical Association's (AMA's) Principles of Medical Ethics (American Psychiatric Association 1992b). These principles contain broad statements that pertain to standards of conduct for physicians. Some authors have discussed the need for didactic education about ethical issues to supplement these codes (Webb 1986). More specific policy statements pertaining to managed care are contained in other publications of AMA and APA (American Medical Association 1993; American Psychiatric Association 1992a). A review of these documents, as well as questions, complaints, and personal contacts from APA members, places the current dilemmas in the following general categories: confidentiality, informed consent, conflicts of interest, double agentry, honesty, and interference in the doctor-patient relationship. There are additional problem areas related to changing roles for psychiatrists and relationships with other mental health professionals.

Although many of the dilemmas encountered by psychiatrists parallel those of other physicians, there are unique problems for psychiatrists because of the intensely personal nature of much psychiatric treatment. What follows is a general discussion of these areas, including some case examples brought to our attention. Although each case could generate considerable discussion, the cases are presented to give general guidance in this emerging area of medical and psychiatric ethics.

CONFIDENTIALITY

Confidentiality concerns have been prominent in discussions about managed care. The literature on confidentiality with respect to managed care is limited; however, some guidance can be gained from APA (American Psychiatric Association Committee on Confidentiality 1987). The issues are also addressed in articles about general medicine (Siegler 1982). These concerns have increased as utilization review and requests for information from employers and other third parties have become more aggressive and sometimes intrusive. The underlying ethics pertaining to the confidential doctor-patient relationship, although unchanged, become strained under pressure for outside review and justification for ongoing treatment. Psychiatrists are asked, with patient consent, to divulge information about history, presenting symptoms, diagnosis, treatment plan, and prognosis. Often information about return to work, danger to self or others, or other highly personal issues is requested. For hospitalized patients, review of charts in total puts the treating psychiatrist and treatment team on notice about the transparency of the record to utilization or quality review. Outpatient records are similarly being requested in some systems.

Although it is ethical to submit one's treatment to peer review, the locus of control and reason for review has shifted. The information in the record may be overly inclusive and unnecessary if cost containment is the primary reason for review. Although the record needs to appropriately reflect the psychiatric treatment rendered, highly personal or sensitive information may not be helpful for review.

What may in the past have been considered "personal notes" are more often being demanded for review. The ethical psychiatrist, under these pressures, needs to maintain confidentiality and only divulge information that the patient has agreed to release. This often entails highly detailed discussions with patients regarding the limits of confidentiality if there is external utilization or quality review.

Often, patients sign blanket release-of-information forms when applying for insurance. This blanket release is not adequate when requests for information are received by the psychiatrist. The specific information to be divulged should be discussed personally with the patient. In addition, the blanket release may be signed by the employed individual rather than by the family member who is the actual patient. The patient has the right to ask the treating psychiatrist not to divulge certain information as long as this request does not create a conflict for the psychiatrist. At times, the psychiatrist may need to decline to divulge any information if there are constraints placed by the patient. The patient may then be in conflict with the insurance company regarding the use of benefits.

Telephone reviews constitute another complicated area. If a patient has agreed to treatment review by a managed care organization, the information divulged over the phone should be reviewed with the patient in advance and in detail. This review is time consuming and may be frustrating for both the psychiatrist and the patient. The primary ethical consideration is to remain the patient's agent in these situations. The psychiatrist should understand the purpose of the review and provide additional information of a sensitive nature only if that information is relevant to the review. If there are any questions about the appropriateness of divulging information, the psychiatrist should review these with the patient and delay the release of information.

It is appropriate for the psychiatrist to know the name and credentials of the reviewing person and to be assured that information given will be treated confidentially. This assurance can be increased by knowing exactly how the review information is processed through the managed care company. Some systems use identifying numbers, rather than patient names, which will provide some additional protection for confidential information. These concerns can become even more complicated when a psychiatrist treating patients for a managed care entity is also a subscriber to that company's benefits and receives psychiatric treatment himself or herself. Separation of the psychiatrist's personal treatment reports from anything having to do with the psychiatrist's contract as a provider for the company can be a perplexing process.

Patient concerns about the withholding of sensitive information during the course of treatment are quite real. The usual resistances to trust may then be complicated by the patient's awareness of the review process. This dilemma may sometimes prevent patients from using their managed care benefit, especially if the managed care company does not maintain adequate safeguards to confidentiality.

Case.   During the course of treatment, a patient confides that he or she occasionally uses cocaine. This issue is addressed during the treatment, and you assist the patient in eliminating this behavior. When the patient's treatment is being reviewed by the managed care company, you are aware that questions about drug and alcohol use will be asked. You inform the patient of this fact and are told not to divulge the cocaine use to the reviewer. What ethics principles are in conflict, and how can you resolve this dilemma?

Discussion.   Here, the principles of beneficence and honesty are in conflict. There are only rare circumstances under which dishonesty would be appropriate (e.g., to save a patient's life). A thorough understanding between yourself and the patient, prior to treatment, about possible utilization review questions may have helped resolve this dilemma. It does not assist the patient or the profession to collude in a dishonest communication. Attempts to help psychiatric patients discriminated against in employment or other situations should be addressed in other ways.

Case.   You are a psychiatrist doing utilization review for a managed care company. During the course of review you learn that the patient was sexually involved with a previous therapist. Do you have an ethical obligation to report the possible ethical breach, and do you need to obtain the patient's consent even though you are not the treating physician?

Discussion.   As the reviewing psychiatrist of a case in which the patient should assume psychiatrist-patient confidentiality, you are under the same ethical constraint as the treating psychiatrist. Unless state law mandates reporting of such information, the better course would be to discuss the issue of reporting the previous psychiatrist with the treating psychiatrist. If the patient gives permission for the treating psychiatrist or you to report, the ethical problem is solved. The fundamental principle here is one of beneficence. Reporting without patient consent may be harmful to the patient. This situation can become more complicated if you hear of the same type of behavior from more than one patient you are reviewing. Here, the ethical obligation you have in reporting of colleagues engaged in unethical or incompetent behavior may supersede the protection of the individual patient. Consultation with your local ethics committee would be helpful in this type of case.

CONFLICTS OF INTEREST

Ethical dilemmas revolving around conflicts of interest are especially apparent in those managed care systems where levels of payment are directly affected by the number of professional services rendered. Issues related to choice of treatment and potential conflicts between the physician and the patient because of differing value systems are discussed in articles related to general medicine and psychiatry (La Puma and Schiedermayer 1989; Sider 1984). Under capitated systems, for example, reimbursement to the psychiatrist may be increased if less psychiatric treatment is provided or if hospital utilization is lessened. Any system of this type has the potential for providing incentives to the psychiatrist to withhold needed care. If the psychiatrist is not the beneficiary of these incentives, but rather the managed care entity is, there still may be pressures on the psychiatrist to withhold care primarily because of fiscal considerations. The managed care or insurance company should inform its enrollees of any such system, and the psychiatrist may then assume adequate informed consent for the patient has been provided. It is incumbent on the psychiatrist to inform the patient of any such potential conflict if the insurance company has not done so.

Any system that provides incentives based on individual treatment decisions or over a short period of time places the psychiatrist in an even more conflicted situation and should be avoided. For example, higher payments to the psychiatrist for the first five sessions of treatment followed by decreased payment thereafter is a highly conflicted situation for the psychiatrist. The psychiatrist has an ethical obligation to place the necessary and effective treatment of the patient first. However, if the patient or patient group is informed of the potential for conflicts of interest and has agreed to that system, it is ethical to provide services to those patients. Indeed, if financial incentives serve to increase access to and quality of care, the ethical psychiatrist may be providing a benefit to the community. As long as care can be provided at the lowest cost without a decrease in quality, there is no ethical problem. In the current climate of disagreement regarding what constitutes quality, there will be ongoing discussion and tension among psychiatrists, patients, and managed care companies.

Psychiatrists working in or for managed care companies administratively or clinically should avail themselves of outside consultation or peer review. These could ensure that concerns for cost containment or financial incentive do not override or undermine patients' trust that decisions regarding their mental health benefits are fairly and scientifically implemented with their full awareness and consent. These ethical obligations for the managed care company cannot be mandated by psychiatrists. However, an ethical managed care company should be interested in areas of its operation where conflicts of interest may affect patient and provider satisfaction. An ethical psychiatrist should inform a contracting company about ethical concerns that place the psychiatrist at jeopardy within the profession.

Utilization review systems that provide incentives to staff for decreasing psychiatric services are operating with a significant potential for conflict of interest. Psychiatrists who perform these functions should avoid salaries or incentives derived in such a way as to tie decreased utilization directly to financial reward. On the other hand, subjecting one's work to peer review is ethical. Psychiatrists can serve important and appropriate peer review functions in their capacities in administration, utilization review, or quality assurance. Payment to the psychiatrist for these services should be on a fixed basis or based on incentives relating to quality of care, or both. If funds are saved within a system to enhance appropriate treatment for a patient, there may be no conflict of interest. Indeed, case management of high-cost treatment should improve treatment of patients while providing cost containment as a secondary goal.

Questions have been raised by psychiatrists in administrative positions about their ethical obligation to report colleagues engaged in fraudulent or incompetent practice. Here, there may be a perceived conflict of interest between the administrative psychiatrist's obligation to the company and his or her obligation to the profession. Unless a psychiatrist is no longer functioning in a medical capacity, the medical-ethical obligation should always supersede other considerations. In reality, the psychiatrist will help the company by striving for high professional ethical standards and protecting the insured population from unethical practitioners.

More and more systems of psychiatric care are developing selected panels of providers that adhere to certain treatment and utilization procedures. Although this method may lessen conflict, there must be adequate safeguards established or approved by psychiatrists, in any system in which they work, to minimize conflicts of interest. At the very least, psychiatrists should be assured that patients are aware of conflicts when they exist.

Case.   A managed care company has an outpatient mental health benefit of 20 outpatient psychiatric visits per year. As part of its contract with you (the psychiatrist), the company asks you to accept a lump sum payment of $500 per patient, regardless of how many visits you have with that patient. Is this ethical, and if not, how could you solve your dilemma?

Discussion.   This situation places the treating psychiatrist in a highly conflicted situation. Clearly, the payment per session will be substantially less if the maximum number of sessions is used. If the company has a thorough and fair utilization process, thus preventing truncation of treatment solely for financial gain, there may be an ethical way to accept such a contract. However, both the company and you should provide patients with adequate informed consent regarding the financial parameters of their treatment. This type of situation, placing the psychiatrist at risk for individual cases, should be discouraged.

Case.   If you are working as utilization reviewer for a managed care company and are reimbursed a percentage of the money saved by the company, should you inform both the treating psychiatrist and patient of this situation?

Discussion.   Again, in the spirit of honesty, and recognizing the possibility of conflict of interest, the patient and treating psychiatrist should be informed. This type of payment arrangement should be avoided by psychiatrists.

INFORMED CONSENT

The general issues relating to informed consent have been discussed widely in the literature (Dyer and Bloch 1987; Ende et al. 1989; Winslade 1983). If the psychiatric profession comes to some consensus on treatment that is only marginally beneficial or not effective, it is ethical to inform patients of this opinion. If a managed care system makes these determinations, they should be based on guidelines established by psychiatrists and should not be primarily related to cost factors. Groups of patients may choose systems of care that provide circumscribed mental health benefits and should be fully informed of these benefit limits. Patients have the right to give up certain benefits regarding access or choice by choosing certain systems of care. Psychiatrists, however, must inform patients when needed care is not available within the benefit limits of the insurance plan or when qualified providers for specialized needs are not available. It is ethically incumbent that appropriate referral is made outside of the system to ensure proper care.

Because there are already mental health benefit limitations in most indemnity and managed care plans, it is important to inform patients of options for treatment that may extend beyond the benefit. Although certain treatment philosophies (especially related to short-term therapy or crisis intervention) may be molded to conform to benefit limitations, psychiatrists should be mindful of the lack of consensus on outcome measures within the field at the present time. Treatment guidelines and outcomes of many comparative therapies will assist us in providing appropriate information to patients. In the interim, treatment philosophies geared to benefit limits (with informed consent) are no more or less ethical than treatment of patients with unlimited resources. Our ethical obligation should be to provide medically necessary and effective treatment in a manner consistent with the financial realities for the individual patient. If some treatment is not considered medically necessary, patients should have a right to avail themselves of that treatment, while recognizing that it may not be covered in the benefits of their managed care plan. Some managed care companies offer mental health benefits that are not linked to medical necessity. It remains to be seen whether these approaches will survive the implementation of cost-containment options in health care reform.

Case.   You are treating a patient with major depression that does not respond to medication and psychotherapy. Because the illness continues to be severe, you recommend a course of electroconvulsive therapy. You find out that the patient's managed care providers do not have a competent psychiatrist to provide these services. Should you inform the patient of this fact and recommend seeking treatment with an out-of-plan provider?

Discussion.   Yes. You are ethically obligated to provide competent medical treatment. Part of that obligation is to ensure that the patient receives care under a reasonable standard in the community. It should be the obligation of the managed care company to ensure that competent care is delivered either within the plan or outside the plan, if necessary.

Case.   As a provider for a managed care company that only provides limited outpatient mental health benefits, are you obligated to inform patients of the possible benefits (if you believe there are any) of longer-term treatment that would far exceed the insurance limit?

Discussion.   Yes. Honesty again supersedes any other principle, and your obligation to provide competent medical service should not be diminished. Although others may disagree with your opinion in a specific case, you are ethically correct in making your own recommendations.

Case.   You are a utilization reviewer for a managed care company. You do a brief personal interview with a patient on a psychiatric inpatient unit. The patient asks you what criteria you will use to determine approving any additional hospital benefit. Are you ethically obligated to provide that information?

Discussion.   Yes. Utilization review criteria, as part of the ongoing assessment of treatment, should be available to the patient on request. Although there may be concerns about patients and physicians colluding to manipulate the system, your obligation as a physician is to be honest.

DOUBLE AGENTRY

The traditional role of the physician working only for the best interests of the individual patient is undergoing significant change in managed care systems. Indeed, the physician often has a position or role within the managed care company, belongs to a group that contracts with the company, or in some way needs to communicate with and work within the procedures of the company. In these ways, the psychiatrist could potentially be in a double-agent position, trying to serve the needs of the patient as well as the needs of the company or group. Informed consent may go a long way toward solving these potential dilemmas. Criteria for benefit limitation, utilization review, quality review, and other parameters that may affect the treatment rendered should be openly available to patients and psychiatrists. Such openness would serve to minimize the effects of double agentry or, at the very least, to provide adequate information to the patient about the potential for double agentry. Just as physicians must adapt to these changing systems (should they choose to be involved in them), so must our patients adapt and understand how their insurance plan administers and regulates their benefits.

Case. As a full-time psychiatrist in a managed care company, you realize that your treatment decisions are being affected by your fiduciary relationship with the company. How much of this double relationship should you reveal to the patients you treat?

Discussion. If it is not possible to reconcile treatment decisions you make for your patients with your fiduciary obligations to your company, you should either inform your patients of this dilemma or seek means within your company to ensure that services are being rendered for the best interest of the patients. If there is full disclosure of the financial pressures that influence medical decisions for the insured patients and a fair method of appeal, there is an ethical middle ground achievable as new systems of care are utilized.

Case. You are in an administrative position with a managed care company. A patient requests treatment with a higher-cost provider in your system and you believe the treatment can be provided equally well with a lower-cost provider. You are also cognizant that this less-expensive treatment will save your company money. Should you discuss this with the patient?

Discussion. Yes. Even as an administrator, you are obligated to uphold the same ethical principles as you would if you were directly treating a patient. If you believe competent medical services of similar quality can be delivered to a patient at lower cost, you have a strong ethical position. If the primary reason for using the lower-cost provider is to save money, however, your ethical position becomes questionable at best.

HONESTY

Honesty is fundamental to the doctor-patient relationship, especially the psychiatrist-patient relationship. One survey of physicians showed that most physicians would use some type of deception if they thought it would be beneficial to their patients (Novack et al. 1989). Therefore, at least in some surveys, physicians will tend to choose beneficence over honesty. Most health care philosophers and ethicists, however, would disagree and see only rare justification for dishonesty. There should be no compromise on this fundamental principle whether one works within or contracts to a managed care company.

One area related to honesty that has received considerable discussion concerns utilization review criteria. These criteria should be available to clinicians who will be reviewed and should not be secret. Likewise, psychiatrists should be honest when providing information to utilization reviewers. There is no place for "gaming the system" on either side. That only leads to an ever-widening circle of dishonesty, mistrust, and eventual interference in treatment and treatment decisions. Any type of collusion with the patient to falsify records, reports, or other communication to the outside also diminishes our ability to maintain the trust of the community. Those in administrative positions in managed care, although understandably having concerns about honesty, must act in a collegial fashion to ensure honest give and take. When there is uncertainty about the "truth" or sense of need to bend the truth, consultation with colleagues or peer discussion with the managed care company would be the ethical high ground to follow. If a psychiatrist thinks that a managed care company's policies are dishonest, he or she should protest to the company or to the appropriate regulatory body.

Case. Should you ever alter clinical data so that a patient's benefits will not be denied? Is there any altering of clinical data that would be seen only as an emphasis on certain aspects of a patient's condition and not as a fundamental distortion or dishonest alteration?

Discussion. The answer to the first question is no. The dilemma between honesty and beneficence again would favor honesty, except in the most extraordinary circumstances. Although a physician should advocate for what (in his or her view) is in the best interest of the patient, altering facts would not be ethically acceptable. Accentuating aspects of the patient's condition that would support your recommendation would be appropriate and expected.

INTERFERENCE IN THE DOCTOR-PATIENT RELATIONSHIP

In times past, there was an underlying assumption that the psychiatrist-patient relationship was highly personal and private. With managed care, this assumption has changed dramatically. For inpatient treatment, in particular, there is massive interference in the dyadic relationship (Sider 1987). It is much more likely that the patient's treatment will be reviewed by several additional people concerned with how the insurance benefit is being administered. These people might include those involved in claims processing for the doctor or the patient, those in utilization review and quality assurance, possibly the patient's employee assistance program or employer, and reviewers within groups contracting with insurance programs. Thus, although the ethical psychiatrist will attempt to do the best for the patient, there may be subtle or not so subtle interference by these outside sources. In some circumstances, it is argued that this interference could improve the quality of care. On the other hand, it is not absolutely clear whether these interferences will be detrimental to patient treatment. Unfortunately, there are no scientific studies that clearly give us direction on this issue. Outcome studies may help to address these areas of concern.

In addition to the daily interferences are the larger issues related to whether the individual psychiatrist is considering what is best for the individual patient or balancing that with the interests of a larger group of patients. If decisions are made with a larger group of patients in mind, it is crucial, as noted above, that the individual patient is aware of this fact. Some systems of care, such as the Harvard Community Health Plan, have clearly informed and gained concurrence from their insured patients regarding these justice decisions. In that system, patients with more severe conditions, as defined by the plan, have a lower copayment (less out-of-pocket cost) than those patients considered to have less severe conditions. It is not yet clear how this arrangement will affect outcome, patient or psychiatrist satisfaction, and other markers for quality of care.

The eventual and real nature of the doctor-patient relationship will be determined by whether the psychiatrist's primary internally and externally identified allegiance is to the patient or the managed care company. Some systems have generated such psychiatrist or patient animosity that any reasonable ongoing treatment is subject to an intolerable degree of interference. These may be systems with extremely tight cost considerations that override treatment considerations. If the individual psychiatrist is faced with such a system, it would be ethically appropriate to opt out if changes in the system will not take place to assure the psychiatrist that ethical treatment is rendered.

The potential interference in the doctor-patient relationship may be especially troublesome in those types of treatment that rely on the understanding of the transference or countertransference phenomenon. Those psychiatrists doing psychodynamic psychotherapy have always recognized the need to address external realities as they affect the therapeutic process. Psychiatrists should work with managed care companies to minimize these interferences while acknowledging the legitimate functions of managed care to meet realistic cost-containment and utilization review requirements.

Case. In your work with a patient who has a managed care benefit, you are required to discuss the patient's treatment with a utilization reviewer after every five visits. You become aware that the review itself occupies your thoughts during the course of your treatment sessions with the patient. How can you handle this interference, and should you discuss your concerns with the patient, reviewer, managed care company, or all three?

Discussion.   This issue should be addressed at every level. The patient needs to be informed when intrusive utilization review interferes with your provision of services. The reviewer should be advised of inappropriate intrusiveness, and the managed care company should seek other methods of review that do not fundamentally interfere with appropriate treatment. If it is not possible to influence the type and intrusiveness of the review, it would be ethical to discontinue your participation in the review and thereby with the particular company, as you would consider the intrusiveness too damaging to your treatment.

Case.   In your work with a difficult borderline patient, you confront certain aspects of the patient's behavior with limit setting. The patient complains to the managed care company, and you are questioned by the administrative staff of the company. This event leads to your assessment that the patient is splitting you and the administrative staff, but the company does not understand your clinical assessment of the situation. How can you handle this ethical, therapeutic, and administrative problem without extreme frustration, which might then get directed back to the patient in an antitherapeutic fashion?

Discussion.   Psychiatrists have an ethical obligation to consult with colleagues, other mental health professionals, and the public. If you are able to educate the administrative staff (and hopefully the medical department of the plan) about the treatment problems encountered with this type of patient, you will have taken an important first step. It is possible, however, that certain patients, because of their psychopathology, will provide unique treatment challenges in a managed care setting. Because many of these patients will be in the high-cost case management group, a well-integrated and well-managed treatment plan available to appropriate administrative staff may help to support appropriate treatment. The psychiatrist should not feel hampered in limit setting when that is a necessary part of the treatment and should develop sufficient lines of communication with the managed care company to ensure proper treatment.

RELATIONSHIPS WITH OTHER MENTAL HEALTH PROFESSIONALS

Some additional ethical concerns have emerged in managed care systems that are much like those in public systems of care. These include relationships with colleagues, appropriate supervisory or administrative functions for psychiatrists, and how the role of psychiatrists may be changing. It is essential from an ethical point of view that the psychiatrist not delegate to nonmedical mental health professionals duties that only a physician should perform. Psychiatric nurses may, within the constraints of their licensure, perform certain medical functions with proper physician oversight. Local regulations need to be reviewed to ensure ethical and legal practice. In addition, a psychiatrist should not work with, supervise, or consult with other mental health professionals not capable—because of training or experience—of providing clinical or other services. Likewise, a psychiatrist should not perform tasks outside of his or her licensure or training. It is ethical for a psychiatrist to attempt to bring these other mental health professionals up to appropriate standards; however, if the psychiatrist cannot be ensured of cooperation in these improvements, the only appropriate ethical course may be to leave the system.

The role of the psychiatrist in relation to other mental health professionals is covered in detail in other APA documents ("Guidelines for Psychiatrists in Consultative, Supervisory, or Collaborative Relationships With Non-Medical Therapists" 1980). The psychiatrist working with or for managed care companies will no doubt be involved in consultation, supervision, or cotreatment with others and should understand the ethical and medical-legal implications of this involvement. Legal consultation may at times also be critical. Many of these ethical problem areas have been part of public systems of care for decades, and consultation with colleagues in these systems would be invaluable.

Case.   A psychologist working in the same managed care company as yourself asks you to call in a prescription for a benzodiazepine for a patient in crisis. You have not yet personally examined the patient. Is this ethical?

Discussion.   No. This would essentially be delegating a medical decision to a nonmedically trained mental health professional. It is your ethical obligation to personally examine the patient or ensure that a physician does an appropriate medical and psychiatric examination before prescribing.

Case.   A managed care company you work for asks you to leave signed prescription blanks for use by nurses in the system. Without written protocols for the nurses, is this ethical? What requirements of the medical and nurse practice acts need to be followed in similar situations?

Discussion.   In the described situation, you would be used as a figurehead, which would be unethical. With appropriate protocols and in compliance with the medical and nurse practice acts in the state in which you reside, there are ethical systems utilizing nurses as physician extenders. Your primary ethical obligation in this situation would be to ensure that competent medical services are provided. At a minimum this obligation would require your personal examination of the patient and adequate supervision of the nurse.

Case.   A managed care company asks for your opinion on the validity of certain psychological tests it is running on patients. You have had no formal training in psychological testing. Is it ethical for you to give such opinions, or to give them only with adequate disclaimers?

Discussion.   You should only provide opinions in areas in which you are competent. If you have had no formal training in psychological testing, the opinions you render would not be based on scientific knowledge, which is a requirement for competent practice. It would be best to recommend that the company engage the services of a competent psychologist to provide these opinions.

All of the above-noted areas of ethical conflict will become more or less intensified as new systems of care develop and funding for mental health care, as a part of health care reform, becomes more clear-cut. The essential principles of ethics do not change, but the psychiatrist must both adapt and understand the limits to which he or she should be willing to adapt. New situations may require a closer look at some underlying ethical assumptions. These will require explication and ethical decision making, utilizing the best thinking of health care philosophers and clinicians. It is only through this process that the public can be assured of the profession's commitment to fundamental principles of medical ethics. Additional ethical issues are raised when opportunity for treatment is rationed because of concerns about mental health and substance abuse costs. The impact of this rationing on patients is the final issue of discussion in this chapter.

MENTAL HEALTH COSTS AND THEIR IMPACT ON PATIENTS

Specific concerns have been raised about mental health and substance abuse costs. These come from many employers who have experienced large increases in mental health and substance abuse expenses in recent years. Their concerns have led to specific changes in mental health benefits, including the redesign of benefits and managed care consisting of selective contracting and utilization management of mental health and substance abuse treatment.

A recent study examined closely the issue of the cost of mental health and substance abuse care (Frank et al. 1991). This study utilized data from a large nationwide sample of employees and dependents from the years 1986 through 1989. Substance abuse and mental health treatments were covered by a variety of health insurance plans during the study period. Benefits did not change significantly between 1986 and 1988, but in the beginning of 1989, benefits did change as limits were introduced on mental health and substance abuse care. Over half of the population studied had their benefits curtailed during that year alone.

During the 1986–1988 period, the charges for mental health and substance abuse treatment rose at rates above the rate for all other health care. These disproportionate increases were due to two major factors: 1) the increase in inpatient utilization by children and adolescents (which accounted for 72% of the increase), and 2) increases in the charges for inpatient treatment of substance abuse. On the other hand, charges for general inpatient as well as outpatient treatment did not increase at a significant rate.

It should be noted that in the early 1990s, a number of scandals occurred in for-profit psychiatric hospitals involving the inappropriate hospitalization of children and adolescents. These hospitals have increased rapidly in number around the country since the early 1980s and cater specifically to adolescents. In some jurisdictions, economic incentives were introduced in a competitive market to inappropriately recruit and hospitalize patients, leading to civil and criminal penalties, more oversight from state regulatory bodies, and cutbacks in insurance coverage. In 1989, sharp declines in inpatient use by children and adolescents began as benefit limits were imposed on this particular population. Substance abuse costs, however, continued to rise.

Another critical issue for mental health care is the special status of the public provision of care. For over 100 years, state government has been the primary source of support for the treatment of the most severely mentally ill patients. Ever since Dorothea Dix embarked on her remarkable campaign to get state governments to support asylums for the insane, public psychiatry has been the dominant force in American psychiatry. It is only in the last 20 years that the private sector has grown in terms of the expansion of private health insurance benefits to include the treatment of mental illness and substance abuse. The public system has been cut back in many jurisdictions. It has become quite fragmented and is less available as a safety net for individuals with long-term and catastrophic illness. Most inpatient psychiatric care today takes place in general hospital psychiatric units, whether publicly or privately funded. The number of state hospital beds has been in decline for nearly two decades (Foley and Sharfstein 1983).

Case.   A 37-year-old lawyer with severe treatment-resistant bipolar disorder was facing financial catastrophe. After 3 years of multiple hospitalizations and unsuccessful outpatient treatment, he had to be rehospitalized in the context of an acute manic episode. At this point, his health insurance benefits were exhausted, the family had mortgaged their home to the hilt, and there was no source of funding for needed treatment. The state hospital loomed as a distinct possibility, but it was becoming apparent that this would only be a stopgap measure. Without resources to pay for either inpatient or outpatient treatment, this patient faced a clinical as well as a financial catastrophe.

Discussion.   With the pressures of cost containment in the private sector, many individuals are having their benefits cut and are resorting to treatment in the public sector. With managed care, we are witnessing the deinstitutionalization of middle-class patients and the movement toward community-based services without the private insurance benefits to support those services. This movement has been particularly troubling for many individuals with acute catastrophic mental illness (Sharfstein 1989).

Case.   A 29-year-old self-employed truck driver became quite concerned when, after returning from a short trip, he found that his wife had taken an overdose of over-the-counter sleep medication. A psychiatric consultation revealed the presence of a major depression, and the recommendation was for a short hospital stay. Because he was self-employed, he had no health insurance except the "bare bones" policy made available to self-employed individuals in his state. This policy contained no inpatient or outpatient mental health benefits. It was estimated that a short-term hospital stay would cost between $5,000 and $10,000.

Discussion.   Because of the historic discrimination in insurance coverage, many more Americans lack access to private care for the treatment of mental illness and substance abuse than for the treatment of other medical conditions. It is estimated today that there are between 35 and 37 million Americans without health insurance. If one looks at those Americans without mental health insurance, the figure nearly doubles. This lack of access has been exacerbated by the push to managed care and cost containment (Frank 1989).

Case.   A 17-year-old depressed and substance-abusing adolescent was hospitalized after a nearly successful suicide attempt. After 24 hours in the hospital, a managed care reviewer began to press for discharge within a few days of admission. The reviewer insisted on long conversations every day to establish the necessity of a continued hospital stay and only granted 1-day-at-a-time extension of benefits. The family became exasperated with this process and sought to transfer the patient out of the private facility and into a state program.

Discussion. Another important issue for mentally ill patients is the high cost and intrusiveness of utilization management of private health benefits. Many patients who have traditional fee-for-service reimbursement are subject to case-by-case review by an outside reviewer in an effort to control costs. Utilization management is distinguished by the emphasis on prior review and recognizes the central role of physicians in the decision-making process regarding treatment. Therefore, utilization management has focused on the physician. It has been described as the application by a third-party payer of a "clinical means test" for the necessity of treatment and the appropriateness of a service. Many psychiatrists have objected to the intrusiveness of this review process, which is often conducted on a daily or every-third-day basis for patients in the hospital, and is conducted with increasing frequency in office practice as well. The intrusion on professional decision making and the autonomy of practice has been particularly disquieting for physicians (Sharfstein 1990).

Case. A 42-year-old man has a 20-year history of chronic paranoid schizophrenia. Mostly treated in and out of state hospitals, he managed (with the help of a psychosocial rehabilitation program) to secure a job with good insurance benefits. When he became acutely agitated and paranoid and needed to be hospitalized, he had his first encounter with a private care system, which included a continuum of care consisting of day treatment, residential care, and individualized case management. After discussions with the insurance company's case manager, it was decided to move this patient, after a few days in the hospital, into a day program and to the group home despite the fact that the insurance benefits did not precisely cover these services. Within 1 month of this patient's relapse, he was back to gainful employment.

Discussion. One specific application of utilization management is of benefit for psychiatric care and therefore is highly ethical. This approach, called high-cost case management, concentrates on the relatively few people in any group who are likely to generate very high expenditures. High-cost case management determines whether extra assistance through planning, arranging, or coordinating a specialized treatment plan outside of the hospital will permit appropriate, less costly, and possibly higher-quality care. If an individual's insurance plan does not cover these alternatives, utilization management can provide extra contractual benefits and will provide necessary day treatment, residential services, and outpatient visits (Sharfstein 1992).

CONCLUSION

The current era of managed costs and care creates ethical dilemmas based on economic constraints and incorporation of principles of distributive justice. Traditional ethical concerns related to confidentiality, conflicts of interest, double agentry, and honesty are complicated by interference in the doctor-patient relationship caused by intrusive utilization management. Arbitrary benefit restrictions have a similar impact on denying necessary treatment or shifting care to an impoverished public sector. National health reform must take these issues seriously if the "cure" promised by such reform efforts is not to be worse than the disease. The challenge for psychiatrists is to adapt to these constraints without losing sight of traditional medical ethical positions.

REFERENCES

Abrams FR: Patient advocate or secret agent? JAMA 256:1784–1785, 1986

American Medical Association: Guidelines for the Conduct of Managed Care. Chicago, IL, American Medical Association, 1993

American Psychiatric Association Committee on Confidentiality: Guidelines on confidentiality. Am J Psychiatry 144:1522–1526, 1987

American Psychiatric Association: Ethics Newsletter, Managed Care. Washington, DC, American Psychiatric Association, 1992a

American Psychiatric Association: The Principles of Medical Ethics With Annotations Especially Applicable to Psychiatry. Washington, DC, American Psychiatric Association, 1992b

Brennan TA: Ethics committees and decisions to limit care: the experience at the Massachusetts General Hospital. JAMA 260:803–807, 1988

Clouser K-D: A critique of principalism. J Med Philos 15(2):219–236, 1990

Daniels N: Just Health Care. Cambridge, MA, Cambridge University Press, 1985

Dougherty CJ: Mind, money, and morality: ethical dimensions of economic change in American psychiatry. Hastings Cent Rep 18(3):15–20, 1988

Dyer AR: Ethics and Psychiatry: Toward a Professional Definition. Washington, DC, American Psychiatric Press, 1988

Dyer AR, Bloch S: Informed consent and the psychiatric patient. J Med Ethics 13:12–16, 1987

Ende J, Kazis L, Ash A, et al: Measuring patients' desire for autonomy: decision making and information-seeking preferences among medical patients. J Gen Intern Med 4:23–30, 1989

Engelhardt HT, Rie MA: Morality for the medical-industrial complex: a code of ethics for the mass marketing of health care. N Engl J Med 319:1086–1089, 1988

Fink PJ: Presidential address: on being ethical in an unethical world. Am J Psychiatry 146:1097–1104, 1989

Fleetwood J, Arnold RM, Baron RJ: Giving answers or raising questions? the problematic role of institutional ethics committees. J Med Ethics 15:137–142, 1989

Foley HA, Sharfstein SS: Madness and Government: Who Cares for the Mentally Ill? Washington, DC, American Psychiatric Press, 1983

Frank RG: The medically indigent mentally ill: approaches to financing. Hosp Community Psychiatry 40:9–12, 1989

Frank R, Salkever D, Sharfstein S: A new look at rising mental health insurance costs. Health Aff (Millwood) 10:116–123, 1991

Furrow BR: The ethics of cost-containment: bureaucratic medicine and the doctor as patient-advocate. Notre Dame Journal of Law, Ethics, and Public Policy 3(2):187–225, 1988

Gillon R: Justice and medical ethics. BMJ 291:101–190, 1985

Goldfield N: Why we cannot agree on the direction of health care reform: an exploration of American values. Physician Executive 4:16–22, 1992

Guidelines for psychiatrists in consultative, supervisory, or collaborative relationships with non-medical therapists. Am J Psychiatry 137:1489–1491, 1980

Hundert EM: A model for ethical problem solving in medicine, with practical applications. Am J Psychiatry 144:839–846, 1987

La Puma J, Schiedermayer DL: Outpatient clinical ethics. J Gen Intern Med 4:413–420, 1989

Lomasky LE: Public money, private gain, profit for all. Hastings Cent Rep 17(3):5–7, 1987

Lynn J: Conflicts of interest in medical decision making. J Am Geriatr Soc 36:945–950, 1988

May WE: On ethics and advocacy. JAMA 256:1786–1787, 1986

Novack DH, Detering BJ, Arnold RA, et al: Physicians' attitudes toward using deception to resolve difficult ethical problems. JAMA 261:2980–2985, 1989

Pellegrino ED: The metamorphosis of medical ethics: a 30-year retrospective. JAMA 269:1158–1162, 1993

Pellegrino ED, Siegler M, Singer PA: Future directions in clinical ethics. J Clin Ethics 2(1):5–9, 1991

Perkins HS, Saathoff BS: Impact of medical ethics consultations on physicians: an exploratory study. Am J Med 85:761–765, 1988

Povar G, Moreno J: Hippocrates and the health maintenance organization: a discussion of ethical issues. Ann Intern Med 109:419–424, 1988

Rawls J: A Theory of Justice. Cambridge, MA, The Belknap Press of Harvard University Press, 1971

Relman AS: Dealing with conflicts of interest. N Engl J Med 313:749–751, 1985

Relman AS: What market values are doing to medicine. The Atlantic Monthly, March 1992, pp 99–106

Schiedermayer DL, La Puma J, Miles SH: Ethics consultations masking economic dilemmas in patient care. Arch Intern Med 149:1303–1305, 1989

Sharfstein SS: The catastrophic case: a special problem for general hospital psychiatry in the era of managed care. Gen Hosp Psychiatry 11:268–270, 1989

Sharfstein SS: Utilization management: managed or mangled psychiatric care? (editorial). Am J Psychiatry 147(8):965–966, 1990

Sharfstein SS: Managed mental health care, in American Psychiatric Press Review of Psychiatry, Vol 11. Edited by Tasman A, Riba MB. Washington, DC, American Psychiatric Press, 1992, pp 570–584

Sider RC: The ethics of therapeutic modality choice. Am J Psychiatry 141:390–394, 1984

Sider RC: Ethical issues in inpatient practice. Psychiatr Med 4:445–454, 1987

Siegler M: Confidentiality in medicine—a decrepit concept. N Engl J Med 307:1518–1521, 1982

Stoline A, Weiner JP, Dans P, et al: The New Medical Marketplace: A Physicians Guide to the Health Care Revolution. Baltimore, MD, Johns Hopkins University Press, 1988

Tancredi LR, Edlund M: Are conflicts of interest endemic to psychiatric consultation? Int J Law Psychiatry 6:293–316, 1983

Todd JS: Professionalism at its worst (editorial). JAMA 266:3338, 1991

Veatch RM: Physicians and cost containment: the ethical conflict. Gerometrics Journal 30(4):461–482, 1990

Webb WL: The doctor-patient covenant and the threat of exploitation. Am J Psychiatry 143:1126–1131, 1986

Webb WL: Ethical psychiatric practice in a new economic climate. Digest of Neurology and Psychiatry September–October 1990, pp 207–213

Winslade WJ: Informed consent in psychiatric practice: the primacy of ethics over law. Behavioral Sciences and the Law 1:47–56, 1983

U.S. Department of Commerce: Health and medical services. US Industrial Outlook 49:1–6, 1990

Chapter 17

Nonsexual Boundary Violations in Psychiatric Treatment

Donna Elliott Frick, M.D.

Sexual boundary violations have received considerable attention in recent years and are widely acknowledged as damaging to doctor-patient relationships. In contrast, relatively little attention has been devoted to nonsexual boundary transgressions, which have been less sensationalized. Therefore, the frequency and consequences of nonsexual violations, as well as the extent of their negative impact on patients and on psychiatric treatment, tend to be less well appreciated and understood by patients and practitioners alike. It is important for psychiatrists to attempt to define appropriate treatment boundaries and to learn to recognize and anticipate possible boundary violations. These are often complex issues that challenge the treatment decisions of all practicing psychiatrists. They are also issues about which there are sometimes legitimate differences of opinion within the psychiatric profession. An understanding of the principles of medical ethics on which to base those decisions is essential for all practicing psychiatrists.

BOUNDARIES AND NONSEXUAL BOUNDARY VIOLATIONS

A universally acceptable definition of appropriate treatment boundaries is elusive. Although clinicians may instinctively understand the concept, they are challenged by attempts to succinctly discuss it and by the application of theory to practice (Gutheil and Gabbard 1993). Moreover, considerable variations of acceptable therapy techniques and accompanying ground rules exist among different mental health professionals in various settings. For example, drug and substance abuse programs, inpatient settings, and cognitive and behavioral disciplines may all differ significantly in terms of the treatments offered and the boundaries that are considered to be acceptable (Simon 1992). Specific ground rules may vary according to technique and setting, but the guiding ethical principle of doing no harm to patients remains constant across all types of practice.

Generally speaking, treatment boundaries can be defined as the set of rules that establishes the professional relationship as separate from other relationships and protects the patient from harm. A patient who seeks medical or psychiatric treatment is often in a uniquely dependent, anxious, vulnerable, and exploitable state. In seeking help, patients assume positions of relative powerlessness in which they expose their weaknesses, compromise their dignity, and reveal intimacies of body or mind, or both (Pellegrino 1987). Psychiatric treatment boundaries define the limits of that professional relationship, and it is the psychiatrist's responsibility to establish and maintain those boundaries (Simon 1992). In doing so, the physician creates a safe and predictable environment in which the patient can focus exclusively on the task of therapy. Changing or ambiguous boundaries will jeopardize the success of treatment because the patient's trust and feeling of safety may be threatened.

Successful psychiatric treatment requires a delicate balance of professional restraint and emotional intimacy between the patient and doctor within the parameters of the therapeutic relationship. Indeed, it is this dynamic balancing act that is the essence of the art of practicing psychotherapy (Mogul 1992).

Boundary Crossings

It appears that nonsexual boundary transgressions often occur on a continuum ranging from appropriately timed, single, minor departures from standard practice patterns to more serious breaches that may become repetitive and increasingly dangerous for the patient and that can result in overt sexual exploitation of the patient. The descriptive convention adopted by Gutheil and Gabbard (1993) to distinguish between relatively harmless boundary "crossings" versus more damaging boundary "violations" is a useful one.

Boundary crossings fall into the gray area of clinical decisions in which the best course of action may not be readily apparent. It may be in the patient's best interest to adhere strictly to established treatment ground rules, because to do otherwise might be damaging to the therapeutic relationship or risk entry onto the slippery slope toward clear boundary violations. On the other hand, an individual decision to deviate from the standard may enhance the therapeutic alliance, especially if properly examined within the therapy. Examples of boundary crossings within this gray area include requests for appointment changes, extension of payments, small gifts to the psychiatrist, and requests from the patient for disclosure of bits of personal information by the psychiatrist (Mogul 1992). Ethical decisions regarding these questions can only be made in the context of individual patient dynamics and often require simultaneous exploration with the patient and personal reflection by the psychiatrist.

Boundary Violations

Boundary violations falling along the slippery slope of the continuum are generally less likely to have neutral or positive consequences for the patient. In addition, these violations are apt to be forerunners of more serious transgressions. Examples include decisions based on feelings by the psychiatrist that an individual patient is somehow special and discussion by the psychiatrist of personal problems or feelings with the patient (Mogul 1992). Again, it is important for the psychiatrist to carefully examine the meaning of such decisions both for the patient and for himself or herself.

When does a boundary crossing become a boundary violation, and when does a violation become unethical? These are important questions not only for ethics committees charged with investigating complaints against fellow psychiatrists, but also for psychiatrists to consider throughout the course of clinical work with patients. Any action by a psychiatrist is clearly unethical when information or emotions derived from treatment are used to benefit the psychiatrist and treatment goals are not advanced. The patient in such a case may suffer either direct or indirect harm. Examples include the acceptance of special services or favors from patients, socializing with patients, and extensive self-revelation by the psychiatrist, including discussion of sexual feelings about the patient (Mogul 1992).

The Exploitation Index (see Table 17–1) is a questionnaire designed by Epstein and Simon (1990) to alert practitioners to slippery-slope behaviors that might prove counterproductive to treatment goals. Forty-three percent of survey respondents indicated that at least one item on the questionnaire alerted them to potentially problematic behaviors, and 29% reported changes prompted by the survey (Epstein et al. 1992).

Single, nonrepetitive, nonsexual transgressions, if properly examined, are unlikely to irreparably damage the therapeutic relationship. However, when clearly exploitative breaches occur, repair of the therapeutic relationship can be difficult, especially because such actions rarely occur as isolated events, but rather as part of an escalating pattern of boundary transgressions (Simon 1989). Constant vigilance against harmful boundary violations and immediate attempts to repair any breaches in a clinically supportive manner are the responsibility of the psychiatrist and will ensure that the ongoing safety and integrity of the therapeutic relationship are maintained (Simon 1992).

Table 17–1. Text of the Exploitation Index questions

1. Do you find yourself doing any of the following for your family members or social acquaintances: prescribing medication, making diagnoses, offering psychodynamic explanations for their behavior?
2. Are you gratified by a sense of power when you are able to control a patient's activity through advice, medication, or behavioral restraint? (e.g., hospitalization, seclusion)
3. Do you find the chronic silence or tardiness of a patient satisfying as a way of getting paid for doing nothing?
4. Do you accept gifts or bequests from patients?
5. Have you engaged in personal relationships with patients after treatment was terminated?
6. Do you touch your patients? (exclude handshake)
7. Do you ever use information learned from patients, such as business tips or political information, for your own financial or career gain?
8. Do you feel that you can obtain personal gratification by helping to develop your patient's great potential for fame or unusual achievement?
9. Do you feel a sense of excitement or longing when you think of a patient or anticipate her or his visit?
10. Do you make exceptions for your patients, such as providing special scheduling or reducing fees, because you find the patient attractive, appealing, or impressive?
11. Do you ask your patient to do personal favors for you? (e.g., get you lunch, mail a letter)
12. Do you and your patients address each other on a first-name basis?
13. Do you undertake business deals with patients?
14. Do you take great pride in the fact that such an attractive, wealthy, powerful, or important patient is seeking your help?
15. Have you accepted for treatment persons with whom you have had social involvement or whom you knew to be in your social or family sphere?
16. When a patient has been seductive with you, do you experience this as a gratifying sign of your own sex appeal?
17. Do you disclose sensational aspects of your patient's life to others? (even when you are protecting the patient's identity)
18. Do you accept a medium of exchange other than money for your services? (e.g., work on your office or home, trading of professional services)
19. Do you find yourself comparing the gratifying qualities you observe in a patient with the less gratifying qualities in your spouse or significant other? (e.g., thinking "Where have you been all my life?")
20. Do you feel that your patient's problem would be immeasurably helped if only he/she had a positive romantic involvement with you?
21. Do you make exceptions in the conduct of treatment because you feel sorry for your patient, or because you believe that he/she is in such distress or so disturbed that you have no other choice?
22. Do you recommend treatment procedures or referrals that you do not believe to be necessarily in your patient's best interests, but that may instead be to your direct or indirect financial benefit?
23. Have you accepted for treatment individuals known to be referred by a current or former patient?

Table 17–1. Text of the Exploitation Index questions *(continued)*

24. Do you make exceptions for your patient because you are afraid she/he will otherwise become extremely angry or self-destructive?
25. Do you take pleasure in romantic daydreams about a patient?
26. Do you fail to deal with the following patient behavior(s): paying the fee late, missing appointments on short notice and refusing to pay for the time (as agreed), seeking to extend the length of sessions?
27. Do you tell patients personal things about yourself in order to impress them?
28. Do you find yourself trying to influence your patients to support political causes or positions in which you have a personal interest?
29. Do you seek social contact with patients outside of clinically scheduled visits?
30. Do you find it painfully difficult to agree to a patient's desire to cut down on the frequency of therapy, or to work on termination?
31. Do you find yourself talking about your own personal problems with a patient and expecting her/him to be sympathetic to you?
32. Do you join in any activity with patients that may serve to deceive a third party? (e.g., insurance company)

Source. Reprinted with permission from the *Bulletin of the Menninger Clinic,* Volume 56, Number 2, pp. 165–166. Copyright 1992, The Menninger Foundation.

ETHICAL PRINCIPLES RELEVANT TO PSYCHIATRIC TREATMENT BOUNDARIES

A working knowledge of the principles of medical ethics is essential for any practicing physician. This knowledge may be particularly important for the psychiatrist because the nature of psychiatric treatment is such that the patient will, at some point during the therapy, almost inevitably challenge the ground rules outlining treatment boundaries. When that occurs, considerable skill and expertise are required from the psychiatrist. Development of that expertise depends on awareness and understanding of six key ethical principles on which the parameters of the psychotherapeutic relationship are established: 1) the delivery of competent medical care, 2) the contractual arrangement between doctor and patient, 3) the fiduciary nature of the doctor-patient relationship, 4) honesty, 5) respect for human dignity, and 6) confidentiality.

The following excerpts from *The Principles of Medical Ethics With Annotations Especially Applicable to Psychiatry* (American Psychiatric Association 1993) clearly state the ethical principles relevant to treatment boundaries:

Section 1

A physician shall be dedicated to providing competent medical service with compassion and respect for human dignity.

Section 1, Annotation 1

The patient may place his/her trust in his/her psychiatrist knowing that the psychiatrist's ethics and professional responsibilities preclude him/her gratifying his/her own needs by exploiting the patient. The psychiatrist shall be ever vigilant about the impact that his/her conduct has upon the boundaries of the doctor/patient relationship, and thus upon the well-being of the patient. These requirements become particularly important because of the essentially private, highly personal, and sometimes intensely emotional nature of the relationship established with the psychiatrist.

Section 2

A physician shall deal honestly with patients and colleagues, and strive to expose those physicians deficient in character or competence, or who engage in fraud or deception.

Section 2, Annotation 2

The psychiatrist should diligently guard against exploiting information furnished by the patient and should not use the unique position of power afforded him/her by the psychotherapeutic situation to influence the patient in any way not directly relevant to the treatment goals.

Section 2, Annotation 5

Psychiatric services, like all medical services, are dispensed in the context of a contractual arrangement between the patient and the treating physician. The provisions of the contractual arrangement, which are binding on the physician as well as on the patient, should be explicitly established.

Section 4

A physician shall respect the rights of patients, of colleagues, and of other health professionals, and shall safeguard patient confidences within the constraints of the law.

An appreciation for the above principles and how they relate to clinical practice will assist the psychiatrist in establishing appropriate treatment boundaries and in responding constructively in the face of challenges to those parameters. Treatment boundaries based on these principles create a safe therapeutic environment, which will ultimately enhance the probability of successful treatment outcomes.

ETHICAL PRINCIPLES AND CHALLENGES TO PSYCHIATRIC TREATMENT BOUNDARIES

Contractual Agreement for Competent Medical Care

Competent medical care is provided in the context of a contractual relationship between a patient and physician. With the practice of medicine evolving and new psychiatric treatments becoming available, psychiatric physicians are delivering services to patients in varied settings and in innovative ways. If we consider psychotherapy to be the prototypical vehicle for the delivery of psychiatric care, it becomes a useful standard against which to measure and explore the psychodynamic implications of boundary issues in any doctor-patient relationship. When deviations from that standard are contemplated, the following precautions may be useful to protect the psychiatrist's therapeutic intent from being misconstrued: review of the available body of professional literature, development of a clear clinical rationale, documentation, and consultation (Gutheil and Gabbard 1993).

Langs (1973) describes the framework for psychotherapy as dependent on ground rules or boundaries that, whether stated or implied, define the parameters of the professional relationship and constitute an essential part of the contractual agreement between the psychiatrist and patient. The parameters of the treatment relationship are further defined by the ground rules regarding the respective roles of the patient and psychiatrist and by arrangements for the time, place, and financing of contracted services. The patient's understanding of and response to the ground rules will often become the catalyst for understanding significant resistances, transference issues, and realistic responses to the therapist. The psychiatrist, therefore, should be ever vigilant regarding the significance of boundaries for patients and always prepared to deal appropriately with challenges to boundaries as they arise. To do otherwise may seriously undermine the therapy. Given the emotional vulnerability of all psychiatric patients, the maintenance of appropriate boundaries is important regardless of the psychiatric treatment or technique employed.

Roles of the patient and psychiatrist.   The patient's role and responsibility in psychotherapy are not easily defined. It is not uncommon for the patient to use therapy to express highly rationalized resistances, as well as both transference-based and reality-based hostile and erotic fantasies about the therapist. Patients will also often use the therapeutic setting to test the therapist's honesty, fairness, and consistency (Langs 1973). The context of the patient's testing and resistance is, of course, the therapeutic exploration of the symptoms and difficulties that motivated the person to seek treatment. In exchange for the treatment provided by the psychiatrist, the patient contracts to pay an agreed amount for services rendered.

The psychiatrist's role is to establish and maintain appropriate parameters for the professional relationship and to set appropriate limits on patient behaviors during treatment, thereby safeguarding proper examination of the patient's concerns. Gutheil and Gabbard (1993) cited the following example:

> A middle-aged borderline patient, attempting to convey how deeply distressed she felt about her situation, leaped from her chair in the therapist's office and threw herself to her knees at the therapist's feet, clasping his hand in both of her own and crying, "Do you know how awful it's been for me?" The therapist responded gently, "You know, this is really interesting, what's happening here—but it isn't therapy; please go back to your chair." The patient did so, and the incident was explored verbally. (p. 190)

Therapists who either fail to establish any boundaries or who set idiosyncratic ones are apt to provide negligent treatment (Simon 1992). Failure to set limits gives tacit approval to the patient for filling that void with his or her own agenda (Peterson 1992). That can be especially risky for both patient and physician when previous boundary crossings or violations fuel the patient's dependent or erotic fantasies about the psychiatrist.

Time. Regularly scheduled appointments are almost always an essential aspect of the "therapeutic frame." A possible exception might involve the psychiatric management of a severely ill or disorganized patient. Ordinarily, however, the psychiatrist's respect for a patient's scheduled time is "so important that there should be no need to mention it." It is simply a matter of courtesy and respect (Bruch 1974).

Although it may occasionally be necessary and appropriate to accommodate a patient's need for special appointment times, the psychiatrist must be certain that any such decision is truly in the patient's best interest and not because the professional is developing a sense of the patient as "special." End-of-the-day appointments that then easily extend beyond usual time lengths can be a precursor to unquestionable boundary violations. At the very least, such actions may have significant meaning for the patient, so care should be taken to explore the meaning of any special allowances with the patient.

> A young woman entering treatment for the first time with a male psychiatrist was unusually careful to end her sessions at exactly the agreed-on time. After one session that was prolonged by several minutes, the patient commented on the extension and apologized for delaying the psychiatrist. She later expressed feelings of attraction toward the physician and described a seductive relationship with her father. She also discussed the anxiety she experienced when the psychiatrist failed to strictly adhere to the established time frame for her sessions.

Place. Either the psychiatrist's office or a room on a hospital unit is usually the acceptable site for psychotherapy. Meeting patients in other settings usually indicates a boundary crossing, but it may be appropriate in some cases. For example, visiting a homebound patient, seeing a patient in a hospital after an overdose or other medical problems, or visiting a patient in jail after an arrest may be necessary and proper crossings (Gutheil and Gabbard 1993). Additionally, alternative settings may be appropriate and necessary for the success of some behavior therapy techniques.

Occasionally, charges of unethical conduct will include a challenge regarding the use of cars as the location for legitimate therapy sessions. Typically, the psychiatrist later reports that he or she, for whatever reasons, provided a ride home for the patient and continued the therapeutic discussion in the car. "From a fact finder's viewpoint, many exciting things happen in a car, but therapy is not usually one of them" (Gutheil and Gabbard 1993).

Fees. Money and fees are an essential part of the boundaries of psychiatric treatment in that financial arrangements underscore and define the business nature of the professional relationship. It is arguable that monetary reward is the only acceptable form of gratification from clinical work (Gutheil and Gabbard 1993).

Fees are usually one of the most sensitive aspects of the treatment contract, so their negotiation can be filled with numerous pitfalls. The real, transference, and countertransference aspects of money can have profound implications for the success or failure of the treatment (Langs 1973). It is, therefore, extremely important that the treatment contract adequately address this issue at the outset and that the procedures for submitting insurance claims and the patient's financial responsibility for the treatment be clearly understood.

Although it may be common practice to negotiate fees that are reasonable and acceptable to individual patients, decisions regarding exceptional variations in fees should be made with considerable caution.

Extreme deviations from usual fees and payment schedules have tremendous potential for altering both the patient's and the psychiatrist's expectations for the therapy.

It is the patient's responsibility to pay the psychiatrist, and it is the psychiatrist's duty to see that the patient honors that commitment. When the psychiatrist fails to confront the issue of unpaid fees, competent care cannot be delivered and the patient may be exploited as his or her needs are obscured by the therapist's conflicts over money.

The question of bartering inevitably arises in discussions about the financial arrangements for psychiatric treatment. Because of the potential for impairing the treatment relationship, this practice is strongly discouraged (American Psychiatric Association 1992). However, exceptions to this opinion must be considered when, as reported in some rural areas, patients can only afford treatment through the exchange of goods (or sometimes services) for psychiatric services. The key issues involved include the establishment of a fair market price for goods and careful attention to the potential for exploitation of the patient.

Fiduciary Responsibility and Nonsexual Exploitation

As a matter of law, the physician-patient relationship has been defined as fiducial (Simon 1992). An understanding of the fiduciary nature of this professional relationship is essential for a full appreciation of the potential for exploitation that exists when treatment boundaries are compromised. Commonly used in reference to legal arrangements, the term *fiduciary relationship* refers to "a special relationship in which one person accepts the trust and confidence of another to act in the latter's best interest" (Feldman-Summers 1989, p. 193).

Inherent in any relationship of trust is the risk of abuse of the power afforded by that trust. Psychiatrists who minimize the impact of their power in therapy relationships are at increased risk for creating or allowing boundary violations (Peterson 1992). It is, therefore, incumbent on physicians to fully appreciate the significance and extent of the power entrusted to them in order to avoid abusing it. When the psychiatrist fails to honor that trust, the potential for harm to both the patient and the profession is great.

The same human needs that enhance the psychiatrist's capacity for empathic response to the patient also leave the physician vulnerable in the treatment setting to the stimulation of those needs by the patient and to the patient's transference projections onto the therapist. Not infrequently, patient exploitation is unintentional and is the result of the psychiatrist's failure to think about the issues involved (American Psychiatric Association 1990). The stage may then be set for an infinite variety of situations in which there is a potential for placing the patient's needs secondary to those of the physician, thereby violating patient trust that the psychiatrist's actions are for the benefit of the patient.

Categories of Nonsexual Exploitation

Epstein and Simon (1990) developed the most comprehensive categorization to date of examples of nonsexual exploitation. Their categories include eroticism, friendliness, enabling, greediness, overinvolvement with patients, excessive self-disclosure, power seeking, and gratification of the therapist's needs. Two additional types of potential exploitation are the use of language (Gutheil and Gabbard 1993) and patient referral (American Psychiatric Association 1990). Awareness and discussion of these categories and the protean manifestations of potential boundary violations should be useful for all physicians, especially psychiatrists.

Eroticism. Eroticism is a type of exploitation referring to private thoughts and fantasies about patients by physicians. Unbidden feelings and thoughts will arise naturally and inevitably during the course of any human interaction. Their sustained and unexamined presence in the doctor-patient relationship, however, is unethical because even covert gratification of the physician's needs poses a threat to the fiduciary relationship. Competent treatment relies heavily on the psychiatrist's objectivity, and that objectivity can be severely impaired in the face of ongoing fantasies and longings regarding a patient.

Friendliness. Boundary crossings under the guise of friendliness may become ethical violations if the physician's actions misrepresent the professional nature of the relationship and the patient subsequently suffers. For example, the use of first names between the psychiatrist and patient (although not always harmful and sometimes very appropriate), as well as the physician's revelation of personal information to the patient, may imply a pseudointimacy that can be used by both parties to avoid dealing with the patient's reasons for being in treatment (Epstein and Simon 1990).

> A 45-year-old woman who had experienced severe childhood physical and sexual abuse by her family sought treatment for her symptoms of chronic depression. She requested that the psychiatrist call her by her first name, and although quiet and withdrawn during many of her early sessions, she gradually began to reveal her history of extensive abuse. A pattern developed in which the patient's sessions would begin with a period of "chitchat." As the initially brief periods of pleasantries grew longer, the patient acknowledged that she enjoyed the social moments but was avoiding important issues. The psychiatrist, in turn, recognized that she was also avoiding the difficult work of dealing with

the patient's painful history by initially allowing the periods of chitchat to go unexamined.

Prohibition against all physical contact beyond occasional handshakes is a controversial issue. Some treatments and procedures may call for clinically correct touching, and occasional hugs or handshakes might arguably represent therapeutic human responses. However, physicians must be extremely wary of gratuitously touching patients (Simon 1992). Such actions appear to be especially common forerunners of sexual boundary violations and, even when not intended as such, may be misinterpreted by the patient.

Enabling.   Enabling is a failure to set limits for the patient in order to avoid the patient's anger or self-destructiveness. It allows the patient to avoid confrontation of destructive behavior patterns and often creates a situation in which the psychiatrist may ultimately feel helpless and intimidated. A "mutual exploitation society" may result (Epstein and Simon 1990). Gabbard observed that therapists who fall within this category often succumb to the sexual demands of patients in an effort to avoid confrontation of their own angry feelings (Gabbard, in press).

Greediness.   Greediness is a form of exploitation in which the psychiatrist derives financial gain, other than that agreed on by the contractual fee arrangement, from the patient. Examples include the referral of patients for procedures that may benefit the treating psychiatrist either directly or indirectly but that may not be in the patient's best interests, and the use by the psychiatrist of financial investment tips offered by the patient (Epstein and Simon 1990). The latter activity may also be illegal, as illustrated by the following:

> A patient who was employed as an executive of a publicly owned company discussed confidential information about a promising new product being developed by his company. The treating psychiatrist bought shares in the company based on this "insider" information and was subsequently convicted for violation of Security and Exchange Commission regulations. (American Psychiatric Association 1990)

Overinvolvement with patients.   Exploitation by overinvolvement with patients suggests a blurring of the separate roles of the physician and patient. Examples may include pride in the accomplishments of current patients and posttermination friendships with patients (Epstein and Simon 1990). The risk of "living through a patient," and hence exploiting the patient's trust that therapy will focus only on treatment goals, is increased in these situations, as illustrated in the following vignette:

A psychiatrist who was a frustrated athlete treated a college freshman who had considerable athletic ability. The young man, however, was ambivalent over whether he would devote his energies to sports or to his growing love of literature. Guided by his own interests, the psychiatrist subtly influenced the direction of the patient's treatment sessions toward an increasing focus on sports events at the university. The patient subsequently sought and won a place on the university basketball team. (American Psychiatric Association 1990)

Self-disclosure. Self-disclosure by psychiatrists to patients is a complicated issue. Although potentially useful for some patients as a supportive measure, disclosures by the physician may unnecessarily burden the patient, and even minimal self-disclosure may indicate the need for careful self-scrutiny by the physician regarding his or her motivation for doing so (Gutheil and Gabbard 1993). Certainly, sexual fantasies or dreams and details of the psychiatrist's personal life should not be shared (Simon 1992).

Power seeking. Power seeking by physicians in relationships refers to the gratification of one's own sense of power through control of the patient's activities (Epstein and Simon 1990). The goals of any psychiatric treatment should include maximum enhancement of the patient's capacity for autonomy and self-determination. When the psychiatrist uses the patient's ongoing dependence on him or her as reassurance of the psychiatrist's own sense of superiority, the patient is exploited (Bruch 1974). Gratification of one's own sense of power through control of the patient's activities is a breach of the patient's trust in the therapeutic relationship and is unethical.

Gratification of the therapist's needs. In either social or professional settings, reference to or discussion of a patient's notoriety or accomplishments exploits the patient if that information is used to enhance the psychiatrist's sense of competence and prestige (American Psychiatric Association 1990; Epstein and Simon 1990). Additionally, it may also violate the patient's confidentiality.

Use of language. The use of language in psychotherapy has potential for exploiting patients. Although the use of first names versus last names in professional relationships has already been discussed, the word tone and word choice must also be considered. Intimate, seductive tones, as well as angry and confrontational ones, are likely to have serious ramifications for a patient and may disrupt the therapeutic process (Gutheil and Gabbard 1993). Similarly, verbal abuse under the guise of constructive and therapeutic confrontation exploits the patient and is disrespectful (Gutheil and Gabbard 1993; Simon 1992).

Patient referrals. Ethical and appropriate patient referrals may be affected by a number of factors, including personal friendships, family relationships, social aspirations, and the physician's wish to extend or receive favors (Wood and Wood 1990). Regardless of what secondary issues may be present, the needs of the patient are the only ethically justifiable considerations when referring patients for services.

> On completion of her training as a psychologist, the wife of a psychiatrist opened her office in her husband's office suite. The psychiatrist had previously used psychological testing only very sparingly with his patients. Wishing, however, to bolster his wife's self-confidence and income, he began to routinely order psychological testing on all of his patients. A group of his peers subsequently challenged him, saying that he had a conflict of interest. (American Psychiatric Association 1990)

The above categories and examples of exploitation represent a number of potential nonsexual boundary transgressions, but the list is by no means exhaustive. The common denominator in each example is that the patient's needs have not been given priority over those of the physician. Consequently, fiduciary trust has been violated and a patient has been exploited.

Honesty and Respect for Human Dignity

Respect through honesty. Honesty and respect for human dignity are implied in any relationship of trust—perhaps especially in the doctor-patient relationship. Lying to or deceiving patients denies them due respect and implies that they are incapable of understanding, accepting, and controlling their situations. In short, it is an affront to patients' dignity (Bakhurst 1992). Why, then, do physicians have a history of lying to patients (Modell 1988)? "Benevolent deception" has long been an integral part of medical practice. Indeed, the physician's duty to truthfulness is not mentioned in the Hippocratic oath, and it was only in 1980 that reference to "dealing honestly with patients and colleagues" was included in the American Medical Association's Principles of Medical Ethics (American Medical Association 1979, 1980; Jackson 1991).

A questionnaire by Novak et al. (1989), designed to assess physicians' attitudes toward the use of deception to resolve ethical problems in medical practice, was sent to 407 physicians. Of the 52% who responded, most indicated some willingness to engage in some form of deception regarding their patients. Their decisions were justified in terms of possible consequences for the patient, and higher value was placed on patient welfare and confidentiality than on truth telling for its own sake. Obviously, competing values can and do create conflicts for physicians attempting to decide what information to relate to patients, families, and third parties.

Regardless of value conflicts, however, a fundamental duty of physicians is to promote health and to respect the autonomy of their patients. Professional knowledge and expertise give physicians an advantage in the doctor-patient relationship, but that advantage is accompanied by a responsibility to use their knowledge on behalf of patients. Deception designed to benefit the physician at the expense of the patient exploits the imbalance of power in the relationship and is unethical. Exploitative deception can include explicit lying, deception by implication, and deception by omission of information needed by patients to make decisions that are in their own best interests (American College of Obstetrics and Gynecology 1990). For example, when a physician refers a patient to an outside facility in which he or she has a financial interest, the patient deserves to be informed that such ownership exists and may affect the objectivity of the referral. Otherwise, the physician risks damage to the fiduciary relationship with the patient either by acting from self-interest or by appearing to do so (Relman 1992).

Honesty and financial considerations.   As it is in all medical practices, the question of honesty as a boundary or ground rule in psychiatric treatment frequently arises around money and insurance matters. Dishonesty in billing matters is a serious boundary violation that is guaranteed to have negative consequences for the patient's treatment (Simon 1992). Care should be taken to bill patients only for the amount contractually agreed on for the type of service rendered.

Questions frequently arise in regard to submission of insurance claims for patients. Irregularities in dealings with third-party payers may be only one aspect of concurrent boundary violations in treatment (Simon 1992). Any suggestion of dishonesty in interactions with third parties is likely to introduce an element of distrust into the professional relationship and may disrupt the treatment. For example, failure of the psychiatrist to clarify with insurance companies the psychiatrist's billing procedures regarding missed appointments may create the appearance of collusion with the patient against the insurance carrier (Simon 1992).

"Gaming the system" or "fudging" on the severity of the patient's symptoms or illness to secure reimbursement or services for a patient is also a hazardous practice. Though sometimes tempting, gaming is dishonest and can harm patients and society as well as violate basic medical principles of contractual and distributive justice (Morreim 1991). The psychiatrist maintains the integrity of the doctor-patient relationship by dealing honestly with third-party payers and actively advocating for needed services and fair reimbursement for patients.

Many psychiatrists occasionally waive copayments and deductibles for patients who cannot afford to pay their portions of their bills. Some may advertise the fact that they do this routinely. In 1988 the Aetna Insurance Company called this practice fraud, reasoning that the insurance company is then paying 100% of the fee rather than its lower contractual percentage (Barton 1990). Under certain circumstances, the practice may indeed be fraudulent. Consider the following: The psychiatrist indicates to the insurance company that the patient has made payment that in fact has not been made; the psychiatrist misrepresents the facts, causing the insurance company to make payment that would not otherwise have been made; or the psychiatrist presents an inflated bill to the insurance company to reclaim lost patient revenue. In each of these cases, the psychiatrist has dealt dishonestly with the third party.

Confidentiality

Confidentiality is a fundamental and long-standing principle of medical ethics and represents an essential boundary or ground rule in psychotherapy. No less than 11 annotations of the *The Principles of Medical Ethics With Annotations Especially Applicable to Psychiatry* refer to issues of confidentiality (Webb 1986). This topic is covered in depth elsewhere in this volume, but it is important to note that progressive boundary violations in psychotherapy frequently include charges of breaches of confidentiality. Indeed, reviews of American Psychiatric Association ethics cases indicate that breach of confidentiality is a distressingly common phenomenon. Practitioners who become involved in romantic relationships with patients are especially likely to discuss with the sexually exploited patient information about multiple other patients in treatment.

CONCLUSION

Psychiatrists in all types of clinical practice face daily decisions regarding appropriate treatment boundaries. This decision making is one of the constantly challenging aspects of clinical work, and as such, it deserves our serious consideration. Otherwise, we may fail to establish and maintain appropriate boundaries, and individual patients may suffer. When one patient is harmed, the integrity of the psychiatric profession is undermined, and other potential patients may then fail to seek needed treatment.

Differences of opinion may exist regarding specific boundary decisions in various clinical settings. In addition, practitioners within the same setting must be prepared to determine when crossing established boundaries may be beneficial for individual patients. Management of appropriate psychiatric boundaries requires adequate training in psychodynamics, psychopathology, professional identity and roles, and issues related to gender and power differentials (Bishop 1992). Training in medical and psychiatric ethics will enhance the practitioner's understanding of all of the above issues and will facilitate difficult clinical decision making. The ethical principles of professional competency, contractual arrangements for services, fiduciary responsibilities of the psychiatrist, respect, honesty, and confidentiality form the fundamental foundation on which all boundary decisions can be wisely and safely based.

The vast majority of psychiatrists do not sexually exploit patients, but the nature of psychiatric treatment leaves all clinicians vulnerable at times to nonsexual boundary violations. It is, therefore, incumbent on all of us to understand the function of boundaries in the doctor-patient relationship and to learn to establish and maintain appropriate ones with patients. An appreciation for the potential for progressive nonsexual boundary transgressions and an awareness of the need to deal constructively with minor violations in treatment relationships are also necessary. Treatment boundaries are essential for the integrity of the doctor-patient relationship and deserve our ongoing consideration.

REFERENCES

American College of Obstetricians and Gynecologists: Committee on Ethics Opinion. Washington, DC, American College of Obstetricians and Gynecologists, 1990

American Medical Association: Opinions and Reports of the Judicial Council. Chicago, IL, American Medical Association, 1979

American Medical Association: Opinions and Reports of the Judicial Council. Chicago, IL, American Medical Association, 1980

American Psychiatric Association: Non-sexual exploitation of patients. Ethics Committee Newsletter, Vol 6, No 2, 1990

American Psychiatric Association: Opinions of the Ethics Committee on the Principles of Medical Ethics With Annotations Especially Applicable to Psychiatry. Washington, DC, American Psychiatric Association, 1992

American Psychiatric Association: The Principles of Medical Ethics With Annotations Especially Applicable to Psychiatry. Washington, DC, American Psychiatric Association, 1993

Bakhurst D: On lying and deceiving. J Med Ethics 18:63–66, 1992

Barton HM III: Waivers of insurance deductibles—charity or crime? Tex Med 86:64–65, 1990

Bishop J: Guidelines for a nonsexist (gender-sensitive) doctor-patient relationship. Can J Psychiatry 37:62–65, 1992

Bruch H: Learning Psychotherapy. Cambridge, MA, Harvard University Press, 1974

Epstein RS, Simon RI: The Exploitation Index: an early warning indicator of boundary violations in psychotherapy. Bull Menninger Clin 54:450–465, 1990

Epstein RS, Simon RI, Kay GG: Assessing boundary violations in psychotherapy: survey results with the Exploitation Index. Bull Menninger Clin 56:150–166, 1992

Feldman-Summers S: Sexual Contact in Fiduciary Relationships. Edited by Gabbard GO. Washington, DC, American Psychiatric Press, 1989, pp 193–209

Gabbard GO: Psychotherapists who transgress sexual boundaries with patients. Bull Menninger Clin (in press)

Gutheil TG, Gabbard GO: The concept of boundaries in clinical practice: theoretical and risk-management dimensions. Am J Psychiatry 150:188–196, 1993

Jackson J: Telling the truth. J Med Ethics 17:5–9, 1991

Langs R: The Technique of Psychoanalytic Psychotherapy, Vol I. New York, Jason Aronson, 1973

Modell EM: Telling patients the truth: a matter of respect. The Pharos, Spring 1988, pp 13–16

Mogul KM: Grey areas, slippery slopes and boundary violations. Paper presented at the annual meeting of the American Psychiatric Association, Washington, DC, May 1992

Morreim EH: Gaming the system. Arch Intern Med 151:443–447, 1991

Novak DH, Detering BJ, Arnold R, et al: Physicians' attitudes toward using deception to resolve difficult ethical problems. JAMA 261:2980–2985, 1989

Pellegrino ED: Altruism, self interest, and medical ethics. JAMA 258:1939–1940, 1987

Peterson MR: At Personal Risk. New York, WW Norton, 1992

Relman AS: "Self-referral"—what's at stake? New Engl J Med 327:1522–1524, 1992

Simon RI: Sexual exploitation of patients: how it begins before it happens. Psychiatric Annals 19:104–112, 1989

Simon RI: Treatment boundary violations: clinical, ethical, and legal considerations. Bull Am Acad Psychiatry Law 20:269–288, 1992

Webb WL: The doctor-patient covenant and the threat of exploitation. Am J Psychiatry 143:1149–1150, 1986

Wood EC, Wood CD: Referral issues in psychotherapy and psychoanalysis. Am J Psychother 44:85–93, 1990

Chapter 18

Sexual Misconduct

Glen O. Gabbard, M.D.

There is a broad consensus within the field of psychiatry that sexual contact of any kind between psychiatrist and patient is unacceptable under any circumstances. *The Principles of Medical Ethics With Annotations Especially Applicable to Psychiatry* (American Psychiatric Association 1993) is unequivocal in this regard:

> The requirement that the physician conduct himself/herself with propriety in his/her profession and in all the actions of his/her life is especially important in the case of the psychiatrist because the patient tends to model his/her behavior after that of his/her psychiatrist by identification. Further, the necessary intensity of the treatment relationship may tend to activate sexual and other needs and fantasies on the part of both patient and psychiatrist, while weakening the objectivity necessary for control. Additionally, the inherent inequality in the doctor-patient relationship may lead to exploitation of the patient. Sexual activity with a current or former patient is unethical. (Section 2, Annotation 1, p. 4)

Although psychiatry was the first of the medical specialties to adopt an ethics code that explicitly prohibited sex between doctor and patient, the prohibition has recently been expanded to all medical specialties. In 1991 the American Medical Association's Council on Ethical and Judicial Affairs reviewed the ethical implications of sexual or romantic relationships between physicians and patients. The council concluded that "sexual contact or a romantic relationship concurrent with physician-patient relationship is unethical" (Council on Ethical and Judicial Affairs 1991, p. 2741). Our colleagues in the other major mental health professions, such as psychology and social work, have established similar standards of conduct.

Despite these clear prohibitions, sexual misconduct continues to be one of the leading causes of malpractice litigation in the mental health professions. In addition, 113 members of the American Psychiatric Association were suspended or expelled from the organization during the last decade, most because of charges involving sexual transgressions

I would like to express my appreciation to Linda Jorgenson, Kenneth Pope, and Gary Schoener for their helpful comments on this manuscript.

(Lazarus 1992). This figure undoubtedly represents only the tip of the iceberg, because many cases of sexual misconduct go unreported (Schoener et al. 1989).

PREVALENCE

The exact prevalence of sexual contact between psychiatrist and patient is unknown. Because many patients refuse to report the therapist who sexually exploited them, and because many therapists will not report sexual activity with a patient even in anonymous surveys, our knowledge of the actual extent of this type of behavior is tentative at best. Most of the relevant data on prevalence comes from the eight national self-report surveys of mental health professionals using questionnaire methodology that have been published in the professional literature (see Table 18–1).

Although Table 18–1 presents data from the various studies on sexual relations with patients, comparing the percentages should be done with considerable caution. First of all, in many cases the studies involved different mental health disciplines. Several studies (Akamatsu 1988; Holroyd and Brodsky 1977; Pope et al. 1979, 1986, 1987) involved psychologists only. Gartrell et al. (1986) surveyed psychiatrists only, whereas the subjects of the Gechtman (1989) study were exclusively social workers. The study reported by Borys and Pope (1989) was unique in that all three major mental health professions—psychiatry, psychology, and social work—were included. A particularly significant finding in this latter study was that the three professions "did not differ among themselves in terms of . . . sexual intimacies with clients before or after termination" (Borys and Pope 1989, p. 283).

Some of these studies did not provide sufficiently detailed data for this table; in such cases, the investigators supplied the data necessary for consistency across studies. For example, the senior author of the Holroyd and Brodsky (1977) article confirmed through personal communication that the study's findings were that 12.1% of the male and 2.6% of the female participants reported having engaged in erotic contact (whether or not it included intercourse) with at least one opposite-sex patient (Pope 1993). The senior author also confirmed that 4% of the male and 1% of the female participants reported engaging in erotic contact with at least one same-sex patient. Also, in response to a separate survey item, 7.2% of the male and 0.6% of the female psychologists reported that they had "intercourse with a patient within 3 months after terminating therapy" (Holroyd and Brodsky 1977, p. 846).

The studies generally were not uniform in presenting data on posttermination sexual involvement. It is possible that some clinicians included sex with former patients when responding to questions about

Table 18–1. National self-report studies of sex between mental health professionals and patients

Reference	Sample size	Polled groups	Return rate (%)	% Reporting sex with patients	
				Male therapists	Female therapists
Holroyd and Brodsky 1977	1,000	Psychologists	70	12.1	2.6
Pope et al. 1979	1,000	Psychologists	48	12.0	3.0
Pope et al. 1986	1,000	Psychologists	58.5	9.4	2.5
Gartrell et al. 1986	5,574	Psychiatrists	26	7.1	3.1
Pope et al. 1987	1,000	Psychologists	46	3.6	0.4
Akamatsu 1988	1,000	Psychologists	39.5	3.5	2.3
Gechtman 1989	1,000	Social workers	54	1.4	0.0
Borys and Pope 1989	4,800	Psychologists, psychiatrists, and social workers	49	0.9	0.2

"sex with patients." The figures in Table 18–1 from the Gechtman (1989) survey represent percentages of "sexual intercourse . . . during the course of therapy" (p. 30). However, the study also found that an additional 0.6% of the male and none of the female social workers reported sexual contact after termination. In the survey of psychiatrists (Gartrell et al. 1986), responses indicated that "the sexual contact occurred *only* after termination . . . in 63% of the cases" (p. 1128). The 1987 survey by Pope et al. included a question about sexual involvement with former patients; 14% of the male and 8% of the female respondents acknowledged sexual involvement with a former patient. The 1988 Akamatsu survey also asked about involvement with former patients and found that 14.2% of male and 4.7% of female psychologists reported such involvement. Finally, the percentages of male and female therapists engaging in sexual activity with a former patient were not published in the 1989 Borys and Pope article, but one of the authors provided the following data: posttermination sexual activity was reported by 6.5% of male and 2.7% of female psychiatrists, 10.5% of male and 2.0% of female psychologists, and 1.3% of male and 0% of female social workers (K. S. Pope, personal communication, August 1993).

As noted previously, questionnaire surveys are fraught with methodological problems. Some clinicians who have had sex with patients will lie about their activities in such surveys, and others will simply fail to return the questionnaire. The apparent decline in prevalence figures between the late 1970s and the late 1980s is probably more apparent than real. Sanctions from licensing boards and ethics committees became increasingly common and more severe during the 1980s, and a number of states criminalized therapist-patient sex. The stiffening of the sanctions may have deterred the same therapists who acknowledged sexual contact on the surveys done in the 1970s from answering the questions honestly when they were surveyed 10 years later. Others may have reverted to the rationalization that the contact occurred only after termination, which might explain the fact that the percentages of posttermination sex observed in the late 1980s are fairly similar to those observed in the late 1970s. In any case, all the American studies have focused on practitioner reports rather than on consumer surveys, so the limitations of that source must be taken into account.

All the data point to a greater prevalence among male therapists than among female therapists. By far the most common gender configuration is a male therapist sexually involved with a female patient. In the study that focused exclusively on psychiatrists (Gartrell et al. 1986), 88% of the respondents who identified both the psychiatrist's and the patient's gender indicated that the sexual involvement was between a male psychiatrist and a female patient, 3.5% specified a female psychiatrist and a male patient, and 1.4% indicated a same-sex dyad of females. Although the majority, 66.7%, had been involved with only one patient, all psychiatrists who admitted contact with more than one patient were male.

Although the vast majority of the literature has focused on heterosexual involvement between therapists and patients, more recent contributions (Benowitz 1991; Gonsiorek 1989; Lyn 1990) have recognized that same-sex dyads are by no means uncommon and that such involvements result in similar sequelae. In a review of 93 ethics committee sexual complaints against psychiatrists, Mogul (1992) found that 8 were filed against women clinicians; 6 of the 8 were for homosexual behavior.

The fact that male patients make relatively few complaints to ethics committees and licensing boards may reflect sex-role stereotypes in the culture. Because men are generally regarded as the seducers and women the seduced, male patients are less likely to feel victimized by sexual involvement with female therapists (Gabbard, in press; Gutheil and Gabbard 1992; Mogul 1992). Indeed, in one study of sexual transgressions, when female therapists were involved with male patients, the male patients were often viewed as responsible and blameworthy for their behavior, whereas the female therapists were viewed as their victims (Averill et al. 1989). Some male patients actually feel triumphant over their "conquest" of the therapist and therefore do not report the sexual involvement to any agency and do not enter into litigation.

PROFILE OF VULNERABLE PATIENTS

Any consideration of the profile of vulnerable patients must begin with one caveat—a patient can never be *blamed* for sexual transgression by a therapist. It is always the therapist's responsibility to act ethically, even when the patient is overtly seductive or demands sexual contact with the therapist. Nevertheless, it behooves the clinician to be aware that certain patients tend to erotize relationships as the result of being victims of childhood sexual abuse. As Kluft (1989) observed, patients in psychotherapy who are incest victims often put themselves in situations in which they are repeatedly revictimized and therefore are "sitting ducks" for sexual exploitation by therapists.

Patients with borderline personality disorder are another group that may be at high risk for exploitation (Gabbard 1993; Gabbard and Wilkinson 1994; Gutheil 1989; Simon 1992). Many of these patients experience a specific form of entitlement that results in their demanding exceptions to the usual professional boundaries. They may insist on self-disclosure by the therapist, physical contact in the form of hugs, and other forms of undue familiarity with the therapist. If their demands are not met, many will escalate by threatening suicide. Indeed, many therapists who have been charged with sexual misconduct insist that the patient would have committed suicide if they had not deviated from their usual practice (Eyman and Gabbard 1991). The high incidence of childhood sexual abuse in the backgrounds of borderline patients also may contribute to the erotization of the therapeutic relationship in the same way it operates with incest victims who do not have borderline personality disorder (Gabbard and Wilkinson 1994). Pope and Bouhoutsos (1986) identified several common characteristics of patients who are at high risk for sexual exploitation by therapists: a history of prior psychiatric hospitalizations, alcohol or drug addiction, a history of suicide attempts, and diagnoses of major psychiatric disorders.

There is some degree of controversy over the validity of these profiles. G. R. Schoener (personal communication, July 1993) has been unable to identify any high-risk characteristics in a sample of 2,000 cases he has studied at the Walk-In Counseling Center in Minneapolis, Minnesota. My own impression in studying numerous cases of sexual misconduct is that the relevance of patient characteristics varies in a manner that is directly related to therapist characteristics. For example, predatory male psychotherapists may attempt to seduce any attractive female patient regardless of her psychological profile. On the other hand, the essentially ethical therapist who is under great stress in his or her personal life may be more susceptible to excessive demands for intimacy by patients who are incest victims or who have borderline psychopathology.

PROFILE AND PSYCHODYNAMICS OF THERAPISTS

As previously noted, patients can never be regarded as responsible or blameworthy for sexual involvement with the therapist. Even with extraordinarily seductive patients, the majority of clinicians appear to act ethically and professionally in preserving the professional boundaries of the relationship. Hence, any attempt to understand the phenomenon of sexual misconduct requires a detailed examination of the characteristics of therapists who have become involved in sexual transgressions. A fair-minded and scientific assessment of these therapists has been hindered in recent years by the increasing politicization of the problem of sexual misconduct. In some segments of the mental health professions there is an insistence on a "politically correct" view of the phenomenon that ascribes all sexual misconduct to evil and thoroughly corrupt male therapists (Gabbard, in press; Gutheil and Gabbard 1992). This perspective may have a particular appeal to other practitioners of psychotherapy, who can reassure themselves that those colleagues who transgress sexual boundaries have characteristics that set them apart from all other therapists. The problem can thus be solved by eliminating these "bad apples" from the various professions.

This politically correct model depends on the projective disavowal of the universal vulnerability to sexual transgressions that is inherent in anyone who practices in the mental health professions. The most sensible approach is to assume that we are all at risk for boundary violations under certain circumstances and to monitor our own countertransference carefully for early warning signals. Rutter (1989), who shares this view, courageously described his own vulnerability with one particular patient. All systematic studies of psychotherapists who have been involved in sexual boundary violations indicate that sexual misconduct occurs among a diverse group of clinicians who become involved with patients for a variety of reasons. Any attempt to lump all the transgressing therapists into one politically correct category is reductionistic and misguided. There have been numerous attempts to identify various groups of therapists and their associated descriptive and psychodynamic features (Apfel and Simon 1985; Averill et al. 1989; Gabbard 1991, in press; Olarte 1991; Pope and Bouhoutsos 1986; Schoener and Gonsiorek 1989; Simon 1992; A. A. Stone 1984; Twemlow and Gabbard 1989).

Schoener and Gonsiorek (1989) based their classification on extensive evaluations of accused therapists, from which they developed six clusters that are useful in assessing the therapist's potential for treatment and rehabilitation: 1) uninformed and naive, 2) healthy or mildly neurotic, 3) severely neurotic and socially isolated, 4) impulsive character disorder, 5) sociopathic or narcissistic character disorder, and 6) psychotic or borderline personality. The first two groups may respond well to education, treatment, and supervision, whereas the last four groups have a much more guarded prognosis, with therapists who have impulsive, sociopathic, and narcissistic character disorders having the worst potential for rehabilitation.

Pope and Bouhoutsos (1986) presented their classification in terms of 10 common scenarios: 1) role trading, in which therapists begin self-disclosing and take on the "patient" role; 2) sex therapy, in which the therapist fraudulently depicts sexual relations as a valid treatment for the patient's sexual problems; 3) as if . . ., in which therapists respond to positive transference as though it is not the result of the therapeutic situation; 4) Svengali, in which therapists deliberately create and exploit extreme dependency in the patient; 5) drugs, in which therapists encourage the use of alcohol and both legal and illegal drugs in the service of seduction; 6) rape, in which therapists apply physical force, intimidation, or threats; 7) true love, in which therapists rationalize their sexual transgression as the outgrowth of true love and dismiss the professional nature of the relationship; 8) it just got out of hand, in which therapists do not effectively deal with the emotional closeness that therapy fosters; 9) time out, in which therapists do not acknowledge that the therapeutic relationship persists outside the boundaries of the scheduled session or the therapist's office; and 10) hold me, in which therapists exploit the patient's desire to be touched or held in a nonerotic physical way.

From his work in forensic psychiatry, Simon (1992) identified five groups at risk for sexually exploiting patients: 1) therapists with a character disorder, including borderline, narcissistic, and antisocial subtypes; 2) therapists with a sexual disorder, which includes those who have paraphilias such as pedophilia and frotteurism; 3) incompetent therapists who are simply poorly trained; 4) impaired therapists who may be alcoholic, drug addicted, or mentally ill; and 5) situational reactors who may be experiencing marital discord, the loss of an important relationship, or a professional crisis. The first two groups are likely to be repeat offenders, whereas the last three are not.

Averill et al. (1989) reviewed personnel files and medical records that shed light on staff-patient sexual relationships in an institutional setting. They delineated two typical profiles. The first group consisted of young staff members in the psychiatric hospital who simply continued an exploitative pattern that had been typical of relationships outside the hospital. The second group involved middle-aged and isolated individuals with personal difficulties that made them extremely needy. Female staff members often experienced intense rescue fantasies about male patients, whereas male staff members often experienced disillusionment about and resentment toward the institution in which they worked.

A comparison of these different classifications suggests considerable convergence and overlap among the different conceptualizations. These different points of view can be subsumed under four psychodynamically based categories linked more to underlying psychological characteristics than to specific diagnostic categories (Gabbard 1991, in press).

Psychotic Disorders

This first category is by far the rarest. Profound loss of reality testing is the unifying theme in this group of therapists. Relevant delusional ideas may range from the notion that the therapist's semen will confer eternal salvation on the patient to the belief that through sexual bonding the therapist's personality can exorcise demons that have inhabited the patient (Gabbard 1991, in press).

Predatory Psychopathy and Paraphilias

This category is not limited to DSM-IV antisocial personality disorders (American Psychiatric Association 1994). It also includes severe narcissistic personality disorders with prominent antisocial features. This grouping addresses the behavior and the accompanying psychological characteristics rather than a specific diagnosis. Paraphilias are included in this rubric with the full awareness that all therapists who suffer from paraphilias are not psychopathic predators or antisocial personalities. However, those therapists who involve their *patients* in their paraphiliac activities have severely compromised superego structures accompanied by character pathology on the narcissistic to antisocial continuum. Therapists in this category are often involved with numerous patients and may be masters at manipulating the legal system so that they escape severe legal or ethical consequences for their behavior.

These therapists generally have experienced profound impairment of internalization during childhood development so that there is massive failure of superego development. They lack the fundamental capacity to experience empathy for their victims, so they rarely feel remorse or guilt about any harm they might have done to the patient. The primary mode of object relatedness is sadistic bonding with others through the exercise of power and destructiveness (Meloy 1988). Many also have childhood histories of profound neglect or abuse and are attempting to achieve active mastery of passively experienced trauma by exploiting others (Schwartz 1992).

Lovesickness

In the 1986 survey of psychiatrists (Gartrell et al. 1986), 65% of those who had been in a sexual relationship with a patient described themselves as in love with the patient. These therapists may be associated with a broad range of diagnostic categories. Some suffer less severe forms of narcissistic personality disorder and are desperately needy for validation and idealization from their patients as a way of regulating their own self-esteem. Some have problems in the neurotic range, whereas still others are essentially psychiatrically healthy but are in the midst of a devastating personal or professional crisis. Indeed, the most common scenario is that of a middle-aged male therapist who falls in love with a much younger female patient while he's experiencing divorce, separation, disillusionment with his own marriage, or the loss of a significant person in his life (Brodsky 1989; Gabbard 1991, in press; Twemlow and Gabbard 1989).

Psychodynamic themes are many and varied in this category (Gabbard 1991, in press). Often there is an unconscious reenactment of incestuous experiences from the patient's past. In such cases there is a collusion with the patient's wish to reenact a sexual relationship with a forbidden object from the past instead of interpreting the unconscious wish and helping the patient understand it. Other psychodynamic themes include the confusion of the therapist's needs with the patient's needs, the perception of the patient as an idealized version of the self, the misperception of the wish for maternal nurturance as a wish for genital sexual relations, and a manic defense against mourning and grief at the time of termination. Indeed, the ending of a psychotherapy relationship is a high-risk time, because neither the patient nor the therapist wishes to deal with the loss of the relationship. One method of defending against feelings of loss is to begin a new relationship of a personal nature at the time the professional relationship is ending.

Sadism and hatred often lie just beneath the surface of lovesickness. In many instances, these aggressive feelings are fueled by the therapist's perception that the patient is deliberately thwarting the process. Some therapists resort to sexual relations out of despair at the patient's frustration of the omnipotent strivings to heal (Searles 1979). In the midst of a stalemate or impasse, the therapist may unconsciously attempt to bypass negative feelings through an erotic relationship designed to sustain an idealizing transference (Celenza 1991). Self-hatred and a history of sadomasochistic interpersonal relationships are also common (Strean 1993) in these therapists. In addition, therapists who violate sexual boundaries may be acting out anger at the institution at which they work as a way of embarrassing persons in the institution who are targets of revenge.

The majority of the female therapists who transgress sexual boundaries fall into the lovesick category. When the patient is male, they often are acting on rescue fantasies toward a young man with characterological symptoms including impulsivity, substance abuse, and action orientation (Gabbard 1991, in press). The female therapist may harbor an unconscious fantasy that her love and attention will somehow "straighten up" this young man, who simply needs the right woman to settle him down. When the patient is female, some female therapists transgress sexual boundaries as a way of dealing with conflicts around their own sexual orientation. In a study of 15 female therapist–female patient liaisons (Benowitz 1991), only 40% of the therapists involved clearly identified themselves as lesbian in their sexual orientation. In a detailed psychodynamic study of four therapists (of both genders), Strean (1993) observed that bisexuality and sexual-identity difficulties were marked characteristics in all four.

Masochistic Surrender

Therapists in this category are profoundly self-destructive and allow themselves to be intimidated and badgered by a patient into a situation of escalating boundary violations until they find themselves tormented day and night by the patient. They typically cannot deal with their own aggression, so that they are unable to set limits on the patient's demands. They use reaction formation to defend against the growing resentment and hatred of the patient. In other words, they repeatedly gratify demands for boundary transgressions—such as concrete demonstrations of love, desires to be held, discontinuation of the fee, extended hours, and phone calls at all times of the night—as a way of denying their anger. As the therapist gratifies the patient's demands, he or she becomes tormented by the seemingly bottomless nature of the patient's neediness. Such therapists often overidentify with the patient because of their own histories of abuse and feel "dragged down" by the patient. These therapists may also masochistically turn themselves in to licensing boards or ethics committees after one sexual transgression because they are overwhelmed with guilt and wish to receive help and supervision.

SANCTIONS AGAINST ACCUSED THERAPISTS

For the patient who has been victimized by a sexually exploitative therapist, several different courses of action are available, all of which result in sanctions against the therapist (Jorgenson and Schoener, in press; Perr 1989; Schoener et al. 1989; Simon 1992). Most of these available actions and the sanctions resulting from them involve malpractice litigation, civil and criminal statutes, professional licensing boards and disciplinary procedures, and ethics committee complaint procedures.

Malpractice Litigation

To pursue a malpractice suit successfully and receive monetary damages, the patient must establish (in most states) that the therapist was negligent and that negligence caused harm to the patient. Malpractice claims are subject to the statute of limitations, but in some states there is a trend to view the time period as one that begins when patients discover that they have been harmed by the therapist's sexual misconduct (Jorgenson and Appelbaum 1991; Jorgenson and Randles 1991). Another recent development in this area is the decision of most malpractice insurance companies to exclude or limit coverage for sexual misconduct claims. In such cases, attorneys may focus on other acts of negligence committed by the therapist that involve nonsexual boundary violations (Jorgenson and Sutherland 1993).

Civil and Criminal Statutes

As this volume goes to press, five states have civil statutes that eliminate the need for patients to establish that sexual contact with their therapists constituted malpractice (Jorgenson and Schoener, in press).

Malpractice is automatically assumed once the charge of sexual contact is confirmed. In addition, a total of 12 states have criminalized therapist-patient sex, and several other states are currently considering such laws. Although the criminal statutes vary from state to state, in all jurisdictions but one the consent of the victim is removed as a defense. Six states have also included prohibitions against sexual contact after termination (Jorgenson and Schoener, in press). Criminal sanctions are highly controversial within the mental health professions (Strasburger et al. 1991). Some argue that criminalization will make it less likely that patients will want to report their therapists, whereas others contend that ethics committees and licensing boards have not done an adequate job in policing the mental health professions so the task must be taken out of their hands. Advocates of criminalization also stress that it is the only way to close the loophole on unlicensed therapists.

Licensure Boards

Boards of healing arts and licensing boards are usually state government agencies that regulate practitioners such as physicians, psychologists, and social workers. A board of peers reviews allegations reported to the licensing board. Sanctions involve reprimands, suspension or revocation of licensure, supervision of the therapist's practice, limitations on the therapist's practice, or required psychotherapy (Jorgenson and Schoener, in press). An attorney is not required for the complainant, and all legal work is done by a prosecutor. No statute of limitations applies in most jurisdictions, and no monetary compensation is provided as a result of hearings. The majority of complaints are generally settled without a hearing or a trial.

Ethics Committees

If the practitioner is a member of a state or national professional organization, such as the American Psychiatric Association or the American Psychological Association, a patient may report the therapist's behavior to the ethics committee of the professional organization. Although many local ethics committees are highly effective in dealing with complaints, the majority lack the legal expertise that is generally available to licensing boards (Jorgenson and Schoener, in press). They also have rather limited sanctions, such as suspension or expulsion from membership in the organization or informal reprimand. In addition, the American Psychiatric Association Ethics Committee can require that the therapist be supervised. It also might request that therapists accept limitations on their practice or enter psychotherapy. The American Psychiatric Association recently decided to send press releases to media in the therapist's immediate geographic area to inform the public of expulsions from the organization.

Although these four sanctions are by far the most commonly used, the patient who has been victimized by a sexually exploitative therapist may also consider other actions. If the transgression occurred while the therapist was under the employment of a clinic or institution, the patient may wish to report the therapist to the institutional employer. Also, in some cities a mediation process is available, whereby the patient meets with the transgressing therapist in the presence of an expert consultant to process what happened (Schoener et al. 1989).

POSTTERMINATION RELATIONSHIP

Although there is uniform agreement that sexual relations between a therapist and a current patient are unethical, there is less consensus on the issue of posttermination sexual relations. Both the American Psychological Association and the American Association for Marriage and Family Therapy have enacted a prohibition on sexual contact with former patients for a 2-year period only. The American Psychiatric Association, on the other hand, recently adopted a new annotation to the ethics code that declares sexual contact with *any* former patient to be unethical, no matter when the termination occurred.

Advocates of a time limit on the posttermination prohibition (Appelbaum and Jorgenson 1991) argue that constitutional rights of privacy and freedom of association are infringed on by a permanent ban. They also argue that stronger evidence of harm from posttermination sexual contact is needed to justify such extreme actions. Those clinicians who argue in favor of an absolute prohibition (Gabbard 1992; Gabbard and Pope 1989) argue that transference is instantly reestablished even years after termination if therapist and patient meet again, and therapists would be wise to assume that they will have continuing professional responsibilities for their patients because many patients recontact their therapists in times of crisis years after termination (Hartlaub et al. 1986). The other compelling reason to impose a permanent ban is that any future possibility of a sexual relationship would profoundly contaminate the psychotherapy relationship. Patients might conceal shameful or embarrassing material to make themselves more sexually desirable, and therapists might foster idealization and avoid unpleasant confrontation to preserve the possibility of a future sexual relationship.

Although there are scant data on marriages between therapists and former patients (Lazarus 1992), anecdotes involving both disastrous and blissful outcomes abound. Marriage, however, is just as irrelevant to ethical considerations as whether or not the therapist and patient are "in love." For many years, marriage conferred sanction on a number of crimes, including rape and assault, until society became enlightened to the fact that the marriage vows do not provide license to break the law. In regard to the argument involving the constitutional right of freedom to associate with whomever one likes, many professional organizations have ethics codes that reflect higher standards of conduct than those prescribed by the Constitution; for example, therapists agree to abide by the principles of confidentiality, despite their constitutional rights to freedom of speech. As far as evidence of harm from posttermination sexual contact is concerned, the burden of proof lies on those who advocate such relationships to demonstrate that *no harm* results from such behavior. Although the controversy continues in the literature, the majority of practitioners clearly favor an absolute prohibition on posttermination sexual relationships. In three different surveys (Borys and Pope 1989; College of Physicians and Surgeons of British Columbia 1992; Herman et al. 1987), nearly two-thirds of the clinicians surveyed do not think sex with a former patient is acceptable under any circumstances.

TREATMENT OF SEXUALLY EXPLOITED PATIENTS

Well-informed estimates suggest that over one-half of all therapists will treat patients who have been sexually involved with prior treaters (Pope and Bouhoutsos 1986). Hence, therapists must be educated about the destructive effects of therapist-patient sexual relations and the common difficulties encountered in the subsequent treatment of such patients. Numerous case studies and a variety of research efforts have documented the harm inflicted on patients by therapists who transgress sexual boundaries (Benowitz 1991; Bouhoutsos et al. 1983; Burgess 1981; Butler 1975; Chesler 1972a, 1972b; D'Addario 1977; Feldman-Summers and Jones 1984; Gabbard 1989; Noel and Watterson 1992; Pope and Bouhoutsos 1986; L. G. Stone 1980; Walker and Young 1986; Williams 1992). Pope (1989) observed a distinct clinical syndrome, which he termed *therapist-patient sex syndrome,* that has much in common with posttraumatic stress disorder. The patient experiences ambivalence, guilt, emptiness and isolation, sexual confusion, impaired ability to trust, suppressed rage, cognitive dysfunction, increased suicidal risk, identity and role reversal, and emotional lability or dyscontrol. Many patients who have been sexually exploited by therapists have made serious suicide attempts or successfully killed themselves, and one of the first orders of business for the subsequent therapist is to assess the patient's suicide risk. Although some observers (Williams 1992) have raised questions about the specific link between the sexual exploitation and harm, Pope et al. (1993b) have persuasively dealt with those questions. Others (Gutheil and Gabbard 1993; Schoener et al. 1989) have stressed that boundary violations that are *not* sexual may be equally damaging.

All patients do not manifest the characteristics of the therapist-patient sex syndrome, however, and the subsequent therapist must approach the patient with an open mind, recognizing that many patients will continue to experience intense feelings of attachment to the exploitative therapist. If the patient professes continued love for the therapist and minimizes any destructive effects of the relationship, some therapists may react by colluding with the denial and minimization of the harm or by imposing attitudes or feelings on the patient to make the patient fit the expected reaction (Sonne and Pope 1991). The therapist must not assume a priori knowledge of what the patient is feeling. Feelings must be allowed to unfold in a spontaneous fashion that allows the patient freedom of expression.

In addition to the assessment of suicide risk, several other issues require attention early in the psychotherapy. First, the therapist must provide a "safe place" for the patient. The boundaries of the relationship should be clear and unambiguous. The patient should understand that there will be no physical contact of any kind in the therapy and that the relationship is a professional one that does not involve meetings outside the office or mutual self-disclosure. It is often useful to allow such patients the freedom to sit anywhere they wish in the therapist's office so that the optimal distance between therapist and patient is established by the patient, not by the therapist.

The therapist must also respect these patients' difficulty in trusting a subsequent therapist (Pope and Gabbard 1989). Some patients respond well to an honest, empathic acknowledgment from the therapist that there is no reason that the patient should trust a stranger, particularly in light of the fact that a previous therapist has not been trustworthy. Subsequent treating therapists should also ask the patient for clarification regarding the current status of the relationship with the previous therapist, because many of these relationships are "on again, off again" situations that can lead the patient to ride an emotional roller coaster.

A third issue is to inform the patient early on about the limits of confidentiality if he or she should mention the name of the psychotherapist. It is incumbent on therapists to know the reporting laws in their state. In Minnesota, for example, therapists are required to report sexually exploitative therapists unless they have gained the knowledge while seeing the offending therapist in the role of a patient. In Texas, the therapist must report a colleague who has had sex with a patient both to the local district attorney and to the licensing board. In states that do not require reporting, the therapist may risk a lawsuit for defamation of character or breach of confidentiality if the patient is not willing to come forth and acknowledge the transgression to a licensing board or ethics committee. The decision to report or not to report in states where there are no requirements is a complex ethical and legal dilemma. The wisest course is to consult with a knowledgeable attorney or colleague, or both, before making a final decision.

Even experienced psychotherapists struggle with intense countertransference feelings when treating the victim of a sexually exploitative therapist. The intense anger evoked by the act of a colleague may lead them to become zealous about the patient's need to file a complaint. One cannot be both a therapist and an attorney for the patient, and a basic principle in these situations is to remember that only the patient can ultimately decide whether to report the therapist. The patient needs information, such as the possibility that his or complaint. According to one chapter of the California Business and Professions Code, the psychotherapist must provide the patient with a brochure that delineates the rights of patients who have been sexually involved with their psychotherapist and the courses of action available. In other states, the therapist may wish to inform the patient of sources of information or to refer the patient to a colleague to discuss his or her options. Many patients have compared the complaint process to a rape trial and thought that they would have been better off keeping quiet, so the therapist must help the patient weigh the pros and cons of any course of action.

Another problematic countertransference reaction is the wish to be the perfect psychotherapist to make up for the damage that the previous therapist did (Pope and Gabbard 1989; Sonne 1989). This type of countertransference may lead the therapist to make special concessions and exceptions to the usual boundaries of psychotherapy in an effort to prove to the patient that the therapist "really cares" (Schoener et al. 1989). Before long, the therapy will become just as boundary free as the previous treatment was because of the therapist's failure to set limits and deal with the aggression in both members of the dyad. Erotic countertransference is also frequently encountered because the patient may erotize the relationship in the same way that the previous relationship was sexualized. Finally, the therapist may become so consumed with the damage done by the exploitative colleague that the original problems the patient sought treatment for are ignored. These problems must all be assessed, along with the destructive effects of the sexual transgression.

Schoener et al. (1989) cited two factors as most important to patients who have been sexually exploited by their therapists in terms of the patients' own perception of the recovery process. The first is taking some sort of action, whether filing a complaint, informing the therapist's employer, or confronting the professional personally. The second is talking with other patients who have been sexually exploited by their therapists. Indeed, group psychotherapy and support groups have been shown to have highly beneficial effects on exploited patients (Luepker 1989; Sonne 1989). Support groups have sprung up in many major cities, where patients can work through their grief and anger in the context of a group of peers who understand their difficulties.

ASSESSMENT AND REHABILITATION OF ACCUSED THERAPISTS

Before a particular therapist's potential for rehabilitation and treatment is assessed, an investigation of the allegations is usually undertaken by an ethics committee, a licensure board, or at times a hospital clinical risk management committee. Punishment or discipline is determined by those agencies, and the evaluation of the therapist for a rehabilitation plan must be clearly separated from the disciplinary measures. If the allegations are substantiated and the accused professional continues to deny sexual misconduct, there is little point in proceeding with a rehabilitation assessment (Schoener et al. 1989). Any plan developed for someone who steadfastly maintains innocence will be a charade.

The overriding principle in assessing accused therapists is that an individualized treatment and rehabilitation plan must be determined on the basis of a thorough psychiatric evaluation (Gabbard, in press; Schoener et al. 1989). One should be wary of "cookie cutter" or "assembly line" approaches that treat all offending therapists with the same program. The causes of the sexual misconduct must be identified, and a determination needs to be made regarding whether rehabilitation is worth the effort. In cases of predatory psychopathy, paraphilias, or severe character pathology, rehabilitation plans are not likely to be successful, and the therapist should be advised to consider a career change.

In those cases where return to practice seems possible, the findings of the assessment should be reviewed both by the accused professional and by the licensure board or other agency that requested the assessment (Schoener et al. 1989). If all parties agree to the findings of the assessment, a rehabilitation plan that may have any combination of the following elements should be implemented (Gabbard, in press; Pope 1989; Schoener et al. 1989):

Pharmacotherapy. By the time many practitioners are assessed, they may be seriously depressed and require antidepressant medication. For the small group that are psychotic, lithium carbonate or antipsychotic medication may be needed. In addition, some lovesick therapists may be fending off depression through a desperate sexual relationship with a patient. This subgroup also may need antidepressants. In most cases, however, pharmacotherapy should be regarded primarily as an adjunct to other interventions.

Assignment of a rehabilitation coordinator.   This individual should be thoroughly informed of all the details of the sexual misconduct and every aspect of the rehabilitation plan. He or she will meet regularly with the accused therapist and make reports to the licensure board. The rehabilitation coordinator should *not* be the psychotherapist, and all roles must be clearly differentiated in any plan.

Personal psychotherapy.   The assessment of whether psychotherapy would be useful requires a careful evaluation of the accused therapist's motivation. Psychotherapy is not surgery—it requires active collaboration by the patient and cannot be imposed when motivation is lacking. Otherwise, the psychotherapist will be in a "police officer" role that makes treatment impossible. Psychotherapy requires confidentiality, so the psychotherapist should not be the person reporting to the agency monitoring the accused therapist (Pope 1989; Strean 1993). If the therapist is perceived as an agent of the licensing board or an enforcer of the law, treatment will be unsuccessful. The therapist's main investment must be in providing understanding for the patient (Strean 1993). Also, in any rehabilitation plan, someone other than the accused therapist should select the person who will be the designated psychotherapist. This person should have no other personal or professional connection with the offending therapist. If accused therapists are free to select whomever they wish, they may select colleagues who are personal friends or who are known to have lenient attitudes about boundary transgressions.

Psychotherapists of transgressing colleagues will have to struggle with formidable countertransference feelings. Feelings of moral superiority and contempt for the accused professional are common and stem from a wish to disidentify with a colleague who has acted on feelings that the rest of us fight within ourselves. Psychotherapists of such patients will also find themselves repeatedly tested regarding the boundaries of the professional relationship. Scrupulous monitoring of the frame of the psychotherapy is essential. Psychodynamic issues in such treatments have been outlined by Gabbard (in press) and by Strean (1993).

Practice limitations.   A variety of limitations on the accused therapist's practice are possible. These may include no treatment of women, restriction of practice to a hospital setting with close supervision, and limitations of time spent with a patient. In many cases it is advisable to have the accused therapist avoid all psychotherapy and shift professional activities to pharmacotherapy (if a psychiatrist), administration, or other alternative practice modes.

Supervision.   In almost every rehabilitation plan, supervision should be built into any continued work in which the therapist is involved. The supervisor, like the rehabilitation coordinator, should make regular reports to the responsible agency.

Further education and training.   Some therapists have had very little training in issues of erotic transference-countertransference, professional boundaries, and prevention of sexual misconduct. Attendance at didactic workshops on these subjects may be useful.

Reassessment of the rehabilitation plan's effectiveness should be undertaken at the point when the clinician seeks to reenter unsupervised practice.

PREVENTION

Any discussion of prevention must begin with the realistic and sober prediction that because of the nature of the therapist-patient relationship, it is unlikely that sexual misconduct can ever be completely eliminated. However, a number of approaches have been found useful; these can generally be subdivided into institutional and individual strategies.

Institutional Strategies

Hospitals and clinics must regard the practice of hiring as one of the most important preventive measures. Schoener et al. (1989) constructed a comprehensive checklist of administrative safeguards that include hiring practices, staff policies, avenues of complaints, staff education, staff supervision, and peer review. Every applicant for a position should have a careful history screening that includes personal contact with previous employers. The institution should also have clearly stated policies that prohibit all sexual contact between staff and patients. Regular educational meetings on sexual boundaries, erotic transference and countertransference, and sexual misconduct should be offered for all new employees, including the whole range from mental health technicians to psychiatrists. The leaders of hospital units should create a cultural norm regarding the sharing of countertransference feelings. Intense feelings about patients should be regarded as useful information about the treatment to be shared in staff meetings and meetings with supervisors. Distinctions should be made between having feelings and acting on them.

Many states now have risk management laws that stipulate the method of investigation within institutions. If not, there should be fair policies established involving investigation of complaints so that a swift decision is reached, taking both the patient's and the staff member's interests and concerns into account. In hospitals and clinics, there should be ongoing peer review and supervision built into the workweek so that no practitioner becomes isolated. Finally, patient education is useful. Many clinics have written guidelines describing psychotherapy that could be distributed to new patients along with information on patients' rights and similar materials.

Individual Strategies

For practitioners who see patients in a private office, prevention is more problematic because it depends on the therapist's own initiative. Education is of paramount importance. Courses in the handling of erotic transference and countertransference and the maintenance of professional boundaries should be offered in medical school, graduate school, and residency training, as well as in continuing education courses attended throughout the clinician's career (Gabbard 1994; Pope et al. 1993a). A key component of this education is to identify minor boundary violations that are precursors to sexual exploitation (Epstein and Simon 1990; Gutheil and Gabbard 1993; Strasburger et al. 1992). Clinicians should be knowledgeable about the "slippery slope" phenomenon of minor transgressions leading to major transgressions. Early signs of problematic countertransference include extending the hour well beyond its usual allotted time, self-disclosure of the therapist's problems, hugging the patient at the end of sessions, discontinuing the fee, meeting the patient outside the office, and switching to the use of the patient's first name (Gutheil and Gabbard 1993).

Although personal analysis or psychotherapy is certainly not a guarantee of future ethical behavior, most clinicians find that therapeutic examination of their psychological conflicts is of enormous value in understanding countertransference reactions with difficult patients. Also, an underutilized means of prevention is regular consultation with a respected colleague. Any case in which therapists find themselves dealing with intense sexual feelings (either their own or the patient's) should warrant regular consultations with a trusted colleague who will not judge but rather help the therapist understand and master the feelings aroused in therapy.

Peer supervision groups have sprung up around the country as a way for solo practitioners to deal with the professional isolation of psychotherapy practice. These groups meet once weekly or once monthly to discuss difficult cases and the countertransference problems they encounter. Finally, although it should be obvious that attention to one's own intimate personal relationships is an essential part of any preventive approach, many therapists neglect their marriages and partnerships to an alarming extent. In many cases, psychotherapists pay more attention to their patients than they do to their spouses. Strean (1993) noted that none of the transgressing therapists he treated had warm, close, and spontaneous relationships. All practitioners of intensive psychotherapy should be sure that their personal relationships are gratifying their emotional needs so that these needs do not require gratification by patients.

REFERENCES

Akamatsu TJ: Intimate relationships with former clients: national survey of attitudes and behavior among practitioners. Professional Psychology: Research and Practice 19:454–458, 1988

American Psychiatric Association: The Principles of Medical Ethics With Annotations Especially Applicable to Psychiatry. Washington, DC, American Psychiatric Association, 1993

American Psychiatric Association: Diagnostic and Statistical Manual of Mental Disorders, 4th Edition. Washington, DC, American Psychiatric Association, 1994

Apfel RI, Simon B: Patient-therapist sexual contact, I: psychodynamic perspectives on the causes and results. Psychother Psychosom 43:57–62, 1985

Appelbaum PS, Jorgenson L: Psychotherapist-patient sexual contact after termination of treatment: an analysis and a proposal. Am J Psychiatry 148:1466–1473, 1991

Averill SA, Beale D, Benfer B, et al: Preventing staff-patient sexual relationships. Bull Menninger Clin 53:384–393, 1989

Benowitz MS: Sexual exploitation of female clients by female psychotherapists: interviews with clients and a comparison to women exploited by male psychotherapists (unpublished doctoral dissertation). Minneapolis, University of Minnesota, 1991

Borys DS, Pope KS: Dual relationships between therapist and client: a national study of psychologists, psychiatrists, and social workers. Professional Psychology: Research and Practice 20:283–293, 1989

Bouhoutsos J, Holroyd J, Lerman H, et al: Sexual intimacy between psychotherapists and patients. Professional Psychology: Research and Practice 14:185–196, 1983

Brodsky AM: Sex between patient and therapist: psychology's data and response, in Sexual Exploitation in Professional Relationships. Edited by Gabbard GO. Washington, DC, American Psychiatric Press, 1989, pp 15–25

Burgess AW: Physician sexual misconduct in patients' responses. Am J Psychiatry 138:1335–1342, 1981

Butler S: Sexual contact between therapists and patients (unpublished doctoral dissertation). Los Angeles, California School of Professional Psychology, 1975

Celenza A: The misuse of countertransference love in sexual intimacies between therapists and patients. Psychoanalytic Psychology 8:501–509, 1991

Chesler P: The sensuous psychiatrists. New Yorker Magazine, June 19, 1972a, pp 52–61

Chesler P: Women and Madness. New York, Avon Books, 1972b

College of Physicians and Surgeons of British Columbia: Crossing the Boundaries: The Report of the Committee on Physician Sexual Misconduct. Vancouver, College of Physicians and Surgeons of British Columbia, 1992

Council on Ethical and Judicial Affairs, American Medical Association: Sexual misconduct in the practice of medicine. JAMA 266:2741–2745, 1991

D'Addario L: Sexual relations between female clients and male therapists (unpublished doctoral dissertation). Los Angeles, California School of Professional Psychology, 1977

Epstein RS, Simon RI: The exploitation index: an early warning indicator of boundary violations in psychotherapy. Bull Menninger Clin 54:450–465, 1990

Eyman JR, Gabbard GO: Will therapist-patient sex prevent suicide? Psychiatric Annals 21:669–674, 1991

Feldman-Summers S, Jones G: Psychological impacts of sexual contact between therapists or other health care practitioners and their clients. J Consult Clin Psychol 52:1054–1061, 1984

Gabbard GO (ed): Sexual Exploitation in Professional Relationships. Washington, DC, American Psychiatric Press, 1989

Gabbard GO: Psychodynamics of sexual boundary violations. Psychiatric Annals 21:651–655, 1991

Gabbard GO: Once a patient, always a patient: therapist-patient sex after termination. The American Psychoanalyst 26:6–7, 1992

Gabbard GO: An overview of countertransference with borderline patients. Journal of Psychotherapy Practice and Research 2:7–18, 1993

Gabbard GO: Psychotherapists who transgress sexual boundaries with patients. Bull Menninger Clin (in press)

Gabbard GO: Psychodynamic Psychiatry in Clinical Practice: The DSM-IV Edition. Washington, DC, American Psychiatric Press, 1994

Gabbard GO, Pope KS: Sexual intimacies after termination: clinical, ethical, and legal aspects, in Sexual Exploitation in Professional Relationships. Edited by Gabbard GO. Washington, DC, American Psychiatric Press, 1989, pp 115–127

Gabbard GO, Wilkinson SM: Management of Countertransference With Borderline Patients. Washington, DC, American Psychiatric Press, 1994

Gartrell N, Herman J, Olarte S, et al: Psychiatrist-patient sexual contact: results of a national survey, I: prevalence. Am J Psychiatry 143:1126–1131, 1986

Gechtman L: Sexual contact between social workers and their clients, in Sexual Exploitation in Professional Relationships. Edited by Gabbard GO. Washington, DC, American Psychiatric Press, 1989, pp 27–38

Gonsiorek JC: Sexual exploitation by psychotherapists: some observations on male victims and sexual orientation issues, in Psychotherapists' Sexual Involvement With Clients: Intervention and Prevention. By Schoener GR, Milgrom JH, Gonsiorek JC, et al. Minneapolis, MN, Walk-In Counseling Center, 1989, pp 113–119

Gutheil TG: Borderline personality disorder, boundary violations, and patient-therapist sex: medicolegal pitfalls. Am J Psychiatry 146:597–602, 1989

Gutheil TG, Gabbard GO: Obstacles to the dynamic understanding of therapist-patient sexual relations. Am J Psychother 46:515–525, 1992

Gutheil TG, Gabbard GO: The concept of boundaries in clinical practice: theoretical and risk-management dimensions. Am J Psychiatry 150:188–196, 1993

Hartlaub GH, Martin GC, Rhine MW: Recontact with the analyst following termination: a survey of 71 cases. J Am Psychoanal Assoc 34:895–910, 1986

Herman JL, Gartrell N, Olarte S, et al: Psychiatrist-patient sexual contact: results of a national survey, II: psychiatrists' attitudes. Am J Psychiatry 144:164–169, 1987

Holroyd JC, Brodsky AM: Psychologists' attitudes and practices regarding erotic and nonerotic physical contact with patients. Am Psychol 32:843–849, 1977

Jorgenson LM, Appelbaum PS: For whom the statute tolls: extending the time during which patients can sue. Hosp Community Psychiatry 42:683–684, 1991

Jorgenson LM, Randles RM: Time out: the statute of limitations and fiduciary theory in psychotherapist sexual misconduct cases. Oklahoma Law Review 44:181–225, 1991

Jorgenson LM, Schoener GR: Sexual exploitation in psychotherapy and counseling: regulation in the USA, in Patients and Victims: Sexual Abuse in Psychotherapy and Counseling. Edited by Jehu D. London, Wiley (in press)

Jorgenson LM, Sutherland PK: Psychotherapist liability: what's sex got to do with it? Trial, May 1993, pp 22–25

Kluft RP: Treating the patient who has been sexually exploited by a previous therapist. Psychiatr Clin North Am 12:483–500, 1989

Lazarus JA: Sex with former patients almost always unethical. Am J Psychiatry 149:855–857, 1992

Luepker ET: Time-limited treatment/support groups for clients who have been sexually exploited by therapists: a nine-year perspective, in Psychotherapists' Sexual Involvement With Clients: Intervention and Prevention. By Schoener GR, Milgrom JH, Gonsiorek JC, et al. Minneapolis, MN, Walk-In Counseling Center, 1989, pp 181–194

Lyn L: Life in the fishbowl: lesbian and gay therapists' social interactions with clients (master's thesis). Carbondale, Southern Illinois University, 1990

Meloy JR: The Psychopathic Mind: Origins, Dynamics, and Treatment. Northvale, NJ, Jason Aronson, 1988

Mogul KM: Ethics complaints against women psychiatrists. Am J Psychiatry 149:651–653, 1992

Noel B, Watterson K: You Must Be Dreaming. New York, Poseidon, 1992

Olarte SW: Characteristics of therapists who become involved in sexual boundary violations. Psychiatric Annals 21:657–660, 1991

Perr IN: Medicolegal aspects of professional sexual exploitation, in Sexual Exploitation in Professional Relationships. Edited by Gabbard GO. Washington, DC, American Psychiatric Press, 1989, pp 211–227

Pope KS: Rehabilitation of therapists who have been sexually intimate with a patient, in Sexual Exploitation in Professional Relationships. Edited by Gabbard GO. Washington, DC, American Psychiatric Press, 1989, pp 129–136

Pope KS: Licensing disciplinary actions for psychologists who have been sexually involved with a client: some information about offenders. Professional Psychology: Research and Practice 24:374–377, 1993

Pope KS, Bouhoutsos JC: Sexual Intimacy Between Therapists and Patients. New York, Praeger, 1986

Pope KS, Gabbard GO: Individual psychotherapy for victims of therapist-patient sexual intimacy, in Sexual Exploitation in Professional Relationships. Edited by Gabbard GO. Washington, DC, American Psychiatric Press, 1989, pp 89–100

Pope KS, Levenson H, Schover LR: Sexual intimacy in psychology training: results and implications of a national survey. Am Psychol 34:682–689, 1979

Pope KS, Ketih-Spiegel P, Tabachnick BG: Sexual attraction to clients: the human therapist and the (sometimes) inhuman training system. Am Psychol 41:147–158, 1986

Pope KS, Tabachnick BG, Keith-Spiegel P: Ethics of practice: the beliefs and behaviors of psychologists as therapists. Am Psychol 42:993–1006, 1987

Pope KS, Sonne JL, Holroyd J: Sexual Feelings in Psychotherapy: Explorations for Therapists and Therapists-in-Training. Washington, DC, American Psychological Association, 1993a

Pope KS, Butcher JN, Seelen J: The MMPI, MMPI-2, and MMPI-A in Court: A Practical Guide for Expert Witnesses and Attorneys. Washington, DC, American Psychological Association, 1993b

Rutter P: Sex in the Forbidden Zone: When Men in Power—Therapists, Doctors, Clergy, Teachers, and Others—Betray Women's Trust. Los Angeles, CA, Jeremy P Tarcher, 1989

Schoener GR, Gonsiorek JC: Assessment and development of rehabilitation plans for the therapist, in Psychotherapists' Sexual Involvement With Clients: Intervention and Prevention. By Schoener GR, Milgrom JH, Gonsiorek JC, et al. Minneapolis, MN, Walk-In Counseling Center, 1989, pp 401–420

Schoener GR, Milgrom JH, Gonsiorek JC, et al: Psychotherapists' Sexual Involvement With Clients: Intervention and Prevention. Minneapolis, MN, Walk-In Counseling Center, 1989

Schwartz MF: Sexual compulsivity as posttraumatic stress disorder: treatment perspectives. Psychiatric Annals 22:333–338, 1992

Searles HF: Countertransference and Related Subjects. Madison, CT, International Universities Press, 1979

Simon RI: Clinical Psychiatry and the Law, 2nd Edition. Washington, DC, American Psychiatric Press, 1992

Sonne JL: An example of group therapy for victims of therapist-client sexual intimacy, in Sexual Exploitation in Professional Relationships. Edited by Gabbard GO. Washington, DC, American Psychiatric Press, 1989, pp 101–113

Sonne JL, Pope KS: Treating victims of therapist-patient sexual involvement. Psychotherapy 28:174–187, 1991

Stone AA: Law, Psychiatry, and Morality: Essays and Analysis. Washington, DC, American Psychiatric Press, 1984

Stone LG: A study of the relationship among anxious attachment, ego functioning, and female patients' vulnerability to sexual involvement with their male psychotherapists (unpublished doctoral dissertation). Los Angeles, California School of Professional Psychology, 1980

Strasburger LH, Jorgenson L, Randles R: Criminalization of psychotherapist-patient sex. Am J Psychiatry 148:859–863, 1991

Strasburger LH, Jorgenson L, Sutherland P: The prevention of psychotherapist sexual misconduct: avoiding the slippery slope. Am J Psychother 46:544–555, 1992

Strean H: Treating Therapists Who Have Sex With Their Patients. New York, Brunner/Mazel, 1993

Twemlow SW, Gabbard GO: The lovesick therapist, in Sexual Exploitation in Professional Relationships. Edited by Gabbard GO. Washington, DC, American Psychiatric Press, 1989, pp 71–87

Walker E, Young PD: A Killing Cure. New York, Holt, Rinehart & Winston, 1986

Williams MH: Exploitation and inference: mapping the damage from therapist-patient sexual involvement. Am Psychol 47:412–421, 1992

Afterword to Section III

Jeremy A. Lazarus, M.D., Section Editor

This section, taken as a whole, provides a composite of ethical thinking and suggested behavior for the psychiatrist in the most crucial current areas of psychiatric ethics. It is not intended to be a rule book;
rather, it provides historical background and information on current
ethical thinking. Unlike scientific study, it also incorporates value systems that are not universal; indeed, there are many differences in other
countries or cultures. When looked at in the context of a therapeutic
relationship, this section provides guidelines on the ethical practice of
psychiatry and psychotherapy, as well as ethical guidelines for the forensic or research psychiatrist. Once this ethical framework is solidly
integrated into the everyday thinking of each practicing psychiatrist,
ethical dilemmas that arise will be less problematic. The interested
reader should consider several texts and bibliographies on psychiatric
ethics for additional reviews (Anzla and Puma 1991; Bloch and
Chodoff 1981; Dyer 1988).

To consider a more comprehensive overview of ethical decision
making and ethical theory would require additional chapters. However, the reader might consider the philosophical contributions of
Hippocrates and Maimonides, as well as those of the utilitarian and
deontological philosophers. The source of much of the framework of
our medical ethics is rooted in the work of these philosophers, and a
review would benefit the enthusiastic reader.

Much of what troubles psychiatrists in contemporary practice has
less to do with past frustrations about the scientific validity of our work
than with the intrusions into the traditional doctor-patient relationship. Those who entered psychiatry because of an intense interest in
human behavior and motivation often find that resources do not allow
sufficient exploration of the underlying causes from a psychological
point of view. Instead, treatment is under the scrutiny of third parties,
and our society has expectations for predictable outcomes in our treatments. Although this is an appropriate expectation, it places burdens
on the treatment relationship that can be frustrating. Hospitals and academic centers, in their search for funding, may find creative methods
of marketing and financing that can place the psychiatrist in compro-
mising situations. These methods have led to abuses in certain hospital
systems and academic centers. As psychiatrists and other physicians
work more in systems of care and less as autonomous practitioners,
these potential conflicts will continue to emerge. Medicine, when defined by some as a business, is expected to follow business ethics, a set

of guidelines that does not always parallel professional ethics.

Although Dr. Frick's chapter on boundary violations represents a very conservative viewpoint, it serves as a stepping-off place from which any psychiatrist can carefully consider the effects of altering the boundaries of the psychiatrist-patient relationship. What might be entirely appropriate in other settings can have detrimental effects on a patient. On the other hand, the psychiatrist's obligation to develop a therapeutic treatment alliance may necessitate nonexploitative boundary crossings.

In his chapter on sexual misconduct, Dr. Gabbard discusses the misbehavior of a small but noticeable percentage of psychiatrists. Its frequency of occurrence and the negative impact on the patient make this an issue warranting particular attention. Incidents of sexual misconduct also are dramatically received by the media, causing yet another level of potential public mistrust in psychiatry. The American Psychiatric Association (APA) has done more than any other professional organization not only in investigating complaints of sexual misconduct and sanctioning its members, but also in educating both its members and the public about this problem. Other medical organizations, mental health groups, and the clergy have used the extensive experience of the APA to develop educational programs and investigatory procedures. Dr. Gabbard accurately describes the APA's changes in ethical thinking—especially the change in the ethics annotation about sexual relationships with former patients. Not all psychiatrists subscribe to the position of the APA, but this area has received wide coverage (Lazarus 1992).

The themes of several recent presidents of the APA have reflected the deep concerns in our profession for ethics and values. Without a solid grounding in ethics, psychiatrists and other physicians risk losing the public's trust. Ironically, although we are now able to do more for our patients from a scientific point of view, we are viewed with less respect than in previous centuries. It is not enough, however, just to read these chapters. A critical examination of those ethical areas where conflict has been experienced in one's own work is crucial. Psychiatrists are no less prone to greed, conflict of interest, or sexual misbehavior than other professionals. Even the best treated or best analyzed psychiatrist, under the proper circumstances, can misbehave. For this reason, our continuing education in this area is of utmost importance.

Psychiatric training has begun to incorporate guidelines for practice and an expectation for cost-effective treatment. The more pronounced emphasis on the biological basis for human behavior and psychiatric illness has sometimes caused training in ethical physician behavior to have a lower priority. With malpractice claims in psychiatry skyrocketing, concerns about legal exposure have surpassed ethical discussions. As malpractice insurance rates climb and risk management assumes a more prominent role in treatment planning, the openness of therapeutic exploration in the psychiatrist-patient relationship comes under stress. What was presumed to be good ethical training for physicians falls short in actuality in terms of a comprehensive and consistent commitment to teaching or in enforcing ethical principles.

In the remainder of this decade, we will witness significant changes in health care delivery. These changes may enable psychiatry to achieve some parity with other medical specialties, but new systems of care will undoubtedly place the treatment of psychiatric patients under even greater scrutiny, with the goal of providing cost-effective and beneficial care. The ethical commitment of physicians should be to deliver the best quality care at the lowest cost. When coupled with demands of access for all, however, the equation is unsolvable without massive expenditure of societal funds. One goal of psychiatric treatment is for patients to develop a realistic assessment of their life. Likewise, when faced with a health care quagmire, psychiatrists must be able to reexamine their own ethical principles. Although it is crucial to stand firm on certain fundamentals of physician ethics, incorporation of the ethical principle of justice will be necessary. The uniqueness of and trust in the doctor-patient covenant need the firm support of all those interested in the physical and mental health of society. Although business ethics may need to play a role in the financing of health care, business ethics should not supersede medical ethics for physicians. This flexible approach, within ethical constraints, will serve the psychiatrist and patient best as we move into the next century.

REFERENCES

Anzla D, Puma J: An annotated bibliography of psychiatric medical ethics. Academic Psychiatry 15:1–17, 1991

Bloch S, Chodoff P (eds): Psychiatric Ethics. Oxford, England, Oxford University Press, 1981

Dyer AR: Ethics and Psychiatry: Toward a Professional Definition. Washington, DC, American Psychiatric Press, 1988

Lazarus JA: Sex with former patients almost always unethical (editorial). Am J Psychiatry 149:855–857, 1992

IV

Psychotherapy With Children and Adolescents

IV

Psychotherapy With Children and Adolescents

Section IV

Psychotherapy With Children and Adolescents

Foreword

Clarice J. Kestenbaum, M.D., and Owen Lewis, M.D.,
Section Editors

In the twentieth century, psychotherapy of children and adolescents closely followed its adult counterpart and evolved, for the most part, from psychoanalysis. Freud developed an entire theory of personality development and maladaptation from the reminiscences of adult patients, their free associations, and their dreams as they attempted to reconstruct their own childhoods. He did not treat children directly (the case of Little Hans was reported to Freud by the child's father, who served as parent-therapist under Freud's supervision). It was not until Anna Freud and Melanie Klein actually observed children and played with them, substituting doll play and fantasies for adult free associations and dreams, that psychotherapeutic work with children began to have a burgeoning place in the psychoanalytic literature.[1]

The basic principles of the psychoanalytic (psychodynamic) paradigm are the same for children and adults: 1) behavior is motivated and related to basic needs or drives; 2) the organism tends to avoid pain and seeks pleasure; 3) there exists an unconscious mind beyond conscious awareness; 4) conflicting motivations are the basis for neurotic action; 5) behavior has its origins in childhood experience and is continuous; and 6) symptoms have a defensive purpose.

Freud's view is rooted in biology and was deeply influenced by Darwin's discoveries. Freud's theory served as the base on which several deeply influential developmental paradigms were developed—namely, the psychosocial theory evolved by Erik Erikson and the ego psychology–object relations theory.

Psychoanalytic theory, however, was not the only developmental theory promulgated during the past 50 years. Behaviorism, or the stimulus-response paradigm, originated in the laboratory study of animal

---

[1] For an informative historical review of the treatment of mentally ill children, see Group for the Advancement of Psychiatry 1982.

learning at the turn of the century. John Watson popularized the doctrine of methodological behaviorism (classical conditioning), which was at the forefront of American psychology from the 1930s through the 1950s and which led to B. F. Skinner's profound influence. Under Skinner's leadership, the operant conditioning paradigm attempted to explain human behavioral change: a system of rewards is established for producing desired effects. Hull and Bandura further contributed to developmental theory within the stimulus-response paradigm with the introduction of learning theory and modeling behavior. Therapeutic interventions used by behavior therapists follow carefully planned treatment regimens.

A third developmental model that has exerted a fundamental influence in terms of cognitive development is Jean Piaget's genetic epistemology. Piaget attempted to answer the question "How is knowledge acquired?" He hypothesized that intellectual development begins with progressive modification of reflexive behavior, which then serves to promote progressively more adaptive techniques until a stage of abstract thinking is achieved by late adolescence. Cognitive-behavior therapy is a treatment designed to change distortions of thinking; it was described by Aaron Beck (1976) for treating depressed individuals and has been adapted for the treatment of depressed adolescents.

Finally, the ethological paradigm, which originated in Darwin's naturalistic studies of animal behavior and was expanded by John Bowlby, promulgated the hypothesis that human attachment functions much as attachment does in nonhuman primates. Independently, Sullivan (1953) developed an interpersonal approach to psychotherapy. Interpersonal therapy adapted for adolescents (Mufson et al. 1993), based on Bowlby's and Sullivan's work, focuses on the style and effectiveness of interpersonal relationships.[2]

With so many divergent developmental theories, it is no wonder that therapists find themselves in opposing camps. Students well grounded in a certain theoretical framework are often unfamiliar with the work being generated in other areas. To date, there is not one unifying developmental theory or set of ideas that explains developmental observations to the satisfaction of all the researchers in the various developmental arenas. Moreover, dozens of other therapeutic models have been developed from four basic paradigms, including family therapy, systems theory, and group therapy, to name but a few. Pharmacotherapy has added to the armamentarium of therapists from all disciplines.

Until recently, child and adolescent therapists did not have a body of research data from controlled studies with which to demonstrate the long-term benefits or lack of benefit from treatment. The choice of ther-

---

[2]For a review of the developmental paradigms, see Lewis 1991.

apeutic modality often reflected the therapist's particular training and bias and was not related to the patient's diagnosis or cognitive developmental level. The last two decades, however, have brought a change in research methodology examining the effect of therapeutic interventions in adults. The last decade has produced a growing body of data concerning the effectiveness of child and adolescent therapies—as well as a deepening knowledge base concerning the biological foundations of many psychiatric disorders.

R. Joffree Barrnett, M.D., and associates (1991) formulated the question concerning the effectiveness of psychotherapy well: "Which set of procedures is effective when applied to what kind of patient with what kind of problems as practiced by what sort of therapist?" (p. 2). Barrnett's introductory chapter to this section, Chapter 19, "Research Update," is a continuation of his 1992 article concerning this question and describes the current research findings with respect not only to particular treatments but also to the efficacy of combined treatment approaches.

This section attempts to deal with the psychotherapy of children and adolescents in the modern world. As O'Brien (1992) pointed out, "There are marked differences between adult and child and adolescent psychotherapy. Adult therapy generally consists of a two group, the therapist and the patient. This is not the case in child or adolescent work; parents are continuously involved" (p. xiii), as, we might add, are housekeepers, teachers, pediatricians, and all those involved in the life of a still-developing individual. The goal of therapy is to get the deviant child back on the normal developmental track.

In Chapter 20, "Neurosis and Conduct Disorders," Efrain Bleiberg, M.D., presents the heart and soul of psychodynamic psychotherapy. One of his basic premises is that "a psychodynamic perspective can provide the glue that holds together psychotherapeutic, pharmacological, cognitive-behavior, and family interventions in a coherent and integrated treatment plan and that such integration results in a significant enhancement of both clinical effectiveness and conceptual sophistication." His case vignettes demonstrate a combined treatment approach predicated on the notion that family interventions are an integral part of child psychotherapy.

In Chapter 21, "The Neuropsychiatric Disorders: ADHD, OCD, and Tourette's Syndrome," Robert A. King, M.D., and Donald J. Cohen, M.D., deal with childhood neuropsychiatric disorders. They also describe a complex multifaceted treatment intervention that includes medication, family and school involvement, and combined psychodynamic and behavior therapy.

Owen Lewis, M.D., and Irene Chatoor, M.D., in Chapter 22, "Eating Disorders," describe work with the mother-child dyad, the need for medical intervention including hospitalization, and again the combined management approaches in working with anorexic and bulimic patients. In these latter conditions, therapy has been organized along interpersonal lines.

In Chapter 23, "Psychotic and Prepsychotic Disorders," Clarice J. Kestenbaum, M.D., illustrates the multidisciplinary work with psychotic and prepsychotic children, particularly involving psychoeducational and milieu therapy. Clinical vignettes describe in detail the process of psychotherapy with severely disturbed children and adolescents.

Finally, in Chapter 24, "Victims of Child Abuse," Arthur H. Green, M.D., deals with the victims of dysfunctional parents, abused children, and the variety of treatment approaches necessary to engage deeply troubled families.

Throughout the section, illustrative vignettes describe specific types of one-on-one psychotherapeutic techniques. As we noted earlier, just as dreams are considered to be the royal road to the unconscious for the adult, so play and imagination (mental play) are considered to be the pathways toward understanding the repressed wishes and unconscious fantasies of the child.

> The healthy child plays out universal fantasies, giving full vent to his rich imagination; the neurotic child plays out personal fantasies in an attempt to resolve unconscious conflicts and master an earlier psychic trauma. What is often difficult for psychiatrists who deal with adults (whose "stock in trade" is verbal interpretation) to understand is how children can play out fantasies and work through areas of conflict without much more than a hint from the therapist. When a child pummels a father doll unmercifully or smashes a clay ball with a mallet the result is more than merely a release of tension. Fantasies are being enacted, games won, villains conquered in the safety of the familiar office with an understanding adult nearby. (Kestenbaum 1985, p. 483)

Inventive child therapists have found myriad different therapeutic approaches such as doll play, painting, woodwork, puppet play, squiggles (as described by Winnicott 1968, 1977), and storytelling (Kestenbaum 1985).

This section highlights the importance of careful diagnostic assessment so that the therapist can select the specific treatment modalities best suited to help the child and his or her family achieve the best possible therapeutic result.

REFERENCES

Barrnett RJ, Docherty JP, Frommect GM: A review of psychotherapy research since 1963. J Am Acad Child Adolesc Psychiatry 30:1–14, 1991

Beck AT: Cognitive Therapy and the Emotional Disorders. New York, International Universities Press, 1976

Group for the Advancement of Psychotherapy: The history of child treatment in Western culture, in The Process of Child Psychotherapy, Vol 3. New York, Brunner/Mazel, 1982, pp 9–45

Kestenbaum CJ: The creative process in child psychotherapy. Am J Psychother 39(4):479–489, 1985

Lewis M (ed): Child and Adolescent Psychiatry: A Comprehensive Textbook. Baltimore, MD, Williams & Wilkins, 1991, pp 87–144

Mufson L, Moreau A, Weissman MM, et al: Interpersonal Psychotherapy for Depressed Adolescents. New York, Guilford, 1993

O'Brien JD: Introduction, in Psychotherapies With Children and Adolescents: Adapting the Psychodynamic Process. Edited by O'Brien JD, Pilowsky DJ, Lewis OW. Washington, DC, American Psychiatric Press, 1992, pp ix–xxi

Winnicott DW: The squiggle game. Voices, Spring 1968, pp 140–151

Winnicott DW: The Squiggle: An Account of the Psychoanalytic Treatment of a Little Girl. New York, International Universities Press, 1977

Chapter 19

Research Update

R. Joffree Barrnett, M.D.

The field of psychotherapy research has generated a great deal of controversy since the 1950s. The effectiveness of psychotherapy was initially questioned (Eysenck 1952, 1960, 1966), which precipitated a vigorous response in rebuttal that stimulated a large body of research that continues to expand today (Garfield and Bergin 1986; Luborsky et al. 1988; Smith et al. 1980). Some studies examining child psychotherapy were part of the data that, when analyzed, produced the initial negative findings regarding the effectiveness of psychotherapy, but these studies were not addressed separately in detail. Specific examination of child psychotherapeutic literature followed shortly after Eysenck's initial report, and Levitt (1957, 1963) reached similar conclusions that psychotherapeutically treated children showed no increased improvement compared with those who had not received therapy. As before, this conclusion generated rebuttals and reevaluations that contended that clear conclusions about the effectiveness of treatment could not be made because of problems with the method of analysis, diagnostic criteria, and the quality of the research reviewed (Barrett et al. 1978; Heinicke and Goldman 1975; Heinicke and Strassman 1975; Hood-Williams 1960; Saxe et al. 1986).

As an outgrowth of the controversy regarding the effectiveness of psychotherapy, there has been an expansion of the varieties and forms of psychotherapeutic intervention (Kazdin 1988). Adult psychotherapy has progressed quite rapidly and gone well beyond the initial concerns regarding the effectiveness of psychotherapy per se. Important advances in psychotherapy research have been made by developing the application of the clinical trial model (American Psychiatric Association 1993; Williams and Spitzer 1984). Studies are now required to demonstrate an acceptable level of competence and skill for all therapists, equivalent skills among all therapists, consistency in applying the skills throughout the treatment trial, and fully described procedures that are similarly applied by all therapists.

By using the clinical trial research format, researchers in adult psychotherapy are able to examine 1) specific issues in relationship to the process of therapy and 2) outcomes of specific therapeutic treatments for particular problems. Examples include comparison studies of the effectiveness of different psychotherapies for depression (Elkin et al. 1989); physiological, behavioral, and cognitive interventions for panic disorder (Barlow 1988; Michelson 1984); the effectiveness of combined treatments (e.g., Conte et al. 1986; Hogarty et al. 1988); and the importance of therapeutic alliance for outcome (Frank and Gunderson 1990; Marziali 1984). The growth of research in adult psychotherapy has also allowed more traditional psychodynamic forms of therapy to delineate important psychological structures that occur in the process of research (e.g., Dahl 1988; Horowitz et al. 1989; Luborsky 1984).

In the area of child psychiatry, behavioral and cognitive psychotherapeutic treatments have advanced methodologically (Harris 1983; O'Leary and Carr 1982; Ollendick 1986; Ollendick and Cerney 1981). Individual child psychotherapy that does not employ behavioral or cognitive techniques per se has not enjoyed as much research examination.

A recent review addressing child and adolescent nonbehavioral or noncognitive individual psychotherapy examined reports between 1963 and 1989 (Barrnett et al. 1991). This study reviewed 43 clinical trials of psychotherapy, assessing each for basic methodological adequacy in four areas: 1) inclusion and exclusion criteria, 2) specification of therapy, 3) matching procedures in control groups, and 4) measurements and outcome evaluations. Table 19–1 presents the results. Using a box score method, the authors found methodological flaws in all of the studies. This included defects in basic research structures in the areas of inclusion or exclusion criteria, specification of therapy or therapists, matching or control groups, and standardized measurements or outcome assessments. The authors concluded that it would be premature to draw hard-nosed scientific conclusions from this body of research due to the number of methodological flaws among the research studies reviewed (Barrnett et al. 1991).

Table 19–1. Type and number of methodological flaws in psychotherapy studies

Type of flaw	No. of studies with flaws/ total no. of studies
Area of methodology	
Poor inclusion or exclusion criteria	40/43
Unspecified details about therapy and therapists	40/43
Poor matching or control groups	36/43
Poor measurements or outcome assessments	25/43
No. of areas with methodological flaws per study	
4	22/43
3	9/43
2	11/43
1	1/43

Source. Adapted from Barrnett et al. 1991.

The purpose of this chapter is to review the research developments in individual child and adolescent psychotherapy since 1989 that take the form of controlled clinical trials. Individual child and adolescent psychotherapy as defined here refers to one-on-one psychotherapy with children and adolescents, using a verbal or play mode of treatment. Not included in this evaluation are behavioral or cognitive-behavioral forms of treatment. The rationale for focusing on the area of individual psychotherapy is that the majority of practicing child psychiatrists and psychologists appear to use this form of therapy and see it as being most effective (Kazdin et al. 1990). Additionally, this area of psychotherapy study has lagged behind in refinements of research methods.

REVIEWS OF CHILD AND ADOLESCENT PSYCHOTHERAPY

Several recent reviews have examined various aspects of child and adolescent psychotherapy research. These reviews evaluate individual psychotherapy in conjunction with other modes of treatment.

One technique utilized to evaluate groups of studies is meta-analysis. Meta-analysis is a method of statistically summarizing and integrating information from a variety of different studies. It entails calculating a measure called the effect size (see, e.g., Smith et al. 1980). The effect size is obtained by dividing the mean difference in outcome scores between the treatment and control groups by the standard deviation (usually) of the control group. The resultant statistic is essentially a difference in standard (Z) score means. The effect size is thus comparable for outcome measures originally expressed in the percentile of distribution of the control patients in which the average (that is, the patient at the 50th percentile of the experimental group) would fall after treatment. A positive effect size indicates that treated subjects as a group achieved a better outcome than control subjects. This method has been used in a variety of different areas such as the assessment of the effect of social class on achievement, the effect of class size on attainment, and the effect of sex differences on conformity.

Shirk and Russell (1992) reviewed a sample of 24 nonbehavioral studies of child psychotherapy drawn from a previous meta-analytic review by Weisz and Weiss (1987). Not all of the studies examined individual psychotherapy. They examined the following three issues: 1) Is there evidence for a relationship between methodological quality and estimates of effectiveness in child psychotherapy? 2) Are estimates of effectiveness independent of the bias of the therapeutic allegiance of the investigator? 3) Does existing research on child psychotherapy adequately represent the practice of nonbehavioral child treatment?

Independent raters coded each of the 24 studies for the presence or absence of eight methodological problems and assessed the theoretical allegiance (behavioral or nonbehavioral) of the study's authors as outlined in criteria suggested by Berman et al. (1985). Utilizing meta-analysis, they determined the effect size and compared the studies. Their conclusions indicated that studies with more serious methodological problems yielded smaller estimates of therapy effectiveness. The average effect size of behavioral-allegiance studies was significantly smaller than the average effect size of nonbehavioral-allegiance studies. This suggested that measures of effectiveness were not independent of the investigators' allegiance to their respective paradigms.

Shirk and Russell (1992) also compared community practice patterns of delivering therapy to the rates of use of different types of therapy in these clinical research samples. They found that client-centered treatment was used three times as often in the clinical research samples compared with community practice patterns. Twenty of the 29 studies used group treatment, whereas this mode is used much less often in community practice. One-third of the studies used 20 or fewer sessions of treatment. Community practice patterns typically engage patients in treatment for longer periods. It was therefore surmised that these clinical samples are likely to diverge substantially from the typical community treatment sample. The authors concluded that all three factors contribute to inaccurate research estimates in child psychotherapy and made recommendations for improving research.

An additional review addressed the impact of other methodological factors on child psychotherapy outcome research (Weiss and Weisz 1990). These authors attempted to address critics of meta-analysis who questioned the results of meta-analytic findings due to the methodological shortcomings of the studies that are included in reviews. The authors reviewed 105 studies of various psychotherapeutic paradigms, including behavior, cognitive, group, and more traditional individual child psychotherapy, and they rated aspects of internal and external validity.

Dimensions of internal validity included experimental attrition, subject assignment, measurement technology, rater blindness, and subject blindness. Dimensions of external validity involved whether the subject would have been in some form of treatment irrespective of the research, the professional level of the therapist, the setting, and the type of control group.

Together, all of these areas of validity accounted for two-thirds as much variance as other substantive factors, such as the type of therapy or age, in the original meta-analyses. This result suggested that relative to therapy and child-characteristic variables, methodological factors have a substantial, though smaller, impact on meta-analysis results.

The hypothesis that methodologically weak studies have led to an overestimate of therapy effects was not supported. Increased experimental rigor was related to larger effect sizes. The validity factors having the most effect included subject assignment (randomization or matching) and measurement technology. The external validity factors appeared to have relatively little influence on outcome. Last, significant interactions were not found between validity factors and predictors of outcome. This led the authors to suggest that previous meta-analyses of studies examining outcome and other variables are not likely to be distorted by the validity factors that they assessed here. These findings were related to the entire sample of child psychotherapies. The authors did not attempt to differentiate among the paradigms of behavioral, cognitive, and traditional psychotherapy.

Mann and Borduin (1991) conducted a critical review of psychotherapy outcome using adolescent patients. Their review examined studies over a 10-year period and is included here because it does incorporate individual psychotherapy in its evaluation of multisystem therapy. However, the focus of this review is on social skills and assertiveness training, cognitive self-instruction and problem-solving skills training, moral reasoning training, family systems therapy, behavior and communication skills family therapy, and peer group interventions. The multisystem therapy, which included individual therapy, revealed positive outcomes over extended lengths of treatment. Other briefer treatments showed positive short-term outcomes. The long-term results of these treatments were thought to be undetermined.

Fauber and Long (1991) reviewed the relative effectiveness of family therapy versus individual child therapy. In examining the previous literature, their conclusion was that both appear to be moderately effective. However, the data would not allow comparisons of the relative effectiveness of the treatments, nor would the data allow specific recommendations regarding when one approach might be preferentially used over the other. After identifying family factors in the evolution of family pathology, Fauber and Long argued that there was a need for an increased focus on family process variables that might contribute to children's difficulties.

In two reports, Kazdin (1990, 1991) reviewed psychotherapy for children and adolescents as a whole. The focus of his reviews is primarily on research issues and several well-designed series of programmatic research that demonstrate effective treatment using cognitive, behavioral, social skills, or family techniques. In his first article (1990), he touched on two analytically based studies of psychotherapy. One (Heinicke and Ramsey-Klee 1986) evaluated psychoanalytic treatment for 7- to 10-year-old children referred for school problems and compared groups differentiated by the frequency of treatment. Both groups gained in adaptation, self-esteem, capacity for relationships, and reading, although the group that was seen more often evidenced greater gains. The second study consisted of psychoanalytic attempts to help children and adolescents control diabetes (Moran and Fonagy 1987a, 1987b). The treatment program focused on disturbances of psychosexual development or object relations, or both; the underlying hypothesis was that these disturbances were expressed indirectly through impaired glucose control. In one single case and another group comparison study, intensive psychoanalytic treatment improved control of diabetes. These two studies are discussed in more detail in a review of psychoanalytic child psychotherapy by Marans (1989). Although psychoanalytic child psychotherapy is a minor focus of these two reviews, they are included here because, compared with many earlier investigations, they delineate research into traditional psychotherapeutic interventions with children that was done with more methodical integrity.

Kazdin (1990, 1991) also spelled out a variety of other important areas of research that go well beyond the issue of effectiveness of psychotherapy. Kazdin delineated numerous priority areas: 1) the lack of use of clinical samples (e.g., Heinicke and Ramsey-Klee 1986), 2) ignoring comorbidity, 3) underserved populations at risk or populations with special needs, 4) understudied techniques (such as psychoanalytic), 5) combined therapeutic modalities, 6) outcome evaluations that would assess broader aspects of social functioning as opposed to simply decreased symptomatology, and 7) the issue of clinical versus statistical significance.

Kazdin (1991) also outlined critical methodological issues, including 1) the need to specify clinical dysfunction in a standardized way, 2) the maintenance of treatment integrity, 3) the timing of follow-up assessments that allow for appropriate evaluation of the impact of treatment, and 4) the issue of statistical power to detect group differences. He concluded that there has been a remarkable increase in the last three decades of the number of studies, the quality of the evidence, and the range of techniques, but indicated that further work needs to be done on the identification of effective treatments and the extension of these services despite the high cost and slow progress that any program of psychotherapeutic research would require.

In summary, these reviews clearly add to the previous calls for methodological rigor in the implementation of clinical trials of psychotherapy. The meta-analytic studies of psychotherapy have been useful in estimating the broad strength of effects. Unfortunately, more detailed conclusions based on meta-analysis have been difficult to reach. Thus, the conclusions remain very general: that psychotherapy is better than no treatment and that behavioral treatments may have a slight edge in effectiveness compared with nonbehavioral treatments (Kazdin 1990). The field of psychotherapy research has embraced meta-analysis as an effective analytical tool. Unlike computer enhancement of a fuzzy picture, however, one must question meta-analysis's capacity to yield a better "picture" if the methodology of the sample that generated the picture is unsound. This is particularly true of traditional individual child and adolescent psychotherapy studies (Barrnett et al. 1991). Based on this, acknowledging an edge to behavior therapy may be premature.

SPECIFIC STUDIES

The medical and psychological abstracts were reviewed for specific studies related to child and adolescent treatment. Only six controlled trials were found involving nonbehavioral or cognitive individual child and adolescent psychotherapy.

The first study compared structural family therapy with individual child psychodynamic therapy (Szapocznik et al. 1989). This study compared boys ages 6–12 years from two-parent families. The subjects were screened to eliminate those who had evidence of organicity, previous mental health care, medication, or suicidal ideation. Sixty-nine boys completed therapy: 26 in structural family therapy and 26 in individual psychodynamic child therapy. Seventeen were in a control condition that controlled for nonspecific or expectancy placebo effects and that essentially was a recreational activity where the boys received warm, supportive supervision. The total length of treatment was from 12 to 24 hours. Each treatment condition was outlined and videotaped. Two clinicians independently assessed adherence to therapy, and the κ statistic was 0.89 for their level of agreement. The therapists were advocates of their assigned form of therapy and consisted of one psychologist and one social worker for each treatment condition. The control group workers had no clinical experience or training. The five outcome measures were attrition rate, standardized behavior ratings, self-report, a theoretically based psychodynamic scale, and structural family systems ratings.

The results indicated little difference among the groups (Szapocznik et al. 1989). The control group was slightly younger, and the socioeconomic status of the psychoanalytically treated patients was higher. In terms of attrition, two-thirds of the dropouts were in the control group. There was no difference in the treated groups in terms of the dropout rate. Patients in both treatment groups and in the placebo group improved over time. The two treatment groups were equivalent in reducing behavioral and emotional problems based on parent and self-reports and were relatively equivalent on psychodynamic ratings. There was increased improvement in family functioning in the group treated with structural family therapy and a decrease in family functioning in the group treated with individual psychoanalysis. Family functioning in the control group remained the same. The authors concluded that these results support underlying hypotheses about the way illness is expressed in disturbed family systems. The identified patient expresses symptoms as a means of holding the family together to avoid other problems. Thus, an improvement in symptomatic function of the analytically treated child would lead to decreased family functioning. This explanation, however, does not address why the control condition family function remained stable despite symptom improvement.

The methodology of this study in general is far superior to those previously reviewed (Barrnett et al. 1991). The integrity of the treatment conditions was monitored closely. Multiple outcome measures were used. However, it is not clear how the subjects were assigned to treatment. Only 69 of 102 patients completed treatment and 58 returned for follow-up. The diagnoses were varied and included conduct disorders, anxiety disorders, and adjustment reactions. There is no report of how these differentially diagnosed subjects were loaded into the three treatment conditions. This loading may have significantly altered the outcome.

The second study (Pelkonen 1990) consisted of a follow-up of inpatient adolescents. In this study, 58 of 61 adolescents were followed up from 4 to 9 years after their first-time admission to the hospital. In this study there were no standardized assessments. Diagnostic assessment was made by a semistructured interview with only one rater. The patients' mental status and Global Assessment Scale level were assessed by two raters. All of the inpatients received individual, group, and family psychodynamic therapy. The inpatients were divided into two groups: 15 in short-term therapy (less than 3 months) and 43 in long-term therapy (more than 3 months). Follow-up assessments were made from a semistructured interview and criminal records. Adolescents treated over the long term were better able to evaluate their problems, were able to develop a closer therapeutic relationship with the case manager, developed improved peer relations, and attended school more, and their mental status improved somewhat during hospitalization. On discharge, only 14% of the total sample had a good mental status. However, on follow-up, 41% had an improved mental status. This improvement appeared to correlate with a positive attitude toward therapy and positive rapport with the case manager.

Although this study does not exclusively examine individual psychotherapy, it does include that mode of treatment. At best, it compares lengths of treatment where individual psychotherapy is one of multiple components. It is very similar to many previous reports reviewed (Barrnett et al. 1991). It does not specify treatments, does not use well-defined comparisons of groups or matching procedures, exhibits poor diagnostic inclusion and exclusion criteria, and only uses one standardized rating instrument. On the basis of these methodological problems, it is difficult to extrapolate conclusions relevant to individual psychotherapy.

The third study (Davidson et al. 1987) examined the relative efficacy of treatments for juvenile offenders by nonprofessionals with respect to reducing delinquent recidivism. Two hundred and thirteen juvenile offenders were treated with four types of therapy: a behavioral contract with the juvenile; a behavioral contract with the family; a behavioral contract with the court; and a relationship that involved aspects of the typical psychotherapeutic relationship including empathy, unconditional positive regard, help with communications skills, and genuineness. A fifth placebo group was given attention only. Subjects in a sixth control group were returned to court for processing. The investigators used measures of adequacy of training and assessed the implementation of training, and they reported good internal integrity of the experimental treatment conditions. Further offenses, degree of the offenses, and a self-report of delinquency were used to assess outcome. Results indicated that the behavioral contracting with the juvenile and the relationship condition (the one most like individual psychotherapy) had equally positive outcomes that were better than the outcomes for the other conditions.

This study made a concerted attempt to maintain the integrity of the treatment conditions and random assignment. Unfortunately, there was no attempt to investigate the subjects diagnostically. The outcome may have been influenced by various subject psychopathological variables or other external variables (such as degree of family support or family integrity) that were not assessed or controlled for. Outcome assessments focused only on the dimension of delinquency and not on other aspects of functioning. Not all the treatment conditions were implemented over the entire 5-year course of the project. The relationship condition (the one most like psychotherapy) was only used for 1 year. Thus, the sample sizes were very skewed, ranging from 76 in the juvenile behavioral contract condition to 12 in the relationship condition. This limits the statistical power of comparisons among groups (Kazdin 1991).

The fourth study (Culp et al. 1991) examined maltreated children's self-concepts in a comprehensive treatment program. The treatment involved a day program organized around typical preschool activities with individual play therapy, speech therapy, physical therapy, and parent treatment. The subjects were 34 maltreated children, 17 in the day program and 17 on a waiting list. There was no difference between the groups in age, sex, race, or intake category (abused or neglected). The mean age was 4 years, 8 months, with a range from 3 years, 9 months, to 5 years, 9 months. Fifteen were female, and 19 were black. Fourteen were physically abused. Twenty were neglected without physical abuse. Assessment measures included a self-concept scale that involved subject self-report, teacher ratings, and a standardized developmental profile.

Culp and his colleagues made two comparisons. First, they compared children in active treatment with children on the waiting list. After 9 months of treatment, children in active treatment differed significantly from those on the waiting list in cognitive competency, peer acceptance, and maternal acceptance but not in physical competence. In the second comparison, they examined differences between pretreatment and posttreatment scores, looking at within-individual change among all treated children. These scores differed statistically on all measures (cognitive competence, peer acceptance, physical competence, and maternal acceptance). In addition, teacher ratings before and after treatment were significantly different on measures of cognitive competence, peer acceptance, and physical competence. On the basis of the standardized developmental assessment, there was a significant increase in areas of cognition, perception, fine motor skills, and social and emotional functioning for all treated children.

This study did not specifically examine individual psychotherapy. It examined the effects of a broad intervention program versus no intervention. Unfortunately, it is difficult to assess the relative impact of individual play therapy among all the other interventions. This study did not have explicit inclusion and exclusion criteria other than abuse and failed to indicate diagnostic assessments. Thus, it is not clear whether the children in the study were a clinical population. The nature of the treatments was not elaborated on, nor was their relative contribution examined. Outcome measures were partially standardized.

Weisz and Weiss (1989) attempted to determine whether the recent, slightly positive assessments of the effectiveness of controlled clinical studies of psychotherapy approximated real-life clinical practice patterns. They examined data from an outpatient clinic–referred sample of 6- to 17-year-olds and compared those who dropped out of treatment with those who participated in treatment. Standardized rating instruments and clinician assessments were done at intake. Rating instruments filled out by parents and teachers were used as outcome measures at 6 months and at 1 year. The treatment conducted was not controlled in any fashion. The results showed no difference between treatment dropouts and treatment participants except that females who continued in therapy showed more improvement than dropouts, according to ratings by their parents. This improved rating was seen only at the 1-year assessment, and the difference became nonsignificant when the investigators controlled for therapist training. The authors reviewed and dismissed a variety of issues that might have tainted the outcome of data analysis, such as excessive variability of the data, reliance on parent reports that might bias the findings, the psychological condition of the dropouts, and the requirement of voluntary participation by subjects, which might preselect a skewed study sample. A final possibility discussed was that these results were a valid reflection of the results of child psychotherapy as it typically occurs. They suggested that the positive results that were observed in previous reviews of psychotherapy treatment occurred as a function of the careful arrangement and control of therapy, as would be done in a clinical trial. The suggestion then is that without careful control and precision of treatment, effective results are less likely.

The sixth study involved a report presented at Institute VI of the 1992 meeting of the Academy of Child and Adolescent Psychiatry (Fonagy and Target 1992). The authors examined the outcome of child psychoanalysis. This presentation was the first in an ongoing program to examine children treated with psychoanalysis at the Anna Freud Center during the past four decades. The center's sample consisted of closed treatment files of 763 cases; 76% of the patients received intensive (four to five times a week) psychotherapy, whereas the remainder were treated once or twice a week. Thirty-six percent of the therapists were experienced analysts, and the others were trainees. The Anna Freud Center's data are remarkable in that in 54% of the cases, the observations had been systematized in the form of analytic diagnoses based on Anna Freud's work (1954). Treatment was described in two-page, weekly process reports.

The initial presentation examined the therapeutic outcome in a sample consisting of 135 children with disruptive behavior disorder; DSM-III-R diagnoses (American Psychiatric Association 1987) consisted of 79 cases of oppositional disorder, 11 cases of attention-deficit hyperactivity disorder, 31 cases of conduct disorder, and 14 cases with a V code of antisocial behavior. The subjects' ages ranged from 3 years, 3 months, to 17 years, 5 months. Seventy-five percent were boys, and 56% were from social classes I and II. Seventy-one percent of the children were offered and accepted intensive psychoanalytic treatment. The remainder were seen one to three times per week.

The mean Child Global Assessment Scale (CGAS) score of the group with disruptive behavior disorder was 54. This group was individually matched with 135 children treated for emotional disorder. Matching was made on the basis of age, gender, socioeconomic status, number of sessions per week, CGAS score, and family structure. Ninety-five percent of the cases yielded a perfect match. Five percent yielded a stringency of three matching criteria.

The reported results indicated that the treatment led to significant improvements in psychiatric symptomatology in both groups. The number of diagnosable cases decreased from 100% at the beginning of treatment to 35.6% at termination. However, 39% could not be diagnosed because of insufficient information. The average improvement in CGAS score was 14.6 points in the emotional disorder group and 7.8 points in the disruptive disorder group. The children with disruptive disorders had a differential response to treatment. Forty-nine percent of the children with oppositional defiant disorder, compared to 33% of the children with attention-deficit hyperactivity disorder and 25% of the children with conduct disorder, showed very marked improvement, with CGAS scores increasing more than 10 points.

The study also examined predictors of improvement by using a stepwise multiple regression. Disruptive children with good outcomes participated in treatment longer, started with more intensive treatment, and exhibited anxiety as an additional complaint. Children with poorer outcomes were more likely to have specific learning disabilities, to be from lower socioeconomic classes, to be underachievers, and to have mothers with anxiety symptoms. For the group with poorer outcome, the initial level of adaptation as defined by the CGAS did not influence the likelihood of good outcome. For the emotional disorder group, marked improvement was associated with a relatively low CGAS score, the absence of enuresis, a high general adaptive rating of the mother, and provision of parental guidance during therapy.

In their conclusions, the authors cautioned that their study was not an outcome study of child analysis and cannot claim to show analysis to be effective or cost-effective. They thought that the study did identify potentially useful indicators for this type of treatment. Although the authors noted that the validity of archival records creates problems and raises doubts because of the lack of standardized methods of data collection, the advantage of the Anna Freud Center's data set in comparison to others was that it was standardized early on, and there were few changes in theoretical position or in the form of treatment offered over the decades that the children were treated.

This examination appears to have been very carefully crafted, with the major limitation being the reliance on past record keeping. These authors outlined aspects of treatment that indicated a high likelihood that the therapy integrity was maintained and consistently applied to all subjects. Standardized diagnoses (DSM-III-R) were made, with reliability of judgments yielding a κ of 0.8–0.9. Symptoms were recorded on standardized rating instruments, and the study utilized matching to improve comparisons between the two groups. Outcome measures were also standardized. This study represents an important step forward in the research into traditional individual psychotherapy. The Anna Freud Center's data base will be an important source of results for comparative review of other modes of individual therapy.

DISCUSSION

These six studies evidence a relative upswing in the frequency of reports of clinical trials of child and adolescent psychotherapy. Previously it had been reported (Barrnett et al. 1991) that the number of published clinical trials dramatically decreased after 1973; between 1973 and 1989, no more than two studies were published in 1 year and only five studies were published worldwide in the English-written scientific literature. Six studies published in 4 years represent an increase and improvement in the attention being paid by psychotherapeutic researchers to the collection of data on child and adolescent individual psychotherapy.

Previous reviews of child and adolescent individual psychotherapy have argued for a move away from a focus on the simplistic question of whether child and adolescent individual psychotherapy is effective (Barrnett et al. 1991). The field as a whole clearly needs to identify specific patient, therapist, and therapy variables relevant to appropriate treatment and treatment outcomes rather than maintaining a general or superficial focus (Kazdin 1991). Of the six studies examined previously, those with more standardized methodology do evidence this turn to a molecular focus. This turn suggests a more positive direction for the field of child and adolescent individual psychotherapy research as a whole.

It is important to note that adherence to methodological standards is the primary basis for a positive assessment of the direction this area of therapy research is taking. The biggest improvement in methodology, as evidenced by these specific studies, is the increased adherence to the integrity of treatment (Davidson et al. 1987; Fonagy and Target 1992; Szapocznik et al. 1989). The use of poorly controlled aspects of treatment intervention has been hypothesized to generate ineffective outcomes of therapy (Weisz and Weiss 1989).

There is also an increasing attempt to utilize standardized assessments and rating instruments. All of the reviewed studies included at least one previously published measuring instrument. Many of the instruments that were used were well standardized, particularly the checklists. The majority of the studies appeared to attempt to employ matching or randomization, procedures designed to ensure that the comparison groups were reasonably similar. Diagnostic specificity or clear inclusion and exclusion criteria were not always attended to. Only one study clearly delineated diagnosis as it relates to outcome (Fonagy and Target 1992).

Despite these improvements in methodology, this small group of studies will not allow specification of critical issues related to therapy, therapist, and patient variables beyond the isolated findings within each of them. Due to some of the methodological weaknesses, each of these findings will require further replication and more detailed study. The field, then, requires continued adherence to more rigorous, basic methodological approaches in order to develop a broader generation of studies that will inform clinicians.

Previously, suggestions have been made for the development of models of traditional psychotherapy that would allow specific evaluation of various kinds of subject, therapist, therapy, and outcome variables (Barrnett et al. 1991). One potentially promising step forward that has yet to produce published results of a controlled clinical trial is to use interpersonal psychotherapy with adolescents (Moreau et al. 1991). However, developmentally appropriate models of psychotherapy (i.e., those that use some form of some play or activity therapy) still need to be developed for younger children.

Other methodological refinements relate to the inherent complexity of the pathogenesis of psychopathology and the process of recovery. The timing and nature of outcome assessments become critical issues in relationship to this complexity. The pathogenesis of and recovery from psychopathology in children and adolescents have been noted to be confounded with issues related to general development (Kazdin 1990). Certain behaviors that might be part of the constellation of the disorder may well change as a function of the natural growth and development of the child, as opposed to the strength of any particular treatment intervention. Refinement of age-appropriate developmental measures to use in conjunction with psychopathological indices might reduce this confound by allowing researchers to examine how development proceeds as patients with illnesses recover.

A second confound related to the pathogenic process of a disease is that not all child psychopathology is stable over time (Cantwell and Baker 1989). In disorders that are inherently remitting and relapsing, one needs to take into account the average duration of the illness as a means to gauge the appropriate length of treatment intervention. For example, outcome assessments made far too late for the average length of duration of the disorder may not be accurately assessing the effectiveness of treatment but merely the natural tendency of the disorder to disappear. Similarly, to measure the strength of a treatment in delaying recurrence, follow-up assessments of short-duration interventions would need to be done well after the last session for patients with illnesses that tend to persist.

A third confound embedded in the pathogenic or recovery process is related to comorbidity of illnesses within one child. Up to half of patients in epidemiological samples exhibit characteristics of other disorders (Bird et al. 1988). In the present review, comorbid factors clearly produce differential outcomes. The presence of anxiety with disruptive disorders predisposed patients to a better outcome, whereas learning disability in association with disruptive disorders predisposed patients to a poorer response to psychoanalysis (Fonagy and Target 1992). Measuring diagnosis comprehensively and carefully and using matching procedures or randomization become very important factors in research design to help sift out these important influences on the response to treatment.

An alternative way of conceptualizing comorbidity is the evolution of one presentation of an illness into the presentation of another illness within the same individual over time. For example, children with attention-deficit hyperactivity disorder might begin with an illness presentation of hyperactivity, impulsivity, and inattention, go on to present as oppositional and defiant, and then evolve into conduct disorder patients who abuse drugs and alcohol (Werry 1992). An individual with this form of illness would theoretically have a differential response to psychoanalysis at different points in time. Fonagy and Target (1992) outlined the differential response rates to psychoanalysis of patients with attention-deficit disorder, oppositional defiant disorder, and conduct disorder. One conclusion that might be drawn from the above evidence is that for individuals who experience this lengthy illness process, appropriate treatment might not be wedded to a rigid therapeutic formulation or treatment application; rather, it may require a complicated array of combined or sequential treatments, used when most appropriate at a particular time. The research solution for the dilemma of comorbidity necessarily lies in studies using combined treatments, an area of child psychotherapy research that is lacking (Kazdin 1991). Theoretically, combined treatment could involve a complicated algorithm of therapeutic intervention that might include pharmacotherapy, individual psychotherapy, family therapy, various skills training, and group techniques.

The complexity of the pathogenesis of disease and the evolution of recovery also require the pairing of appropriate treatments to appropriate treatment outcome targets. It is quite likely that our array of different psychotherapies will have differential effects on the way individuals function. It is important, then, to ask what should change and whether this change is relevant to the intervention under study or relevant to the study population under examination. Outcome measures that focus purely on resolution of specific symptoms may not yield a true picture of outcome, and a more comprehensive assessment of multiple dimensions of outcome functioning might reveal other improvements. Kazdin (1990) noted that, in comparison with symptom reduction, other aspects of functioning are rarely assessed at outcome. In the area of schizophrenia, it has long been known that evaluation of other aspects of functioning besides symptom expression is important to obtain a comprehensive, valid assessment of outcome (Carpenter et al. 1978). A related issue is that statistically significant change (change that occurs beyond chance) in response to treatment does not necessarily reflect clinically significant change. That is, statistically significant symptom reduction may not produce or correlate with improved social or academic function. Jacobson (1988) outlined four possible approaches to the identification of clinical significance. Incorporation of these approaches into outcome assessments would greatly improve the application of research findings to clinical practice.

The degree of change to expect in response to a particular duration of treatment of a particular therapeutic paradigm for a specific clinical condition is a crucial issue that needs to be defined by psychotherapy research. Dramatic changes are occurring in the way psychotherapeutic practice is conducted in the community due to the influence of external economic factors. Inequities in the pattern of third-party reimbursement for mental health services versus other medical services (National Advisory Mental Health Council 1993; Peterson et al. 1992) have increased the focus on brief treatments and utilizing managed care. As a result, the community practice patterns of therapists are likely to move away from a longer-term, more traditional model of therapy. Accordingly, the finding of Weisz and Weiss (1989) that generic uncontrolled outpatient clinic treatment results in little improvement in functioning might be viewed as support for a managed care review process. Like the clinical trial model of research, managed care requires problem specification, delineation of goals and treatment plans, and a treatment-monitoring process established over the course of treatment to ensure appropriateness of intervention and better outcome. Unfortunately, insurers and managed care companies have implemented standards for treatment and expectations regarding outcome that show a great deal of variability.

Although national standards have been developed in response to the outcry for standardized utilization review (National Utilization Review Standards 1991), not all states require their use. Psychotherapy can be sanctioned by managed care groups in a variety of different ways. For example, patients may receive permission to participate in treatment every few sessions with reviews occurring frequently, or treatment may be capped at a yearly maximum length of 20 sessions. Alternatively, treatment can be left relatively unmonitored over a 1- or 2-year period until it reaches some lifetime maximum. These limits are often applied irrespective of the problem and mode of treatment. None of these guidelines for delineating the amount of treatment coverage or for monitoring psychotherapeutic intervention appears to be based on any scientific standards.

In comparison, a recent longitudinal study of depressive disorders in school children (Kovacs et al. 1984) delineated the length of illness over time. The average durations of adjustment disorder with depressed mood and major depressive disorder were 25 and 32 weeks, respectively, whereas dysthymia had a mean length of duration of 3 years. The maximal recovery rate for adjustment disorder (90%) was reached at 9 months. The maximal recovery rate for major depressive disorder (92%) was reached at 18 months, and the maximal recovery rate for dysthymic disorder (only 89%) was reached at 72 months. When one compares treatment standards as outlined by these various insurance and managed care companies with the natural history of depressive disorders, it is clear that many children are likely to be left untreated if treatment ends because of either the managed care process or limits on insurance company benefits. This restriction will create an ever-expanding pool of partially treated children with no additional resources for treatment. Their future will be grave.

There is a great deal of concern about incentives given to treatment providers by insurance or managed care companies. The quality of treatment may be threatened by encouraging inappropriate reduction of services (General Accounting Office 1988). A recent study of depressed patients receiving care financed by prepayment found less detection and treatment in that group compared with similar depressed patients receiving fee-for-service care (Wells et al. 1989). If researchers set standards for improvement similar to the expectations for treatment held by insurance companies and managed care corporations, it might not be surprising to find that psychotherapy continues to be assessed as ineffective by outcome measures.

A recent report titled *Psychotherapy in the Future* by the Committee on Therapy of the Group for the Advancement of Psychiatry (1992) presents a dismal prognosis but emphasizes the critical need for education of the public and business community to moderate the outside influence on appropriate practice of psychotherapy. It is crucially important that psychotherapy researchers redouble their efforts to generate a wide body of data that outline appropriate treatments of appropriate lengths for specific illnesses in light of the fact that the entire field of managed care (i.e., monitoring the implementation of treatment in the community) has moved forward in the absence of or ignoring scientific data. To address this situation, psychotherapeutic researchers in child and adolescent psychiatry require much more grant support to fund more studies to really delineate this field.

In summary, the recent developments in the area of individual, nonbehavioral, and noncognitive psychotherapy represent a modest but positive turn in the development of the field of child and adolescent treatment. These developments include increasing adherence to more sophisticated methodological standards, such as maintaining the integrity of treatment, using standardized assessments and rating instruments, using procedures to control similarity of comparison groups, and using standardized diagnostic assessments or clear inclusion and exclusion criteria. However, the field of child and adolescent individual psychotherapy has not yet attained the level of sophistication that adult psychotherapy has. Researchers in child and adolescent psychotherapy would clearly benefit from following the adult model and asking similar or related questions regarding children and adolescents who are participating in treatment. The field requires a systematic effort to develop an empirical base to further inform clinicians about their treatment and to inform society as a whole about expectations for treatment and the need for supportive financial resources for treatment. Previously, it was concluded that there had been multiple decades of anecdotal evidence of the usefulness of child psychotherapy and several decades of developing attempts to establish scientific legitimacy (Barrnett et al. 1991). The better methodologically conducted studies reviewed here represent a legitimate attempt to establish adequate data by using current research standards.

REFERENCES

American Psychiatric Association: Diagnostic and Statistical Manual of Mental Disorders, 3rd Edition, Revised. Washington, DC, American Psychiatric Association, 1987

American Psychiatric Association: Psychosocial Treatment Research in Psychiatry: A Task Force Report of the American Psychiatric Association. Washington, DC, American Psychiatric Association, 1993

Barlow D: Anxiety and Its Disorders. New York, Guilford, 1988

Barrett CL, Hampe IE, Miller LC: Research on child psychotherapy, in The Handbook of Psychotherapy and Behavior Change: An Empirical Analysis, 2nd Edition. Edited by Garfield SL, Bergin AE. New York, Wiley, 1978, pp 411–435

Barrnett RJ, Docherty JP, Frommelt GM: A review of psychotherapy research since 1963. J Am Acad Child Adolesc Psychiatry 30:1–14, 1991

Berman JS, Miller CR, Massman PJ: Cognitive therapy versus systematic desensitization: is one treatment superior? Psychol Bull 9:451–461, 1985

Bird HR, Canino G, Rubio-Stipec M, et al: Estimates of the prevalence of childhood maladjustment in a community survey of Puerto Rico: the use of combined measures. Arch Gen Psychiatry 45:1120–1126, 1988

Cantwell D, Baker L: Stability and natural history of DSM-III childhood diagnoses. J Am Acad Child Adolesc Psychiatry 28:691–700, 1989

Carpenter WT, Bartko JI, Strauss JS, et al: Signs and symptoms as predictors of outcome. Am J Psychiatry 135:940–945, 1978

Conte H, Plutchik R, Wild K, et al: Combined psychotherapy and pharmacotherapy for depression: a systematic analysis of the evidence. Arch Gen Psychiatry 43:471–479, 1986

Culp RE, Little V, Letts D, et al: Maltreated children's self-concept: effects of a comprehensive treatment program. Am J Orthopsychiatry 61:114–121, 1991

Dahl H: Frames of mind, in Psychoanalytic Process Research Strategies. Edited by Dahl H, Kachele H, Thoma H. Heidelberg, Germany, Springer-Verlag, 1988

Davidson WS, Redner R, Blakely CH, et al: Diversion of juvenile offenders: an experimental comparison. J Consult Clin Psychol 55:68–75, 1987

Elkin I, Shea T, Watkins JT, et al: National Institute of Mental Health Treatment of Depression Collaborative Research Program: general effectiveness of treatments. Arch Gen Psychiatry 46:971–984, 1989

Eysenck HJ: The effects of psychotherapy: an evaluation. Journal of Consulting Psychology 16:319–324, 1952

Eysenck HJ (ed): The effects of psychotherapy, in Handbook of Abnormal Psychology: An Experimental Approach. London, Pitman Medical Publishing, 1960, pp 697–722

Eysenck HJ: The Effects of Psychotherapy (With Commentary). New York, International Science Press, 1966

Fauber RL, Long N: Children in context: the role of the family in child psychotherapy. J Consult Clin Psychol 59:813–820, 1991

Fonagy P, Target M: Predicting the outcome of child psychoanalysis: the relative success of child psychoanalysis with disruptive and emotional disordered children. Paper presented at the annual meeting of the American Academy of Child and Adolescent Psychiatry, Washington, DC, October 1992

Frank AF, Gunderson JG: The role of the therapeutic alliance in the treatment of schizophrenia: relationship to course and outcome. Arch Gen Psychiatry 47:228–236, 1990

Freud A: The widening scope of indications for psychoanalysis: discussion. J Am Psychoanal Assoc 2:607–620, 1954

Garfield SL, Bergin AE (eds): Handbook of Psychotherapy and Behavior Change, 3rd Edition. New York, Wiley, 1986

General Accounting Office: Medicare physician incentive payment by prepaid health plans could lower quality of care (GAO/HRD-89-29). Washington, DC, U.S. Government Printing Office, 1988

Group for the Advancement of Psychiatry: Psychotherapy in the future (GAP Report 133). Washington, DC, American Psychiatric Press, 1992

Harris SL: Behavior therapy with children, in The Clinical Psychology Handbook. Edited by Hansen M, Kazdin AE, Bellark AS. Elmsford, New York, Pergamon, 1983

Heinicke CM, Goldman A: Research on psychotherapy with children: a review and suggestions for further study. Am J Orthopsychiatry 30:561–588, 1975

Heinicke CM, Ramsey-Klee DM: Outcome of child psychotherapy as a function of frequency of session. J Am Acad Child Adolesc Psychiatry 25:247–253, 1986

Heinicke CM, Strassman LH: Toward more effective research on child psychotherapy. J Am Acad Child Adolesc Psychiatry 3:561–588, 1975

Hogarty GE, McEvoy JP, Munetz MD, et al: Dose of fluphenazine, familial expressed emotion, and outcome in schizophrenia. Arch Gen Psychiatry 45:797–805, 1988

Hood-Williams J: The results of psychotherapy with children: a reevaluation. Journal of Consulting Psychology 24:84–88, 1960

Horowitz LM, Rosenberg SE, Ureno G, et al: Psychodynamic formulation, consensual response method, and interpersonal problems. J Consult Clin Psychol 57:599–606, 1989

Jacobson NS (ed): Defining clinically significant change (special issue). Behavioral Assessment 10(2), 1988

Kazdin AE: Child Psychotherapy: Developing and Identifying Effective Treatments. New York, Pergamon, 1988

Kazdin AE: Psychotherapy for children and adolescents. Annu Rev Psychol 41:21–54, 1990

Kazdin AE: Effectiveness of psychotherapy with children and adolescents. J Consult Clin Psychol 59:785–798, 1991

Kazdin AE, Siegel TC, Bass D: Drawing upon clinical practice to inform research on child and adolescent psychotherapy: a survey of practitioners. Professional Psychology: Research and Practice 21:189–198, 1990

Kovacs M, Feinberg TL, Crouse-Novak MA, et al: Depression disorders in childhood, I: a longitudinal prospective study of characteristics and recovery. Arch Gen Psychiatry 41:229–237, 1984

Levitt EE: The results of psychotherapy with children: an evaluation. Journal of Consulting Psychology 21:189–196, 1957

Levitt EE: Psychotherapy with children: a further evaluation. Behav Res Ther 60:326–329, 1963

Luborsky L (ed): An example of the case conflicted relationship theme method: its scoring and research support, in Principles of Psychoanalytic Psychotherapy: A Manual for Supportive-Expressive Treatment. New York, Basic Books, 1984, pp 199–228

Luborsky L, Crits-Cristoph P, Mintz J, et al: Who Will Benefit From Psychotherapy? Predicting Therapeutic Outcomes. New York, Basic Books, 1988

Mann BJ, Borduin CM: A critical review of psychotherapy outcome studies with adolescents: 1978–1988. Adolescence 26:505–538, 1991

Marans S: Psychoanalytic psychotherapy with children: current research and trends. J Am Acad Child Adolesc Psychiatry 28:669–674, 1989

Marziali E: Three viewpoints on the therapeutic alliance: similarities, differences and associations with psychotherapy outcome. J Nerv Ment Dis 172:417–423, 1984

Michelson L: The role of individual differences, response profiles and treatment consonance in anxiety disorders. Journal of Behavioral Assessment 6(4):349–368, 1984

Moran GS, Fonagy P: Insight and symptomatic improvement. Paper presented at the Workshop on Psychotherapy Outcome Research with Children, National Institute of Mental Health, Bethesda, MD, 1987a

Moran GS, Fonagy P: Psychoanalysis and diabetic control: a single-case study. Br J Med Psychol 60:57–72, 1987b

Moreau D, Mufson L, Weissman MM, et al: Interpersonal psychotherapy for adolescent depression: description of modification and preliminary application. J Am Acad Child Adolesc Psychiatry 30:642–651, 1991

National Institute of Mental Health: Health care reform for Americans with severe mental illnesses: report of the National Advisory Mental Health Council. Bethesda, MD, National Institute of Mental Health, 1993

National Utilization Review Standards. Washington, DC, Utilization Accreditation Commission, June 1991

O'Leary KD, Carr EG: Childhood disorders, in Contemporary Behavior Therapy. Edited by Wilson GT, Franks C. New York, Guilford, 1982

Ollendick TH: Child and adolescent and behavior therapy, in Handbook of Psychotherapy and Behavior Change, 3rd Edition. Edited by Garfield SL, Bergin AE. New York, Wiley, 1986, pp 525–564

Ollendick TH, Cerney JA: Clinical Behavior Therapy With Children. New York, Plenum, 1981

Pelkonen M: Inpatient psychiatric adolescents function better than expected after discharge: a follow-up study. Acta Psychiatr Scand 81:317–321, 1990

Peterson MS, Christianson JB, Wholey D: National survey of mental health, alcohol and drug abuse treatment in HMOs: 1989 chartbook. Excelsior, MN, Interstudy Center for Managed Care Research, 1992

Saxe LM, Cross T, Silverman N: Children's mental health: problems and services (background paper). Washington, DC, U.S. Government Printing Office, 1986

Shirk SR, Russell RL: A reevaluation of estimates of child therapy effectiveness. J Am Acad Child Adolesc Psychiatry 31:703–708, 1992

Smith ML, Glass GV, Miller TI: The Benefits of Psychotherapy. Baltimore, MD, Johns Hopkins University Press, 1980

Szapocznik J, Rio A, Murray E, et al: Structural family versus psychodynamic child therapy for problematic Hispanic boys. J Consult Clin Psychol 57:571–578, 1989

Weiss B, Weisz JR: The impact of methodological factors on child psychotherapy outcome research: a meta-analysis for researchers. J Abnorm Child Psychol 18:639–670, 1990

Weisz JR, Weiss B: Assessing the effects of clinic-based psychotherapy with children and adolescents: a meta-analysis for clinicians. J Consult Clin Psychol 55:542–549, 1987

Weisz JR, Weiss B: Assessing the effects of clinic-based psychotherapy with children and adolescents. J Consult Clin Psychol 57:741–746, 1989

Wells KB, Hays RD, Burnam A, et al: Detection of depressive disorder for patients receiving prepaid or fee for service care. JAMA 266:3298–3302, 1989

Werry JS: History, terminology and manifestations at different ages, in Attention Deficit Hyperactivity Disorder (Child and Adolescent Psychiatric Clinics of North America, Vol 1, No 2). Edited by Weiss G. Philadelphia, PA, WB Saunders, 1992, pp 297–310

Williams JBW, Spitzer RL (eds): Psychotherapy Research. New York, Guilford, 1984

Chapter 20

Neurosis and Conduct Disorders

Efrain Bleiberg, M.D.

Surveys of child and adolescent psychiatrists indicate that individual child psychotherapy is a major component of their practice (Silver and Silver 1983). Such practice is rooted in a rich tradition, largely nurtured by psychodynamic principles and based on the use of talk and play to explore children's experiences and effect therapeutic change. This tradition's claim to legitimacy relies heavily on case reports that, however moving or dramatic, tend to be highly resistant to objective assessment and controlled scrutiny. As the old quip goes, psychodynamically oriented therapists have failed to realize that data is *not* the plural of anecdote.

This quip ignores the vigorous efforts made over the last 20 years to bring methodological rigor to the assessment of adult psychodynamic psychotherapy (Crits-Cristoph et al. 1988; Hartley and Strupp 1983; Luborsky 1976; Luborsky et al. 1981). Nonetheless, psychodynamic child psychotherapy research lags behind (Barrnett et al. 1991; Kazdin 1993) and still largely asks global questions such as "Is psychotherapy effective?" instead of addressing the more focused inquiries of contemporary research: "Which set of procedures is effective when applied to what kind of patients with what kind of problems as practiced by what sort of therapist" (Barrnett et al. 1991, p. 2). Lack of specificity in both research and clinical practice has rendered individual psychodynamic child psychotherapy vulnerable to charges of ineffectiveness in comparison with competing therapeutic approaches, such as cognitive-behavior procedures, pharmacotherapy, and family therapy.

Yet none of these competing paradigms addresses the realms of children's subjective experience, coping and defense mechanisms, and interpersonal relationships as clearly as psychodynamic psychotherapy does. Basic premises of this chapter are 1) that a psychodynamic perspective can provide the glue that holds together psychotherapeutic, pharmacological, cognitive-behavioral, and family interventions in a coherent and integrated treatment plan, and 2) that such integration results in a significant enhancement of both clinical effectiveness and conceptual sophistication.

THE CONCEPT OF PSYCHONEUROSIS IN CHILDREN AND ADOLESCENTS

The concept of psychoneurosis is central to psychoanalytic theory and therapy. In the classic psychoanalytic formulation, neurotic symptoms (i.e., obsessions and compulsions, phobias, conversions, and other hysterical manifestations) represent an unconscious compromise formation between conflicting forces: forbidden wishes, whose origins are infantile derivatives of sexual and aggressive drives, and the defensive counterforces mobilized by the ego to prevent the expression of these wishes (Fenichel 1945).

Symptoms are thus conceptualized as having specific meaning: they represent an internal struggle, largely fought outside of conscious awareness. The neurotic compromise allows the individual to achieve an internal equilibrium, albeit an unstable one and at the price of a restriction in functioning and some degree of psychic pain. Secondarily, neurotic symptoms may acquire additional purposes when they serve to secure advantages to neurotic individuals in their relationship with the environment.

For Freud and his followers (Nagera 1966), the adult's neurosis repeats a compromise reached in childhood—the infantile neurosis—which children develop largely to cope with the problems associated with the Oedipus complex. Freud (1924/1961) thought that children feared the same-sex parent's retaliation for their hostile, competitive strivings that are, in turn, fueled by the children's sexual wishes for the other-sex parent. Children resolve the dilemma of whether to strive for or to give up forbidden satisfactions by internalizing the parent's prohibition against Oedipal gratification and by identifying with the same-sex parent. Identification with the same-sex parent allows children to postpone sexual gratification and provides them with an ideal—a road map to guide the development of sexual roles and sexual choices. The superego, which Freud described as "the heir to the Oedipus complex," is a psychic system with limit-setting and direction-giving functions (Hartman and Loewenstein 1962) that results from internalizing parental authority. The superego prompts the ego to block the awareness and expression of Oedipal wishes by mobilizing an array of defensive mechanisms, but with repression as the basic mechanism. The "shape" of the neurotic symptom, in turn, depends on the "choice" of defense mechanism; in other words, repression and displacement lead to phobias or cognitive-emotional isolation, and repression and reaction formation generate obsessive-compulsive symptoms.

The case of little Hans (Freud 1909/1955) is a classic example of the Freudian formulation. According to Freud, little Hans feared horses as a displacement of his fear of his father, who had become a menacing figure because of the boy's own hostility toward him. Fear of horses restricted little Hans's functioning but allowed him a better interpersonal and intrapsychic accommodation than he could have achieved had he faced more directly his rage at his father and the related fears of parental retaliation.

Thus, in the Freudian paradigm, the psychoneurosis came to be conceptualized as 1) a compromise formation between forbidden Oedipal wishes and defense mechanisms mobilized to prevent their expression, and 2) a category of mental disorders characterized by particular symptoms and an underlying structure—the infantile neurosis. This paradigm has come under attack from both within and without psychoanalysis since the 1960s.

Psychoanalytic writers have noted the problems with the concept of neurosis. Freud (1924/1961) believed that every person produces an infantile neurosis as the price humans pay to traverse the Oedipus complex and live in civilized society. Yet obviously not everyone develops neurotic symptoms, and the distinction between normal and pathological development becomes muddled in the Freudian paradigm. Furthermore, as the focus shifted in the psychoanalytic literature to pre-Oedipal development and, to a lesser extent, to post-Oedipal development, questions were raised about the obligatory link between neurosis and Oedipal issues. Tysson (1992) questioned the correlation between "Oedipal" and "neurotic" and proposed instead that the central factors of neurotic disorders are 1) an internalized conflict, 2) some capacity for affect regulation, and 3) capacity for self-responsibility. To Tysson's triad I would add 4) a predominance of defenses centered on repression and 5) the ability to process and communicate experience at a symbolic level.

Outside of psychoanalysis, the concept of neurosis has been assaulted with much greater ferocity. The concept of neurosis has been discredited by the trend toward descriptive clarity and reliability in diagnosis; theoretical, operational definitions of psychiatric disorders; and biological explanations of pathogenesis. Described as vague, unreliable, impossible to verify empirically, overinclusive, and tied to an obsolete theory, neurosis was excluded from psychiatry's official diagnostic classifications.

Despite this slight, neurosis refused to disappear altogether. Empirical studies of psychiatric symptoms in children (Achenbach and Edelbrock 1978) support a dichotomy between internalizing—or emotional—disorders and externalizing—or conduct—disorders. In an oversimplified way, this dichotomy distinguishes children who make themselves miserable (i.e., those who experience their symptoms as ego-dystonic) from children who make everyone but themselves miserable (i.e., those who experience their symptoms as syntonic). Clinically, children with the internalizing disorders resemble the anxious, inhibited children for whom psychodynamic child therapy was invented: internalizing disorders can be roughly described as neurosis shorn of its theoretical baggage.

Although the internalizing-externalizing dichotomy seems to capture meaningful dimensions of children's psychopathology, an easy distinction between inner suffering versus outwardly directed misery does not stand up well to close clinical scrutiny. Aggressive, delinquent, and hyperactive children experience much suffering and inner turmoil (Katz 1992; O'Brien 1992), just as surely as anxious and inhibited youngsters can entrap their parents in a tight web of control and misery.

CONDUCT AND PERSONALITY DISORDERS IN CHILDREN AND ADOLESCENTS

However imprecise, the category of "conduct disorder" has become firmly entrenched in psychiatric usage, achieving the status of the most commonly utilized diagnosis in child and adolescent psychiatry (Kazdin et al. 1990). Its popularity notwithstanding, the concept of conduct disorder remains controversial (Lewis et al. 1984).

By the early 1950s, a number of psychoanalytic writers inspired by Aichhorn (1935) had proposed a variety of ideas to understand "wayward," impulsive youngsters. Redl and Wineman (1957) described the failure of ego controls underlying the difficulties of "children who hate." Johnson and Szurek (1952) examined the adolescents' enactment of their parents' unconscious delinquent tendencies. Winnicott (1958) interpreted the "antisocial tendency" as an effort to test and secure relationships. Such contributions stirred up hope and therapeutic enthusiasm. Yet over the next three decades, enthusiasm gave way to widespread disillusionment with the effectiveness of psychoanalytically oriented approaches in general and psychotherapy in particular for youths with conduct disorders.

Such waning of therapeutic enthusiasm can hardly be surprising. Conducting psychotherapy with youngsters with conduct disorders presents unique challenges to clinicians' skill, sensitivity, and compassion. Aggressive, manipulative, arrogant, defiant, and apparently unconstrained by guilt, these children are far more likely to elicit feelings of anger and helplessness than of empathy and concern. Furthermore, their seeming lack of suffering, motivation for change, or serious psychiatric impairment strains treaters' ability to justify the necessity for a tortuous, lengthy, and often unsuccessful treatment. Last, but not least, these youngsters expose the limits of psychoanalytic perspectives, making clear that this vantage point cannot optimally cover some central dimensions of human functioning.

Beginning in the early 1960s, other approaches have attempted to address the questions raised by youngsters with conduct disorder: 1) sociocultural models (i.e., Cloward and Ohlin 1960; Rutter and Giller 1983), which identify the significance of socioeconomic class, family size, access to social, medical, and psychiatric services, child-rearing and socializing practices, and modes of exposure to alcohol and drugs; 2) family interaction models (i.e., Patterson 1982; Patterson et al. 1992), which emphasize the importance of parental violence and physical abuse, marital discord, and parental inadequacies in providing structure, supervision, and emotional involvement; and 3) neurological models (i.e., Christiansen 1977; Lewis 1983), which stress genetic influences, neuropsychiatric vulnerabilities, attention-deficit hyperactivity, learning disabilities, and depression.

These studies make abundantly clear that conduct disorder is a diagnostic label encompassing an array of biopsychosocial vulnerabilities, intermixed in various combinations, rather than a homogeneous combination. Subdividing these youngsters in ways that help make sense of the heterogeneity offers the potential to provide a firmer base from which to conceptualize psychotherapeutic approaches.

Yet subtyping of conduct disorders has been fraught with difficulty. Rutter and Giller (1983) concluded that the most meaningful distinction was along the lines of socialized versus undersocialized. According to Rutter and Giller (1983), the capacity to form enduring, affectionate bonds and experience concern for others is a psychological dimension associated with a more benign outcome. Almost in passing, they questioned whether the most significant differentiation is between degrees or types of personality disturbance rather than between symptoms of conduct disorder.

Unfortunately, Rutter and Giller's suggestion has, with some notable exceptions, gone largely unheeded. DSM-III-R (American Psychiatric Association 1987) classifies the conduct disorders among the "disruptive behavior disorders" and includes a solitary aggressive type, a group type, and an undifferentiated type but fails to link these youngsters' pervasive behavioral patterns with relatively enduring patterns of experiencing, coping with, and relating to others, except for the superficial attention given to whether disruptive behavior occurs in the context of belonging to a group or as a solitary pursuit.

It is still in dispute whether children and adolescents should be given a diagnosis of personality disorder. Nonetheless, much greater therapeutic, particularly psychotherapeutic, specificity could be gained by looking at children with conduct disorders against the background of their developing personality organization. Along these lines, Marohn et al. (1979) conducted a factor analysis study of a sample of juvenile delinquents that yielded four psychological subtypes: 1) the impulsive, 2) the narcissistic, 3) the empty-borderline, and 4) the depressed borderline. Marohn et al.'s sophisticated analysis of personality types contrasts with the oversimplistic notion that "character" disorders equate with psychopathy, which in turn is shorthand for individuals devoid of scruples, concern for others, or motivation for treatment.

The personality types associated with conduct disorder are linked to histories of trauma—particularly physical and sexual abuse and early losses—interacting with a broad range of genetic and constitutional vulnerabilities, including mood disorders, attention-deficit hyperactivity disorder, and learning disabilities (Gunderson and Zanarini 1989). Traumatic antecedents, joining with a constitutional proclivity to hyperarousal, promote a way of organizing experience and coping with stress that is heavily reliant on dissociation, emotional isolation, numbness, splitting, and projection. This array of coping and defensive mechanisms induces fragmentation of experience and concreteness and contrasts with the symbolic elaboration that repression permits. This crucial difference shapes differences in the technical approaches used with neurotic youngsters and those with conduct disorders.

In this chapter, I contrast psychotherapeutic strategies applicable to children who are largely inhibited and conflicted, who are capable of—in fact haunted by—an inordinate sense of self-responsibility, and who experience distress about their symptoms with approaches better suited for youngsters who rigidly insist on imposing their misery on the environment and are generally less prepared to acknowledge their inner turmoil.

BEGINNING PSYCHOTHERAPY WITH NEUROTIC CHILDREN

The clinical literature reports a strong consensus that the initial goal of psychodynamic psychotherapy is to create a context in which a therapeutic alliance can emerge (Greenson 1967). Therapists initially direct their interventions to promote in their patients the notion that a collaborative activity with the treater is possible, safe, and potentially helpful.

Neurotic children may approach the therapist filled with dread, haunted by shame, or tormented by guilt, yet they are generally endowed with a "basic trust" (Erikson 1963) that hope and help can be derived from relationships with others. Pained by their symptoms, neurotic children generally long for help and are at least somewhat motivated to overcome the restrictions in their functioning.

> Mary, a pretty 6-year-old, was referred to therapy because of encopresis, constant worrying, fears of dying, lack of friends, and poor performance in school despite obvious intelligence and eagerness to do well. The

daughter of two hard-working, rather shy, and obsessional physicians, Mary developed normally during the first 3 years of her life and had achieved bowel and bladder control before age 3. A bladder infection at that point and the catheterization she underwent as part of the diagnostic workup proved rather traumatic for her. From that point onward, she became constipated and experienced both diurnal and nocturnal enuresis. As her parents treated the constipation with mineral oil, she began to "leak" fecal matter. Anxiously, she began to talk of her concern of being attacked by a snake.

Her worries became more generalized as she got older. Often, she spoke of her fears of dying. Fears of growing up also plagued her, as she associated growing up with dying. Repeatedly, she expressed the wish to turn into a baby just like her sister Anne, 3 years younger.

The birth of this sister strained Mary's relationship with her parents. She became bossy and argumentative with her father, insisting that he put her to bed at night but also demanding loudly that he refrain from hugging her or kissing her. With her mother, she talked about her plans to marry her father "after mother dies." Her mother's death also preoccupied her, and she had developed an elaborate fantasy about her mother's funeral.

Kindergarten was a source of great distress for Mary. Shy and lonely, she would sit still, not daring to move, unable to participate in games or activities, preoccupied with the idea that the smell of her soiling would be detected by other children and would turn her into the object of ridicule and derision.

On starting therapy, Mary seemed eager to form a relationship, yet she signaled her need to proceed cautiously. She started every session by lining up a number of puppets, dolls, and animal figures until she was satisfied that they were in the "right" position. Before the end of the session, she asked for a 5-minute warning so she could meticulously rearrange the toys to the position she had assigned them at the beginning of the hour.

After a few sessions of observing this sequence, I commented on how frightening it must be when things change and seem to get out of control and how reassuring it must be when somehow everything could be returned to its original state. She responded to this comment with greater freedom in her play, and an elaboration of play themes centered on losses. All of the animals, puppets, and dolls were orphans or had otherwise lost their parents.

I then inquired about the circumstances of such losses, which brought to the fore that the reason the animals had lost their parents was linked to their greed and hostility. With increasing ease she began to play out how the animals felt so hungry and competitive and, for the first time, introduced human figures into the play. Human figures, mainly two girl dolls, appeared in her play, ensuring that the animals stayed within a fenced space or responded to an elaborate system of commands and instructions. I commented on the fear of the animals escaping and going wild but wondered if we could find out more about their hunger, neediness, and anger. Perhaps then the animals would need less vigilance.

Parallel with these developments in the sessions—about 3 months into the therapy—her parents reported at one of the meetings scheduled with them every 3 or 4 weeks that Mary seemed much improved both at home and in school. She was less frightened of dying, appeared less anxious and more able to work in school, and had dramatically decreased the number of encopretic accidents.

This vignette illustrates a number of points regarding the early phase of the therapy of neurotic children:

- Parents are capable of striking a reasonably good alliance with the therapist and can respect the boundaries of the treatment and support the child's participation in it. Regularly scheduled sessions with the parents are designed to 1) obtain information about the patient's life circumstances, 2) promote a sense of collaboration with the parents, and 3) assess family interactional patterns that maintain or reinforce the child's psychopathology.
- Conflictive themes pervade children's experience and limit their developmental opportunities and interpersonal relationships. Mary struggled with anger and rivalry; her wishes to eliminate her rivals conflicted with fears of deprivation, loss, and retaliation.
- Early comments are designed to help children recognize and put into words their fears and conflicts while gently challenging their defenses. Comments are generally kept in the metaphor of the play theme rather than translated into their explicit meaning (Hoffman 1993) and refer both to the issues the child seems to be struggling with and to the resistances in expressing and exploring those struggles. Children respond to these interventions with an enhancement of the alliance and greater freedom in their play or verbalizations, or both. This point, based on clinical experience, parallels the data drawn from adult psychotherapy research (Hartley and Strupp 1983; Luborsky 1976), which show that in patients capable of a good alliance, exploring conflicts and negative feelings—including those directed toward the therapist—fosters the alliance and improves outcome, whereas failure to address these feelings undermines the alliance and yields poor results.
- Diagnostically, neurotic children tolerate clarification of their struggles, fears, and conflicts without becoming disorganized or resorting to destructive and distancing defenses.
- The therapist's comments communicate that the sessions have a purpose: 1) that play, as well as words, can serve to express thoughts, feelings, conflicts, fears, and concerns; and 2) that the goal of the therapist's observations and participation is to help the child make sense of his or her experience and conflicts so that inner struggles can be mastered more effectively.

CREATING A THERAPEUTIC CONTEXT FOR CHILDREN WITH CONDUCT DISORDER

Faced with the frequently intimidating and typically deflating challenge of treating youngsters with conduct disorders, therapists have often despaired of finding basic principles to guide their interventions. An important contribution by P. Kernberg and Chazan (1991) described in detail a "trio of therapies": individual, supportive-expressive play psychotherapy; parent training; and play group psychotherapy specifically designed for children of elementary school age with mild to moderate conduct disorders.

P. Kernberg and Chazan indicated that their approaches are intended for children who demonstrate a capacity for social bonding, as manifested by at least two of the following four characteristics: 1) the ability to form and sustain peer group friendships for at least 6 months, 2) the capacity to extend themselves to others, 3) the potential for feeling at least a minimum of guilt, and 4) the possibility of experiencing loyalty toward companions and showing some concern for the welfare of others.

The three therapeutic modalities described by P. Kernberg and Chazan can be used separately or in combination. The treatment approach presented in this chapter is predicated on the notion that the treatment of youngsters with conduct disorders should *always* integrate individual and family interventions. This notion is based on the premise that children with conduct disorders organize their experience of themselves and the world in rigid and stereotypical ways and then are equally rigid in their insistence on inducing interpersonal responses that validate and reinforce their internal "model" of reality. A perverse cycle typically evolves in which youngsters evoke interpersonal dysfunction in their families that, in time, reinforces their intrapsychic pathology. Thus, much greater therapeutic leverage can be achieved by carefully coordinating individual psychotherapy and family treatment.

Patterson (1982) and Kazdin et al. (1992) delineated specific approaches to help parents of delinquents become consistent limit setters and effective promoters of prosocial behavior, as well as become better prepared to minimize the coercive parent-child interaction that escalates children's aggressive and antisocial behavior. P. Kernberg and Chazan (1991) advocated a similar approach in a four-phase program of parental guidance: in the first phase, the parents' management techniques are assessed and agreement is reached on how to modify these techniques; during the second phase, parents are taught general principles of development and modification of behavioral problems; the third phase focuses on specific approaches for parents to apply with their children; and the fourth phase helps parents learn how to maintain their children's behavior at home and how to provide input to the therapist.

Structural-strategic family therapists (Minuchin and Fishman 1981) emphasize the importance of interventions and assignments designed to establish clear generational boundaries and extricate symptomatic children from the roles they play within the family, often precisely through their disruptive behavior. For example, disruptive behavior can detour one parent's hostility onto the child instead of the other parent.

From a psychotherapeutic vantage point, family interventions such as those described by Minuchin and Fishman introduce what Horowitz (1987) called a "representational mismatch," that is, an interpersonal reality that contradicts rather than supports the child's intrapsychic model of reality. A review of the clinical literature (Bleiberg 1987, 1989; Marohn 1991, Marohn et al. 1980; Masterson 1988; Rinsley 1989) reveals that although authors conceptualize their interventions differently, they all agree that the treatment of children with conduct disorders cannot take place without first establishing effective limits to impulsive, manipulative, and destructive behavior.

From a clinical standpoint, the crucial considerations in deciding between a residential setting or an outpatient plan are 1) the capacity of the youngsters' parents to establish and maintain a consistent representational mismatch; 2) the extent of the youngster's need for containment, support, and structure; and 3) the availability of community resources and services to support the family's containment.

Faced with parental efforts to set limits and provide structure, children with conduct disorders react blatantly or subtly to sabotage adult competence. In so doing, they attempt to re-create an interpersonal context characterized by the caretakers' ineptitude, inconsistency, and unreliability and by adult reliance on children's power, instead of one in which children can count on protection.

Pseudocompliance and pseudoinsights are frequent maneuvers to preserve the status quo. Seductive efforts to sexualize therapeutic relationships or become "buddies" with the treaters can render treatment ineffective. Open defiance, threats, assaults, contempt, or manipulation instigate chaos in the family, school, or the residential treatment center.

A consistent representational mismatch is a prerequisite to achieve the initial goals of treatment, which include 1) challenging the youngster's pathological defenses enough to induce therapeutically useful anxiety; 2) establishing the adults, both parents and treaters, as reliable protectors and limit setters; and 3) promoting the children's capacity to share some aspect of their subjective experience with the treater.

Children with conduct disorder who have prominent narcissistic features require an environment that, although challenging their sense of omnipotence and curtailing their efforts to derail treatment, also avoids unnecessarily exposing their vulnerability. Borderline and impulsive children need structure and support. Specific pharmacological agents such as stimulants or mood stabilizers can be important elements in these youngsters' treatment. Yet perhaps the most critical factor in determining therapeutic success is the alliance established between parents and clinician.

BEGINNING PSYCHOTHERAPY WITH CHILDREN WITH CONDUCT DISORDER

Achieving a sense of collaboration with children who have conduct disorder is hardly a simple task. These children fail to engage in symbolic play and are unable to utilize symbolic means of communication (Katz 1992). Therapists typically contend instead with an opening phase in which the patient's behavior is marked by ruthless tyranny, aloofness, suspiciousness, demands for control of the sessions, or attempts to reduce the therapist's role to that of captive audience for an elaborate show.

Older school-age and adolescent narcissistic patients often present themselves as "hotshots" filled with bravado and pretentious self-sufficiency, bent on demeaning the therapist. On the other hand, they may appear grateful and seemingly compliant, brimming with intellectual insights or seductively communicating to therapists that they find them exceptionally sensitive, brilliant, and attractive.

Borderline youngsters can fall madly in love with their therapist and are eager to declare their good fortune in having found the perfect person to love—and to be loved by. Impulsive children play aggressively and destructively, but those who have experienced significant trauma or who are depressed often present a narrow range of verbal and emotional involvement and concrete, repetitive, joyless play themes. These initial gambits provide a window into the subjective experience and characteristic defensive maneuvers of these children.

> Robert, a 15-year-old hospitalized adolescent with a mixture of borderline and narcissistic features, began therapy with a superficial eagerness to solve his problems. Such therapeutic zeal soon gave way to rather flamboyant expressions of contempt for the hospital, the hospital's treatment team, and me. He had expected that a famous clinic would provide him with a therapist perfectly suited to treat him—a "perfect match." He had some hope (on first meeting me) that I was such a match because he noticed we both had blue eyes and blond hair. He was quickly disappointed, however, especially when he heard my obviously foreign

accent. He could not understand why he had been subjected to the ignominy of having a "spic" (his reference to my Hispanic accent) for a therapist. I commented that he seemed to experience my accent as a put-down—a flaw with which he would be embarrassed to be associated.

"Not bad for a spic," he replied, quickly turning to his doubts about whether "spics" could understand the concerns of someone of obvious Nordic descent, such as he was. At that point I mentioned that, if I heard him right, he seemed to be saying that if we were not identical—not only in our looks but in our backgrounds as well—I would not be able to understand him and appreciate him. "Not bad for a spic," was again his response. Yet I could detect some budding relatedness in his mocking compliment.

Such relatedness, of course, was only tentative. Nonetheless, he then could confide his concerns that if he trusted me, I would find a way to sabotage his plans to "behave appropriately" and maintain a "positive attitude." Such behavior would, he was sure, convince the clinical staff and his parents that he was ready to return to his beloved home state, instead of enduring the disgrace of rotting in dreadful Kansas. This comment, of course, betrayed Robert's own questions about how effectively manipulation and pretense could serve to solve his problems. Not picking up on this issue, I commented instead that I appreciated his concern about what would happen to him if he trusted me, even a bit (again, what would happen if I "could hear him right"). Would it help him or would it hinder him?

This clinical vignette illustrates how initial interventions should focus on clarifying the patient's subjective experience ("Let me see if I understand what you are saying—am I hearing you right?"), with the primary goal of helping the patient find an area of subjective experience that can be safely shared, either verbally or in play. The therapist should avoid prematurely interpreting the patient's envy, sadness, vulnerability, or rage, as well as the related defenses of grandiosity, dissociation, denial, and projective identification. In other words, the therapeutic intent is to facilitate the establishment of a beachhead, an area of self-other relatedness.

Prematurely confronting the patient's defenses before this beachhead is established only exacerbates the need for distance, control, or devaluation of the therapist and the therapy.

Elliot, an 11-year-old boy with a narcissistic conduct disorder, responded to my premature inquiry into his feelings of pain and sadness by frantically denying any dysphoric experiences. He proceeded to launch into a tirade that explained how "any idiot knows that babies only learn to feel pain when their mothers get all hysterical" after they injure themselves. Without such "hysteria," he claimed, babies would never learn to feel pain. He, fortunately, had been forced to rely on his own resources by his parents' self-absorption, so he had been spared the need to learn to feel vulnerable. Instead, his task was to monitor his mother's mood and to keep her amused and buoyant. Disappointment, particularly the failings of an unavailable husband, threw this chronically depressed woman into a suicidal despair from which only Elliot could rescue her.

Bent on convincing me of his power—and his lack of familiarity with either pain or vulnerability—Elliot began to lose his grip on reality. His tirade became more desperate, as he insisted on proving the power of his mind over ordinary matter. Before long, he was telling me how once he had wished to fly so badly that he had been able to defy the laws of gravity. Then he grew anxious, keenly aware that maintaining an illusion of omnipotence was requiring him to treat reality in an ever more arbitrary fashion.

Helping Elliot at this juncture presented me with a dilemma. To acknowledge my mistake in addressing his vulnerability before he was ready would only add the insult of implying that he was not tough enough to the injury of exposure. I offered him a compromise: I asked, "Are you saying that when you really put your mind to something, no matter how impossible it may seem, you can accomplish it?" He agreed, but only after dismissing my formulation ("No, that's not it"). A moment later, however, he replied, "What I really mean is that when you really put your mind to it, you can accomplish just about anything. You can even learn to fly in an airplane." Elliot was thus able to save face, regain his grip on reality, maintain his sense of omnipotence unchallenged, and use my help without having to acknowledge it.

Interventions that help these youngsters save face can pave the way for a therapeutic alliance. That is, therapists help their patients to maintain a sense of control even when confronted with the blow of the family's or inpatient staff's growing capacity to provide a holding environment. Such face-saving help facilitates patients' ability to accept their representational mismatch and the implicit "humiliation" of therapy itself. As the case of Elliot illustrates, such tasks involve a delicate balance between fostering more adaptive solutions to life's demands, maintaining a semblance of control, and keeping anxiety and shame within manageable limits. Therapists, for example, can discuss how youngsters might respond more adaptively to their parents'—or the inpatient staff's—limits on manipulative or provocative behavior or to the enraging, anxiety-provoking prohibition on using drugs and alcohol. Cognitive-based treatments can reduce aggression and antisocial behavior (Kazdin et al. 1990, 1992), thus reducing social pressure and helping these youngsters gain a measure of control.

Not only the patients' reactions require careful attention, however. Perhaps the greatest therapeutic obstacle is the therapist's countertransference. Therapists often experience dread of the sessions; concern about being fooled by the patient; wishes to show who "really is in charge"; feelings of worthlessness, helplessness, defeat, and irritation; urges to reject these patients; and boredom or indifference. O. Kernberg

(1975) pointed out the usefulness of countertransference reactions as invaluable clues to the patient's rejected self-experiences being evoked in the therapist. Kohut's (1971) contributions enhanced therapists' awareness of the necessity of paying minute attention to patient's feelings of disappointment in the therapist. Kohut's stress on empathy highlights the importance of respecting the need to feel powerful and in control without prematurely interpreting warded-off feelings. This clinical observation is consistent with the research findings that to explore and express negative and conflictive feelings with poorly motivated patients undermines the development of an alliance (Hartley and Strupp 1983).

MIDDLE PHASE IN THE PSYCHOTHERAPY OF NEUROTIC CHILDREN

The middle phase of therapy with neurotic children is marked by the emergence of transference material that can be amenable to therapeutic use. As children gain greater confidence and freedom in the sessions, the currents of their feelings, thoughts, and conflicts begin to coalesce and be experienced in the context of the relationship with the therapist.

Transference is facilitated by 1) the therapist's implicit offer of help and relatedness coupled with a basic stance of acceptance, encouragement to express thoughts and feelings, attention to resistances, and attunement to the child's predicaments; and 2) a therapeutic structure that emphasizes regularity, consistency, and the specialness of the hours (Chethik 1989). Every action of the therapist conveys to the child that the time and space of the session is set aside to better understand what bothers the child.

> In Mary's case, an interruption in the therapy when I informed her that I would be away for a month after 4 months of treatment brought transference material to our attention. She was first sad, said how much she would miss me, and poignantly remarked that her life "had gotten so much better" since she started seeing me. But sadness soon gave way to anger, at least in the metaphor of her play. She staged vicious fights between dinosaurs, insisting that I play the role of the meat-eating dinosaur while she played the plant-eater's role. She accused me, as a meat eater, of lying and cheating. A sense of betrayal dominated her play and associations, but she agreed to make a plan to deal with the dinosaurs' hunger and rage during my absence. She identified a number of sources of food, including fast food restaurants, pizza parlors, and grocery stores, where the beasts could find nourishment without killing each other until I returned.

It should be noted that all comments and interpretations derived from the play were kept within the context of the play situations about the play figures. Clinical experience suggests that interpreting the play in reference to the patient's "real" feelings in actuality only disrupts the child's communication (Feigelson 1977). Thus, I did *not* link her reference to cheating, vicious meat eaters to her disappointment at my departure and her anger projected onto me.

Therapy resumed after a 4-week interruption. While I was away, she soiled frequently and became rather belligerent with her parents and sister. She seemed, however, eager to start right back where we had left off and let me know that despite her difficulties she had kept in mind her "plan" to soothe the dinosaurs.

Mary shared a fantasy about my absence: I had left to have babies. This fantasy was expressed in the metaphor of the play: one of the dinosaurs became pregnant and would soon give birth to four babies. This "birth" gave us an opportunity to examine feelings of rivalry and deprivation and related fears of abandonment and punishment. One of the babies, wishing to have mother dinosaur all to herself, was viciously attacked by her siblings.

At a meeting with her parents, we planned together a token economy program to address the encopresis, which greatly bothered them. Mary could get a small item—she chose little plastic dinosaurs—by going to the bathroom on her own. Her parents could thus simultaneously structure and nurture, helping her gain control while providing gratification linked to her own metaphorical vehicle.

Encopresis and enuresis improved greatly, but a new symptom developed: an insect phobia. She was afraid that a bug would crawl onto her. I did not address the possible sexual aspects of her phobia or of her concerns about my babies. Aggression was clearly close to her conscious awareness, whereas sexuality was not. Thus, I commented over a number of sessions on how thinking of me having babies made her angry and concerned that she would be punished for her angry thoughts—abandoned and left with no food or hurt in another way. As she acknowledged this interpretation, I could point out to her how she tried to avoid this predicament by either keeping everything, especially her anger, under tight control, or when that failed, she wished to pretend that she could go back to being a messy baby herself, pooping in her pants but innocent of hostile and competitive intentions.

She responded to these interventions by developing a new play theme centered on how dangerous animal mommies become after they have a baby: not only do they need to find food for themselves, but also for their babies. Mary made herself the link between the play and her competitive feelings toward her mother. She remembered her sister's birth and her father taking her to the hospital to visit. She was demonstrating at this point, about 7 months after the beginning of therapy, 1) that she identified with the basic task of understanding and 2) that she felt that her anger and rivalry had become safe enough that she could explore them without relying so extensively on repression and other associated defense mechanisms.

Exploring the theme of the "dangerous mommy" allowed us to examine the dangers of turning to father for comfort and maybe having babies of her own. As we talked and played about these issues, the paternal transference intensified. She mistakenly called me daddy during the sessions and coyly and excitedly planned to cook meals for me.

These ventures into Oedipal relatedness alternated with forceful displays of her own independent strength. A puppet whale, for example, whose spout had been "bent" and who had lost the power to squirt with it, recovered this capacity and learned to leap high into the sky. Her greater confidence carried into other areas of her life outside of the sessions. Ten months after beginning treatment, she began the first grade with enthusiasm, quickly excelling in reading and writing and even showing some comfort and joy in playing with peers.

The excitement and success were not devoid of anxiety. She equated the "fullness" in her stomach after a pretend meal she had cooked for me to the satisfaction of hunger but also to the fullness associated with fecal retention and to the thoughts she had about how it would feel to be pregnant. As we explored these themes, she worried about getting hurt or hurting me. After one "meal," when we both ate until we were totally full, she became concerned that she would get heartburn and wondered whether heartburn can lead to heart attacks. In a more symbolic way she reported that the "whale" had a dream: it wished to rest on my foot, yet in the end it bites me and hurts me.

As her anxiety mounted, she would return to obsessive concerns and wishes to control and line up animals in precise ways. If her anxiety escalated even more, she would become preoccupied with themes of hunger, deprivation, and raw aggression, typically played out by dinosaurs. This sequence, from humans to contemporary animals to dinosaurs, correlated with the intensity of her anxiety linked to specific stressors, mainly interruptions in the therapy. Yet her functioning outside of the sessions was not, by and large, affected by the fluctuations in her "status" in the evolutionary scale.

Mary demonstrates how the major themes in neurotic children's lives come to be concentrated in the therapeutic relationship, which opens the possibility of correcting distortions; mastering conflicts and anxieties; overcoming repression; gaining information that interrupts maladaptive interactions; and, more generally, taking advantage of developmental opportunities like school and friends.

Regression and progression alternate as children struggle to face conflicts and anxieties without undue repression. Yet they retain the capacity for the symbolic transformation of their experience, which allows them to communicate in metaphorical ways and utilize interpretations. Their ability to bring their concerns out of the metaphor and link their actual experience to their play signals a major step forward in the therapeutic alliance and the internalization of the therapeutic attitude to solving problems.

MIDDLE PHASE IN THE PSYCHOTHERAPY OF CHILDREN WITH CONDUCT DISORDER

The readiness of children with conduct disorders to enter the middle phase of therapy is signaled by two indicators: the obvious appearance of anxiety and the beginning of a therapeutic alliance. Anxiety is generated largely by the representational mismatch created by the holding environment—whether the parents' greater competence or the limits of the inpatient milieu. To some degree, however, anxiety also can be traced to the children's own wishes for closeness with their therapists and the dawning conviction (fraught with uncertainty and fears of being subjugated, destroyed, or humiliated) that hope and help can be derived from therapeutic relationships. Only rarely can these youngsters openly acknowledge their attachment to their therapists. More commonly, children can demonstrate some embryonic collaboration in the form of sharing experiences with the therapists or in using their treaters to find face-saving solutions to the adults' "conspiracy" to deprive them of their usual coping mechanisms.

The presence of some form of collaborative relationship allows therapists to gently encourage their patients to consider an expansion in the range of "shareable" experiences. Narcissistic youngsters are invited to share their experiences of vulnerability, depression, pain, helplessness, and dependency. Borderline and impulsive children are introduced to the notion of continuity of the self and relationships. Depressed patients are encouraged to look at the restrictions in their play and emotional range.

> Jimmy, a 10-year-old narcissistic boy, created a play theme in which his father was the president of the United States. This pathetic father-president, however, could barely function without Jimmy's guidance. Jimmy instructed the therapist to play the role of the father and relished ordering him around, barking directives for the country. The therapist began to point out the child's desire to share in the power of an exalted, yet secretly diminished, ruler. If he could share in such power, maybe he would not have to feel little, vulnerable, or envious of anyone else.

Only at this point can therapists attempt to systematically confront children's characteristic defenses and begin the exploration of the motives and functions of those defenses. However, as children face their vulnerability, pain, and depression, they are filled with stark panic. Jimmy, for example, became extremely anxious when the therapist pointed out his defensive need to cover up fears of helplessness and vulnerability. Yet this vignette illustrates also a tentative foray into the realm of symbolization.

Not surprisingly, a heightened reliance on old defensive mechanisms becomes apparent: efforts to control, devalue, intimidate, manipulate, or seduce the therapists; rejection of help; running away; abuse of drugs; intensified antisocial behavior outside of the sessions; or attempts to pit parents and therapists against each other.

Joe, a 13-year-old borderline narcissistic boy, had been subjected to brutal physical and sexual abuse by an alcoholic father, while his mother pursued her theatrical career. Almost in spite of himself he began to feel more comfortable with me, even to look forward to the sessions. Yet desires for closeness were almost unbearable for him. Thus, he began to carefully look for "mistakes" (e.g., interrupting him or "invading" his space while walking), which triggered hateful barrages. He let me know of his plans to run away from the hospital and find out my house's location ("I have good sources, you know") so he could set it on fire after raping my wife and murdering my children with slow, intravenous injections of cocaine. He would spare my life, but only to ensure that I would suffer the devastation of the loss of everything I hold dear.

Joe's tirade spoke volumes about what closeness meant to him: a painful, destructive invasion of his house-fortress, a rape, and a painful penetration of his body and bloodstream that could evoke burning, devastating feelings leading to total collapse; the envy of my possessions and my relationships and the associated rage at his own deprivation and abuse; and the wish to eliminate all possible rivals for my love but also the desire to leave me as deprived, lonely, and needy as him.

Obviously, such outbursts evoke rather intense countertransferential responses in the treaters. Interestingly, while attempting to weather the storm of Joe's vindictive rage, I felt neither threatened nor cut off from him. I wondered whether he wished to provoke me yet remain connected to me, all the while denying any attachment. He seemed to tell me that he did not love me. In fact, he hated me. I was a pedantic, know-it-all, rich shrink who could not possibly understand someone steeled by a life in the mean streets of the big city.

Sensing his desire to maintain a relationship while overtly disowning it, I commented on the meanness and cruelty of his imagery. Where did that come from? He looked at me with a mix of contempt and amusement and proceeded to describe, in a wildly exaggerated fashion, the toughness of his neighborhood and its brutal gang wars. He was sure that my wimpy, nerdy self had been shielded from such roughness.

Together with contempt and devaluation, I sensed an inviting, playful teasing in Joe's account of his gang escapades. In effect, he had grown up in the far more sedate environment of an upper-middle-class community in New England. His interest in and knowledge of gangs had mostly been acquired through extensive reading on the subject. Before his outburst he had brought to the sessions magazines and tapes glorifying the Bloods, the Latin Kings, and other equally unsavory characters.

I picked up (perhaps with more hope than conviction) on the implied teasing and replied with an even more fantastic account of my own heroic battles as a gang kingpin—a secret identity hidden behind my deceptively mild appearance.

He seemed to enjoy this gambit, and over the next few sessions we engaged in a good deal of increasingly more good-natured bantering. Only after we reestablished our relationship at a distance that he could more readily tolerate did I return his attention to the rage he had experienced and the abuse he had inflicted on me.

This vignette illustrates how these youngsters often require a transitional area of relatedness akin to Winnicott's (1953) transitional experience. In this transitional, as-if area (often jointly created by patient and therapist) standing between fantasy and reality, patients can both own and disown their rejected feelings and experiences and test out the therapist's attunement, respect, and responsiveness to the vulnerable aspects of the self.

Younger narcissistic patients often introduce, as a transitional relationship, a play theme involving an imaginary twin. The twin typically embodies the "weak," dependent, sad, helpless experiences these children find unbearable. Another version of the transitional experience, common to all children with conduct disorders, is somatic complaints. These complaints offer a way of requesting help without acknowledging it and of reconnecting with feelings of pain and inadequacy while keeping open the possibility of disowning such feelings.

Borderline youngsters fight mightily to prevent a disruption of their transitional space. They create play themes so vivid and absorbing that they, and at times their therapists, can no longer tell the difference between fantasy and reality. They come to life in their play theme while adamantly refusing to let reality intrude and thereby question the arbitrariness they need to impose on their life and relationships.

Cory, a Taiwanese-born 8-year-old girl, was adopted as a baby by a Caucasian family from the Midwest. Threats of separation from her adoptive mother triggered dramatic disruptions in Cory's reality contact as well as raging outbursts, stealing, and disruptive behavior in school. The possibility of a separation, such as when mother visited her own mother in a nearby town for a few days, prompted Cory to hold on to an elaborate fantasy about her biological mother, whom she "knew" was an Asian princess.

The fantasy was extraordinarily vivid for Cory and animated her lashing out at the world, where reality failed to appreciate her entitlement to royal prerogatives. Yet even without reality's assistance, a dream of a bad thought typically sufficed to disrupt the idyllic fantasy. In her dreams and play the Asian princess would be replaced by a witch, a vicious vixen whose features combined Asian and Caucasian traits. This woman would taunt Cory and try to drag her to a bottomless pit, leaving the child with no choice but to strangle the witch in self-defense. Cory herself changed. Without the love and protection of the princess, she would become a "Chinese bitch." These play themes were soon incorporated into her therapy.

As the vignette illustrates, the transitional sphere of the play's theme provides the illusion of a perfect, magical union with the therapist. At the same time, the split-off, threatening aspects of both the patient's self and of the real world are kept safely apart.

Tooley's (1973) "Playing It Right: A Technique for the Treatment of Borderline Children" is a beautiful account of how the therapist can more closely attempt to align borderline children's play and fantasy to reality's constraints. Gradually, children are nudged to introduce small modifications in their play to better encompass the complexities, limitations, conflicts, and frustrations of reality. The transitional space of play and fantasy becomes a stage in which to try out new identifications, to practice imagined solutions to life's dilemmas, to explore new ways of being in the world and relating to others, and to test behavior that promises greater mastery, more effective coping, and increased pleasure and adaptation. In particular, it offers borderline children the magic of anonymity in which to attempt to bring together split-off representations of the self and others.

In the safe haven of the transitional sphere of relatedness, therapists can confront children with the systematic exploration of the youngsters' pathological defenses and the motives for such defenses. In particular, they can examine, as in Cory's case, the advantages of splitting, that is, of keeping the hated and hateful image of the witch carefully disconnected from the memory of the loving and lovely princess. Thus, in a transitional space children can be invited to consider that a whole section of their experience stands unlived, so to speak—never owned or shared.

Therapists' acknowledgment of the utter terror children feel as they enter into a rejected, dissociated, denied aspect of their lives and relationships can prevent therapeutic stalemates and limit regression. Therapists should always point out the many advantages of *not* changing—in effect, the price children would pay if they were to give up their maladaptive, but often life-saving, defenses. Ultimately, therapists present to their patients, implicitly or explicitly, a therapeutic "bargain": relinquishing pathological defenses and the illusion of control and safety they provide for the far more exposed and laborious process of attempting to achieve real mastery and meaningful relationships.

Such a bargain is unlikely to prove appealing unless a number of factors are operant in the children's interpersonal world. Thus, it is essential for the psychotherapist to maintain close and ongoing contact with the hospital or residential treatment staff and the family therapist. Such meetings provide invaluable information to both the psychotherapist and the staff regarding the child's subjective experience, the realities of his or her life, and the ways that milieu, family treatment, and psychotherapy can be effectively aligned. Family treatment must address the powerful coalitions often apparent between one of the parents and the symptomatic child. It is particularly imperative to extricate these children from their roles as saviors, confidants, or special partners of one of the parents (typically the other-sex parent). At the same time, opportunities should be provided to foster the relationship between children and the same-sex parent while promoting the ability of that same-sex parent to function as a model to the children (a relationship that requires the other parent's sanction).

The family therapist gives the individual psychotherapists access to a vantage point from which to assess the consequences to the family of the patients' relinquishment of symptoms and the anxieties that the children's changes may trigger in the family. Bringing the parents into the treatment serves to address a major source of resistance to treatment: the children's overwhelming anxiety that their growth and change will shatter the family and cause the parents to hurt one another, divorce, commit suicide, or abandon the children.

Educational programs and activity and occupational therapy provide opportunities to promote real mastery and competence, thus lessening children's need to rely on illusory solutions. Yet teachers and other therapists need to sensitively approach children's fears of exposing their limitations and the gaps in their knowledge. Cognitive approaches are useful in the individual sessions to increase children's ability to anticipate ways of relating to peers and to provide new sources of support and identification.

Interventions that change children's interpersonal context help bring to the fore material that is usefully pursued in individual psychotherapy. Themes of dependency, safety, autonomy, envy, rage, and vulnerability become available for exploration, often mixed with items of Oedipal competition, fears of loss of body integrity, and unconscious guilt over destructive wishes. Just as important as the attunement to feelings of real pain and vulnerability is the therapist's sharing in the real joy, renewed hope, and genuine pride children experience as a result of their growth, increased competence, and comfort with their feelings.

TERMINATION PHASE: MOURNING AND RESUMING DEVELOPMENT

The harbingers of termination for both neurotic and conduct disorder children are found both within and without the therapy process. Naturally, sustained amelioration of symptomatic behavior is a hopeful sign. For children with conduct disorders, the development of nondelinquent peer relationships and interests is perhaps more significant than the simple absence of overt antisocial activities. Changes in family interaction and school functioning are particularly important. Children's growing ability to utilize their parents and other nondelinquent adults as sources of protection and comfort and as models of identification bodes the end of the psychotherapeutic process. When children can approach parents and teachers for help in solving problems in reality, the beginning of termination is in view.

Within the therapeutic process itself, therapists recognize other clues of impending termination: children's open acknowledgment of missing the therapist during interruptions and vacations; youngsters' expressions of gratitude for help received; patients' spontaneously bringing to the sessions their sense of how they utilize something they learned in therapy outside of the sessions; and—perhaps the most sensitive clue—patients' bringing to the sessions their sense of loss about missed or botched opportunities and life's unfairness.

The final stage of psychotherapy offers a chance to test children's readiness to relinquish pathological defenses. Beginning to discuss with patients and parents a termination date fuels anxiety and often brings about a reactivation of symptoms in the patient and of dysfunctional interaction patterns in the parents.

Jill, a 10-year-old girl in residential treatment, began attending public school. This move meant clearly that discharge from the residential treatment center and termination of psychotherapy were looming. This narcissistic girl proceeded—as was characteristic of her before beginning treatment—to alienate her classmates with her petulance and manipulativeness, tall tales about extraordinary accomplishments, and demands to be the center of everyone's attention. Along with this return of old patterns, Jill attempted to present in therapy a rosy picture of her adaptation to the world outside of the residential treatment center. She was liked by her peers, she said, was eagerly sought out as a playmate, and could count two or three girls as her best friends.

Only a school report brought home the true picture of Jill's struggles. Confronted with the discrepancy, Jill could speak of her fears of disappointing me, the residential unit staff, and her parents. She wondered whether her progress was all contingent on the therapy and the staff's support, and worried whether she could sustain it without such a protective envelope. She was skeptical as to whether her parents and I would really appreciate her if she was anything less than a perfect, smashing success. Could she be loved if she was just a regular girl? Only after much work did another dimension of the girl's regression emerge: her difficulties in dealing with the sadness and loss associated with termination.

Mourning the anticipated loss of the therapy and the therapist is an essential task of the termination phase. Just as important is the opportunity to work through children's disappointments: with their own shortcomings, with the adults that never measured up to their expectations, with everything they could not achieve in therapy, and with the therapists' limitations.

For Mary, termination brought back some anxiety about the future and fears of dying. She was able, however, to talk of her "old" fear of growing up now without my help. Here again, she was demonstrating how capable she was of carrying the therapeutic attitude within herself. More importantly, Mary evidenced a capacity to undo the transference relationship and to appreciate our relationship as having had a specific function that was now close to completion. She gave herself a birthday party as termination approached and spoke confidently of the future. In her play, parental figures became more helpful and competent in assisting children.

But regardless of whether or not regression and symptomatic reactivation occur, the termination phase requires a relaxation of supervision, particularly for children with conduct disorders. Naturally, such a stance is not without risk.

Adam offers an example of the vicissitudes that can be encountered during termination.

Adam, a 12-year-old boy, had found himself in the state's custody after repeated desertions by his mother. His unremitting destructiveness and defiance landed him in a residential treatment center. There he explained to his therapist, in the metaphor of his play, the reasons for his hatred: the therapist, who was the leader of the "Irans" (this vignette occurred at the time of the Teheran embassy hostage crisis), had kidnapped the mother of "Billy." Billy naturally was bent on revenge and fully intended to rob all the banks in the world and kill people until his mother was released.

Much work went into slowly turning this play theme around until it could encompass the possibilities of maternal abandonment, rage at mother, and the notion that Billy's badness, greed, and neediness had damaged mother and driven her away.

As discharge to a group home was becoming a realistic possibility, Adam ran away. However, he returned on his own a few days later. He had traveled more than 100 miles and had located his mother (a feat that had eluded the investigative powers of the child protective services). Having found her, he said, he had made peace with this distraught and rather limited woman. Soberly, Adam told his mother that "he knew what she had done," and no matter what happened between them, he still loved her and would go on with his life. Anna Freud could not have stated more eloquently the criterion for termination: children's experience of reinstatement into the path of growth and development.

CONCLUSION

This sketchy review fails to do justice to the complexities that are part and parcel of the psychotherapeutic treatment of youngsters with neurosis and conduct disorders. Systematic evaluation of the effectiveness of this and other treatment models is sorely needed before more definitive statements can be made regarding what interventions, in what timing or sequence, predict positive outcomes in children with specific forms of neurosis or conduct disorders.

Developmental research continues to push the boundaries of our understanding of how subjective experience is organized and structured. Family therapists' growing appreciation of individual differences is building new bridges between family and individual psychotherapy. These advances promise to dramatically enhance our conceptual sophistication and clinical effectiveness.

For now, clinical experience suggests that individual psychotherapy can play a pivotal role in helping break the grip that anxiety and vulnerability have fastened on these children.

REFERENCES

Achenbach T, Edelbrock CS: The classification of child psychopathology: a review and analysis of empirical efforts. Psychol Bull 85:1275–1301, 1978

Aichhorn A: Wayward Youth. New York, Viking, 1935

American Psychiatric Association: Diagnostic and Statistical Manual of Mental Disorders, 3rd Edition, Revised. Washington, DC, American Psychiatric Association, 1987

Barrnett R, Docherty J, Frommelt G: A review of child psychotherapy research since 1963. J Am Acad Child Adolesc Psychiatry 30:1–14, 1991

Bleiberg E: Stages in the treatment of narcissistic children and adolescents. Bull Menninger Clin 51:296–313,1987

Bleiberg E: Stages of residential treatment: application of a developmental model. Residential Treatment for Children and Youth 6(4):7–28, 1989

Chethik M: Techniques of Child Therapy: Psychodynamic Strategies. New York, Guilford, 1989

Christiansen KO: A review of studies of criminality among twins, in Biosocial Bases of Criminal Behavior. Edited by Mednick S, Christiansen KO. New York, Gardner, 1977, pp 89–108

Cloward RA, Ohlin LE: Delinquency and Opportunity. Chicago, IL, Free Press, 1960

Crits-Cristoph P, Luborsky L, Dahl L, et al: Clinicians can agree in assessing relationship patterns in psychotherapy. Arch Gen Psychiatry 45:1001–1004, 1988

Erikson E: Childhood and Society. New York, WW Norton, 1963

Fenichel O: The Psychoanalytic Theory of Neurosis. New York, WW Norton, 1945

Feigelson CI: Essential characteristics of child analysis. Psychoanal Study Child 32:353–361, 1977

Freud S: The dissolution of the Oedipus complex (1924), in The Standard Edition of the Complete Psychological Works of Sigmund Freud, Vol 19. Edited by Strachey J. London, Hogarth Press, 1961, pp 173–182

Freud S: The analysis of a phobia in a five-year-old boy (1909), in The Standard Edition of the Complete Psychological Works of Sigmund Freud, Vol 10. Edited by Strachey J. London, Hogarth Press, 1955, pp 3–152

Greenson RR: The Technique and Practice of Psychoanalysis. New York, International Universities Press, 1967

Gunderson JG, Zanarini MC: Pathogenesis of borderline personality. Am Rev Psychiatry 8:25–48, 1989

Hartley, DE, Strupp, HH: The therapeutic alliance: its relationship to outcome in brief psychotherapy, in Empirical Studies of Psychoanalytical Theories, Vol 1. Edited by Masling J. Hillsdale, NJ, Analytic Press, 1983, pp 7–11

Hartman H, Loewenstein R: Notes on the superego. Psychoanal Study Child 17:42–81, 1962

Hoffman L: An introduction to child psychoanalysis. Journal of Clinical Psychoanalysis 2:5–26, 1993

Horowitz M: States of Mind: Configurational Analysis of Individual Personality, New York, Plenum, 1987

Johnson AM, Szurek SA: The genesis of antisocial acting out in children and adults. Psychoanal Q 21:323–343, 1952

Katz CL: Aggressive children, in Psychotherapies With Children and Adolescents: Adapting the Psychodynamic Process. Edited by O'Brien JD, Pilowsky DJ, Lewis OW. Washington, DC, American Psychiatric Press, 1992, pp 91–108

Kazdin AE: Psychotherapy for children and adolescents: current progress and future research directions. Am Psychologist 4836:644–657, 1993

Kazdin AE, Siegel TC, Bass D: Drawing upon clinical practice to inform research on child and adolescent psychotherapy: a survey of practitioners. Professional Psychology: Research and Practice 21:189–198, 1990

Kazdin AE, Siegel TC, Bass D: Cognitive problem solving, skills-training and parent management training in the treatment of antisocial behavior in children. J Consult Clin Psychol 733–747, 1992

Kendall P: Child and Adolescent Therapy: Cognitive-Behavioral Procedures. New York, Guilford, 1991

Kernberg OF: Factors in the treatment of narcissistic personalities. J Am Psychoanal Assoc 22:243–254, 1975

Kernberg PF, Chazan SE: Children with Conduct Disorders: A Psychotherapy Manual. New York, Basic Books, 1991

Kohut H: The Analysis of The Self. New York, International Universities Press, 1971

Lewis DO: Neuropsychiatric vulnerabilities and violent juvenile delinquency. Psychiatr Clin North Am 6:707–714, 1983

Lewis DO, Lewis M, Unger L, et al: Conduct disorder and its synonyms: diagnosis of dubious validity and usefulness. Am J Psychiatry 141:514–519, 1984

Luborsky L: Helping alliances in psychotherapy, in Successful Psychotherapy. Edited by Claghorn JL. New York, Brunner/Mazel, 1976, pp 92–116

Luborsky L, Crits-Cristoph P, Mintz J, et al: Who Will Benefit From Psychotherapy? Predicting Therapeutic Outcomes. New York, Basic Books, 1981

Marohn RC: Psychotherapy of adolescents with behavioral disorders, in Adolescent Psychotherapy. Edited by Slomowitz M. Washington, DC, American Psychiatric Press, 1991, pp 145–161

Marohn RC, Offer D, Ostrov E, et al: Four psychodynamic types of hospitalized juvenile delinquents. Adolesc Psychiatry 7:466–483, 1979

Marohn RC, Dalle-Molle D, McCarter E, et al: Juvenile Delinquents: Psychodynamic Assessment and Hospital Treatment. New York, Brunner/Mazel, 1980

Masterson J: Psychotherapy of the Disorders of the Self. New York, Brunner/Mazel, 1988

Minuchin S, Fishman HC: Family Therapy Techniques. Cambridge, MA, Harvard University Press, 1981

Nagera H: Early Childhood Disturbances, the Infantile Neurosis, and the Adult Disturbances. New York, International Universities Press, 1966

O'Brien JD: Children with attention-deficit hyperactivity disorder and their parents, in Psychotherapies With Children and Adolescents: Adapting the Psychodynamic Process. Edited by O'Brien JD, Pilowsky DJ, Lewis OW. Washington, DC, American Psychiatric Press, 1992, pp 109–124

Patterson G: Coercive Family Process. Eugene, OR, Castilia, 1982

Patterson GR, Reid JB, Dishion TJ: Antisocial Boys. Eugene, OR, Castilia, 1992

Redl F, Wineman D: The Aggressive Child. Glencoe, IL, Free Press, 1957

Rinsley D: Developmental Pathogenesis and Treatment of Borderline and Narcissistic Disorders. New York, Jason Aronson, 1989

Rutter M, Giller H: Juvenile Delinquency. New York, Guilford, 1983

Silver L, Silver B: Clinical practice of child psychiatry. Journal of the American Academy of Child Psychiatry 22:573–579, 1983

Tooley K: Playing it right—a technique for the treatment of borderline children. Journal of the American Academy of Child Psychiatry 12:615–631, 1973

Tysson P: Neurosis in childhood and in psychoanalysis. Paper presented at the annual meeting of the American Psychoanalytic Association, New York, December 1992

Winnicott DW: Transitional objects and transitional phenomena. Int J Psychoanal 34(2):89–97, 1953

Winnicott DW: The antisocial tendency, in Collected Papers. New York, Basic Books, 1958, pp 306–315

Chapter 21

The Neuropsychiatric Disorders: ADHD, OCD, and Tourette's Syndrome

Robert A. King, M.D., and Donald J. Cohen, M.D.

The classification of Tourette's syndrome (TS), attention-deficit hyperactivity disorder (ADHD), and certain forms of obsessive-compulsive disorder (OCD) as *neuropsychiatric* disorders reflects the presumption that these conditions have a primarily neurobiological, rather than psychosocial, etiology. This presumption, however, is not incompatible with the notion that psychological factors may influence the onset, course, and severity of these disorders. All three disorders have primary psychological manifestations, as well as significant secondary effects on the patient's psychosocial development. In addition, patients (and their families) give psychological meanings to the symptoms and to the fact of patienthood. Finally, psychological factors influence patients' engagement with, compliance with, and reactions to all forms of treatment, including pharmacotherapy.

All of these considerations imply that psychological therapies have an important role to play in the management of these childhood neuropsychiatric disorders. The availability of medications that can partially or completely suppress many of the pathognomonic symptoms of these disorders should not obscure the fact that the goal of treatment is not merely symptom suppression. Rather, it is to help individuals move forward successfully with their developmental tasks of establishing gratifying relationships with family and peers, functioning competently at school or at work, and consolidating a positive identity and healthy sense of self-esteem (Towbin et al. 1988).

Despite many contrasting features, TS, ADHD, and OCD share certain commonalities that have important implications for psychological management. These three conditions often have 1) a familial component; 2) a childhood onset; 3) a chronic course, albeit with fluctuations

This chapter distills the collective experience and collaborative efforts of the Specialty Clinic Staff of the Yale Child Study Center, including James F. Leckman, M.D.; Mark A. Riddle, M.D.; Kenneth E. Towbin, M.D.; Sharon I. Ort, R.N., M.P.H.; Larry Scahill, M.S.N., M.P.H.; Phyllis Cohen, Ed.D.; Lawrence A. Vitulano, Ph.D.; Maureen T. Hardin, M.S.N.; and Kimberly A. Lynch, M.S.N.

or developmental shifts in clinical phenomenology; 4) a deleterious impact on social, emotional, cognitive, and family functioning; 5) and a frequent association with anxiety disorders or depression, or both. All three disorders also confront both the patient and others with important but difficult-to-resolve questions: "What is the disorder? What is the self?"

THE CLINICAL DISORDERS

Tourette's Syndrome

TS is defined by the presence of multiple motor and vocal tics, which persist over at least a year, despite fluctuations in location and severity.

TS provides a useful paradigm for other childhood-onset neuropsychiatric disorders in that it is characterized by 1) an apparent genetically determined vulnerability; 2) a changing expression of symptoms with age, reflecting maturational factors; 3) sexual dimorphism; 4) stress-dependent fluctuations in symptom severity; and 5) apparent environmental influences on the phenotypic expression of the underlying genotype (Leckman et al. 1988). (For comprehensive reviews of TS, see Chase et al. 1992; Cohen et al. 1988; King and Noshpitz 1991; and Kurlan 1993.)

Tics may range from *simple* tics (such as blinks, grimaces, arm or head jerks, grunts, throat clearing, sniffing) to more *complex* tics (such as clapping, touching, or blurted-out words or phrases). These tics may occur in a virtually inexhaustible variety of patterns and combinations that typically wax and wane over weeks or months. Their intensity may be so mild that only the patient or a trained observer notices them or so violent as to result in serious damage or self-injury. Tics most frequently first appear between ages 5 and 10 years, with progression from upper to lower parts of the body and from simple to more complex. Fatigue, stress, and excitement often exacerbate tics.

Although the most severe and dramatic cases initially attracted clinicians' notice, recent epidemiological studies reveal that there are a large number of milder cases, many of which may never come to clinical attention (Apter et al. 1992; Zahner et al. 1988).

Some individuals experience their tics as completely involuntary; others report a premonitory urge to perform the tic to which they ultimately submit, although efforts to suppress or resist it may be transiently successful (Bliss 1980; Leckman et al. 1993). For such patients, the distinction between what is actively willed and what is involuntarily experienced is constantly called into question, with an attendant blurring of the boundary between what is the self and what is the disease (Cohen 1990, 1991).

Obsessions and compulsions are common in individuals with TS and their families. Simple compulsions, such as touching, may be difficult to distinguish phenomenologically from complex tics. The OCD symptoms associated with TS, however, may be identical to those found in individuals without tic disorder (Leonard et al. 1992). Family studies suggest that TS and some forms of OCD are alternative phenotypic manifestations of an autosomal dominant trait (Pauls et al. 1991).

ADHD, learning difficulties, irritability, and affective lability are found in as many of 25% of children with TS and are often apparent even before the onset of tics. It is unclear to what extent these difficulties represent part of a genetically determined TS diathesis or an artifact of ascertainment bias in clinical samples, reflecting the greater likelihood that more severe cases or those complicated by comorbid conditions will come to clinical attention (Cohen and Leckman 1993; Cohen et al. 1992).

The degree of functional impairment is not directly related to tic severity per se (Cohen and Leckman 1993). Some individuals with very severe tics function well; in contrast, other children with mild tics, but prominent ADHD and OCD features, may do very poorly, with impaired academic and social functioning and attendant low self-esteem (Stokes et al. 1991).

The impact of puberty on the course of TS is variable. In the majority of cases, tics diminish in severity and number by young adulthood. As tics diminish in significance with age, however, OCD symptoms may come into greater prominence.

Haloperidol, pimozide, and clonidine are the most widely used drugs, but require careful management. Even when effective in reducing tics, these agents may produce psychologically significant side effects. Sleepiness, irritability, and cognitive blunting are potential dose-related side effects of all three agents, and the neuroleptics may produce depression or drug-induced separation anxiety as well (Bruun 1988; Leckman et al. 1991; Linet 1985; Shapiro et al. 1989).

Obsessive-Compulsive Disorder

OCD is defined by the presence of functionally impairing or subjectively distressing obsessions and compulsions that are experienced as ego-dystonic and resisted (American Psychiatric Association 1987). (For a comprehensive review of OCD, see King and Noshpitz 1991 and Rapoport 1989.)

Epidemiological surveys suggest that OCD occurs in 0.35% to 3.6% of adolescents (Flament et al. 1988; Zohar et al. 1992) and represents one end of a continuum of severity that includes many individuals with milder ego-syntonic or nonimpairing obsessions and compulsions. As many as half of adults with OCD report their symptoms began before age 15.

Common obsessions and compulsions include washing and contamination concerns, checking, arranging, touching, counting, doubting, religious scrupulosity, and "evening up." Many patients describe having to repeat a mental or physical act until they get it "just right" (Leckman et al., in press). In young children, ego-dystonicity and the degree of resistance may be difficult to determine.

Follow-up studies suggest that although the exact content of their obsessions and compulsions may change, many individuals with OCD continue to be symptomatic for years (Berg et al. 1989; Rettew et al. 1992).

The personality context in which childhood OCD occurs is variable. At one time, OCD was considered to be an extreme manifestation of a compulsive personality style characterized by perfectionism, excessive meticulousness and rigidity, and emotional constriction (Adams 1973). The majority of children with OCD, however, do not have a compulsive personality and indeed may even be irritable, labile, or impulsive outside the area of their particular symptom (King and Noshpitz 1991; Riddle et al. 1990; Swedo et al. 1989b). However, there does appear to be a subgroup of children whose frank obsessions and compulsions occur against the backdrop of an anxiously perfectionist style, characterized by emotional overcontrol and a burdened scrupulousness.

Many children with OCD are ashamed and furtive about their symptoms, at least with peers and teachers, who may remain unaware of the child's difficulties. At home, however, family life may be severely disturbed by the child's extensive rituals, which may occupy up to several hours a day and entail the parents' coerced participation. Some children become withdrawn and socially isolated as their rituals, obsessive concerns, and social or separation anxieties increasingly interfere with school and peer activities. In such children, depression may be an important component of the clinical picture.

Traditional psychodynamic approaches to OCD have emphasized the excessive, maladaptive use of intellectualization; reaction formation; affective isolation; and other obsessional defenses against conflicts over aggressive or libidinal concerns (Adams 1973). More recent neurobiological paradigms point to the role of genetically determined or acquired dysfunctions of the basal ganglia and serotonergic dysregulation (Rapoport 1989). Many cases of OCD appear to be familial, with an increased prevalence of OCD and tic disorder in the families of some OCD probands and an increased prevalence of anxiety disorder without tics in the families of other OCD probands (Black et al. 1992); still other cases appear to be nonfamilial. Whether these various subtypes of OCD differ in phenomenology or treatment responsiveness is unclear (King et al. 1992).

How to reconcile these competing explanatory paradigms remains a challenge. Many cases of OCD clearly appear to be neurobiological in origin, especially those linked to a TS genetic diathesis or to basal ganglia dysfunction, for example, Sydenham's chorea (Swedo et al. 1989a). Some cases, however, do appear to be more susceptible to psychodynamic formulation and intervention. These include transient obsessional symptoms in toddlers faced with parental demands for increased impulse control, as well as cases involving perfectionist latency-age children or adolescents struggling with phase-specific conflicts over aggression or sexual concerns. Such dynamic formulations are, of course, fully compatible with the possibility that the choice of obsessive-compulsive defenses and symptoms as a coping style may be partially determined by genetic or constitutional factors (Freud 1965).

Effective pharmacological treatment of OCD relies on serotonin reuptake inhibitors such as the tricyclic antidepressant clomipramine or the more specific serotonergic antidepressants fluoxetine, fluvoxamine, sertraline, and paroxetine (King et al. 1992). Behavioral side effects of these agents include disinhibition, agitation, hypomania, and, in rare cases, intrusive self-destructive ideation (King et al. 1991; Riddle et al. 1991).

Attention-Deficit Hyperactivity Disorder

ADHD is defined by symptoms of impulsivity, inattention, and motoric restlessness that have their onset before age 7. Considerable controversy exists about the appropriate diagnostic criteria and the syndromic validity of the condition, given the high prevalence of such symptoms reported by teachers and parents in community samples, the overlap with other syndromes (such as the other disruptive disorders), and wide cross-national differences in diagnosed prevalence. (For a comprehensive review of ADHD, see Barkley 1990 and King and Noshpitz 1991.)

Features frequently associated with ADHD include emotional lability, irritability, learning and language difficulties, and poor social skills. Not surprisingly, depression, anxiety, and conduct disorder are also common concomitant conditions. The low self-esteem of children with ADHD is understandable in light of the cumulative difficulties they encounter at school, with peers, and at home because of their impulsivity, inattentiveness, and poor social judgment.

Although motor restlessness may decrease in adolescence, other core symptoms frequently persist into young adulthood. Long-term follow-up studies of children with ADHD find an apparent increased rate of conduct problems, legal difficulties, and substance use in late adolescence, especially among the substantial number of subjects with persistent ADHD symptoms (Klein and Mannuzza 1991). Although these difficulties may decrease in young adulthood, ADHD subjects as a group attain lower educational and vocational adult status than suitable control subjects.

Etiological speculation has largely centered on constitutional factors of genetic or perinatal origin. Neurochemical, electrophysiological, imaging, and neuropsychiatric studies have attempted to elucidate these hypotheses. Several lines of evidence point to possible dysregulation of monoaminergic neurotransmitter systems, especially those involving dopamine. The recent evidence from imaging studies that cerebral metabolism is reduced in the prefrontal and premotor cortex, left temporal and parietal cortex, and other cortical areas of untreated adults with histories of childhood ADHD suggests a possible neurophysiological basis for the deficits in attention, impulse control, social judgment, and language (Zametkin et al. 1990).

Family studies point to a genetic component to ADHD, but they are inconclusive as to the nature of what is inherited: ADHD per se or a broader vulnerability to impulsiveness, as well as to anxiety and mood disorders (e.g., Biederman et al. 1992).

The most widely used drugs for ADHD are the stimulants methylphenidate, D-amphetamine, and pemoline, which produce dramatic improvement in the core ADHD symptoms and social interactions of up to 70% of affected children. Other agents useful in children who are unresponsive to stimulants or who have comorbid tics include clonidine and the tricyclic antidepressants. Psychologically significant side effects of the stimulants may include perseveration, depression, euphoria, tics, anorexia, and jitteriness. Even children who have a positive therapeutic response may complain of slight dysphoria or feeling "funny." Despite the dramatically beneficial short-term effects of stimulants on attention and behavioral problems, it has been difficult to demonstrate long-term benefits from medication alone.

Despite great theoretical expectations for behavioral and cognitive approaches to ADHD, these techniques have in practice yielded only limited, if any, positive results (Abikoff 1990; Gittelman-Klein and Abikoff 1989) and are best employed as part of a multimodal treatment program, including medication and other psychosocial and educational interventions. Because the generalizability of effects outside the specific treatment setting is often problematic, parent training and consistency across settings may be particularly important.

PSYCHOTHERAPEUTIC CONSIDERATIONS

Because childhood ADHD, TS, and OCD are frequently chronic disorders with far-reaching effects on development, their treatment is best approached in the context of an ongoing relationship with a clinician familiar with both the clinical phenomenology and dynamic aspects of these disorders. Beginning with the initial assessment, diagnosis, and treatment planning, the clinician must remain available to the patient and family over the months and years as the changing vicissitudes of the disorder and development require. At times, the clinical tasks may require frequent meetings (weekly or more often), formally structured as intensive psychotherapy; at other times, contact may be more intermittent, taking the form of periodic checkups on the status of the patient's (and family's) symptoms and adaptation. These variations in the frequency or format of treatment should not obscure the fundamental focus that guides the clinician's overall approach—the facilitation of the child's optimal development.

Psychotherapeutic Aspects of the Evaluation and Diagnostic Process

The initial diagnostic assessment and evaluation has, in itself, important psychotherapeutic components. By the time they come to competent clinical attention, children with these disorders and their families have often suffered much and been frustrated in their efforts to obtain help. The various symptoms have often been a source of pain, rejection, or shame to the child and of frustration, anger, or dismay to the parents. The opportunity to tell their respective stories, to be heard, and to be empathically understood by a clinician knowledgeable about the disorder is an essential element of care.

For individuals with TS or OCD, who may have regarded their symptoms as a form of private madness, there is often immense relief in talking with someone who knows what their symptoms are like. Given the opportunity to discuss the more subtle manifestations of their condition—the driven need to repeat an action until it feels "just right," the feeling of getting stuck or of being unable to be rid of a thought, the internal tension between yielding to or resisting an unwanted impulse—patients may confide that they had never before been able to put the feeling into words or to tell anyone what it was like.

Formulating the child's symptoms in the context of a disorder also helps to "decriminalize" them. Before consultation, children and their parents are often caught up in a vicious circle of reproach and recrimination. Parents and teachers may regard tics or compulsions as fully voluntary acts indulged in as deliberate annoyances or stubborn defiance. Tremendous pressure may be brought on the child with TS or OCD to sit quietly or still in class or church or to suppress a given tic or compulsion. The child with ADHD may have become a pariah both at school and at home. Framing these symptoms in the clinical context of a disorder permits the beginning of a more informed dialogue as to what degree of control over a given symptom can be reasonably expected in various situations. Both the child and family can thus begin to see the child's symptoms as difficulties requiring help and problem solving rather than blame. Aggravated parents can begin to see the child more sympathetically as in need of help rather than as merely bad.

Education is thus an important component in the psychotherapeutic management of this disorder. Education, however, means more than a didactic exegesis of facts about the disorder; it entails helping the child and parent to bring their own experiences of the child's difficulties into relation with what is known about the condition. Furthermore, children and parents all attempt to give psychological meaning to the child's deeply disturbing symptoms. These attempts at understanding are conditioned by the individuals' developmental phase and degree of sophistication and can, of course, serve defensive ends as well as those of mastery. Thus, didactic neurobiological explanations may end up misunderstood, reified, conflated with the child's own private theories, or used defensively. The clinician must therefore remain alert as to whether talking about "OCD," "tics," or "hyperactivity" is serving as a useful form of shorthand or as an unhelpful and obfuscating form of intellectualization.

Learning about the child's private language for his or her symptoms is important. Finding an individually tailored, shared language for discussing the symptoms with the child and parent is a crucial part of the therapeutic task, one that entails exploring and clarifying their understanding of the disorder. Especially in the initial evaluation, it is useful to know what connotations terms such as "Tourette's syndrome" or "OCD" carry, because parents' (or patients') concepts of the disorder may be derived from extreme cases seen on television talk shows.

A 9-year-old boy with TS had tics that were exacerbated by eating, unless the urge to tic was relieved by spitting. The boy explained to his doctor his own theory as to how the "kaka" rising from his stomach collided with the "tics coming down from the brain" and ricocheted about to produce his various symptoms. In his formulation, he struggled to reconcile the explanations he had heard from his doctors with his sense of uncontrollable "bad" impulses within.

An 11-year-old boy with TS who had been exposed to ticks in an area with endemic Lyme disease produced a series of drawings of brightly colored *ticks* that he used to represent and explain his *tic* symptoms, as well as his various emotions.

A 9-year-old boy with ADHD defensively excused having gotten into trouble at an overstimulating birthday party by explaining that he had had "too much sugar."

A 7-year-old girl had come to think of her intrusive obsessions and associated irritability and unhappiness as "Sally Sourmind."

Indications for Formal Psychotherapy

The primary focus of psychodynamic psychotherapy in these disorders is usually not the direct reduction of the severity of the core symptoms, such as tics, compulsions, inattention, or impulsivity. In some cases, however, developing better individual and family coping strategies may have the secondary benefit of reducing stress-induced exacerbations of tics, obsessions, and compulsions (Wolff 1988).

A developmental psychotherapeutic focus extends beyond the core symptoms and attends to how the child is proceeding with the central developmental and adaptive tasks of developing friendships, acquiring a sense of competency at school or at work, maintaining supportive relationships at home, and developing a coherent and positive identity. The decision as to whether and when formal psychotherapy is indicated is based in large part on the child's success or failure in mastering these developmental tasks.

The most common indications for formal psychotherapeutic intervention are low self-esteem; debilitating anxiety or depression; and poor interpersonal relationships with family, teachers, or peers. As noted earlier, all of these may be direct consequences of the child's disorder.

In addition to the developmental burdens imposed by TS, OCD, and ADHD, children and their families are not immune to other psychiatric difficulties or psychosocial adversities. Indeed, these childhood neuropsychiatric disorders are often comorbid with a host of other pathologies (especially anxiety and depression) that may require treatment in their own right. When present, other forms of psychopathology and adversity may exacerbate the impact of the neuropsychiatric disorders and complicate their treatment.

TECHNICAL AND DEVELOPMENTAL ISSUES

Psychodynamic psychotherapy with children who have neuropsychiatric disorders relies on many of the same components of psychotherapy with other children: therapeutic alliance and transference, the growth of insight and mastery through clarification and interpretation, education, and increased capacity for sublimation. Therapeutic work with such children, however, involves various dynamic and technical issues specific to each of the disorders and each developmental phase.

Prepubertal Children

The symptoms of TS and ADHD often first come to clinical attention during the early school years. Although isolated transient tics or hyperactivity may have been noted earlier, it is usually at this age that the pattern of chronic multiple tics characteristic of TS becomes apparent. Similarly, although children with ADHD may manifest motoric hyperactivity and short attention span as toddlers, it is the entry into school, with its growing academic and interpersonal demands, that brings the child's difficulties into sharp focus.

ADHD. For school-age children with ADHD (with or without tics), experiences of failure at school, sports, and social activities and chronic struggles at home frequently result in low self-esteem and feelings of misery and resentment from early on. Such children may develop characteristic, but maladaptive, ways of dealing with these difficulties, including denial, externalization of blame, withdrawal, regression, and bullying or clowning. One goal of psychotherapy with such children is to identify the affective triggers for such reactions and to develop more effective coping strategies.

Unmodified play therapy with markedly hyperactive children is usually neither feasible nor useful. To protect the patient, the treatment setting, or themselves, the therapists must set limits on destructive or disruptive behaviors; such interventions should not be viewed simply as regrettable necessities, but as opportunities to observe and to learn with the child in the therapeutic setting about the difficulties he or she characteristically encounters at school and at home.

In addition to hyperactivity and attentional difficulties, children with ADHD may also have perseverative tendencies, language difficulties, and an impaired ability to "read" interpersonal situations and rules. Therapy with such children thus usually requires a good deal of structure and includes many explicit didactic elements, such as training in social problem-solving skills. Some of the specific modifications of individual psychotherapeutic techniques for working with children with ADHD have been described by O'Brien (1992) and Gardner (1971).

Tourette's syndrome. The indications for psychotherapy in young school-age children with TS more often arise from ADHD-related difficulties (impulsivity, irritability, oppositionality) than from tics per se. (Indeed, young children may be less aware of their tics than their parents are.) By third or fourth grade, however, some children may have tics severe enough to provoke embarrassment, teasing, or adverse reactions from teachers. Such situations may require active intervention at school (see below). In the therapeutic context, however, situations such as these provide a concrete opportunity to explore how these children represent their symptoms to themselves and others and how their interpersonal attempts to deal with the reactions of others may enlist support or provoke further difficulties. It is often a useful therapeutic exercise to work through with TS children the question of how and with whom they will share the secret of their tics.

OCD. For children whose OCD symptoms appear rooted in obsessive-compulsive personality features (such as perfectionism and emotional constriction) or specific internal conflicts, these underlying difficulties may themselves warrant psychotherapeutic attention. For children whose principal difficulties stem from their compulsive character traits, Adams (1973) recommends a flexible interpersonal therapeutic approach that actively uses the therapeutic relationship to 1) help the child clarify his or her feelings in the here and now, 2) encourage more direct communication in lieu of overintellectual obfuscation, 3) support risk taking and tolerance for uncertainty instead of an insistence on magical omnipotent control, and 4) foster increased pleasure in interactions with the therapist and peers.

Expressive therapy techniques may help clarify the structure and context of children's obsessions and compulsions.

> In his initial interview, Richard, an imaginative, nonpsychotic 10-year-old boy with TS and OCD, played a repetitive scenario in which the lone hero finally succeeded in corralling the bad guys into prison; just when he thought he could relax, however, they would break out and attack him, necessitating his beginning all over again. The therapist expressed sympathy for the hero's Sisyphean struggles and wondered whether Richard ever felt himself to be in the same situation. Richard went on to describe the elaborate imaginary world of warring figures he had created to represent his obsessive-compulsive need to count his actions and to "even up." Perry, the King of the Evens, was the good guy, because with Perry's support Richard could feel relief after completing an action an even number of times. Arrayed against them was the evil King of the Odds, who tormented Richard with feelings of incompleteness and urged him "just one more time." Richard confided, however, that he was considering going over to the side of the Odds, because then, perhaps, he might be able to do something only *once* and feel done with it.

Adolescence

Like all adolescents, teenagers with TS, OCD, and ADHD struggle with issues of autonomy and acceptance by peers and members of the opposite sex. By later adolescence, concerns with identity, intimacy, leaving the parental home for college or work, and vocational choice come into increasing prominence. Given the characteristic adolescent propensity to avoid feelings of weakness, defectiveness, or dependency, some adolescents with neuropsychiatric disorders may be wary of any form of therapy. Noncompliance with medication may become a problem because of oppositionality, struggles over autonomy, or the wish not to feel deviant. Resistant adolescents perceive therapy as a narcissistic assault that entails a humiliating admission of weakness or weirdness. In working with such adolescents, it is important to stress the progressive aim of treatment—that of helping the patient to feel *more* in control of his or her own feelings, thoughts, actions, and destiny.

By adolescence, many untreated or treatment-resistant youngsters with ADHD feel embattled and consider themselves failures at school and at home. The relative frequency of late-adolescence conduct difficulties and substance abuse in such youngsters reflects their risk of turning to deviant peer groups or to drug and alcohol use to compensate for feelings of failure, rejection by more adequate peers, and depression. Although stimulant and tricyclic medications may continue to be useful for ADHD in adolescence, some teenagers experience a shift in their responsiveness to previously helpful drugs.

For some perfectionist children with strong obsessive-compulsive traits, adolescence may be a difficult time because of the increased challenges of sexual and autonomous longings. With adolescence, some obsessive-compulsive youngsters develop deviant eating behaviors or even full-blown anorexia nervosa (Kaye et al. 1993).

Adolescents with TS may feel painfully stigmatized or different from their peers. The burden of constant internal vigilance may weigh heavily on some patients due to the felt need to suppress sexually or aggressively charged tics or compulsions. For some adolescents with TS or OCD, perseverative stickiness and struggles against a chronic perceived lack of control may combine with adolescent oppositionality to produce stubborn and stormy confrontations.

Issues of Identity and Locus of Control in Psychotherapy

A generic issue in the psychotherapy of all three disorders is helping children and parents come to a realistic assessment of the disorder's impact on the child's functioning, while still maintaining a positive identity for the child as more than just the victim of a disorder or the bearer of symptoms.

Thus, one important goal of treatment is to help support intact strengths and areas of functioning, including interests or talents. Perhaps the most poignant finding to emerge from Weiss and Hechtman's (1986) long-term follow-up of childhood ADHD was the importance that the most successful of these young adults placed on having had someone—be it a coach, parent, boss, or lover—who saw something special in them. For these adolescents with much-battered self-esteem, this support was crucial for seeing themselves as intact and worthwhile.

FAMILY ISSUES IN PSYCHOTHERAPEUTIC MANAGEMENT

Family issues loom large in the treatment of TS, OCD, and ADHD. The frequent genetic component in these disorders makes it likely that in many cases at least one parent (or other close relatives) may have a similar condition. These commonalities between parent and child have important treatment implications beyond the task of genetic counseling, when requested, for young adult patients and parents (regarding siblings of the child). On one hand, they may be a useful source of empathy and mutual understanding. For example, a father with childhood history of TS may have a unique understanding of his son's inner experience and can serve as a model of successful perseverance in the face of similar challenges. Overidentification, on the other hand, can be problematic. A parent may see his or her own worst self-doubts (or misgivings about a spouse or sibling) reactivated by the appearance of similar symptoms in a child. Where a familial pattern of inheritance is clear, issues of guilt or blame may require therapeutic attention.

Parental symptoms of these disorders may impinge directly on the child. A father with a history of TS or ADHD may himself be reactive, irritable, or impulsive and may have difficulty maintaining the structured environment that his child, with the same difficulty, requires. On the other hand, a parent with rigid, obsessional features may be deleteriously intolerant of a hyperactive, impulsive child or a child with prominent tics. As in other situations, "goodness of fit" may be more fateful than the specific individual temperaments of different family members.

Although children with these disorders may place great demands on parental patience, a high degree of negative parental expressed emotion further burdens the child's development and requires intervention. Attention must be paid to the impact of the child's disorder on overall family functioning, including siblings and the spousal relationship. Where the child's impairment is severe and persistent, parental mourning of unrealizable expectations is a painful, but necessary, task.

Overprotectiveness poses a different set of problems. Whatever the limits are to volitional control of symptoms, children probably do best with an approach that helps to foster an internal locus of control by maintaining reasonable expectations and emphasizing active problem solving.

COLLABORATION WITH SCHOOLS

Given the frequently pervasive effects of these disorders on academic and interpersonal functioning, treatment usually requires active collaboration with school personnel.

Although many school personnel are now familiar with the school-related issues posed by ADHD, teachers and support staff often benefit from information about the less common syndromes of TS and OCD. The written and video materials for educators available from advocacy groups such as the Tourette Syndrome Association, the Obsessive Compulsive Foundation, Children With Attention Deficit Disorder (C.H.A.D.D.), the Attention-Deficit Disorder Association, and the Learning Disabilities Association are useful supplements to the clinician's and parents' discussions with school staff concerning the individual student's needs and difficulties. Such efforts to help school staff understand the pupil's disorder usually reduce parents' fears concerning stigmatization.

For teachers of students with TS and OCD, it is often useful to reframe the child's potentially disruptive difficulties as partially involuntary symptoms rather than as oppositionality. Although difficult decisions may have to be made as to when such symptoms (especially vocal tics) necessitate the child leaving the classroom, such reframing may help to increase teachers' and classmates' tolerance. A sympathetic teacher's carefully planned explanation and discussion of the child's symptoms with the class can be invaluable in terms of decreasing teasing and increasing peer support. Teachers' daily observations are extremely useful for evaluating and monitoring symptoms (especially those of ADHD). A variety of standardized teachers' rating forms for ADHD have been developed, of which the Conners Teacher Rating Scale is the most widely used (Barkley 1990). Teachers' observations are vital in assessing the efficacy of medication and adjusting dosage, especially when short-acting preparations are used.

Children with attentional difficulties usually need individualized educational planning, including small, structured classes; resource room help (especially when there are also concomitant specific learning disabilities); carefully tailored behavioral management; and daily feedback to parents concerning behavior and homework. Behavioral techniques work best when there is continuity and consistency between the approaches used at home and at school.

INTEGRATION OF MULTIMODAL APPROACHES

Although medication, behavioral techniques, and psychotherapeutic interventions may sometimes yield dramatic results, there is no single "magic bullet" for TS, OCD, or ADHD. Given the chronicity and wide-ranging manifestations of these disorders, most patients and families require a flexible, nondoctrinaire approach that draws on a variety of modalities as the symptoms evolve or as the child faces different developmental challenges.

Integrating Diverse Psychological Approaches

When described in theoretical terms, the various psychodynamic, behavioral, and cognitive approaches may appear quite distinct. As actually practiced, however, there are often important commonalities among therapists with nominally different allegiances that extend beyond the nonspecific effects of attention and support (Arkowitz and Messer 1984; Wachtel 1977, 1982). Important shared components of both the behavioral and the psychodynamic approaches to these disorders include self-monitoring, identifying situational and affective antecedents of problematic behaviors, imaginal exposure, encouragement of response prevention, and reframing of expectations and beliefs. One of the most useful contributions of the behavioral perspective to the more psychodynamic approaches is the former's strong emphasis on empirical assessment of behavior and the effects of various interventions.

Combining Pharmacological and Psychotherapeutic Approaches

As described above, medication plays an important role in the treatment of ADHD, TS, and OCD. The impact of medication is mediated by more than its pharmacological effects. The meanings that patients assign to medications and their therapeutic and adverse effects provide an important psychological dimension to the decision to start or stop medication and are crucial determinants of compliance.

Unfortunately, a substantial proportion of children with these disorders show only a limited response to medication. Even when medication is successful in suppressing the symptoms of TS or ADHD, medication alone cannot make up for the social or academic skills that may have been missed, nor can it set right the cumulative effects on the child's self-image and perceived competency; these require the appropriate psychotherapeutic, behavioral, and remedial educational interventions. Furthermore, symptoms often reemerge when medication is stopped, posing difficult questions as to how long to maintain children on potent medications.

·Comparative efficacy studies and studies of multimodal treatment are methodologically difficult and are confounded by the heterogeneity of clinical samples, outcome measures, and research designs

(Abikoff 1990; Kazdin 1988). As Whalen and Henker (1991) have observed, the goal of such research must go beyond either/or questions about the single "best" treatment to deeper theoretical and developmental questions concerning pathogenesis and therapeutic change.

ADHD. The outcome studies by Satterfield et al. (1981, 1987) concluded that long-term, individually tailored multimodal treatment was superior to brief treatment or stimulant medication alone. The multimodal treatment consisted of an individually tailored program of medication plus some combination of educational, individual, group, and family therapy; the parent work included both casework and training in behavioral techniques. A newer generation of outcome studies of multimodal therapy is now under way (Abikoff 1990).

OCD. A limited number of studies comparing psychological versus drug treatment of OCD suggest that the beneficial effects of behavioral treatments may be longer lasting than those of medication (O'Sullivan et al. 1991). Exposure and response prevention are the central techniques for the behavioral treatment of compulsions and related obsessive thoughts; the treatment of pure obsessions (e.g., by thought-stopping techniques) has proven more difficult (Berg et al. 1991; Steketee and Tynes 1991). Defining the subgroup of children with OCD or TS, or both, for whom behavioral treatment is suitable remains a challenge (Baer and Minichiello 1990; King et al. 1993). Such techniques are probably most suitable for children with a relatively small number of stable symptoms.

Psychotherapeutic approaches often incorporate, albeit less formally, many of the components of behavioral analysis, exposure, and response prevention. These include exploring in detail the situational, cognitive, and affective triggers for the rituals or obsessions; constructing a hierarchy of such target situations; examining the patient's beliefs and feelings concerning the symptoms; and identifying family interactions that may maintain the symptoms. Although traditional psychotherapeutic techniques make less use of in vivo exposure during the session, imaginal exposure and encouragement of exposure to the trigger situation outside the hour are often used, as well as encouragement toward response prevention. Family interventions are important to reduce secondary gains and to support other interventions (Bolton et al. 1983; Fine 1973).

> Karen, a 13-year-old honor student, had been troubled for several years with obsessive-compulsive symptoms and traits. An excellent student, musician, and athlete, she had always felt that she never did well enough. Around age 10, she developed a compulsive need to confess "unworthy" thoughts, such as the thought that her father was prejudiced

or that she might have inadvertently hurt someone's feelings. (In fact, both Karen and her family were devout and highly conscientious members of their community, active in many worthwhile causes.) On one occasion, for example, after being given an "I was good today" sticker by her dentist, she became tearful thinking that she wasn't as good as Jesus.

A 9-month trial of fluoxetine markedly decreased Karen's depression and compulsive doubting and confession but had little impact on her perfectionist traits. Coinciding with menarche, Karen developed several new obsessions and compulsions, including intrusive sexual thoughts, doubting, and concerns about her clothes becoming "stretched" (which she feared would make her look fat). Anyone's touch stirred the fear that her clothes would become stretched, which had to be counteracted by immediately laundering her clothes to restore their shape. Soon thereafter she developed frank anorexic symptoms, with an obsessional pursuit of thinness. Careful examination (including a daily journal) of the precipitants of her self-reproaches and expiatory rituals revealed that the situational triggers were often commonplace adolescent impulses or irritations that her strict conscience found unacceptable. Treatment with fluoxetine was restarted, and she began psychotherapy that focused on her intolerance toward her adolescent strivings for autonomy, her nascent heterosexual interests, and her often-conflicted family loyalties. Family work focused on ways that her family had reinforced her perfectionist traits and her intolerance of ambivalent feelings.

Jeff, a 14-year-old boy with ADHD, was the only child of his single, artisan mother and musician father, whose superficial charm covered a long history of difficulties suggestive of childhood ADHD. Although Jeff had above-average intelligence, his impulsivity and short attention span, coupled with specific learning difficulties and poor social skills, resulted in perennially unsatisfactory school performance, isolation from peers, and frequent clashes with his mother. Although stimulants had been effective when Jeff was younger, they had recently lost their effectiveness.

Treatment proceeded on a variety of fronts. Casework with Jeff's mother addressed the contributions of unresolved conflicts with her family of origin and disappointments at the hands of various males in her life, among whom she included Jeff. This parental work helped Jeff's mother feel less reactive to Jeff's irritability and oppositionality and enabled her to utilize more consistently the various behavior management techniques that she, the parent caseworker, and the school jointly developed. Individual therapy with Jeff focused on helping him to develop better social skills with peers and to feel less entangled by his mixed concern and resentment over what he perceived as his mother's depression and inconsistency. In addition, Jeff's ambivalent longings and resentments toward his mother's succession of boyfriends and his largely absent father were explored.

As Jeff became increasingly attached to his male therapist, much of the work took place through the medium of drawing, an activity at which Jeff excelled and on which he was able to concentrate for substantial periods of time. Various mutually planned cartoons and picture books ex-

plored themes of thwarted friendships, rejections, and their possible re-
mediation. Medication was switched to a carefully monitored tricyclic
with beneficial results (and the elimination of a hated lunchtime dose).
Jeff was pleased to have his artwork cherished at school and gradually
developed a small circle of friends. Just as perceived failure had previously led to a vicious circle of withdrawal and antagonism, provoking
further negative responses from those about him, Jeff now took more of
an interest in school and peers, was less reactive to setbacks, and in turn
evoked more positive and less punitive reactions from those around him.

CONCLUSION

The childhood neuropsychiatric disorders are most often chronic conditions, with far-reaching effects on the child and an intergenerational
impact on the family. In such cases, treatment is complex and multifaceted, involving the coordination of multiple perspectives, disciplines,
and techniques in response to the evolving developmental needs of the
patient and family. The challenge for clinical research concerning the
treatment of these disorders is to determine more specifically the indications for different interventions, to characterize more precisely their
respective mutative elements, and to examine more carefully their individual and interactive effects on various aspects of outcome.

REFERENCES

Abikoff H: Combined psychosocial and psychopharmacologic treatments for ADHD
   children: methodologic issues. Paper presented at the NIMH Conference on Combination Psychosocial and Psychopharmacologic Treatments for Mental Disorders,
   Rockville, MD, October 1990
Adams PL: Obsessive Children. New York, Brunner/Mazel, 1973
American Psychiatric Association: Diagnostic and Statistical Manual of Mental Disor-
   ders, 3rd Edition, Revised. Washington, DC, American Psychiatric Association, 1987
Apter A, Pauls DL, Bleich A, et al: A population-based epidemiological study of Tourette
   syndrome among adolescents in Israel, in Tourette Syndrome: Genetics, Neurobiol-
   ogy, and Treatment (Advances in Neurology Series, Vol 58). Edited by Chase TN,
   Friedhoff AJ, Cohen DJ. New York, Raven, 1992, pp 61–66
Arkowitz H, Messer SB: Psychoanalytic Therapy and Behavior Therapy: Is Integration
   Possible? New York, Plenum, 1984
Baer L, Minichiello WE: Behavior therapy for obsessive-compulsive disorder, in Obses-
   sive Compulsive Disorders: Theory and Management. Edited by Jenike MA, Baer L,
   Minichiello WE. Chicago, IL, Year Book Medical, 1990, pp 203–232
Barkley RA: Attention Deficit Hyperactivity Disorder: A Handbook for Diagnosis and
   Treatment. New York, Guilford, 1990
Berg CZ, Rapoport J, Whitaker A, et al: Childhood obsessive-compulsive disorder: a two-
   year prospective follow-up of a community sample. J Am Acad Child Adolesc Psychiatry 28:528–533, 1989
Berg CZ, Rapoport J, Wolff RP: Behavioral treatment for obsessive-compulsive disorder
   in childhood, in Obsessive-Compulsive Disorder in Children and Adolescents. Edited
   by Rapoport JL. Washington, DC, American Psychiatric Press, 1991

Biederman J, Faraone SW, Keenan K, et al.: Further evidence for family genetic risk factors: attention deficit disorder. Arch Gen Psychiatry 49:728–738, 1992

Black DW, Noyes R, Goldstein RB, et al: A family study of obsessive-compulsive disorder. Arch Gen Psychiatry 49:362–368, 1992

Bliss J: Sensory experiences in Gilles de la Tourette's syndrome. Arch Gen Psychiatry 37:1343–1347, 1980

Bolton D, Collins S, Steinberg D: The treatment of obsessive-compulsive disorder in adolescence: a report of fifteen cases. Br J Psychiatry 142:456–464, 1983

Bruun RD: Subtle and underrecognized side effects of neuroleptic treatment in children with Tourette's Disorder. Am J Psychiatry 145:621–624, 1988

Chase TN, Friedhoff AJ, Cohen DJ (eds): Tourette's Syndrome: Genetics, Neurobiology, and Treatment (Advances in Neurology Series, Vol 58). New York, Raven, 1992

Cohen DJ: Tourette's syndrome: developmental psychopathology of a model neuropsychiatric disorder of childhood. Twenty-Seventh Annual Institute of Pennsylvania Hospital Award Lecture in Memory of Edward A. Strecker, Philadelphia, PA, November 19, 1990

Cohen DJ: Tourette's syndrome: a model disorder for integrating psychoanalysis and biological perspectives. International Review of Psychoanalysis 18:195–209, 1991

Cohen DJ, Leckman JF: The child and adolescent with Tourette's syndrome: clinical perspectives on phenomenology and treatment, in Handbook of Tourette's Syndrome and Related Tic and Behavioral Disorders. Edited by Kurlan R. New York, Marcel Dekker, 1993, pp 461–480

Cohen DJ, Ort SI, Leckman JF, et al: Family functioning in Tourette's syndrome, in Tourette's Syndrome and Tic Disorders: Clinical Understanding and Treatment. Edited by Cohen DJ, Bruun RD, Leckman JF. New York, Wiley, 1988, pp 179–196

Cohen DJ, Friedhoff AJ, Leckman JF, et al: Tourette syndrome: extending basic research to clinical care, in Tourette's Syndrome: Genetics, Neurobiology, and Treatment (Advances in Neurology Series, Vol 58). Edited by Chase TN, Friedhoff AJ, Cohen DJ. New York, Raven, 1992, pp 341–362

Fine S: Family therapy and a behavioral approach to childhood obsessive-compulsive neurosis. Arch Gen Psychiatry 28:695–697, 1973

Flament MF, Whitaker A, Rapoport JL, et al: Obsessive-compulsive disorder in adolescence: an epidemiological study. J Am Acad Child Adolesc Psychiatry 27:764–771, 1988

Freud A: Normality and Pathology in Childhood: Assessments of Development. New York, International Universities Press, 1965

Gardner RA: Therapeutic Communication with Children: The Mutual Story Telling Technique. New York, Science House, 1971

Gittelman-Klein RG, Abikoff H: The role of psychostimulants and psychosocial treatments in hyperkinesis, in Attention Deficit Disorder: Clinical and Basic Research. Edited by Sagvolden T, Archer T. Hillsdale, NJ, Lawrence Erlbaum, 1989

Kaye WH, Weltzin T, Hsu LKG: Anorexia nervosa, in Obsessive-Compulsive–Related Disorders. Edited by Hollander E. Washington, DC, American Psychiatric Press, 1993

Kazdin AE: Child Psychotherapy: Developing and Identifying Effective Treatments. New York, Pergamon, 1988

King RA, Noshpitz J: Pathways of Growth: Essentials of Child Psychiatry—Psychopathology, Vol 2. New York, Wiley, 1991

King RA, Riddle MA, Chappell PB, et al: Emergence of self-destructive phenomena in children and adolescents during fluoxetine treatment. J Am Acad Child Adolesc Psychiatry 30:179–186, 1991

King RA, Riddle MA, Goodman WK: The psychopharmacology of obsessive compulsive disorder in Tourette's syndrome, in Tourette's Syndrome: Genetics, Neurobiology, and Treatment (Advances in Neurology, Vol 58). Edited by Chase TN, Friedhoff AJ, Cohen DJ. New York, Raven, 1992, pp 283–291

King RA, Vitulano LA, Riddle MA: The treatment of obsessive-compulsive disorder in Tourette's syndrome, in Handbook of Tourette's Syndrome and Related Tic and Behavioral Disorders. Edited by Kurlan R. New York, Marcel Dekker, 1993, pp 401–422

Klein RG, Mannuzza S: Long-term outcome of hyperactive children: a review. J Am Acad Child Adolesc Psychiatry 30:383–387, 1991

Kurlan R (ed): Handbook of Tourette's Syndrome and Related Tic and Behavioral Disorders. New York, Marcel Dekker, 1993

Leckman JF, Riddle MA, Cohen DJ: Pathobiology of Tourette's syndrome, in Tourette's Syndrome and Tic Disorders: Clinical Understanding and Treatment. Edited by Cohen DJ, Bruun RD, Leckman JF. New York, Wiley, 1988, pp 103–116

Leckman JF, Hardin MT, Riddle MA, et al: Clonidine treatment of Gilles de a Tourette syndrome. Arch Gen Psychiatry 48:324–328, 1991

Leckman JF, Walker DE, Cohen DJ: Premonitory urges in Tourette's syndrome. Am J Psychiatry 150:98–102, 1993

Leckman JF, Walker DE, Goodman WK, et al: "Just right" perceptions associated with compulsive behaviors in Tourette's syndrome. Am J Psychiatry (in press)

Leonard HL, Lenane MC, Swedo SE, et al: Tics and Tourette's disorders: a 2-to 7-year follow up of 54 obsessive-compulsive children. Am J Psychiatry 149:1244–1251, 1992

Linet LS: Tourette syndrome, pimozide, and school phobia: the neuroleptic separation anxiety syndrome. Am J Psychiatry 142:613–615, 1985

O'Brien JD: Children with attention-deficit hyperactivity disorder and their parents, in Psychotherapies With Children and Adolescents: Adapting the Psychodynamic Process. Edited by O'Brien JD, Pilowsky DJ, Lewis OW. Washington, DC, American Psychiatric Press, 1992, pp 109–124

O'Sullivan G, Noshirvani H, Marks I, et al: Six-year follow-up after exposure and clomipramine therapy for obsessive compulsive disorder. J Clin Psychiatry 52:150–155, 1991

Pauls DL, Raymond CL, Leckman JF, et al: A family study of Tourette's syndrome. Am J Hum Genet 48:154–163, 1991

Rapoport JL: Obsessive-Compulsive Disorder in Children and Adolescents. Washington, DC, American Psychiatric Press, 1989

Rettew DC, Swedo SE, Leonard HL, et al: Obsessions and compulsions across time in 79 children and adolescents with obsessive-compulsive disorder. J Am Acad Child Adolesc Psychiatry 31:1050–1056, 1992

Riddle MA, Scahill L, King RA, et al: Obsessive compulsive disorder in children and adolescents: phenomenology and family history. J Am Acad Child Adolesc Psychiatry 29:766–772, 1990

Riddle MA, King RA, Hardin MT, et al: Behavioral side effects of fluoxetine in children and adolescents. Journal of Child and Adolescent Psychopharmacology 1:193–198, 1991

Satterfield JH, Satterfield BT, Cantwell DP: Three-year multi-modality treatment study of 100 hyperactive boys. J Pediatr 98:650–655, 1981

Satterfield JH, Satterfield BT, Schell AM: Therapeutic interventions to prevent delinquency in hyperactive boys. J Am Acad Child Adolesc Psychiatry 26:56–64, 1987

Shapiro ES, Shapiro AK, Fulop G, et al: Controlled study of haloperidol, pimozide, and placebo for the treatment of Gilles de la Tourette syndrome. Arch Gen Psychiatry 46:722–730, 1989

Steketee G, Tynes LL: Behavioral treatment of obsessive-compulsive disorder, in Current Treatments of Obsessive-Compulsive Disorder. Edited by Pato MT, Zohar J. Washington, DC, American Psychiatric Press, 1991

Stokes A, Bawden HN, Camfield PR, et al: Peer problems in Tourette's disorder. Pediatrics 87:936–942, 1991

Swedo SE, Rapoport JL, Cheslow DL, et al: High prevalence of obsessive-compulsive symptoms in patients with Sydenham's chorea. Am J Psychiatry 146:246–249, 1989a

Swedo SE, Rapoport JL, Leonard H, et al: Obsessive-compulsive disorder in children and adolescents. Arch Gen Psychiatry 46:335–341, 1989b

Towbin KE, Riddle MA, Leckman JF, et al: The clinical care of individuals with Tourette's syndrome, in Tourette's Syndrome and Tic Disorders: Clinical Understanding and Treatment. Edited by Cohen DJ, Bruun RD, Leckman JF. New York, Wiley, 1988, pp 329–352

Wachtel PL: Psychoanalysis and Behavior Therapy: Toward an Integration. New York, Basic Books, 1977

Wachtel PL: Resistance: Psychodynamic and Behavioral Approaches. New York, Plenum, 1982

Weiss G, Hechtman LT: Hyperactive Children Grow Up: Empirical Findings and Theoretical Considerations. New York, Guilford, 1986

Whalen CK, Henker B: Therapies for hyperactive children: comparisons, combinations, and compromises. J Consult Clin Psychol 59:126–137, 1991

Wolff EC: Psychotherapeutic interventions with Tourette's syndrome, in Tourette's Syndrome and Tic Disorders: Clinical Understanding and Treatment. Edited by Cohen DJ, Bruun RD, Leckman JF. New York, Wiley, 1988, pp 208–222

Zahner GEP, Clubb MM, Leckman JF, et al: The epidemiology of Tourette's syndrome, in Tourette's Syndrome and Tic Disorders: Clinical Understanding and Treatment. Edited by Cohen DJ, Bruun RD, Leckman JF. New York, Wiley, 1988, pp 79–89

Zametkin AJ, Nordahl TGE, Gross M, et al: Cerebral glucose metabolism in adults with hyperactivity of childhood onset. N Engl J Med 323:1361–1366, 1990

Zohar AH, Ratzoni G, Pauls DL, et al: An epidemiological study of obsessive-compulsive disorder and related disorders in Israeli adolescents. J Am Acad Child Adolesc Psychiatry 31:1057–1061, 1992

Chapter 22

Eating Disorders

Owen Lewis, M.D., and Irene Chatoor, M.D.

Individuals with eating disorders share a disturbance in somato-psychological differentiation: an inability to separate physiological sensations of hunger and fullness from emotional feelings such as anger, fear, anxiety, sadness, loneliness, and feelings of rejection. Somatopsychological differentiation is a developmental process that is established in the first 2 years of life. Infant characteristics and parental behavior can facilitate or impede this developmental process. In addition, depression and intense anxiety frequently blunt the awareness of hunger and fullness, and cultural pressures for thinness induce more and more children and adolescents to "diet"—to regulate their food intake by calorie counts and weight checks instead of relying on their internal signals of hunger and satiety.

The understanding of the eating disorders presented here assumes a developmental model in which various factors such as infant temperament, parental characteristics, the experiences of depression or anxiety, and cultural pressures interact to lead to the expression of various eating disorders at various stages of development of the infant, the child, or the adolescent.

The classification of feeding disorders described in this chapter is more elaborate because DSM-III-R (American Psychiatric Association 1987) describes only reactive attachment disorder of infancy associated with failure to thrive and rumination disorder of infancy. The adolescent eating disorders will follow the DSM-III-R classifications of anorexia nervosa and bulimia nervosa. Obesity will not, however, be discussed in this chapter.

EATING DISORDERS IN INFANTS, TODDLERS, AND CHILDREN

Most of the research on eating disorders has focused on anorexia nervosa and bulimia nervosa in adolescent and adult women. Some studies have described the onset of anorexia nervosa in prepubertal children (Blitzer et al. 1961; Fosson et al. 1987; Hawley 1985; Silverman 1974); however, clear diagnostic criteria for the diagnosis of anorexia nervosa or bulimia nervosa in children have not been established. Other eating disorders in children have been described as food aversion (L. Siegel 1982), posttraumatic eating disorder (Chatoor et al. 1988a), and food phobia (Singer et al. 1992).

The lack of a generally accepted classification for eating disorders in infants and toddlers has led to a confusing array of labels for feeding problems and failure to thrive (FTT) in this young age group. Whereas FTT has been used primarily by pediatricians to describe the syndrome of inadequate growth and development in infants and young children, behaviorists have focused on associated feeding problems.

Since 1908, when Chapin alerted pediatricians to the failure of growth and development associated with poverty and institutional care of infants and young children, researchers have assumed the existence of an awkward and, in many cases, not useful dichotomy differentiating organic FTT from nonorganic FTT. More recently, several authors have suggested a third FTT category for patients who present with a combination of organic and nonorganic factors in the etiology of their growth disturbance (Budd et al. 1992; Casey et al. 1984; Homer and Ludwig 1981).

Several authors have addressed the multifactorial etiology of the FTT syndrome. Bithany and Dubowitz (1972) proposed a biopsychosocial model that incorporates the complex bidirectional interaction between infant characteristics and psychosocial parental factors. Woolston (1985) suggested the use of a multiaxial system for the diagnosis of FTT. This system includes physical illness, growth failure, developmental delay, caretaker-infant interaction, observation of feeding, age at onset, and the cognitive or financial disability of caretakers. Some authors have taken an interactional approach to understanding and treating FTT (Liebermann and Birch 1985; Linscheid and Rasnake 1985). Drotar (1989) pointed to the heterogeneity of the FTT syndrome and to the difficulties in comparing studies because sample heterogeneity may obscure group differences and contribute to inconsistent findings.

Because of the diversity in etiology, the existence of nonorganic, organic, and mixed types of FTT, and the lack of a standard classification system for childhood feeding disorders, Chatoor et al. (1984, 1985) proposed a developmental classification of feeding disorders associated with FTT. (The term *feeding disorder* is applied to infants and toddlers who cannot yet eat independently.) This classification incorporates an interactional approach to a multifactorial etiology of the FTT syndrome, including various organic and inorganic factors that can create, exacerbate, or be a sequela of an infant's feeding and growth problem.

Although the exact etiology or causes of the various eating disorders are not known, most experts agree with Garfinkel and Garner (1982) that eating disorders are the product of the interplay of a number of forces. For example, there appear to be predisposing factors that combine with precipitating events in an individual's life that lead to dysregulation of eating. Organic factors, such as pain caused by gastroesophageal reflux or fever and malaise, can interfere with the perception of hunger. At the same time, emotional experiences during eating and associations between the external environment and eating can strengthen or weaken the awareness of hunger or fullness. All eating disorders, whether in infants, children or adolescents, appear to be characterized by an acute disruption or a developmental derailment of internal regulation of eating in accord to physiological needs as expressed through signals of hunger and fullness. To treat eating disorders successfully, it is important to identify the factors that interfere with internal regulation of eating—to look at predisposing and precipitating factors as well as those factors that maintain dysregulation of eating. After a thorough evaluation of the individual child, within a developmental framework, a treatment plan needs to be developed to establish internal regulation of eating free from both emotional and external interference.

Two groups of eating disorders in infants, toddlers, and children will be discussed. The first group includes disorders that represent developmental deviations in the regulation of eating. The developmental classification of feeding disorders by Chatoor et al. (1984, 1985) draws on Greenspan and Lourie's (1985) stages of early infant development and Mahler et al.'s (1975) concept of separation and individuation. Chatoor et al. (1984) identified three stages of feeding development in which adaptive and maladaptive behaviors in both the infant and the mother can be identified: 1) homeostasis, 2) attachment, and 3) separation. Considering the developmental progression expressed during feeding, Chatoor et al. (1985) classified feeding disorders on the basis of age at onset and the specific characteristics of each disorder. This classification incorporates the fact that organic and psychosocial factors as well as infant characteristics can contribute to the development of feeding disorders. Anorexia nervosa with prepubertal onset during childhood, as described in DSM-III-R, will not be discussed in this section.

The second group of eating disorders, which are characterized by a more acute disruption in the regulation of eating, has been described by Chatoor et al. (1988a) as posttraumatic eating disorder in children and posttraumatic feeding disorder in infants (Chatoor 1991a).

Feeding Disorder of Homeostasis

The Clinical Picture
In the first few months of life, an infant's primary task is to regulate and establish an eating and sleeping pattern. In feeding, infants need to move from reflex sucking at birth to a situation where they control the beginning and ending of feedings through giving signals of hunger

and fullness to the caregiver. The mother needs to read these signals and respond contingently to allow the infant to develop a regular feeding pattern.

Problems in regulation of feeding at this stage of development are characterized by poor food intake that can vary in quantity and timing from one feeding to the next. Either the infant is too irritable or too sleepy to feed successfully, or the mother might be too anxious or too depressed to read her infant's cues and to help her infant reach a state of calm alertness for feeding. Infants with difficult temperamental traits, central nervous system immaturity, medical illnesses (e.g., cardiac or pulmonary disease), or anatomical abnormalities of the oropharynx or gastrointestinal tract are especially at risk for failing to develop adequate feeding behaviors. Frequently, a combination of infant vulnerability and maternal difficulty leads to dysregulation of feeding at this stage of development.

Treatment

Treatment of these infants needs to be individualized to reflect maternal as well as infant factors that have interfered with feeding. For example, "colicky infants" with a labile autonomic nervous system are vulnerable to overstimulation. Parents can be helped to look at connections between overstimulation and irritability or colic in the infant and to modify the environment to facilitate calmer feeding periods.

Infants with respiratory or cardiac problems frequently have difficulties in coordinating sucking and breathing and are unable to feed successfully. For some infants with medical problems, gavage feedings are necessary for weeks or months to supplement oral feedings because the infants are too weak to drink enough milk to sustain them nutritionally. These early feeding difficulties usually have a strong impact on the mother. For many mothers, feeding is central to their relationship with their infants. Difficulties in feeding evoke feelings of helplessness, anxiety, and depression in the mother (Vietze et al. 1980). The mother's intense emotional arousal during feeding interferes with her ability to read her infant's cues and to provide the infant with a calm environment that facilitates feeding. Frequently, it is necessary to address the mother's emotional state and to treat her anxiety or depression before she is able to successfully feed her baby. This treatment can best be done by observing the mother and infant during feeding and dealing with the mother's difficulties with the baby in the room.

Early regulation of feeding has a significant impact on the overall motivation and drive of the infant (Dowling 1977). Successful self-regulation of the infant lays the foundation for the next stage of development, whereas feeding difficulties early in life frequently leave infant and mother vulnerable for problems during later stages of development.

Feeding Disorder of Attachment

The Clinical Picture

Having achieved some capacity for self-regulation, the adaptive infant is able to mobilize and engage his or her caretakers in increasingly complex interactions. Consequently, between ages 2 and 8 months the infant is ready for the major psychological and affective task of the first year of life—the task of attachment.

Attachment develops within a reciprocal relationship wherein either partner can facilitate or impede the process. Evidence of good attachment behavior includes mutual eye contact and gazing, reciprocal vocalizations, and mutual physical closeness expressed through cuddling and molding. Because many of an infant's interactions with caretakers occur around feedings, the infant's regulation of food intake seems closely linked to his or her affective engagement with the caregiver.

Various authors have indicated that dysfunctional interactional patterns between mothers and infants are associated with dysregulation of feeding and FTT. Vietze et al. (1980) found that mothers of male newborns who subsequently failed to thrive were more likely to terminate their responses to their infants than were mothers of infants who did not develop nonorganic FTT. Bradley et al. (1984) reported that mothers of infants with nonorganic FTT showed lower responsiveness, acceptance, and organization of the physical environment than mothers of healthy infants. Drotar et al. (1990) observed that mothers of infants with nonorganic FTT showed less adaptive social interactional behavior and positive affective behavior and terminated feedings more arbitrarily. Haynes et al. (1984) found three patterns of mother-infant interaction that differentiated the FTT group from the group of thriving infants: benign neglect, incoordination, and overt hostility. Mathisen et al. (1989) noted that infants' deficient ability to signal their needs combined with less encouragement and communication by the mothers was associated with shorter duration of feedings in the group with nonorganic FTT.

Chatoor (1991a, 1991b) described distinct interactional patterns of mothers and infants who fail to regulate their eating successfully and who do not thrive, starting at this stage of development. Observations of these mothers and babies during feeding reveal a general lack of pleasure in their interactions. The mothers appear listless, detached, and apathetic; they hold their babies loosely on their laps without much physical intimacy; and seemingly unaware of the infant's signals, they rarely initiate verbal or visual contact with their babies, who also appear listless and apathetic. Frequently, these babies seem to actively avoid eye contact with the mother. When these babies are picked up, they seem unable to cuddle and mold to the examiner's body. They usually show disturbances in body tone, being floppy or rigid, and many are developmentally delayed.

Evans et al. (1972) distinguished three groups of mothers of FTT infants and classified them along a continuous spectrum of psychopathology. In the first group, the mothers had experienced the loss of an important person and suffered from acute depression. The second group of mothers had experienced repeated personal loss, lived in deprived conditions, showed severe depression, and appeared helpless and overwhelmed. The third group showed the most severe psychopathology: the mothers were openly hostile and very angry in their interactions with their infants. Fraiberg et al. (1975) pointed to the lack of nurturing in the mother's own infancy and childhood and the lack of a satisfying relationship with another emotionally supportive person as leading to the mother's inability to nurture her infant. More recently, Main and Goldwyn (1984) systematically explored the mother's attachment behaviors from her childhood into adult life and found that the mother's experience of rejection by her own mother was related to specific distortions in her cognitive processes, to rejection of her infant, and to the infant's avoidant insecure attachment as observed in the laboratory. Drotar and Eckerle (1989) suggested that the manner in which a traumatic or deprived childhood experience can influence the mother-infant relationship is affected by the current context of family life.

Treatment
Treatment of attachment disorders is very difficult and time consuming, and feeding problems cannot be easily separated from the larger context of the mother-infant relationship. Because of the complexity of the issues involved, a multidisciplinary team composed of a pediatrician, nutritionist, physical or occupational therapist, social worker, and child psychiatrist is generally required to identify the pathology that may have led to the attachment problems in both the mother and the infant. Some mothers can be helped in the attachment process by early identification of difficult temperamental characteristics or hypersensitivities of the infant. Other mothers may need psychotherapy for their depression; some may further need medication to mobilize their depression and to make them more available to their infants. Mothers with severe character pathology who have suffered deprivation or abuse during their own childhood will frequently avoid health care professionals and are difficult or impossible to treat in an office setting. However, nurturing the mother is a first critical step in the treatment to facilitate her potential to nurture the infant (Fraiberg et al. 1975). Frequently, hospitalization is necessary to thoroughly assess the infant, the social environment, and the potential for intervention and may be critical in starting nutritional rehabilitation.

During hospitalization, a number of specialized infant-directed interventions can be carried out. They include nutritional rehabilitation, developmental stimulation, and emotional nurturing. It is important to assign a primary care nurse and limit the number of alternative caretakers as much as possible to facilitate a special relationship between the primary caregiver and the infant.

Because mothers frequently present with a variety of social and psychological disturbances, their problems need to be explored while treatment proceeds with the infant. The mother's emotional availability may be assessed in videotaping feeding and play sessions between her and her infant, which may be used diagnostically and therapeutically. The therapist can view the tapes together with the mother and point out any positive affective interchange between infant and mother. The therapist needs to approach the mother in a kind and empathic way even if the mother appears hostile and avoidant. The goal is to reach her and explore the "ghosts in the mother's nursery" described so well by Fraiberg et al. (1975). Hospitalization of the infant is critical in assessing whether the mother can be engaged in a therapeutic relationship or whether the infant needs to be placed in alternative care. The establishment of a mutual attachment relationship is critical for the infant to regulate his or her feeding and to thrive physically as well as emotionally in the future.

Feeding Disorder of Separation (Infantile Anorexia Nervosa)

The Clinical Picture
From age 6 to 36 months, coinciding with rapid gains in locomotion and fine motor skills, language acquisition, and capacity for symbolic representation, an infant becomes more aware of himself or herself as an individual. With the development of this emerging aspect of an infant's sense of self—and the new demands he or she places on the environment—mother and infant must negotiate general issues of autonomy and parental control. While an infant is in transition to self-feeding, mother and infant need to negotiate in particular who is going to put the spoon in the infant's mouth. This is a critical developmental period during which the infant not only learns to self-feed, but also learns to regulate his or her eating internally in response to hunger and fullness. Both mother and infant contribute to the child's successful learning of somatopsychological differentiation, the ability to differentiate physical hunger from the emotional need for affection and from anger and frustration. The infant needs to signal emotional versus physiological needs, and the caretaker needs to differentiate whether the infant is hungry or needs a hug and whether the infant is full or refuses to open his or her mouth out of anger or frustration. Infants who do not give clear signals and caretakers who respond noncontingently, who offer the bottle when the infant is distressed or force the

infant to eat everything on the plate, will encounter difficulties during this stage of development.

In 1983, Chatoor and Egan published a clinical report on the diagnosis and treatment of an eating disorder that may start during this developmental period of separation and individuation and that is characterized by food refusal or extreme food selectivity and undereating. They called it a separation disorder; later, because of its similarities to anorexia nervosa, it was called infantile anorexia nervosa (Chatoor 1989; Chatoor et al. 1988b). Other authors (Liebermann and Birch 1985), who also placed the root of FTT in a transactional impasse between the infant and the caregiver, described a similar developmental disorder associated with growth failure. Others, such as Linscheid and Rasnake (1985), described two types of nonorganic FTT differentiated on the basis of the child's age and the nature of the caregiver-child interaction. Their type I resembles the disorder described in DSM-III (American Psychiatric Association 1980) as reactive attachment disorder and correlates with the attachment disorder described above by Chatoor (1991a, 1991b). Type II has the characteristics of the separation disorder described as infantile anorexia nervosa in this classification by Chatoor et al.

Chatoor and Egan (1983) described the onset of infantile anorexia nervosa between ages 6 months and 3 years, with a peak onset around age 9 months. The parents report a history of the infant's food refusal or extreme food selectivity and undereating despite all efforts to increase food intake. The feeding difficulties stem from the infant's thrust for autonomy, with mother and infant embroiled in conflicts over autonomy and control, primarily during feeding. This leads to a battle of wills over the infant's food intake. Characteristically, parents mention that they have tried "everything" to get the infant to eat, including coaxing, cajoling, bargaining, distracting, or forcing food into the infant's mouth. However, the conflict over the infant's food intake interferes with the development of somatopsychological differentiation, and the infant confuses emotional hunger for affection and the experience of anger and frustration with physiological sensations of hunger and fullness. As a result, the confusion of somatic and psychological needs leads the infant to be controlled by emotional experiences rather than physiological needs. The infant fails to develop internal regulation of eating, which leads to FTT. Initially, the infant fails to gain or may lose weight, linear growth is gradually impaired, and eventually these children may become dwarfed. Interestingly, despite marginal physical development, the cognitive development of these infants does not seem affected by their poor nutrition.

The study of the interactional patterns of mothers and infants with infantile anorexia (1988) led to the following hypotheses about the etiology of this feeding disorder:

1. Infantile anorexia nervosa is a relationship disorder that is characterized by intense conflict between mother and child over issues of control, autonomy, and dependency, with feeding being the primary battleground. This conflict in turn leads to confusion of emotional versus physiological needs by the infant and interferes with internal regulation of eating in accord to hunger and fullness.

2. The infant's characteristics of intense interpersonal sensitivity combined with stubbornness evoke conflicts over control and limit setting in a vulnerable mother who has experienced extremes of parental discipline in the form of either overcontrol or permissiveness while she was growing up. The mother's insecurity in regard to limit setting leads to inconsistency of her responses and fuels conflict with her temperamentally provocative infant. (These temperamental characteristics of assertiveness and stubbornness are postulated to result in onset of anorexia nervosa during the early period of separation and individuation in infancy, as opposed to during the later period of separation and individuation in adolescence.) The mother's childhood conflicts about control frequently involved parental management of eating as well and resulted in her difficulty in interpreting her own signals of hunger and satiety and in reading her infant's signals correctly.

Treatment

Treatment of infantile anorexia nervosa is based on the developmental model outlined above. The goal of the treatment is to facilitate the infant's internal regulation of eating through learning somatopsychological differentiation.

Empowerment of the mothers (Bromwich 1990; Chatoor et al. 1992) is the first goal of treatment, proceeding from the first contact. Without this empowerment, the evaluation and psychoeducational interventions may not occur. These interventions include helping parents understand the child's temperament and developmental level. Parents must be reassured that in these cases, malnutrition does not affect cognitive development. The therapist then explores the mother-infant conflict from the developmental perspective, educating parents about the normal aspects of the conflict between autonomy and dependency at this stage.

At this point, specific behavioral techniques are provided to the parents to allow the infant more autonomy during feedings while limiting maladaptive behaviors. These include 1) regular meals with only planned snacks, 2) limiting meals to 30 minutes, 3) praise of self-feeding without comments about the quantity of food, 4) cleaning up only at the end of the meal, 5) eliminating use of food as a reward, 6) limiting distracting games at meals, 7) time-out for anger, and 8) ending meals if child plays with food.

Working through these stages can require from three to eight meetings with the parents and the infant. Parents who are able to support one another usually succeed in changing the infant's eating pattern within a few weeks. However, parents who are in conflict with one another or mothers who continue to struggle with unresolved issues of control stemming from their own childhood may have difficulties following these behavioral instructions. In these cases, the second phase of treatment can involve couples therapy to address unresolved marital conflicts or individual psychotherapy for the mother to deal with her struggle over control by bringing out the "ghosts" from her childhood, as Fraiberg et al. (1975) described.

For older toddlers able to engage in symbolic play, play therapy using dolls to reenact feeding and sleeping of the baby can be helpful to explain that the baby doll eats when he or she feels hungry in his or her "tummy," and that he or she stops eating when the tummy is full. Contingent behaviors can be modeled by the therapist through play with the doll baby.

Mary is a 15-month-old toddler who was referred by her pediatrician for a psychiatric evaluation because of food refusal and FTT. Both parents were college educated. The father holds a high-level managerial position, whereas the mother has interrupted her career since Mary's birth. The mother reported that Mary was a full-term baby, had been breast-fed since birth, and was thriving well until age 9 months. When Mary was introduced to cereal and baby food, she showed strong preferences for certain types of food. She would spit out food or refuse to open her mouth if she did not like it. However, Mary was quite inconsistent. She refused a certain type of food one day but took it the next day. The mother felt confused by Mary's behavior. She tried to please Mary by offering her a variety of foods of different taste, by preparing baby food herself, and by coaxing, cajoling, and distracting Mary to get her to eat. Despite all her mother's efforts, Mary ate very little and relied primarily on breast-feeding for her nutrition, but also for comfort.

The parents reported that Mary was still sleeping in their bed, that the mother had to breast-feed Mary to settle her to sleep, and that Mary woke up a couple of times during the night to breast-feed. The pediatrician had suggested that the mother wean Mary from the breast, and the mother felt guilty that she had been unable to do so.

During exploration of the parents' difficulty in setting limits on Mary's demanding behavior, Mary's mother revealed that her own mother had been unmarried and destitute, rejected by her parents when Mary's mother was born. Forced to earn money to survive, Mary's grandmother had placed Mary's mother in the care of various nannies. When she was around, however, Mary's grandmother was very forceful with Mary's mother to get her to eat. Mary's father reported that in his family his mother expressed her affection through food and was very offended if he did not eat. He stated that his younger sister had been struggling with anorexia nervosa since her teens and was quite ill at the time. Both sets of Mary's grandparents were very concerned about Mary's lack of weight gain and growth and had encouraged her parents to get Mary to eat by force-feeding her.

Observation of mother and infant during feeding and play revealed that Mary was a strong-willed little girl who took the lead in the interactions with her mother. Mary seemed very curious about everything in the room and showed little interest in the food her mother offered to her, although she had not eaten for several hours. Shortly into the feeding, Mary refused to open her mouth and grunted and whined until the mother took her out of the high chair and allowed her to explore the room. The mother followed Mary with the food and spoon, coaxing and begging her to eat. Occasionally, Mary allowed her mother to slip some food into her mouth, but Mary's interest was clearly directed toward exploration of the room and having mother follow her leads.

After this evaluation, the therapist helped the parents understand that Mary was a very perceptive, curious, and strong-willed little girl who seemed to have a primary interest in mastery of her environment and little awareness of her internal cues of hunger. The therapist explained that these temperamental characteristics had facilitated external regulation of eating to meet Mary's physiological needs; then the parents were provided with the "food rules." The overall goal of these rules was explained to center on strengthening Mary's hunger cues by providing her with food only at regular times and by not allowing her to drink from the breast or snack in between meals, which could blunt her appetite.

Each of the rules was discussed with regard to its implementation, and the difficulties the parents anticipated were explored. Considerable time was spent on how to limit breast-feeding and how to deal with Mary's protestations and provocative behaviors if she could not have her way. The mother's difficulty in saying "no" to Mary was linked to the harshness with which her own mother had treated her around eating when the mother had been a child. The parents agreed to limit breast-feeding to bedtimes only to facilitate transitioning Mary into sleep. Although the father would have preferred to put Mary into her own crib, the parents agreed with each other to focus on the feeding first and to allow Mary to continue sleeping in their bed. The parents asked for 3 weeks to work on the new food rules.

During the follow-up visit, mother reported that Mary had settled into a regular feeding pattern and that her appetite seemed greatly improved, although she continued to have some mealtimes when she ate little. The mother felt that Mary seemed to enjoy feeding herself and that she had gained some weight. Her parents were delighted that they had been able to help her establish a regular feeding pattern and were ready to tackle the next developmental task, to wean Mary from breast-feeding and to transition her to sleep in her crib in a separate room.

Posttraumatic Eating Disorder

The Clinical Picture

The term *posttraumatic eating disorder* was first coined by Chatoor et al. (1988a) in a paper on food refusal after an incident of choking. That paper described five latency-age children who experienced episodes of choking and who later refused various foods for fear of choking again. Their symptoms resembled those commonly associated with posttraumatic stress in that the children were preoccupied with the fear of dying because of choking or were afraid of choking in their sleep and dreamed of choking and dying. Food refusal and the fear of dying was reported by Solyom and Sookman (1980) in four adult cases. L. Siegel (1982) reported on the treatment of a 6-year-old with symptoms described as "food aversion." Bernal (1972) treated a 4-year-old whose eating problem started at age 9 months after the child choked on a string bean. These articles were primarily concerned with behavioral management techniques and did not address the psychodynamic or developmental issues involved. Recently, Singer et al. (1992) described three boys ages 6–8 years with what they called "food phobia." The symptoms of food refusal started acutely after an incident of choking in one child and in association with acute medical illnesses in the other two children.

Food refusal after an episode of choking, as described by Chatoor et al. (1988a), presented as a phobic symptom in children who were struggling with developmental difficulties involving separation and individuation, which set the stage for these children to respond to a relatively minor trauma of choking with severe symptoms such as nightmares about choking and dying. The children experienced intense anticipatory anxiety when they thought of eating, and they scrupulously avoided eating foods they feared would lead to choking. In most cases, these were foods they had to chew, but a few children developed such an intense fear of swallowing liquids that they had difficulty swallowing their own saliva. One child was frightened to go to sleep out of fear that one of her teeth would loosen and choke her to death. When forced to eat, the children would go into a panic state with crying, screaming, gagging, general agitation, and combativeness.

The children's eating disorder and concomitant weight loss had a powerful impact on the parents, who became very solicitous in trying to relieve their children's anxiety. The mothers spent much time preparing special foods and then coaxing and begging their children to eat. At other times, the parents felt so frustrated that they unsuccessfully resorted to force to get the child to eat. The children withdrew from peers and their usual activities, and several stopped going to school. They became increasingly dependent on their parents, some even sleeping in bed with a parent because of their fear of bad dreams and fear of choking to death at night. Several parents left work or took leave to be with their child, reflecting persistent anxiety about the child's eating patterns despite the fact that all the children were healthy and, in three cases, overweight before the onset of the food refusal.

The children's reactions to the episode of choking were similar to the reactions of those who experience a severe trauma and develop a posttraumatic stress disorder. What clearly sets this posttraumatic eating disorder apart from posttraumatic stress disorder is the nature of the trauma. An episode of choking is not likely to evoke significant symptoms of distress in almost anyone, which is the first criterion needed to make a diagnosis of posttraumatic stress disorder. The children's reactions to the episodes of choking, however, were similar to the reactions seen in persons with posttraumatic stress disorder. Specifically, all of the children reexperienced the choking episode by recurrent recollections of the event or recurrent dreams of the event, or both. In addition, they withdrew from their usual activities and developed new symptoms not present before the trauma. Several developed sleep disturbances, and all of the children avoided activities that aroused recollection of the traumatic event by avoiding any food they might choke on. In addition, several of the children avoided events that might symbolize or resemble the choking episode: one child wouldn't play jacks for fear one would fly into her mouth and choke her, and another child would not touch his pet because of fear of getting hair in his mouth and choking on it.

The question arises as to why these children responded to the choking episode as if it were a major traumatic event. In her study of the effects of psychic trauma on children after the school bus kidnapping in Chowchilla, Terr (1983) noted that symptom severity was related to the child's prior vulnerability, family pathology, and community bonding. A similar concept was developed by Furst (1967), who concluded that the response to a traumatic event depended on the content and intensity of the original trauma, the strength of the ego, and the subsequent life experience. Developmental, social, and family history of the children described by Chatoor et al. (1988a) revealed that many of the children had experienced some loss and had shown evidence of separation anxiety and overdependence on the parents that predated the onset of the disorder.

All of the children lost weight because of their food refusal, which created significant concern and anxiety in the parents. The children received much solicitous attention and special treatment because of their symptoms, thus increasing the secondary gain and demonstrating the power of their symptoms to control their parents and the environment. These children also received much attention from doctors and medical personnel during repeated medical workups. All of these factors created a "subsequent life experience" that mitigated toward continuation rather than resolution of the symptoms.

Treatment

Treatment of these children involves three components. In the initial phase of treatment, the child's nutritional needs have to be addressed. Then, the child's anticipatory anxiety about eating and choking is treated through in vitro and in vivo desensitization procedures. Concurrently, the child and the family are seen in family therapy to address the familial context in which the disorder developed.

As a first step, the parents and child must be clearly reassured that the child will begin to eat again on a gradual basis. The parents should be seen in family therapy to help them understand the role that the shared anxiety about separation played in the development and maintenance of the food refusal symptoms, and they should then be helped to appropriately separate from the child and to disengage from the child's anxiety about the eating process. Parents should not discuss eating with their child or prepare special food for the child. They should be taught to treat mealtimes in a neutral manner and not to plead with or attempt to coax the child to eat, a process of disengagement that proves very difficult for many parents.

Simultaneously, the child should be engaged in a food desensitization program that focuses on gaining control over the phobic symptoms, an approach that has also been used in the treatment of school phobia (Croghan 1981). The child is taught self-hypnosis to help him or her overcome the anticipatory anxiety of eating and choking and then is assisted in the development of a hierarchy of food groups beginning with the least feared and moving to the most feared. Next, the child is involved in an in vitro desensitization procedure, during which he or she imagines eating foods of increasing texture and learns to control the associated anxiety. After some success with the in vitro procedure, an in vivo desensitization procedure begins; when the child is successful in eating the foods in one level of the hierarchy, he or she advances to the next level of the hierarchy.

There are similarities between the treatment of food refusal and the recommended treatment of school phobia. In both disorders, the focus is on the child's mastery of his or her anxiety as quickly as possible and resuming the feared activity. In addition, it seems crucial to both treatments that the parents understand the role that the shared anxiety about separation plays in the development and maintenance of the symptoms.

Posttraumatic Feeding Disorder

The Clinical Picture

Food refusal can often be seen in infants and toddlers after an incident of choking, after painful manipulation of the oropharynx by insertion of tubes and vigorous suctioning, or after vomiting. Because of the feeding dependency of the infant or toddler and the resemblance of symptoms of this disorder to the posttraumatic eating disorder in children, Chatoor (1991a, 1991b) described this type of food refusal as posttraumatic feeding disorder. Numerous papers describe this feeding disorder under labels such as food refusal (Linscheid et al. 1987; Ramsay and Zelazo 1988; Singer et al. 1991), food phobia (Singer 1992), food aversion (L. Siegel 1982), and feeding resistance (Geerstma et al. 1985). Many of these cases involved infants who had severe medical illnesses associated with painful symptoms in the oropharynx or gastrointestinal tract, such as gastroesophageal reflux (Shepard et al. 1987), cleft palate (Richard 1991), cystic fibrosis (Singer et al. 1991), short gut syndrome (Linscheid et al 1987), and dumping syndrome (Hirsig et al. 1984). These infants appeared to associate anything related to feeding with pain, and they showed fear in anticipation of feedings. In severe cases, this disorder is characterized by refusal to put anything in the mouth, and in milder cases it is characterized by refusal to chew or swallow solid food. The infant seems to have no awareness of hunger and experiences severe distress if he or she is force-fed, becoming even more fearful at subsequent feedings.

In time, secondary complications of this posttraumatic feeding disorder develop. If the infant refuses to put anything in his or her mouth over weeks or months, he or she does not get any practice in sucking, chewing, and swallowing. In addition, as the infant matures cognitively, he or she becomes more aware of cause and effect in caretaker interactions, learning to anticipate certain of the caretaker's emotional responses. Food refusal usually arouses such intense feelings of anxiety, anger, or frustration in the parents that they try anything to get the infant to eat. The infant learns to exercise control over the parents' emotions and behaviors through feeding behavior. These secondary complications perpetuate the feeding disorder.

Treatment
Treatment occurs in three stages. A multidisciplinary team is usually necessary to treat this disorder. In severe cases, an infant's nutrition has to be managed through nasogastric or gastrostomy tube feedings to allow the behavioral treatment to be carried out.

1. It is important to help parents understand the dynamics of a posttraumatic feeding disorder so that they can become active participants in the treatment. The first stage of treatment is desensitization of the infant to the fear of eating. This is best done after thorough exploration of what seems to trigger anticipatory anxiety about eating: whether the sight of the bottle, food, or high chair is sufficient or whether the trigger is the infant's being touched around the mouth. Gradual exposure of the infant to the sight of

the bottle or pleasurable touching of the oral area should occur until the infant is able to open his or her mouth, mouth a toy, or take a spoon without fear. Once the infant is able to mouth toys without fear, food can be introduced.

2. Introduction of food is begun with water rather than milk to avoid previous unpleasurable associations with milk and to minimize the risk of choking. It is important that a professional assess the infant's oromotor coordination and work with the infant directly on chewing and swallowing semisolids before any type of food that can lead to choking is introduced. Again, a hierarchy of solid foods should be established, with meats introduced last due to their texture. For older infants or toddlers, learning to drink from a cup instead of the feared bottle or participating in the feeding with a second spoon helps the infant gain a sense of control and overcome fear. During this stage the emphasis is on teaching the infant oromotor skills. There should be no emphasis on the amount of food consumed.

3. Once the infant has fairly good feeding skills, experiencing hunger becomes an important goal. The infant's tube feedings should be decreased, particularly during the day, to produce hunger at feeding time. It is important that the parents not pressure the infant to eat more and that they allow him or her to learn how to regulate intake according to physiological needs.

In summary, posttraumatic feeding disorder has become a new challenge in the treatment of severely ill infants. Many intertwining factors contribute to this severe feeding disorder, which frequently requires an integrated, multidisciplinary team approach for successful intervention.

EATING DISORDERS IN ADOLESCENTS: ANOREXIA NERVOSA AND BULIMIA NERVOSA

Anorexia nervosa and bulimia nervosa have generally been considered disorders of adolescence and young adulthood. In both of these disorders, there is a preoccupation with weight and food. There are, however, many significant symptomatic and psychological differences between the disorders that shape the therapy.

Age at Onset

Halmi and co-workers (1979) reported a bimodal distribution of age at onset of anorexia with peaks at ages 14 and 18, clearly establishing its adolescent onset. Garfinkel and Garner (1982) reported that 83% of subjects in their study had an onset of anorexia before age 20. In a more recent study of patients seen in a tertiary referral center, Woodside and Garfinkel (1992) reported an earlier onset of bulimic symptoms compared with anorexic symptoms. Almost 90% of both pure bulimic patients and those bulimic patients with a prior history of anorexia had an onset of bingeing before age 20, whereas fewer than 60% of the anorexic patients had achieved their lowest weight (considered by the authors to be the onset of the disorder) by age 20. The authors concluded that anorexic and bulimic symptoms have fairly consistent and independent patterns of onset, regardless of whether they occur together in the same person or separately in different people. They noted, however, that onset of the disorders might alternatively be defined as the first appearance of specific psychological symptoms such as weight preoccupations. It would seem that this latter approach, although more difficult to define operationally, has more clinical utility.

Anorexia

The Clinical Picture

Anorexia is a condition in which there is a severe restriction of calorie intake leading, by DSM-III-R definition, to at least a 25% loss of body weight. Weight loss may often proceed to life-threatening levels. Associated physical features include loss of menses, hypothermia, bradycardia, and development of lanugo hair. There may be an extreme preoccupation with food and the emergence of bizarre food choices over time. A patient might limit herself,[1] for instance, to only root vegetables. There may also be hoarding of food or excessive handling of food.

Anorexia may be associated with other disorders. Bemporad et al. (1992) found that 43% of anorexic patients had an Axis I diagnosis, predominantly mood disorders, and that 77% of the patients gave evidence of an Axis II disorder, predominantly borderline personality disorder.

There is usually a profound distortion of body image. Patients typically claim to look or feel fat even when emaciated. The relentless pursuit of thinness is accompanied by fears of eating and weight gain. Crisp (1970) described these symptoms as a general weight phobia, but there may be food phobias as well. There is usually a profound denial

---

[1]Given the significantly higher incidence of these disorders among females, the pronoun *she* will be used in this section. It is not meant, however, to indicate that these disorders do not occur in males.

of illness and of nutritional needs. Periods of hyperactivity are also common.

No one single set of psychodynamic factors accounts for the disorder. Bruch (1973) described a pervasive ineffectiveness in these children, who have great difficulties in establishing control and autonomy over their lives. Diet provides an arena of control, and thinness provides a venue for self-esteem. Crisp et al. (1980) discussed anorexia as a means of avoiding the development of a mature female body and an evasion of assuming adult responsibilities. Both of these sets of factors, among others, are usually operative to some degree.

Individual Psychotherapy

Because of the nature of the disorder and its course, anorexia must be treated with a variety of modalities. These need to be integrated and coordinated to effectively care for the patient. Treatment modalities include individual psychotherapy, behavioral and cognitive approaches, family therapy, and effective liaison with a pediatrician and an inpatient unit. Individual psychotherapy is central to the treatment and serves to encompass and organize the other treatments.

One of the most persuasive approaches to the anorexic patient was described by Davis (1992). According to him, the central task of the individual therapy is to work with what he termed "anorexic resistance." In most cases, the anorexic patient does not want to be in treatment. She sees the therapist as "an enemy, someone who will attempt to prevent her from remaining thin or becoming thinner" (p. 197). She is threatened by any loss of control in her entrenched patterns of maintaining weight control. Her primary relationship is not to people, but to her thinness. The therapist by his or her very presence is a challenge.

Manifestations of the resistance include silence, rejection, and overt hostility to the therapist's approaches. There may also be a superficial compliance with what sounds like "therapeutic" talk; however, this talk in essence reveals nothing.

Davis (1992) noted that "anorexia nervosa may produce more countertransferential responses in trained psychotherapists than any other psychiatric disorder" (p. 198). Therapists must prepare themselves for feeling disconnected, ineffective, and spurned. Davis also noted that there will be no appreciation for the help offered.

A traditional therapeutic stance of neutrality, exploration, and interpretation may only be employed very late in treatment after the illness no longer serves as the prime organizer of experience. The therapist who approaches the task of therapy in terms of understanding his or her patient and communicating this understanding is at cross-purposes with the patient, who is only interested in pursuing thinness. The exploration is highly threatening, and the neutrality will leave the patient in her state of isolation and loneliness.

Davis recommended a very specific therapeutic stance for the early and middle phases of treatment that involves taking a "dynamic, authoritative, and actively caring approach to the patient" (p. 201). This approach not only disarms the anorexic patient's resistance but in essence begins to structure a human relationship for the patient, whose primary relationship is with the illness. Davis stated that in the initial contacts the therapist must present himself or herself as a friendly authority who asks knowing questions—about which foods are safe, about the inner voices who talk about the patient's eating, or about the magic number beyond which she cannot gain.

Attention to the symptomatic details is the only empathy the patient will allow. The therapist may then proceed to educate the patient about the evolution of her illness, noting the progression from a simple diet to extreme dieting serving to solve life's other problems. When the therapist takes responsibility for the success of the treatment, which essentially means the therapeutic relationship itself, the anorexic resistance is not allowed to exert the same degree of control as it does in the patient's other relationships. By this therapeutic stance, the therapist positions himself or herself as a real entity who is not reactive to the patient's various withdrawals. He or she is a known quantity to be liked or not, trusted or not, befriended or not—in either case, there are real emotions that can lead the patient out of herself and back into the world of relating to other people. As the therapeutic relationship evolves, the therapist must reveal his or her responses to the patient and offer support, compliments, and real advice as the patient begins to reengage herself in relationships and activities.

Weight management should be simple and straightforward. The pediatrician will set a minimum weight. Periodic visits to the pediatrician are necessary for weight and nutritional assessment. If the patient falls below the minimum, she is to be hospitalized, where she is to be managed with the behavioral approach described below. In time, the patient will risk gaining, pound by pound, above her acceptable maximum. At such time, specific advice about normalizing the diet needs to be given. As the patient can enter into a more related involvement with the therapist, so too can she begin to hesitantly enter the risky world between thin and fat.

In the final phases of treatment, the therapist must use more traditional therapeutic techniques not only to elucidate the problems left unsolved by the anorexic solution, but also to help the patient move beyond her reliance on the therapist. Dependence on the therapist may have supplanted the dependence on anorexia. Instead of freely giving advice, the therapist may gently push the patient to attempt her own solutions. What happens when the therapist does this? Can the patient tolerate the anxiety or feel anger at an apparent withdrawal of support? Does she blame an unsatisfactory outcome of a given situation on the therapist? Does she return to a restrictive diet? Her responses must be tracked, and the therapist's stance must be subtly shifted and modified accordingly.

Additional Components of Treatment

The pediatrician. As noted, a pediatrician is essential to the treatment program. His or her role is principally to ensure that a minimal weight is maintained. During the initial stages, a weekly visit is advisable for weighing. The pediatrician's involvement should center on the medical concerns, with only limited inquiries into the patient's emotional well-being. The patient should be instructed not to weigh herself, because minor fluctuations will trigger exaggerated emotional reactions.

The pediatrician will specify a desirable weight in addition to the minimum weight. Movement from the minimum to the ideal weight may be approached through contracting (but not at the initial stage of treatment) and also integrated with the ongoing therapy.

Hospitalization. If the patient's weight falls below the acceptable level, she needs to be hospitalized. In the hospital, a highly structured approach is advised (Eckert and Labeck 1985) in which caloric intake is prescribed and weight gain is rewarded. Meals as presented must be finished in a set period of time, and patients are initially watched after meals to guard against purging. If meals are not finished, liquid meals are prescribed. If weight gain is not accomplished, tube feeding is then required. Weight gain of one-half pound per day is expected, and this gain is rewarded by increasing off-ward privileges.

Family therapy. Work with the families of anorexic patients was pioneered by both Minuchin (1978) and Palazzoli (1978), who reported good results using various family restructuring techniques. Their outcome findings had no control subjects.

Although it is possible that not all anorexic patients may benefit from family therapy, it has been shown that adolescent anorexic patients clearly do. In a large controlled trial of family therapy, Russell and co-workers (1987) demonstrated that those patients who had onset of illness before age 19 and an illness duration of less than 3 years had good or intermediate outcome at 1 year follow-up when family therapy was part of the treatment program. Patients of the same age group treated only with individual therapy had a low rate of good or intermediate outcomes.

Family therapy, of course, may be as diverse as individual therapy and should ideally be specified. Le Grange and co-workers (1992) reported on a pilot study evaluating family treatments in adolescent anorexia nervosa. In this study, conjoint family therapy (with the patient present) was compared with individual therapy plus family counseling during which the patient was not present. The family counseling group actually fared a bit better, but statistically the groups were equivalent. Le Grange and co-workers found that the patients who expressed high levels of dissatisfaction with family life and whose parents were openly critical of them did better with counseling than with conjoint therapy.

Pharmacotherapy.   Although medication may be indicated on a case-to-case basis for associated disorders, there is no established medication used for anorexia nervosa.

> On returning from a family vacation to Mexico, Sally, then 16 years old, developed amoebiasis and, in the 3 weeks until the condition was diagnosed and treated, lost almost 15 pounds. On returning to school she found that she liked the compliments for the weight loss, having been a bit overweight. Sally decided to keep dieting. Her older sister had made a suicide attempt the previous year and had been hospitalized, and the sister had returned home in a state of depression just before the Mexico vacation. Distracted by the sister's problems and Sally's recent gastrointestinal problem, the family did not notice Sally's weight loss until she fainted in school. At this point she was preoccupied by thinness. In the emergency room, the diagnosis of anorexia nervosa was made and she was hospitalized.
>
> Sally was treated in the hospital with a structured behavioral program leading to a minimal acceptable weight gain. Individual sessions revealed her envy of the attention given to her sister, and family sessions led to a shifting of focus to her. Enraged that she might wind up as "emotionally sick" as her sister and determined to prove to everyone that she could maintain the minimal "approved" weight, Sally refused to continue in individual treatment or family treatment after discharge.
>
> For the next 2 years, she did maintain this minimal weight but found herself thinking about food and exercise to the exclusion of much else. The slightest departures from her minimal diet would be corrected with exercise calculated by calorie expenditure. After a nearly "perfect" freshman year, she requested treatment. From this point, she remained in psychotherapy for the next 3 years.
>
> Her initial approach to the therapy was passive. It was the therapist's job to do therapy with her. She wanted easy answers, and she began to notice that when the therapist made suggestions to her she would "zone out." She eventually understood that in this type of interchange she was equating her therapist's suggestions with her father's demands. Being with people meant pleasing them if there was to be a relationship.
>
> Once that issue and other dynamic issues relating to her sense of effectiveness and fear of passion were interpreted, she no longer depended on a thin self to present to the world. She began to desire to have her period back and began to admire, rather than disdain, friends with healthy appetites. At this point, in the third year of treatment, she wanted to see a nutritionist, who helped her plan a weight gain of 1–2 pounds per month.

Bulimia Nervosa

The Clinical Picture
Bulimia nervosa is an eating disorder in which there is a pattern of binge eating that is felt to be irresistible. *Bingeing* is defined as consumption of a large amount of food in a discrete period of time, usually less than 2 hours. The food is usually of high-calorie content, and the eating is done in a solitary, inconspicuous, if not secretive, manner. Each episode of bingeing will usually proceed until terminated by abdominal pain, sleep, an unwanted social interruption, or self-induced vomiting. A state of mounting anxiety and tension precedes the binge, and depression, guilt, and remorse usually follow the binge. Attempts to dispel the ingested food include self-induced vomiting, laxative and diuretic abuse, and obsessive and extreme exercise often exactly calculated to work off the ingested calories. There is an overwhelming fear of becoming fat, and there may be wide fluctuations of weight. There is also a sense that behaviors are out of the individual's control.

There are a number of conditions associated with bulimia nervosa. Rates of depression have been reported to be as high as 75% (Herzog 1982). Impulsivity is also a problem. This impulsivity is seen not only in the bingeing itself but also in shoplifting and sexual behaviors. Drug and alcohol use has been reported in perhaps 30% of patients (Herzog 1982). One report (Herzog et al. 1989) indicated that nearly 25% of patients made a major suicide attempt.

Bulimic behaviors often interfere with the individual's life in terms of work or school performance, social relationships, and family relationships. The bingeing and purging behaviors may occupy many hours each day. The shame about these behaviors isolates the individual further. Interpersonal problems are rarely dealt with directly. Rather, they are coped with through the sequence of eating behaviors.

Central to a psychodynamic understanding of bulimia is the role the eating behaviors play in tension regulation (Herzog et al. 1989). An insistence on solitary symbolic meanings avoids the complexity of the symptom. Bruch (1973) views eating disorders as adaptation to early developmental disruptions when there were no responses to the child's needs. Hamburg (1989) described the multiple structural meanings of bulimia as including oral meanings (hunger, emptiness, painful seeking, food that soothes tension), anality (needs bring humiliation, expulsion of poison, assertions of control), and genitality (sexualized hunger fulfilled in a frenzy, food as stimulation to the deadness within). Noting that the task of late adolescence is consolidating identity, Brisman (1992) wrote, "The defensive position of early adolescence, that of over-idealization and identification, is not relinquished. Instead, a 'foreclosed' identity is assumed in which there is a reliance on fixed, idealized notion of whom one should be" (p. 173). Lewis and Brisman

(1992) discussed three interrelated dynamic features: difficulties with separation, unstable identity, and chronic disappointment in others.

Individual Psychotherapy

Herzog et al. (1989) stressed that the multidimensional nature of bulimia nervosa, particularly for refractory patients, requires an integrative approach comprising elements of psychodynamic psychotherapy, cognitive-behavior psychotherapy, and pharmacotherapy. Brisman (1992) extended this approach and put forth a fully integrated model of psychotherapy for all bulimic patients.

Brisman's basic premise is as follows: The bulimic teenager is rarely interested in self-exploration. Given the potential destructiveness of the symptoms themselves, symptom management is an issue present from the very start of treatment. The adolescent is truly alone with her symptoms—ashamed, despondent, desperate, and endangering herself. She will bring only some version of an idealized self into a relationship, yet she needs to understand all that she finds unacceptable and must hide. A strictly psychodynamic approach misses the point: "The eating disorder itself is the only language the patient has developed to communicate that something is wrong" (Brisman 1992, p. 176). An approach that overly relies on interpretation tends to use a language the patient does not understand and misses the profound impact the disorder has on her day-to-day life. On the other hand, an overreliance on controlling the symptoms will ultimately backfire because both the patient and the therapist will miss what the symptoms are intended to communicate.

The therapy must begin with a detailed inquiry into all factors and circumstances that give rise to the bingeing and purging. It may not have occurred to the patient that any particular feeling state precedes the bingeing. More often than not, binges just happen. Although this type of inquiry sets the stage for the psychoanalytic inquiry that is ultimately necessary, it is rarely helpful at first. In fact, it will often leave the patient feeling more despair and hopelessness.

Certain cognitive-behavioral methods that have documented effectiveness need to be used (Fairburn 1981). Self-monitoring through keeping a diary may offer a modicum of structure to replace that lost as the bingeing and purging sequence is questioned. When internal dysphoric states or external stressors are identified, the patient can be asked not only to delay the binge for whatever time period is agreed on, but also to provide some alternative means of self-soothing. These might include speaking to a friend, listening to music, or taking a bath.

The purpose of these early interventions is to make some experience of anxiety possible, guarding that it does not become overwhelming. Contracting involves some agreement between patient and therapist regarding a delay in the timing of a binge or the frequency of a binge.

Someone who binges three to four times a day might agree to skip a binge every other day.

Such contracts may provide for some immediate symptomatic relief, but that is not the only purpose. The goal "is not merely to set up contracts that the patient can keep, but to understand what gets in the way of her keeping the contracts in the first place, or what allows for successes she was unable to achieve on her own" (Brisman 1992, p. 178). Brisman further noted that the contract provides a vehicle of relatedness necessary for work with the teenager who has learned to avoid the substance of relationships at the cost of her own identity. Contracts are necessarily broken. In the process, the patient's wish for the solution and structure provided by the contract becomes apparent, as does her fear that it will suffocate her, control her, and strip her identity away. Within these vacillations, major themes from the patient's unconscious are played out.

Thus, step by step the patient learns to tolerate anxiety and the "mess" within that she had previously purged away. This new tolerance is developed in the context of a therapeutic relationship that is progressively allowed to contain more of the patient, both messy and perfect. Brisman (1992) cautioned that it is "when the treatment appears to be at its best that the patient may in fact be most defended, most guarded, most withdrawn" (p. 182).

The psychodynamic orientation of the above approach is interpersonal in nature. Attention to the quality and limitations of relatedness and the effect of symptoms on the capacity to relate serves as the main focus of the therapeutic inquiry. Such a stance does not specify neutrality and reconstructive interpretation as central to the technical approach. The symptomatic relief obtainable through various cognitive-behavioral techniques does not work against the psychodynamic inquiry, as held by a traditional approach. Rather, such maneuvers are useful in that they generate new interpersonal situations that ultimately advance the therapeutic inquiry.

Additional Components of Treatment

The previously described model for the individual psychotherapy of bulimic patients integrates cognitive-behavioral and interpersonal psychodynamic approaches. In addition, several other components of treatment may be necessary.

Pharmacotherapy.   The use of antidepressant medications has been extensively reviewed and found to diminish bulimic symptoms, at least in the short term (Garfinkel and Garner 1987). It is not clear whether these drugs work via a separate antibinge mechanism of action or via antidepressant mechanisms of action. As Lewis and Brisman (1992) observed, the positive effects of the medication may cause bulimic patients to reject the medication because of a variety of psychological reactions, including fears of separation (stopping the medication because at some point in the future the medication will have to be stopped), loss of identity (feeling better but changed), or activation of the perennial disappointment in primary objects (the medication helps but does not make all the bad feelings go away). As with the cognitive-behavioral interventions, these kinds of reactions can serve to further the psychodynamic inquiry.

Family therapy.   Although there is no clear consensus about whether a structural family therapeutic approach is superior to parental counseling, the parents of an adolescent bulimic patient need some involvement with the treatment. It is often helpful to give the patient the option of being present for such meetings. M. Siegel et al. (1988) described some of the goals of such counseling or therapy. These included helping parents 1) to understand the disorder, 2) to learn to discuss the disorder with their daughter, 3) to cope with their daughter's denial of illness, 4) to disengage from the eating problems, and 5) to relate to their daughter as an individual with age-specific concerns.

Group psychotherapy.   Group psychotherapy has been advocated as an important adjunct to individual treatments. Given the secretive nature of the disorder, group therapy at the start of treatment is not usually advisable. Groups can be useful in decreasing the isolation and shame of the bulimic patient. In addition, the group may aid the individual in objectifying the obsessive concerns with weight and diet and in seeing their effects in a social context.

Outcome: Anorexia Nervosa and Bulimia Nervosa

Anorexia nervosa has a high mortality rate. The longest follow-up study to date (Theander 1983), during which patients were observed for a total amount of time ranging from 22 to 50 years, found that the mortality from anorexia nervosa and suicide among 94 probands was 18%. Hsu et al. (1979) followed up 100 women for 8 years. At this point the mortality among this sample was 2%, but only 48% had a good outcome as determined by nearly normal weight, regular menstruation, and satisfactory psychosexual and psychosocial adjustment. Eckert (1985) reported that most researchers associate a favorable prognosis with an early age at onset of illness and a less favorable outcome with a later age at onset. Longer duration of illness, frequent hospitalizations, extremely low weight, and mixed syndromes with bingeing, purging, and laxative abuse also predicted poorer prognosis. Extreme distortions of body size, premorbid personality, and family difficulties also predicted poorer outcome. Strong social support has been reported as predictive of good outcome at 3 years (Sohlberg et al. 1992).

Although bulimia nervosa does not tend to have a significant mortality rate, morbidity rates tend to be high. Short-term follow-up studies of pure bulimic patients have shown good immediate results, but longer-term studies show extraordinarily high rates of chronicity and recurrence. Keller et al. (1992) reported on the approximately 3-year follow-up of 30 women and found a 63% cumulative probability of relapse by 78 weeks after recovery. Predictors of good outcome included having less disturbed eating behaviors, less disturbed self- and body images, and good social support.

CONCLUSION

Central to the early childhood developmental eating disorders is a profound disorder of relationships. Treatment of the childhood disorders (excluding the posttraumatic disorders) hinges on correcting the mother's, or caregiver's, ability to tune in to what the child needs. Simply put, if the mother cannot perceive and distinguish these needs, it becomes an impossible task for the infant or toddler to learn, and maladaptive behaviors result. Although different behavioral, family, and educational approaches need to be employed, the psychiatrist's empathy toward the parent is central to the recovery of the mother and her infant or toddler.

The situation is similar with the adolescent disorders, except that therapy is now primarily addressed to the symptomatic patient, not to his or her parents. The patient's ability to receive the empathy and advice of the psychiatrist is central to any cure.

Although the psychotherapy of anorexic adolescents differs from that of bulimic adolescents, there are several shared features. First and foremost is the need to integrate various components of treatment. Within the organizing therapeutic relationship, psychodynamic and cognitive-behavioral approaches can be combined with additional components as necessary. The psychodynamic approach described in this chapter implies an interpersonal orientation, with very particular uses of the therapist's self in the therapy. For anorexia nervosa, the therapist's stance is authoritative regarding the illness and responsible regarding the therapeutic relationship. For bulimia nervosa, the stance involves positioning oneself to be defeated, if not rejected, until the basic need to defeat and reject help can be made apparent to the patient. Central to the therapist's empathy is his or her acceptance of the self-organization that the disorder provides for the patient and the very language of the symptoms themselves. In an in-depth report on 13 women recovering from anorexia nervosa, Beresin and co-workers

(1989) found (and the same would seem to hold true for bulimia nervosa as well) that "the essential therapeutic agent for this lengthy change is the establishment of a relationship. . . . Through the medium of being empathically understood by another person, the anorectic begins to learn who she is" (p. 127).

REFERENCES

American Psychiatric Association: Diagnostic and Statistical Manual of Mental Disorders, 3rd Edition. Washington, DC, American Psychiatric Association, 1980

American Psychiatric Association: Diagnostic and Statistical Manual of Mental Disorders, 3rd Edition, Revised. Washington, DC, American Psychiatric Association, 1987

Bemporad JR, Beregin E, Ratey J, et al: A psychoanalytic study of eating disorders, I: a developmental profile of 67 index cases. J Am Acad Psychoanal 20:509–531, 1992

Beresin E, Gordon C, Herzog D: The process of recovering from anorexia nervosa. J Am Acad Psychoanal 17:103–130, 1989

Bernal ME: Behavioral treatment of a child's eating problem. J Behav Ther Exp Psychiatry 3:43–50, 1972

Bithany WG, Dubowitz H: Organic concomitants of non-organic failure to thrive: implications for research, in New Directions in Failure to Thrive: Research and Clinical Practice. Edited by Drotar D. New York, Plenum, 1972, pp 47–68

Blitzer JR, Rollins N, Blackwell A: Children who starve themselves: anorexia nervosa. Psychosom Med 23:369–383, 1961

Bradley RH, Casey PM, Wortham B: Home environments of low SES non-organic failure to thrive infants. Merrill Palmer Quarterly 30:393–402, 1984

Brisman J: Bulimia in the older adolescent: an analytic perspective to a behavioral problem, in Psychotherapies With Children and Adolescents: Adapting the Psychodynamic Process. Edited by O'Brien JD, Pilowsky DJ, Lewis OW. Washington, DC, American Psychiatric Press, 1992, pp 171–187

Bromwich RM: The interaction approach to early intervention. Infant Mental Health Journal 11:66–79, 1990

Bruch H: Eating Disorders: Obesity, Anorexia, and the Person Within. New York, Basic Books, 1973

Budd KS, McGraw TE, Farbisz R, et al: Psychosocial concomitants of children's feeding disorders. J Pediatr Psychol 17:81–94, 1992

Casey PH, Bradley R, Wortham B: Social and nonsocial home environments and infants with nonorganic failure to thrive. Pediatrics 73:348–353, 1984

Chapin HD: A plan of dealing with atrophic infants and children. Archives of Pediatrics 25:491–496, 1908

Chatoor I: Infantile anorexia nervosa: a developmental disorder of separation and individuation. J Am Acad Psychoanal 17:43–64, 1989

Chatoor I: Diagnosis, mother-infant interaction, and treatment of three developmental feeding disorders associated with failure to thrive, institute II: a developmental perspective on eating disorders from infancy to adulthood. Paper presented at the annual meeting of the Academy of Child and Adolescent Psychiatry, San Francisco, CA, 1991a

Chatoor I: Eating and nutritional disorders of infancy and early childhood, in Textbook of Child and Adolescent Psychiatry. Edited by Wiener J. Washington, DC, American Psychiatric Press, 1991b, pp 351–361

Chatoor I, Egan J: Nonorganic failure to thrive and dwarfism due to food refusal: a separation disorder. Journal of the American Academy of Child Psychiatry 33:294–301, 1983

Chatoor I, Schaefer S, Dickson L, et al: Nonorganic failure to thrive: a developmental perspective. Pediatr Ann 13:829–843, 1984

Chatoor I, Dickson L, Schaefer S, et al: A developmental classification of feeding disorders associated with failure to thrive: diagnosis and treatment, in New Directions in Failure to Thrive: Research and Clinical Practice. Edited by Drotar D. New York, Plenum, 1985, pp 235–258

Chatoor I, Conley C, Dickson L: Food refusal after an incident of choking: a posttraumatic eating disorder. J Am Acad Child Adolesc Psychiatry 27:105–110, 1988a

Chatoor I, Egan J, Getson P, et al: Mother-infant interactions in infantile anorexia nervosa. J Am Acad Child Adolesc Psychiatry 27:535–540, 1988b

Chatoor I, Kerzner B, Zorc L, et al: Two-year old twins refuse to eat: a multidisciplinary approach to diagnosis and treatment. Infant Mental Health Journal 13:252–268, 1992

Crisp AH: Anorexia: feeding disorders, nervous malnutrition or weight phobia. World Rev Nutr Diet 12:452–505, 1970

Crisp AH, Hsu LKG, Harding B: Clinical features of anorexia nervosa: a study of a consecutive series of 102 female patients. J Psychosom Res 24:179–191, 1980

Croghan LM: Conceptualizing the critical elements in a rapid desensitization to school anxiety: a case study. Pediatric Psychology 6:165–170, 1981

Davis W: The anorexic adolescent, in Psychotherapies With Children and Adolescents: Adapting the Psychodynamic Process. Edited by O'Brien JD, Pilowsky DJ, Lewis OW. Washington, DC, American Psychiatric Press, 1992, pp 189–208

Dowling S: Seven infants with esophageal atresia: a developmental study. Psychoanal Study Child 32:215–256, 1977

Drotar D: Behavioral diagnosis in nonorganic failure to thrive: a critique and suggested approach to psychological assessment. J Dev Behav Pediatr 10:48–55, 1989

Drotar D, Eckerle D: The family environment in nonorganic failure to thrive: a controlled study. J Pediatr Psychol 14:245–257, 1989

Drotar D, Eckerle D, Satola J, et al: Maternal interactional behavior with non-organic failure-to-thrive infants: a case comparison study. Child Abuse Negl 14:41–51, 1990

Eckert E: Characteristic of anorexia nervosa, in Anorexia Nervosa and Bulimia: Diagnosis and Treatment. Edited by Mitchell J. Minneapolis, University of Minnesota Press, 1985, pp 3–28

Eckert E, Labeck L: Integrated treatment program for anorexia nervosa, in Anorexia Nervosa and Bulimia: Diagnosis and Treatment. Edited by Mitchell J. Minneapolis, University of Minnesota Press, 1985, pp 152–170

Evans SL, Reinhart JB, Succop RA: Failure to thrive: a study of 45 children and their families. Journal of the American Academy of Child Psychiatry 11:440–457, 1972

Fairburn CG: A cognitive behavioral approach to the management of bulimia. Psychol Med 11:707–711, 1981

Fosson A, Knibbs J, Bryant-Waugh R, et al: Early onset anorexia nervosa. Arch Dis Child 62:114–118, 1987

Fraiberg S, Anderson E, Shapiro V: Ghosts in the nursery. Journal of the American Academy of Child Psychiatry 14:387–421, 1975

Furst S: Psychic Trauma: A Survey. New York, Basic Books, 1967

Garfinkel PE, Garner DM: Anorexia Nervosa: A Multidimensional Perspective. New York, Brunner/Mazel, 1982

Garfinkel PE, Garner DM: The Role of Drug Treatment for Eating Disorders. New York, Brunner/Mazel, 1987

Geerstma MA, Hyams J, Pelletier J, et al: Feeding resistance after parenteral hyperalimentation. Am J Dis Child 139:255–256, 1985

Greenspan SI, Lourie RS: Developmental structuralist approach to classification of adaptive and pathologic personality organizations: infancy and early childhood. Am J Psychiatry 138:725–735, 1985

Halmi KA, Casper R, Eckert E, et al: Unique features associated with age of onset of anorexia nervosa. Psychiatry Res 1:209–215, 1979

Hamburg P: Bulimia: the construction of a symptom. J Am Acad Psychoanal 17:131–140, 1989

Hawley RM: The outcome of anorexia nervosa in younger subjects. Br J Psychiatry 146:657–660, 1985

Haynes CF, Cutler C, Gray J, et al: Hospitalized cases of non-organic failure-to-thrive: scope of the problem and short-term lay health visitor intervention. Child Abuse Negl 8:229–242, 1984

Herzog DB: Bulimia: the secretive syndrome. Psychosomatics 23:481–487, 1982

Herzog DB, Frank DL, Brotman AW: Integrating treatments for bulimia nervosa. J Am Acad Psychoanal 17:141–150, 1989

Hirsig J, Baals H, Tuchschmid P, et al: Dumping syndrome following Nissen's fundoplication: a cause for refusal to feed. J Pediatr Surg 19:155–159, 1984

Homer C, Ludwig S: Categorization of etiology of failure to thrive. Am J Dis Child 135:848–851, 1981

Hsu L, Crisp AH, Harding B: Outcome of anorexia nervosa. Lancet 1(8107):61–65, 1979

Keller M, Herzog D, Lavori R, et al: The naturalistic history of bulimia nervosa: extraordinarily high rates of chronicity, relapse, recurrence, and psychosocial morbidity. International Journal of Eating Disorders 12:1–9, 1992

Le Grange D, Eisler I, Dove C, et al: Evaluation of family treatments in adolescent anorexia nervosa: a pilot study. International Journal of Eating Disorders 12:347–357, 1992

Lewis O, Brisman J: Medication and bulimia; binge/purge dynamics and the "helpful" pill. International Journal of Eating Disorders 12:327–331, 1992

Lieberman A, Birch M: The etiology of failure to thrive: an interactional developmental approach, in New Directions in Failure to Thrive: Research and Clinical Practice. Edited by Drotar D. New York, Plenum, 1985, pp 250–277

Linscheid TR, Rasnake LK: Behavioral approaches to the treatment of failure to thrive, in New Directions in Failure to Thrive: Research and Clinical Practice. Edited by Drotar D. New York, Plenum, 1985, pp 279–294

Linscheid TR, Tarnowski KJ, Rasnake LK, et al: Behavioral treatment of food refusal in a child with short-gut syndrome. J Pediatr Psychol 12:451–459, 1987

Mahler MS, Pine F, Berman A: The Psychological Birth of the Human Infant. New York, Basic Books, 1975

Main M, Goldwyn R: Predicting rejection of her infant from mother's representation of her own experiences: implications for the abused abusing interactional cycle. Child Abuse Negl 8:203–217, 1984

Mathisen B, Skuse D, Wolke D, et al: Oral motor dysfunction and failure to thrive amongst inner city infants. Developmental Medicine and Neurology 31:293–302, 1989

Minuchin S: Psychosomatic Families. Cambridge, MA, Harvard University Press, 1978

Palazzoli MS: Self-Starvation. New York, Jason Aronson, 1978

Ramsay M, Zelazo P: Food refusal in failure to thrive infants: nasogastric feeding combined with interactive behavioral treatment. J Pediatr Psychol 13:329–347, 1988

Richard ME: Feeding the newborn with cleft lip and/or palate: the enlargement stimulate swallow rest (ESSR) method. Journal of Pediatric Nursing 6:317–321, 1991

Russell GFM, Szmukler G, Dove C, et al: An evaluation of family therapy in anorexia nervosa and bulimia nervosa. Arch Gen Psychiatry 44:1047–1056, 1987

Shepard RW, Wren J, Evans S, et al: Gastroesophageal reflux in children. Clin Pediatr 26:55–60, 1987

Siegel L: Classical and operant procedures in the treatment of a case of food aversion in a young child. Journal of Clinical Child Psychology 11:167–172, 1982

Siegel M, Brisman J, Weinshel M: Surviving an Eating Disorder: New Perspectives and Strategies for Family and Friends. New York, Harper & Row, 1988

Silverman JA: Anorexia nervosa: clinical observations in a successful treatment plan. J Pediatr 84:68–73, 1974

Singer LT, Nofer JA, Benson-Szekely LJ, et al: Behavioral assessment and management of food refusal in children with cystic fibrosis. J Dev Behav Pediatr 12:115–120, 1991

Singer LT, Ambuel B, Wade S, et al: Cognitive-behavioral treatment of health impairing food phobias in children. J Am Acad Child Adolesc Psychiatry 31:847–852, 1992

Sohlberg S, Norring C, Borje E: Prediction of the course of anorexia nervosa/bulimia nervosa over three years. International Journal of Eating Disorders 12:121–131, 1992

Solyom L, Sookman D: Fear of choking and its treatment. Can J Psychol 24:30–34, 1980

Terr LC: Chowchilla revisited: the effects of psychic trauma four years after a school bus kidnapping. Am J Psychol 140:1543–1550, 1983

Theander S: Research on outcome and prognosis of anorexia nervosa and some results from a Swedish long-term study. International Journal of Eating Disorders 2:167–174, 1983

Vietze PM, Falsey S, O'Connor S, et al: Newborn behavioral and interactional characteristics of nonorganic failure-to-thrive infants, in High Risk Infants and Children. Edited by Field TM, Goldberg S, Stern D, et al. New York, Academic Press, 1980, pp 5–24

Woodside DB, Garfinkel PE: Age of onset in eating disorders. International Journal of Eating Disorders 12:31–36, 1992

Woolston J: Diagnostic classification: the current challenge in failure to thrive research, in New Directions in Failure to Thrive: Research and Clinical Practice. Edited by Drotar D. New York, Plenum, 1985

Chapter 23

Psychotic and Prepsychotic Disorders

Clarice J. Kestenbaum, M.D.

This chapter focuses on the psychotherapy of psychotic and prepsychotic children and adolescents.[1] The psychoses for the most part occupy two major domains: the schizophrenic syndromes and the major affective disorders, namely, bipolar disorder. The establishment of an accurate diagnosis before embarking on a treatment course is extremely important because the treatment approaches for schizophrenic syndromes and affective disorders are vastly different from one another. In DSM-III-R (American Psychiatric Association 1987), diagnostic criteria for schizophrenia and bipolar disorder were identical for school-age children and adults. Overt psychotic symptoms such as thought disturbance and perceptual distortions had to be present for the diagnosis of schizophrenia. This is no longer the case in the DSM-IV (American Psychiatric Association 1994) classification. In DSM-IV, schizophrenia is classified by the presence of at least two of the following symptoms, each present for a significant portion of time during a 1-month period: delusions, hallucinations, disorganized speech, grossly disorganized or catatonic behavior, negative symptoms (i.e., affective flattening, alogia, or avolition) (Criterion A); social/occupational dysfunction (Criterion B); and duration of symptoms of at least 6 months (Criterion C). Symptoms may be more difficult to ascertain in children than in adults, however, because hallucinations must be differentiated from fantasies and do not necessarily indicate psychosis (Chambers 1986). Thought disorder in preschool children is difficult to assess, especially in the case of language delay or expressive and receptive dysphasia. Global retardation is not always easy to differentiate from a primary developmental language disorder or pervasive developmental disorder. Because of continuing

---

[1]DSM-IV includes the following psychotic syndromes: schizophrenia (all subtypes); schizophreniform disorder; schizoaffective disorder; delusional disorder; brief psychotic disorder (brief reactive psychosis in DSM-III-R); shared psychotic disorder; psychotic disorder due to a general medical condition; substance-induced psychotic disorder; psychotic disorder NOS (not otherwise specified atypical psychosis); bipolar disorder with psychotic features (all subtypes); and major depression with psychotic features (all subtypes).

disagreement about the etiology and diagnosis of early childhood psychotic disorder, the following brief summary is presented.

HISTORICAL OVERVIEW

The concept of childhood psychosis has had a long and varied course, and for decades the term was synonymous with childhood schizophrenia. In the early 1900s, DeSanctis's "dementia praecoccissima" and Heller's "dementia infantilism," originally considered to be early manifestations of schizophrenia, were found to be postencephalitic states resulting in mental retardation (Kestenbaum 1978). The 1940s brought forth several other syndrome complexes, including Bender's childhood schizophrenia, Kanner's early infantile autism, Mahler's symbiotic psychosis, and Bergman and Escalona's "unusually sensitive children"; all were assigned the label "childhood schizophrenia" (Kestenbaum 1978). Bender (1942) described childhood schizophrenia as a prepubertal disorder that "reveals pathology in behavior at every level and in every area of integration of patterning within the functioning of the central nervous system, be it vegetative, motor, perceptive, intellectual, emotional or social" (p. 139). She believed the disorder was organic in nature, was demonstrable before age 2 years, and resulted in uneven development, language deficits, soft signs and motility disturbances, emotional instability, and extreme anxiety.

Kanner (1943) described a similar group of children, whom he called autistic, whose symptoms included desire for sameness, severe disturbance in language, which was echolalic and not communicative, and profound social withdrawal. He believed that the disorder was nonorganic and was brought about by parental "refrigeration" and rejection in constitutionally vulnerable children.

In accordance with Bender's original findings, Barbara Fish (1975) concluded that gross impairment in human relationships and noncommunicative speech were the two symptoms both necessary and sufficient to make the diagnosis, which she considered organic in origin. She proposed that infantile autism and schizophrenic disorder with childhood onset are one and the same pathological entity manifested by different symptoms according to age at onset and severity.

Kolvin and his group (1971) used the age at symptom onset as a primary criterion in classification, dividing the group of children into those with onset between birth and age 3 years, between 3 and 5 years, and after 5 years. The late-onset group is composed of children who manifest the symptoms often associated with adult schizophrenia: formal thought disorder, hallucinations, and delusions. Kolvin (1971) and Rutter (1972) were influential in establishing infantile autism and schizophrenia as two distinct entities, so that in DSM-III-R early forms

of childhood psychoses are now subsumed under pervasive developmental disorders, with autistic disorder considered the prototype of the
developmental disorder, whereas the child with onset after age 5 years
is usually labeled schizophrenic (Kestenbaum et al. 1989).

Autism is a rare disorder. Atypical pervasive developmental disorder (also referred to as atypical personality development or pervasive
development disorder not otherwise specified) refers to children with
some but not all of the features of autism. Available research is in general agreement regarding the prevalence of autism: 2–4 cases per 10,000
population. However, "atypical pervasive developmental disorder not
otherwise specified" is far more common—occurring in 1 of 200 school-
age children; typically, autism is four to five times more common in
boys than in girls (Volkmar 1991). Prevalence rates for schizophrenia
remain approximately 1% for adult-onset schizophrenia. Childhood
schizophrenia appears to be even less common than autism, with 1–2
cases per 10,000 population (Kolvin 1971).

Some researchers suggest that schizophrenia, usually of the poor-
prognosis, nonremitting type, may develop in some individuals who
fulfilled criteria for autism in childhood (Howells and Guirguis 1984;
Tanguay and Cantor 1986). Green (1988) observed that autistic children
who subsequently meet criteria for schizophrenia (i.e., hallucinations
and delusions) possibly compose a small, etiologically distinct subgroup who have significant symptom overlap with autistic disorder;
the pathognomonic symptoms of thought disorder may not appear
until a more mature level of development is reached, enabling the manifestation of florid psychotic symptoms. Van der Gaag (1993) reported
that two adults who met full criteria for autistic disorder in childhood
were diagnosed as schizophrenic in adult life with positive symptoms
of hallucinations and delusions. In addition to language impairment,
which makes diagnosis difficult in preschool psychotic children, intellectual functioning is variable. Although less impaired than autistic
children (whose IQs may range from 20 to above average), many
schizophrenic children were found to have mild to moderate retardation in Green's (1988) sample of schizophrenic children; Kolvin (1971)
had similar findings.

PSYCHOTIC THOUGHT
PROCESSES—SCHIZOPHRENIC RISK

One of the explanations given for the diagnostic confusion has been
difficulty in the assessment of formal thought disorder in young children—a hallmark of psychotic thinking, along with disturbance in the
content of thought. In describing positive and negative signs in schizophrenic adults, Andreasen (1982) noted illogical thinking, loose associ-

ations, incoherence, circumstantiality, overelaborate or vague speech, clanging, neologisms, poverty of content of speech, and derailment of thought, among other examples of thought disturbance. DSM-III-R considered four of these to be pathognomonic for the diagnosis of formal thought disorder: incoherence (usually indicating psychotic breakdown), loose associations (a sign of positive thought disorder), and poverty of content of speech and illogical thinking (signs of negative thought disorder).

Studies of thought disorder in childhood are sparse. However, after review of the literature, Caplan and Tanguay (1991) concluded that two of the DSM-III signs of formal thought disorder were applicable to school-age children with schizophrenia spectrum disorders—illogical thinking and loose associations. They found that "illogical thinking and loose associations appear to be related to different aspects of impaired attention (information processing in children with schizophrenia spectrum disorders)" (p. 312).

Caplan and Tanguay's findings were consistent with those of researchers studying schizophrenic risk who hypothesized that children vulnerable to schizophrenia had difficulty processing stimuli and demonstrated deficits in attention and responsiveness (Caplan and Tanguay 1991; Erlenmeyer-Kimling and Cornblatt 1987; Neuchterlein and Dawson 1984; Rutchmann et al. 1986). The New York High Risk Project (Erlenmeyer-Kimling 1975; Erlenmeyer-Kimling and Cornblatt 1987)—a prospective study of children of schizophrenic, affective disorder, and "normal" parents—had as a primary aim the identification of early indicators of genetic liability for the development of schizophrenic disorders (e.g., in the areas of attentional and informational processing).

A 23-year follow-up of all subjects in the High Risk Project demonstrated that attentional tasks in particular were found to differentiate the high-risk group from the comparison groups. The significance of these findings is that a group of children may be identified as vulnerable to schizophrenia at an early age—before the onset of behavioral deviance. In fact, the high-risk subgroup that was deviant on the laboratory measures also demonstrated increasingly deviant behavior as they got older, a finding that supports the hypothesis that attentional dysfunctions serve as early predictors of later pathology.

The high-risk children subsequently hospitalized for schizophrenia tended to have lower IQ scores, particularly in the verbal subtests; poor performance on composite attentional indices (the attentional span task and the Continuous Performance Test); and poor performance on the Bender-Gestalt psychological examination. (Interestingly enough, high-risk children who subsequently developed paranoid schizophrenia did not demonstrate these findings [Erlenmeyer-Kimling and Cornblatt 1987].) The premorbid clinical picture of boys who subsequently developed schizophrenia included histories of aggression, poor affective control, and social isolation (Asarnow and Goldstein 1986; Watt 1972). Watt (1972) reported a history of shy introversion in females as part of the premorbid adjustment. Carpenter et al. (1991) described a "deficit syndrome" that included the negative symptoms of blunted affect, poverty of speech, diminished sense of purpose, and diminished social drive, which could antedate the onset of positive symptoms in a schizophrenic adolescent.

Sudan and his colleagues (1993) described a 16-year-old male who had been diagnosed as having oppositional defiant disorder with prominent aggressive features 6 years before hospitalization. He was described as socially awkward and isolated, bizarre (e.g., he exhibited himself in class and attempted to throw feces encased in a glass jar from the window), and with flat affect; he also had poverty of speech production and content and impaired concentration. Yet he was not considered schizophrenic until his deterioration compared with his baseline functioning was considered more consistent with schizophrenia than a personality disorder. Mukherjee and his group (1991) found that impairment and poverty of speech content were associated with a childhood history of cognitive deficits and poor school function.

It would seem that schizophrenia is a heterogeneous disorder with extreme variation in symptoms and course (Cloninger 1987). The clinical picture is the result of genetic factors and environmental factors such as a chaotic home environment, child abuse, trauma, and disturbed parental behavior. The concept of a basic core unique to the schizophrenia syndrome involves the existence of a set of measurable lifelong traits that would distinguish schizophrenia from other psychopathological conditions and should be detectable in schizophrenic individuals at all times, independent of a psychotic or nonpsychotic state. Chambers (1986) believes that the clinical significance of hallucinations and delusions in preadolescent children is questionable. Organic conditions such as temporal lobe epilepsy may produce hallucinations, and children with major depressive disorder have experienced hallucinations as well. Eisenberg (1962) reported that children under stress report hallucinations that disappear when the stressors are removed.

PSYCHOTHERAPY WITH CHILDREN WITH EARLY-ONSET SCHIZOPHRENIA

Two problems have hitherto governed the choice of treatment modality for schizophrenic individuals. The first involves the complexity of a treatment plan for a schizophrenic child and has, for the most part, reflected the heterogeneity of the early-childhood schizophrenic population. The second has been the fact that the choice of a treatment modality too often reflects the theoretical orientation of the therapist and not the specific needs of the patient. "Thus treatment modalities used with schizophrenic children have ranged from parentectomy (removal of the child from the family), psychoanalysis for both child and parents, behavior therapy, milieu therapy, family therapy, educational therapy and a variety of psychotherapeutic techniques such as movement and paraverbal therapy—as well as psychopharmacological intervention" (Cantor and Kestenbaum 1986, p. 623). Therefore, it is of the utmost importance to obtain as much information as possible before deciding on a treatment plan, including genetic and developmental history, psychiatric and neurological examinations, neuropsychological testing, language assessment, and tests of psychotic function. Because schizophrenia is a chronic lifetime disorder, therapy will be multidisciplinary and is seldom brief.

Therapy can occur in a variety of settings: a hospital or residential treatment center, a therapeutic nursery, or a psychotherapist's office. Symptom expression and the degree of dysfunction are variable. It is obvious that children who first demonstrate psychotic behavior after age 6 have achieved a higher level of cognitive development than preschool psychotic children. Very young schizophrenic children, as noted, may resemble children with pervasive developmental disorder, particularly when language is delayed. For the majority of preschool schizophrenic children, some form of milieu therapy, as well as individual psychotherapy, will be required throughout the developmental years. The child psychiatrist serves as the team manager who oversees the psychoeducational treatment, language and occupational therapy, and family interactions. The therapist should be prepared to ensure that the child receives the tactile, proprioceptive, and kinesthetic experiences that have been missed. Young schizophrenic children are prone to aggressive outbursts and panic reactions, particularly when separated from their primary caregivers, and have not achieved object constancy. The therapist serves as an auxiliary ego because the children lack the appropriate adaptive mechanisms required for coping with the normal stresses of life. Goldfarb (1970) labeled his therapeutic approach "corrective socialization," which represents an attempt to develop a self-regulating capacity that involves a realistic correction of each child's impairment; the therapist, he noted, "must take into account differences in capacity, motivation, level of communication, and the characteristic substantive features of [the child's] bewilderment" (p. 775).

The therapist must be aware that an outburst of rage may reflect intolerance of being alone, that obsessional rituals may be an attempt to ward off imagined dangers, and that reality testing is, by definition, poor. The schizophrenic child lacks the ability to distinguish fantasy from reality. According to Escalona (1964), therapy with such children in the past has taken two directions: "expressive" and "suppressive."

Expressive therapy, derived from concepts inherent in the psycho-analysis of neurotic individuals, permits the expression of previously unconscious material. Fantasies are seen as meaningful and are inter-preted in the context of the child's reality experience. The relationship between affects and their source, as well as between symptoms and their deeper meaning, is explored.

Suppressive therapy proceeds from a recognition of the fact that psy-chotic children show extreme weakness in ego functioning; hence, they have failed to repress psychic experience that normally should be un-conscious. Thus, therapy would be directed at discouraging the expres-sion and the acting out of fantasies, at providing as much gratification as possible in more realistic pursuits, and at strengthening reality test-ing by all possible means.

Cantor and Kestenbaum (1986) proposed a reality-oriented therapy at all times and stressed the importance of the therapist's serving as a bridge to the real world.

Case Vignette[2]

George, a 5-year-old boy with early-onset schizophrenia and moderate retardation, was referred for inpatient treatment at a psychiatric hospital after a 1-year trial in a therapeutic nursery for severely disturbed chil-dren. George was the second of three children in a family with no known history of mental illness. The parents were middle-class professionals, the 6-year-old sister was extremely bright and friendly, and the 2-year-old brother was quick and outgoing. His mother reported that despite an uneventful planned pregnancy and a full-term normal birth, she noted that George was different from the other children "from the first day." He rarely cried and seemed content to remain in his crib or playpen. She noted that he either felt very soft to pick up—floppy at times—or very stiff, arching his back and seeming to dislike being held. George liked to rock, and smiled when he rocked himself.

At 2 years, he spoke only 15 words. He did cuddle with his mother, to whom he became deeply attached and demanding. "He'd scream a lot, pulling my hand to reach for things he wanted. Away from me he was fearful of anything or anyone new, or of being left alone in his room." Tantrums became a daily occurrence. He was punished at first by being left home alone, "but it made him scream louder." George was very re-sentful of his 2-month-old brother Tim and became more demanding of his mother's attention. The family attributed this resentment to normal sibling rivalry in a sensitive child. The pediatrician assured the family that George was a slow starter and "would outgrow it."

By age 4 it was clear that George was not about to "outgrow" his dif-

---

[2]Adapted from Kestenbaum 1978.

ficulties. He was increasingly withdrawn or, when not clinging to his mother, enraged and out of control each time his desires were frustrated. His vocal production was limited to echolalic imitations and strange noises as if imitating automobile horns, trains, or vacuum cleaners. At times he hallucinated and spoke to figures in the wall, "Bleepey" and "Blooney." He could not play with other children, relating only to his mother and older sister. Declared "retarded," he was sent to a local clinic for a workup. The child psychiatrist noted that he could be absorbed in music for hours, watching the turntable while he listened to records, and also that his speech—unintelligible jargon—was delivered in a monotone. He was preoccupied with turning light switches on and off or with locking doors and pushing elevator buttons.

George was enrolled in a therapeutic day nursery where he made some progress in speaking and comprehension. He always had great difficulty separating from his mother and seemed depressed and fearful much of the time.

Once George pushed his hand through a window during a tantrum that followed his having been refused a second piece of cake. He did not cry, nor did he show any reaction either to the blood streaming down his arm or to the stitches he received in the emergency room.

Although George was untestable by usual criteria, the psychologist noted perceptual deficits and overall retardation but felt he was only "pseudoretarded" and capable of intellectual growth. Although language was delayed, he was able to grasp the concept of pronouns; a primary language disorder was ruled out. A working diagnosis was finally established: schizophrenia—early-onset type with some autistic features.

George was placed in individual psychotherapy, psychoeducational therapy, and an inpatient therapeutic milieu. The family met with the therapist weekly and then with the teacher on a regular basis so that they could reinforce the cognitive training he was receiving. George became attached to his female therapist, but when she became pregnant and left for maternity leave, George began to mutilate himself, scratching his face with his fingernails, and regressed to the point of urinating and defecating on the floor. He would stay alone in his room, rocking, repeating to himself "Daddy's angry." He wouldn't speak to anyone and seemed to be hallucinating.

Treatment Plan for Children With Early-Onset Schizophrenia

The multimodal treatment plan is largely determined by the child's cognitive developmental level, particularly taking into account communication skills. George's initial treatment was similar to that employed with autistic children even though his clinical presentation was different. (He was capable of attachment despite language deficits and used language to communicate.) The first task of the therapist was to establish trust, at first by quietly sitting close to George, on the floor if necessary, until he could develop enough of a bond to share his feelings. Only then was he motivated enough to comply with the ward's structure and the tasks presented to him: body care, school attendance, and self-control. (Thioridazine was the drug selected to control George's psychotic symptoms, particularly hallucinations.) George was given two dolls he called Blooney and Bleepey that substituted for the hallucinated characters who lived in his psychotic world. During doll play, George reenacted events and feelings he would not ascribe to himself, giving detailed accounts of what the dolls thought and felt. New themes emerged involving George's low self-esteem, confused body image, and maladaptive defense mechanisms (chiefly denial and projection). A behavior therapy approach was employed with "time-out" and rewards for compliance—gold stars or cookies.

The ward personnel helped George develop a body awareness and an impression of separateness with the help of mirrors. Eye contact was encouraged. Emphasis on pronouns such as "I," "mine," "you," and "yours" was a focus of the initial therapeutic work. In addition, the special education teacher worked intensively on language acquisition so that George could communicate his needs as well as develop an understanding of his own feelings—anger, sadness, or pleasure. Play therapy was largely educative and reality oriented as the therapist helped stimulate George's interest in the outside world. (Imaginative play with monsters and dragons, for example, is often too anxiety producing for psychotic children.)

One difficulty for families and staff members working with schizophrenic children is the sudden regression under stress. "A quiet corner, a favorite book, music and gross motor therapy can help restore the child to a higher level of functioning. Interpretations of behavior and attempts to heal the child through increasing interpersonal contact are likely to drive the child further into psychotic withdrawal" (Cantor and Kestenbaum 1986, p. 626).

George's family not only met with the social worker for counseling but also with the occupational therapist and teacher so that there could be a continuity between the hospital experience and visits at home. As George's deviant behavior became more understandable to the family, they came to understand his profound fear of abandonment and never again used isolation as a means of punishment.

George was eventually able to return home to a day treatment program but never achieved enough social judgment to be capable of living in an unprotected setting. His parents accepted the fact that schizophrenia is a lifelong condition, but George never again experienced the pain of a psychotic decompensation.

This vignette illustrates the cognitive problems of psychotic and prepsychotic schizophrenic children. Treatment should be specifically tailored primarily to meet the psychoeducational needs of these patients and secondarily to improve their communicative and social skills.

CHILDREN AT RISK FOR AFFECTIVE DISORDERS

Although there is no absolute proof of a genetic mode of transmission for manic-depressive (bipolar) illness, there is consistent evidence supporting the prominent role of a genetically transmitted predisposition for affective illness, especially bipolar illness (Tsuang 1978). Bipolar disorder occurs in 1% of adults, with men and women equally affected. Nurnberger and Gershon (1982) reported that the concordance of mania in monozygotic twins is 65%, compared to 14% in dizygotic twins; bipolar disorders in children are rare. Bipolar disorder has often been underdiagnosed or misdiagnosed as attention-deficit hyperactivity disorder, conduct disorder, or schizophrenia (Carlson and Kashani 1988; Weller et al. 1986).

The characteristics that have been reported in association with children of parents with bipolar disorder who will later develop bipolar illness are very different from those of children vulnerable to schizophrenia. These characteristics include a history of affective lability, periodic outbursts and impulsive behavior, or impulsivity; evidence of discrete depressive episodes in childhood and adolescence; and the presence of prominent personality traits associated with extroversion or dysthymia (Kestenbaum and Kron 1987).

Although retrospective and prospective studies concerned with descriptions of childhood precursors of schizophrenia abound, few studies describe premorbid functioning in bipolar adults (Kestenbaum and Kron 1987). Premorbid functioning is reportedly normal or often superior. The few existing studies hypothesize that children at risk for bipolar disorder show verbal IQ scores significantly higher than performance IQ scores (Decina et al. 1983) and full-scale IQ scores higher than those of children at risk for schizophrenia (Erlenmeyer-Kimling and Cornblatt 1987).

In a controlled sample of children at risk for bipolar disorder, Kron and his colleagues (1982) found that the experimental group was significantly different from the control group with respect to ratings on depression scales, overactivity, and overproduction of florid fantasy. Young children at risk for bipolar illness present with symptoms of irritability and emotional lability (Carlson 1983).

Akiskal and his group (1983) concluded that a spectrum of affective disorders is associated with a positive family history of related behaviors. They observed that patients with cyclothymic disorders fulfilled many of the criteria for borderline personality disorder and had a higher percentage of extroversion, rage outbursts, obsessional symptoms, and bipolar relatives compared with control subjects.

Formal thought disorder in manic adolescents includes positive signs (i.e., loose associations, distractibility, tangentiality, and digressiveness) together with pressured speech, whether or not the adolescent is psychotic (Marengo and Harrow 1985).

Thus, the prodromal symptoms of adolescents who subsequently develop manic episodes are substantially different from those of schizophrenic adolescents, in whom negative signs predominate.

The psychotic state of manic adolescents is essentially the same as that of manic adults: elated mood or irritability, grandiosity, sleeplessness, and bizarre behavior, along with the aforementioned thought disorder, grandiose delusions, and occasionally hallucinations. In addition, adolescents vulnerable to bipolar disorder fail to discriminate normal from abnormal moods. Davenport and his group (1984) observed that the affective instability of adolescents with bipolar disorder shapes their personalities. Maladaptive defense mechanisms, chiefly denial and projection, result in subsequent character pathology such as borderline personality disorder (Kestenbaum and Kron 1987).

In vulnerable children and adolescents, stressful life events resulting in sleep deprivation can precipitate manic episodes. The bipolar diathesis in combination with external life events can result in interruption of normal developmental tasks, particularly in adolescents (Jamison and Goodwin 1983). The adolescent fails to form a unique personal identity, relationships are frequently compromised, and career goals remain fragmented and undefined.

PSYCHOTHERAPY OF CHILDREN AND ADOLESCENTS WITH BIPOLAR DISORDER

Preschool children at risk for bipolar disorder (strong genetic loading, difficulty in self-regulation, affective storms) need careful management: parental understanding of the need for structure and limit setting; a predictably well-structured preschool environment; and psychotherapy, often behavioral, with the goal of self-control. Through doll play, stories, and games the child learns to limit his or her temper tantrums, share toys, lose a game without undue distress (i.e., without attacking the winning child), and identify his or her moods (a tantrum resulting from fear of being alone is vastly different from rage at not having one's own way).

Case Vignette

Charles, age 5 years, was brought for psychiatric consultation because he was unable to conform to classroom routine and exhibited himself to other children. Charles lacked confidence, made no attempt to do new things, and was easily frustrated, giving up without trying. His mother recalled that Charles had been hypersensitive to noise as an infant and was fearful in the presence of strangers. Until age 3, moreover, he sucked his fingers continually and would not leave the house without his favorite pillow. He was teased by his classmates for crying and for having tantrums; his teacher reported he occasionally lost control and struck children and even adults. A psychological test had been performed before the consultation—his full-scale IQ was 112. The family history was positive for bipolar disorder. The therapist considered Charles to be a developmentally immature, depressed child who "gave up" in the face of perfectionist parental demands. The recommendation was for psychoanalytically oriented psychotherapy; a low-pressured, structured first grade with few students and sensitive teachers; and parental counseling on a weekly basis.

During the first therapy session, Charles acted out a story with hand puppets, a scene that appeared and reappeared on numerous occasions. A baby tiger, 5 years old, ran away from his forest cave "because his daddy spanks him and his mother leaves him with a baby-sitter. He hates school and wants to hide in his own cave and never come out. He has no friends. He is always scared."

The play session that followed dealt with similar themes. Charles spent many hours preoccupied with Lego blocks and constructed castles that were safe "with a very strong base." Charles soon constructed a Lego representation of school and home. He created characters similar to those in his own life. There was a curious boy who wondered about girls' genitalia. There was the boy who threw blocks at the teacher and the one who sucked his thumb and sulked when he didn't come in first in the footrace. All interpretations and clarifications were made via the doll characters, such as Doll A, who became upset when Doll B beat him in checkers but was able to control himself anyway.

After several months of therapy, Charles's school reports improved. He had settled into a new school environment where the principal was warm and motherly, yet firm and able to set limits. Charles was soon able to join a group, started to participate in activities, and began to read with comprehension and pleasure. Six months after beginning treatment, Charles was involved in a very positive therapeutic relationship. He spoke more about his past problems.

"There is a bad kid Stevie who makes a lot of noise and has to leave the room."

"Maybe he has a problem like the one you used to have a long time ago?"

"Yes," he replied, "I used to have that problem but that was in the other school; it went away."

In Charles's case, psychodynamic psychotherapy and environmental change were enough to alleviate his symptoms. In other instances, psychopharmacological intervention, including lithium, is recommended to stabilize the child and prevent explosive behavior. Feinstein and Wolpert (1973) noted that children do not exhibit the full-blown characteristics of affective disorder but show specific equivalent behaviors that are the precursors of manic-depressive states of adulthood. They contend that the affective system of patients with manic-depressive illness may display a basic vulnerability that, when over-stimulated, begins a discharge pattern that does not lend itself easily to autonomous emotional control. These patients do not have the capacity for self-regulation, the ability to "dampen down" as Mahler et al. (1975) observed. They need continued intervention by a caretaker sensitive to their needs; otherwise, the separation-individuation stage of develop-ment is incompletely realized, as Greenspan (1981) noted in his re-search with vulnerable infants. Moreover, such children need to take apart and understand the overwhelming emotions with which they are flooded.

Case Vignette[3]

Jody was first seen for psychiatric consultation at age 9 years for a severe depressive reaction after the death of an aunt. She stated that she wanted to die, tried to jump from a second-story window, and threatened to run away. Psychological tests revealed that her IQ was in the superior range, with a 19-point discrepancy between verbal and performance scores. Family history was positive for affective disorder. The paternal grandfa-ther suffered from depression, and the father, a successful businessman, was considered to be domineering and was prone to outbursts of rage. The maternal aunt had been diagnosed as bipolar II (severe depressions with a hypomanic personality in between episodes).

Childhood history revealed that Jody was outgoing, sociable, and precocious; she preferred adults to age-appropriate peers. Although psy-chotherapy was recommended, the family declined. During the next 5 years, Jody began having social trouble, developed anorexia, and abused street drugs. Despite these problems, Jody received honors, was active in extracurricular activities, and was the editor of the school newspaper. At 16, she saw a psychoanalyst because of bouts of depression and suicidal preoccupation, but the treatment was not successful. During her fresh-man year in an out-of-town college, 18-year-old Jody experienced anxiety, depersonalization, and severe suicidal ideation and was hospi-talized. The hospital course was stormy; antidepressant medication was started, but a manic episode ensued. Lithium was added to the regimen, which controlled the manic symptoms (delusions of grandeur and excep-tional powers, insomnia, agitation, outpourings of verse, and stream-of-consciousness essays). She was discharged after 4 months and returned to a local college where she began psychotherapy on a twice-weekly basis. Diagnosis was bipolar disorder with a comorbid borderline per-sonality disorder.

When the treating physician first saw her, Jody was a lovely, well-

---

[3] Adapted from Kestenbaum and Kron 1987.

groomed, slender, somewhat reserved young woman. She was open and responsive as she described her lifelong feelings of being different and out of touch; she hated the tormenting morbid thoughts and painful depressive moods that used to invade her very being, she said. She did not know how to talk to friends who had "normal" lives. She felt constantly alienated from both male and female friends, resulting in vicious verbal attacks when she felt disappointed and let down. She had never had a boyfriend.

The psychotherapeutic approach was twofold: a problem-solving, cognitive approach added to the psychoanalytic therapy. The nature of the bipolar disorder was explained to her (clearly differentiated from unipolar depression by history as well as by the manic response to antidepressants), as was the reason lithium had been prescribed to help her regulate her own emotional states and change her negative view of life. Jody was also taught to be aware of stresses that might upset her delicate balance: work pressures, menses, exhaustion. She kept a diary with notations about mood changes and stressors—a cognitive therapeutic technique. The psychiatrist insisted that she use the therapeutic relationship to help control impulses (by telephone calls between sessions when necessary). Jody was told how she had missed many of the everyday life occurrences her friends had experienced and that it was not too late to discuss friendship, dating, and family relationships. Her analytic therapy—with full interpretation of dreams, associations, and use of the transference—proceeded like any other analysis of a neurotic patient. The dual-track psychotherapeutic approach, plus medication, continued to be successful throughout the treatment course. Jody returned to college and experienced both academic and social success.

EFFICACY OF THERAPEUTIC INTERVENTIONS WITH PSYCHOTIC CHILDREN: PROGNOSIS AND OUTCOME

Follow-up studies are for the most part unreliable and impressionistic, mainly because of three factors: 1) the lack of controlled studies of psychoses in childhood, 2) the dissimilarity of diagnostic criteria used by different researchers, and 3) the rarity of the illness.

When the schizophrenic groups are broken down into subgroups, it is clear that determination of outcome is directly related to the presence or absence of speech by age 5 years, with absence of speech being associated with a poorer prognosis (Bettelheim 1967; Rutter 1972). Rutter believes that IQ has prognostic significance: children having an IQ below 60, for example, have a poor outcome. Pollack (1966) in his review of 13 studies of childhood schizophrenia found that most of the children in the studies had evidence of cerebral dysfunction and low IQ scores. Almost half had IQs lower than 70.

Goldfarb (1974) selected 140 cases, using 65 carefully matched healthy children as control subjects. Forty measured characteristics were divided into two capacities: 1) characteristics that represent capacity levels that may be expected to improve in healthy children solely on the basis of maturation and 2) characteristics that reflect the primary influence of social and educational experience (e.g., social competence).

Goldfarb made the point that, despite significant change, after 3 years the schizophrenic children as a group remained below normal levels on most of the variables tested. Those abnormalities that changed the least were activity level and muscle tone, which may be hypothetically related to the level of integrity of the schizophrenic child's nervous system (Goldfarb 1974). In terms of the efficacy of psychotherapy with bipolar children and adolescents, follow-up studies are sparse and anecdotal. Clinical experience, however, testifies to the great benefit of early intervention (Kron and Kestenbaum 1987).

Many treatment approaches have been used in conjunction with the major treatment strategies for psychotic children and adolescents, depending on the child's age and level of development and the severity of the symptoms. In view of the focused approaches of many different therapies, the literature often does not differentiate clearly among autistic, schizophrenic, and emotionally disturbed children and adolescents. In a review of treatment approaches, Ruttenberg and Angert (1980) include sensorimotor integrative therapy, language therapy, play therapy, art therapy, and music therapy. Nevertheless, they suggested that the best approach is a multidisciplinary one that integrates learning theory, behavioral strategies, psychodynamic therapy, and, when necessary, medication. Recently, there has been increasing interest in approaches that focus on interpersonal cognitive problem-solving deficits. Even though their utility has not been established formally, these approaches have been implemented with emotionally disturbed boys in residential treatment centers (Elias 1979). These interventions focus on the covert thinking processes that underline effective social interactions in children (Kestenbaum et al. 1989).

CONCLUSION

One far-reaching goal of research involving children at high risk for developing schizophrenia and affective disorders is to detect the vulnerable child and to provide competence-enhancing interventions. Interventions are particularly useful when they are specifically directed toward correcting primary problems. Until more is known about the core psychopathology involved in schizophrenia and affective disorders, primary prevention and therapeutic interventions involve much guesswork. The evidence gathered thus far indicates that the pre-schizophrenic child has difficulty filtering stimulus input and has problems in attention that subsequently lead to school difficulties and social problems. Early intervention could include genetic counseling, careful perinatal examination, and frequent pediatric developmental evaluation of at-risk children. Therapeutic nurseries could be made available to children who showed signs of early deviance.

The at-risk child who is bright but not living up to his or her potential should be evaluated as soon as symptoms appear; school failure, attentional problems, social withdrawal, and loss of self-esteem should not be left unnoticed until symptoms become fixed. Special school programs for the child with attentional problems should focus on strengthening existing assets that would enhance self-esteem. Special training in correcting attentional deficits could be provided. Recommendations for family treatment, selection of the proper school or camp, individual psychotherapy, or pharmacotherapy could be tailored to fit the particular needs of each family. For the child at risk for affective disorder, the problem is not one of deficit but of excess; the multitude of unexamined feelings can lead to impulsive behavior. A psychodynamic psychotherapy to help channel the enormous energy in creative and constructive ways (and medication, when indicated) is the treatment of choice for such children and can help them to lead happier and more productive lives (Kestenbaum et al. 1989).

REFERENCES

Akiskal HS, Hirschfield NA, Yerovanian BJ: The relation of personality to affective disorders: an initial review. Arch Gen Psychiatry 40:801–810, 1983

American Psychiatric Association: Diagnostic and Statistical Manual of Mental Disorders, 3rd Edition, Revised. Washington, DC, American Psychiatric Association, 1987

American Psychiatric Association: Diagnostic and Statistical Manual of Mental Disorders, 4th Edition. Washington, DC, American Psychiatric Association, 1994

Andreasen NC: Negative symptoms in schizophrenia: definitions reliability. Arch Gen Psychiatry 39:787–788, 1982

Asarnow JR, Goldstein MJ: Schizophrenia during adolescence and early adulthood: a developmental perspective on risk research. Clinical Psychology Review 6:211–238, 1986

Bender I: Childhood schizophrenia. The Nervous Child 1:138–139, 1942

Bettelheim B: The Empty Fortress. New York, Free Press, 1967

Cantor S, Kestenbaum CJ: Psychotherapy with schizophrenic children. Journal of the American Academy of Child Psychiatry 25:265–630, 1986

Caplan R, Tanguay PE: Development of psychotic thinking in children, in Child and Adolescent Psychiatry: A Comprehensive Textbook. Edited by Lewis M. Baltimore, MD, Williams & Wilkins, 1991, pp 310–317

Carlson EA: Bipolar affective disorders in childhood and adolescence, in Affective Disorders in Childhood and Adolescence—An Update. Edited by Cantwell D, Carlson GT. New York, Spectrum, 1983, pp 61–84

Carlson EA, Kashani JH: Manic symptoms in a non-referred adolescent population. J Affect Disord 15:219–226, 1988

Carpenter WT, Buchanan RW, Kirkpatrick B: Negative Schizophrenic Symptoms: Pathophysiology and Clinical Implications. Edited by Greden JF, Tandon R. Washington, DC, American Psychiatric Press, 1991, pp 3–20

Chambers WJ: Hallucinations in psychotic and depressed children, in Hallucinations in Childhood and Adolescence. Edited by Pilowsky D, Chambers WJ. Washington, DC, American Psychiatric Press, 1986, pp 78–111

Cloninger RC: Genetic principles and methods in high risk studies of schizophrenia. Schizophr Bull 13:515–523, 1987

Davenport YB, Zahn-Wexler C, Adlund M, et al: Early child rearing practices in families with a manic-depressive parent. Am J Psychother 141:230–235, 1984

Decina P, Kestenbaum CJ, Farber S, et al: Clinical and psychological assessment of children of bipolar parents. Am J Psychiatry 140:548–553, 1983

Eisenberg L: Hallucinations in children, in Hallucinations. Edited by West IJ. New York, Grune & Stratton, 1962, pp 11–61

Elias MJ: Helping emotionally disturbed children through pro-social television. Except Child 46:217–218, 1979

Erlenmeyer-Kimling L: A prospective study of children at risk for schizophrenia: methodological considerations and some preliminary findings, in Life History Research in Psychopathology, Vol 4. Edited by Wirt R, Winokor G, Roff M. Minneapolis, University of Minnesota Press, 1975, pp 22–46

Erlenmeyer-Kimling L, Cornblatt B: The New York high risk project—a follow up report. Schizophr Bull 13:451–461, 1987

Escalona S: Some considerations regarding psychotherapy with psychotic children, in Child Psychotherapy. Edited by Haworth MH. New York, Basic Books, 1964, pp 50–58

Feinstein SC, Wolpert EA: Juvenile manic-depressive illness. Journal of the American Academy of Child Psychiatry 12:123–136, 1973

Fish B: Biological antecedents of psychosis in children, in The Biology of the Major Psychoses (Association for Research into Mental Disorders Publ No 54). Edited by Freeman DX. New York, Raven, 1975, pp 49–80

Goldfarb W: Childhood psychosis, in Manual of Child Psychology, Third Edition. New York, Wiley, 1970, pp 765–830

Goldfarb W: Growth and Change of Schizophrenic Children: A Longitudinal Study, New York, Wiley, 1974

Green WA: Pervasive developmental disorders, in Handbook of Clinical Assessment of Children and Adolescents. Edited by Kestenbaum CJ, Williams DT. New York, New York University Press, 1988, pp 469–498

Greenspan SI: Psychopathology and Adaptation in Infancy and Early Childhood: Principles of Clinical Diagnosis and Preventive Intervention. New York, International Universities Press, 1981

Howells JG, Guirguis WR: Childhood schizophrenia 20 years later. Arch Gen Psychiatry 41:123–128, 1984

Jamison KR, Goodwin FF: Psychotherapeutic treatment of manic depressive patients on lithium, in Psychopharmacology and Psychotherapy. Edited by Greenhill MH, Gralnick IT. New York, Macmillan, 1983, pp 53–78

Kanner I: Autistic disturbances of affective contact. The Nervous Child 2:217–250, 1943

Kestenbaum CJ: Childhood psychosis: psychotherapy, in Handbook of Treatment of Disorders in Childhood and Adolescence. Edited by Wolman BE, Egan J, Ross AO. Englewood Cliffs, NJ, Prentice-Hall, 1978, pp 354–384

Kestenbaum CJ, Kron L: Psychoanalytic intervention with children and adolescents with affective disorders: a combined treatment approach. J Am Acad Psychoanal 15:2153–2174, 1987

Kestenbaum CJ, Canino IA, Pleak RR: Schizophrenic disorders of childhood and adolescence, in American Psychiatric Press Review of Psychiatry, Vol 8. Edited by Tasman A, Hales RE, Francis AJ. Washington, DC, American Psychiatric Press, 1989, pp 242–261

Kolvin I: Studies in the childhood psychoses, I: diagnostic criteria and classification. Br J Psychiatry 118:381–384, 1971

Kolvin I, Ounsted C, Humphrey M, et al: Studies in the childhood psychosis, I–VI. Br J Psychiatry 118:385–415, 1971

Kron L, Kestenbaum CJ: Assessment of the child at-risk for psychotic disorder in adult life, in Clinical Assessment of Children and Adolescents: A Biopsychosocial Approach. Edited by Kestenbaum CJ, Williams DJ. New York, New York University Press, 1987, pp 650–672

Kron L, Decina P, Kestenbaum CJ, et al: The offspring of bipolar manic-depressives: clinical features, in Adolescent Psychiatry, Vol 10. Edited by Feinstein SC, Looney JG, Schwartzberg AZ, et al. Chicago, IL, University of Chicago Press, 1982, pp 273–291

Mahler MS, Pine F, Bergman A: Overview, in The Psychological Birth of the Infant. New York, Basic Books, 1975, pp 4–8

Marengo J, Harrow M: Thought disorder: a function of schizophrenia, mania or psychosis. J Nerv Ment Dis 173:35–41, 1985

Mukherjee S, Reddy R, Schnur DB: A developmental model of negative syndromes in schizophrenia, in Negative Schizophrenic Symptoms: Pathophysiology and Clinical Implications. Edited by Greden JF, Tandon R. Washington, DC, American Psychiatric Press, 1991, pp 173–186

Nurnberger IT, Gershon E: Genetics, in Handbook of Affective Disorders. Edited by Paykel ES. Edinburgh, Churchill-Livingston, 1982

Nuechterlein KH, Dawson ME: Information processing and attentional functioning in the developmental course of schizophrenic disorders. Schizophr Bull 10:160–203, 1984

Pollack N: Mental subnormality and "childhood schizophrenia," in Psychopathology of Mental Development. Edited by Zubin J, Jervis G. New York, Grune & Stratton, 1966, pp 39–47

Rutchmann J, Cornblatt B, Erlenmeyer-Kimling L: Sustained attention in children at risk for schizophrenia: findings with two visual continuous performance tests in a new sample. J Abnorm Psychol 14:365–383, 1986

Ruttenberg B, Angert AH: Psychotic disorders, in Emotional Disorders in Children and Adolescents. Medical and Psychological Approaches to Treatment. Edited by Sholivar P, Bensen M, Blinter B. New York, SI Medical & Scientific, 1980, pp 88–110

Rutter M: Childhood schizophrenia reconsidered. Journal of Autism and Childhood Schizophrenia 2:315–338, 1972

Sudan R, Setterberg S, Whitaker A, et al: An emerging schizophrenic syndrome. J Am Acad Child Adolesc Psychiatry 32:1295–1301, 1993

Tanguay PE, Cantor SI: Schizophrenia in children—introduction. Journal of the American Academy of Child Psychiatry 25:591–594, 1986

Tsuang MT: Genetic counselling for psychiatric patients and their families. Am J Psychiatry 135:1465–1475, 1978

Van der Gaag RS: Specifying PPD-NOS: multiplex developmental disorder, a multivariate exploration of a heuristic category. Paper presented at the annual meeting of the American Academy of Child and Adolescent Psychiatry, San Antonio, TX, October 1993

Volkmar FR: Childhood schizophrenia, in Child and Adolescent Psychiatry—A Comprehensive Textbook. Edited by Lewis M. Baltimore, MD, Williams & Wilkins, 1991, pp 499–508

Watt NF: Longitudinal changes in the social behavior of children hospitalized for schizophrenia as adults. J Nerv Ment Dis 155:42–54, 1972

Weller RA, Weller EB, Tucker SE, et al: Mania in prepubertal children—has it been underdiagnosed? J Affect Disord 11:151–154, 1986

Chapter 24

Victims of Child Abuse

Arthur H. Green, M.D.

DEFINITIONS AND INCIDENCE OF CHILD ABUSE

Most state laws in this country define child physical abuse as the infliction of injury on a person under age 18 years by a parent or legally responsible caretaker, or allowing such injury to take place. Sexual abuse, which is considered to be a subtype of physical abuse, is defined as sexual contact between an adult and a child under age 18 in which the child is used for the sexual gratification of the adult. A parent or caretaker who allows another person to have sexual contact with a child is also regarded as sexually abusive. Acts defined as sexual abuse are not limited to genital or anal intercourse but also include a variety of sexual behaviors such as fellatio; fondling of the genitalia, anus, or breasts; and genital exhibitionism.

According to the findings of the national incidence study of child abuse and neglect carried out in 1986 (U.S. Department of Health and Human Services 1988), 5.7 of 1,000 children (or 358,300) were estimated to be physically abused, and 2.5 of 1,000 children (or 155,900) were estimated to be sexually abused. When the prevalence of child neglect (17 per 1,000 children) is included, a total of 1,500,000 children experienced some form of abuse or neglect in 1986. Prevalence data reveal that approximately one-third of all women and one-tenth of all men were sexually abused during their childhood (Finkelhor 1986).

COMPARISONS BETWEEN PHYSICAL AND SEXUAL ABUSE

Physical and sexual abuse are similar to the extent that they involve the intentional misuse or exploitation of a child by a parent or caretaker in the context of a pathological family environment. Both are considered to be offenses by the family court and juvenile court system and must be reported by physicians and other child care professionals to designated child abuse registries. Some cases of alleged sexual or physical abuse, usually those of greater severity, may be prosecuted in the criminal courts.

Physical and sexual abuse are dissimilar because of the differences in the frequency of victimization by the parents. Physical abuse is committed almost equally by mothers and fathers or father surrogates on boys and girls in equal numbers, whereas sexual abuse is primarily inflicted by fathers or father surrogates on female children. Sexual abuse is more likely to escape detection because it is less likely to result in physical injury and less likely to be disclosed by the child or family member because of the greater degree of guilt and stigma associated with sexual victimization, especially by a family member.

PSYCHOLOGICAL IMPAIRMENT IN ABUSED CHILDREN: A REVIEW

The psychopathology, cognitive impairment, and developmental sequelae observed in child victims of physical and sexual abuse reflect the impact of two broad categories of trauma: 1) the acute physical or sexual assault confronting the child with feelings of anxiety, helplessness, and betrayal by a trusted caretaker; and 2) a background of long-term deviant parenting, such as harsh and punitive child rearing, scapegoating, stigmatization, role reversal, and maternal deprivation.

The following symptoms and psychopathology have been frequently described in both physically and sexually abused children: anxiety states and anxiety-related symptoms such as sleep disturbances, insomnia, nightmares, psychosomatic complaints, and hypervigilance; reenactments of the victimization, which may be associated with posttraumatic stress disorder (Goodwin 1985; Green 1985); depression, which may be accompanied by low self-esteem and self-destructive and suicidal behavior (Gaensbauer and Sands 1979; Sgroi 1982); dissociation, characterized by forgetfulness with periods of amnesia, trancelike states, and blackouts; and multiple personality disorder, which is the most extreme manifestation of dissociation (Kluft 1985; Putnam 1985). Additional sequelae of physical and sexual abuse are paranoid reactions and mistrust (Green 1978; Herman 1981); excessive reliance on primitive defense mechanisms such as denial, projection, dissociation, and "splitting" the abuser into "good" and "bad" images (Green 1978); and impaired impulse control. Physically abused children have often been cited for aggressive and destructive behavior at home and in school (George and Main 1979; Green 1978), whereas sexually abused children are typically unable to control their sexual impulses, often exhibiting precocious sexual play with a high level of sexual arousal (Friedrich and Reams 1987; Yates 1982).

There are also sequelae that are primarily associated with either physical or sexual abuse. Physically abused children often display cognitive and developmental impairment (Elmer and Gregg 1967; Oates 1986), delayed language development (Martin 1972), and neurological impairment (Green et al. 1981b). Sexually abused children may exhibit weakened gender identity with a tendency to reject their maleness or femaleness (Aiosa-Karpas et al. 1991) and exhibit an increased incidence of homosexuality (Finkelhor 1984).

LONG-TERM EFFECTS IN ADULT SURVIVORS OF CHILD ABUSE

Controlled studies of adult survivors of childhood physical and sexual abuse offer a longitudinal perspective on the traumatization process and the long-term coping of the victims. The following psychological symptoms and psychiatric disorders of the survivors are similar to those displayed by the children: anxiety symptoms and delayed or chronic posttraumatic stress disorder (Briere and Runtz 1988; Lindberg and Distad 1985), multiple personality disorder (Putnam 1985), and depression and suicidal behavior (Briere and Runtz 1988; Sedney and Brooks 1984). Aggressive and assaultive behavior may be perpetuated by adult survivors of physical abuse, resulting in abusive behavior with their own children (Steele 1983) and criminally assaultive behavior (Alfaro 1977; Geller and Ford-Somma 1984). Adult survivors of sexual abuse are similarly predisposed toward molesting children, as documented by the high incidence of sexual abuse in the backgrounds of male and female child molesters (McCarty 1986; Seghorn et al. 1987). Sexual inhibition, an inability to enjoy sexual activity, or compulsive sexual behaviors are additional sexual problems encountered in adults who were molested as children (Courtois 1979).

Another group of psychiatric disorders appearing in adult survivors of child abuse have their onset in adolescence or in adult life. Drug and alcohol abuse have been frequently reported as long-term sequelae of sexual abuse (Briere 1984; Herman 1981). These substances help to blot out the painful memories and affects associated with the victimization. Eating disorders, which often begin during adolescence and usually reflect underlying problems with self-image, body image, and sexual identity, are often present in survivors of sexual abuse (Oppenheimer et al. 1985). Borderline personality disorder is a common finding in adults (especially women) with a history of sexual and physical abuse (Herman et al. 1989). Herman et al. regarded borderline personality disorder as a posttraumatic syndrome in which the patients fail to perceive a connection between their current symptoms and their abusive childhood experiences and in which the memories of their victimization become integrated in the total personality organization and become ego-syntonic. Somatization disorder has also been described as a frequent long-term sequela of child sexual abuse (Morrison 1989).

INTERVENTION IN CHILD ABUSE

General Principles of Intervention

A conceptual framework that recognizes the difference between acute and long-term traumatic processes operating in abused children and the tendency of abused children to rapidly repress or dissociate from terrifying memories of their victimization will be helpful in designing intervention strategies. Most abused children are not referred for intervention or receive only short-term treatment (Adams-Tucker 1984). After the initial posttraumatic anxiety symptoms subside, the child's psychopathology and suffering might be underestimated if sexual or aggressive acting out is minimal and depressive symptoms are not prominent. Parents or even professionals are often reluctant to recommend treatment out of concern about inflicting additional suffering by confronting the child with the frightening memories of the abuse. If the child's phobic, avoidant defenses and constricted affect predominate, the evaluator may minimize the negative impact of the abuse and regard the child's distress as temporary and easily reversible. In other cases, the initial symptoms of anxiety might be overlooked or absent, so that the child is thought to be relatively unaffected by the abuse. Because there is a long latency period between the childhood abuse and the emergence of symptoms in late adolescence or adulthood in some cases, timely intervention may prevent long-term or lifetime sequelae as well as alleviate current symptoms. Therefore, it is recommended that each physically or sexually abused child receive a thorough psychiatric evaluation to identify the acute and potential long-term effects of his or her victimization and the adequacy of his or her coping mechanisms.

The primary goal of intervention with the abusing family is to protect the child from further maltreatment and to strengthen and support the family unit by providing crisis-oriented services. An effective treatment program must deal specifically with the psychopathology of the child victim, the parental dysfunction, and the environmental stressors that may trigger and perpetuate the abuse. The phases of intervention may be outlined as follows: evaluation and crisis intervention, intervention with the child and parent(s), and postintervention follow-up. A wide variety of psychotherapeutic and educational techniques have been utilized with abused children and their families, including individual play therapy, individual psychotherapy, and group psychotherapy for the children; individual therapy, group psychotherapy, and parenting education for the parents; and family therapy and crisis nurseries for abused preschool children.

Evaluation and Crisis Intervention

Intervention begins as soon as the child discloses the abuse to a professional or is referred from an outside source (e.g., child protective services, pediatric emergency room, pediatrician, schoolteacher, counselor). The major goals of the evaluation are as follows.

Determination of the child's diagnosis and current functioning. The evaluation is designed to assess the nature and extent of the child's psychopathology and the effectiveness of his or her defensive response to the physical or sexual victimization. A careful developmental history should provide an estimate of the child's baseline adaptation before the abuse so that any trauma-induced changes in his or her psychological functioning may be documented. The child's feelings and the significance he or she attaches to the abuse should also be determined. The rendering of a psychiatric diagnosis is essential for treatment recommendations and disposition.

Validation of the abuse. If the maltreatment is ambiguous or questionable because of an absence of physical evidence or the failure of the child to make a disclosure, or both, the evaluation serves to validate or refute the alleged abuse. The evaluator obtains a careful history from the parent and child or other collateral individuals (e.g., a relative, pediatrician, or teacher) to discern the onset, nature, frequency, and duration of the abuse. The evaluator tries to determine whether the emergence of symptoms in the child correlates with the onset of the abuse. Symptoms may be regarded as more or less specific indicators of maltreatment. For example, acute symptoms of anxiety associated with the apparent onset of abuse—such as phobic avoidance of the alleged abuser, clinging, nightmares, and hypervigilance—are more reliable indicators of victimization than nonspecific symptoms of depression or conduct disorder. In sexually abused children, premature and inappropriate sexual behavior may be considered to be reliable evidence of a molestation. In the absence of positive or unambiguous physical findings, the ability of the child to describe the abusive events in a credible and reliable fashion is the most valid indicator that maltreatment has occurred.

Family assessment. The evaluation also includes an assessment of the family, including the parents, siblings, and adult relatives living in the home. Information from the family assessment reveals the child's risk for further abuse. If the father or father surrogate is the perpetrator of physical or sexual abuse, his removal from the home should be promptly effected. The ability of the nonoffending parent to protect and support the child's disclosure of abuse must also be determined. In cases where this parent had knowledge of the abuse but either failed to intervene or collaborated with the perpetrator, the child might have to be temporarily placed outside of the home. The evaluator must also determine whether the siblings of the abuse victim have also been abused and whether they are at risk for future maltreatment. The family assessment should also determine which adult or caretaker is best equipped to support and nurture the abuse victim, and this relationship should be strengthened.

Disposition and Treatment Planning

The diagnostic assessment of the child and family influence the disposition and treatment plan. The evaluator must decide whether it is possible to make the home safe for the child and how to accomplish this. If the abuser admits his or her guilt, accepts responsibility for his or her actions, and agrees to leave the home temporarily and if the nonabusing parent is supportive to the child and cooperates with the treatment plan, the child would appear to be safe remaining at home. If the abuser is threatening and noncooperative, this information should be directed to child protective services or the police.

The child's need for intervention and the most appropriate treatment modalities should be determined during the evaluation. Most abused children are symptomatic and require some crisis intervention with brief psychotherapy. Some abuse victims benefit from long-term intervention, whereas a minority of abused children remain relatively asymptomatic and might not require treatment if they are in a supportive family environment.

Depending on the structure of the treatment facility, the evaluator may or may not assume the role of the child's therapist. Many clinicians recommend that the functions of the evaluator and therapist be separated because the evaluator-therapist's obligation to report his or her observations to the court might contaminate the patient-therapist confidentiality.

Specific Treatment Goals

Intervention must create a safe environment and establish a supportive and positive therapeutic relationship with the child. Treatment must attempt to contain and reverse the pathological sequelae observed in the abused child and strengthen the child's ego functions and defenses to permit a continuation of his or her normal psychological growth and development. The therapist also helps the child validate the abusive experiences and counteracts any misdirected guilt or responsibility for the victimization. Intervention is also designed to support and strengthen the family unit, reduce environmental stress, and improve parenting skills.

After the child is evaluated and protected from further abuse, individual play therapy or psychotherapy may be initiated. Individual therapy is the most common type of child abuse intervention.

MAJOR TREATMENT ISSUES IN INDIVIDUAL PSYCHOTHERAPY

Betrayal and the Establishment of Trust

The experience of sexual exploitation or physical abuse by a parent from whom nurturance and love are expected generates feelings of betrayal and mistrust in the child victim. The child feels easily betrayed by the nonabusive parent for failing to protect him or her from the abuse. Feelings of betrayal and mistrust are easily generalized and are displaced onto other parental and authority figures, and they inevitably intrude into the therapeutic relationship. Abused children provoke and test the therapists by engaging in aggressive or seductive behaviors designed to provoke a punitive or sexual response. Sexual or aggressive acting out by the child with a female therapist might be an attempt to gauge her protectiveness. The therapist can eventually interpret these transference reactions by tracing them back to the child's original feelings of betrayal and disillusionment regarding his or her parents. After a period of testing and provocative behavior, the child is able to relax his or her vigilance and realizes that the therapist is reliable, predictable, and trustworthy. This newly acquired sense of trust may then be extended to extratherapeutic relationships.

Validation of the Victimization

It is important to validate the child's feelings of having been victimized and exploited by a caretaker in the opening phase of psychotherapy. The child's sense of reality about the abuse is compromised by the following elements:

1. Child victims of physical and sexual abuse are taught by their abusers that their beatings or participation in sexual acts are "normal" or beneficial to them.
2. The nonoffending parent often either fails to believe the child when the maltreatment is disclosed or minimizes its importance.
3. Parental attempts to rationalize or deny their abuse are reinforced by the natural tendency of the child to deny, repress, or dissociate from traumatic memories.
4. The reality of the victimization is further undermined by the perpetrator's insistence on secrecy. This insistence is often accom-

panied by threats that the child will be harmed or that the abuser will be incarcerated, leading to the destruction of the family.

The therapist must confirm and identify with the child's genuine feelings of victimization and betrayal and reinforce the concept that the abuse is a deviant act for which the parent must be held accountable. For some abuse victims, the opportunity to testify in court and to successfully convince a judge or jury of their abuse is the ultimate validation of their victimization.

Retrieval and Integration of Traumatic Memories

During the initial stages of treatment, the therapist often encounters episodes of acute anxiety with phobic elements that are obviously linked to the abusive experience and are reenacted in play. These anxiety states often occur in anticipation of revictimization as a manifestation of posttraumatic stress disorder. These states may be triggered by exposure to reminders of the abuse, which may not be evident to the child or the therapist.

The ultimate therapeutic goal is to identify and interpret the unconscious link between the compulsive, repetitive play activity and the original traumatic experience. Once the child is able to make this connection, he or she will be in a position to verbalize the traumatic memories and express the painful affect in words rather than in actions. In some child abuse victims, the initial presentation of the traumatic events may be disguised and less obvious. The child might be relatively nonverbal, and his or her play might appear sterile. It is unwise to pressure such children; they should be allowed to talk about the abuse at their own pace.

> Betty, a seductive and hyperactive 6-year-old girl, lived with her father after the marital separation. He, however, reverted to a homosexual lifestyle and forced Betty to participate in frequent orgies where she was sexually abused by both lesbians and gays, including her father. Betty could not talk about the abusive experiences. Her play appeared to be constricted and compulsive, consisting of scribbling heavy lines in a driven, intense manner. Betty called these primitive drawings "squiggly lines," which had no apparent meaning. After some time, she added heads and bodies to the scribbles, and it became clear that the "squiggly lines" connected the genital areas of the two figures. These lines represented the intense feelings of excitement associated with the genital contact with adults of both sexes experienced during the orgies. After the therapist made this connection, Betty was able to verbalize the feelings she had during these activities, such as fear, disgust, and sexual excitement.

The retrieval of split-off, dissociated traumatic memories, allowing them to be reexperienced and verbalized, the identification and encouragement of expression of the associated painful affects in a controlled and supportive setting, and the reintegration of these memories into the personality are essential in the treatment of children traumatized by physical and sexual abuse.

Use of Primitive Defenses

The use of primitive defense mechanisms such as denial, projection, splitting, and dissociation is common among physically and sexually abused children. These defenses are necessary to maintain the fantasy of having a "good parent," while the "badness" is projected onto some other person or attributed to themselves. The predominance of these defenses impairs the child's ability to integrate the loving and hostile aspects of their parents and others, leading to an overcategorization of objects into "good" and "bad."

The child's polarization of objects is readily extended to new encounters and to the therapeutic relationship. The child's initial mistrust usually gives way to an overidealization of the therapist in response to the latter's acceptance and support. The child attempts to please the therapist by demonstrating his or her skill in games, strength, and intelligence.

However, the enormity of the child's demands compared with the therapist's limited availability as a real object leads to an inevitable sense of betrayal and rejection. The child becomes angry with the therapist, who begins to take on the attributes of the "bad" parent. This shift is enhanced by the projection of the child's anger onto the therapist, with fears of retaliation. The child's ensuing aggressive behavior intensifies his or her negative self-concept and exacerbates his or her own "bad" self-image. The rapid shift in the child's perception of the therapist from an overidealized "good" parent to a hated and feared "bad" parent may be interpreted as a manifestation of the child's anger and frustration at not being gratified. The child's tendency to elicit punishment from the therapist in an attempt to re-create and master the original "bad" parent–"bad" child relationship should also be pointed out.

With the progression of therapy and the child's diminishing fear of victimization, the child effects a positive identification with the therapist and internalizes the therapist's values and attitudes, which leads to the emergence of more effective defenses such as repression, sublimation, and reaction formation. The child is then able to appraise the behavior of his or her parents and others more realistically. Therapeutic interventions must consistently identify and reverse the distortions of reality caused by these primitive defenses.

Donna, a 10-year-old girl who had been a victim of physical abuse, began to express feelings of anger and deprivation because of her therapist's inability to satisfy her insatiable demands for love and attention. She frequently refused to leave the playroom at the end of the session, saying, "If you love me, you'll let me stay." Donna's anger peaked when she saw another child with her therapist. She shouted at the therapist, "You don't like me, and the doll you gave me for Christmas was dirty, and the lollipop you gave me was poison." She threw herself on the floor and asked the therapist to pick her up.

The therapist explained that Donna's anger toward him was connected to her disappointment that he couldn't spend more time with her, which she interpreted as a personal rejection. He reassured her that he liked her and understood the source of her frustration. The therapist also made a connection between Donna's jealousy of the other child and her severe sibling rivalry with two younger sisters who were preferred by the parents.

Stigmatization and Low Self-Esteem

The stigmatization of an abused child through beatings, scapegoating, or sexual abuse results in shame, guilt, and low self-esteem. Feelings of shame and guilt are intensified if the child is blamed by the nonabusing parent for participating in sexual activity or provoking physical abuse. Depression and stigmatization are often associated with feelings of bodily damage. Sgroi (1982) described the "damaged goods syndrome," in which some sexually abused children believe that they have been permanently damaged by the sexual activity. The feeling of damage extends to a belief that they won't be able to marry, get pregnant, or have normal babies. Sexually abused children who sustain genital trauma or a sexually transmitted disease are at greater risk for this syndrome. Victims of physical abuse who are scapegoated are made to feel loathsome and deviant by their parents. Suicidal or self-destructive behavior in these physically abused children often reflects the child's compliance with the parental wishes for his or her destruction or disappearance.

The therapist must challenge the victim's perception that he or she is responsible for beatings or sexual assault inflicted by parents or caretakers. It should be emphasized that the child who is beaten or coerced into sexual activity by an adult can never be regarded as culpable in any way. The child should be informed that the offender's behavior is deviant and inappropriate.

The child's self-esteem in the treatment setting gradually improves during his or her exposure to the warmth and acceptance generated by the therapist. The abused child slowly modifies his or her self-concept to coincide with the therapist's positive view of the child.

Cathy's mother repeatedly hit and humiliated her because of Cathy's poor school performance. Her mother remarked, "I call her dumb and stupid because she is just like I was as a girl; she's passive and has no spunk." In reality, Cathy's IQ was above average, but she had a reading disorder. Her therapist continually reassured her that she was not stupid and that her reading was improving since she had been placed in a special class. The therapist praised her when she read to him. The therapist also challenged Cathy's alleged clumsiness as he complimented her for her skill in throwing and catching a ball in the playroom.

This case illustrates the cardinal feature in scapegoating: the projection of the parent's own unacceptable personality traits onto the child, who is then punished for the parental failure.

Emergence of Repressed Anger

At some point in the treatment setting, the victimized child begins to express anger toward his or her abuser, anger that had been previously denied. This anger is repressed for numerous reasons, such as fear of retaliation and further abuse, dependency on the abuser, and fear of the extent of the unleashed anger. In addition, the awareness of the anger forces the child to deal with the reality of the abusive experience.

The therapist should help the child to gradually remember how and why the original anger about the victimization was suppressed and gradually allow the child to reexperience these angry feelings. Although the emergence of this anger may be frightening to the child, it should be encouraged and justified. The emergence of repressed anger toward the nonabusive parent may also become an issue in treatment. A common cause of this anger is the failure of this parent to protect the child from the abuser or this parent's holding the child responsible for the abuse. The pent-up, repressed anger is often internalized and directed by the child toward himself or herself in the form of depression, self-hatred, and suicidal behavior.

Jenny, a 17-year-old girl, had been sexually victimized by her father, who was a successful businessman and prominent in the community. The molestation, which took place when she was between ages 5 and 12, consisted of vaginal fondling, mutual masturbation, and fellatio. Jenny's mother refused to acknowledge the molestation and acted as if nothing had happened. Jenny finally confronted her parents when she barricaded herself in her room and refused to come out until her father promised to stop abusing her.

Jenny was quite depressed during the initial phases of treatment and allowed the therapist to read her diary, which was full of self-loathing and suicidal ideation. It also contained references to her anger toward both parents. The therapist helped Jenny to gradually acknowledge and verbalize her anger. As her rage mounted, she recalled that she had re-

frained from getting angry in the past because the family had been dev-
astated by the sudden death of one of her older brothers when she was
14 years old. She felt that she had no right to get angry because her parents were depressed and grieving over their loss. Once her anger became
mobilized, she used it adaptively by confronting her parents once again
about their respective roles in the molestation and its cover-up, and she
arranged for a family session to be held in the presence of the therapist.
At this time, using the therapist as a witness and ally, she made a list of
demands: that her parents would acknowledge their wrongdoing, apol-
ogize to her, and seek help for their problems.

Quest for Control and Mastery

Abused children are keenly aware of their feelings of powerlessness
during their victimization at the hands of a powerfully perceived adult
caretaker. To reverse their long-standing feelings of vulnerability, these
children seek to achieve a sense of belated control and mastery in their
relationships with peers and with the therapist, but this quest for mastery often occurs in a maladaptive fashion. This behavior is usually expressed in the transference and often serves as a formidable resistance
during psychotherapy. The therapist is in a good position to interpret
this belated attempt at mastery as a need to reverse the power imbalance originating in the physical or sexual abuse during childhood.

> Jenny (described in the previous case illustration) recalled during her
> psychotherapy that she had attempted to seduce other children in the
> past. When she was 7, she engaged in sex play with the other girls in her
> bunk at summer camp. As she rolled around naked in bed, she recalled
> that she insisted on being "on top." At age 10, she initiated sex play with
> a boy by pulling his pants down, while telling him to keep it a secret. As
> a teenager, Jenny compulsively initiated sexual contact with boys but
> would never respond to a boy who approached her first. These were ob-
> vious attempts to assert mastery and control in sexualized relationships
> so as to prevent a reexperiencing of her vulnerability and powerlessness
> during the molestation by her father. In the treatment setting, Jenny's
> quest for control was expressed by her frequent attempts to change or
> cancel appointments at the last minute and by her constant vacillation
> about whether to have one or two therapy sessions weekly.

Role Confusion

One of the major psychodynamic mechanisms operating in families involved in physical abuse is role reversal, in which the child is expected
to gratify the needs of the parent. These "parentified" children are
often beaten when they fail to perform this role adequately. Therefore,
many physically abused children with severe ego deficits and developmental delays maintain a precocious capacity to perform household

duties such as cooking, cleaning, and infant care. In the treatment setting, these children tend to overingratiate themselves with the therapist by helping to clean up the office or to repair toys or office equipment. Their desperate efforts to please the therapist may be interpreted as a carryover from their need to please and "perform for" their abusing parents. The child may be told that he or she is acceptable to the therapist without having to act as a "servant." Beneath the facade of pseudoindependence lurks a depressed, needy child longing for loving contact but fearing it at the same time.

A child's experiences in an incestuous family easily lead to a similar type of role confusion. In a typical case of incest, a young girl is treated like a spouse or confidante by her father and her mother is psychologically unavailable, and she is made to feel responsible for her father's happiness while simultaneously assuming some of the household responsibilities of her mother. The child is often given the additional responsibility of keeping the family intact. These role reversals are in direct conflict with the child's needs for protection, nurturance, and dependency gratification. The child victim of incest maintains her infantile attachment to the father despite the pseudoadult facade. The therapist should encourage the child to engage in age-appropriate childhood activities and to develop peer relationships. These goals can only be achieved with the cooperation of the mother, who must resume her role as a caretaker and protector of the child.

Problems With Impulse Control

Aggression in physically abused children.   The abused child's aggressive and destructive behavior within and outside of the home is a major cause of referral for psychiatric evaluation and treatment. The abused child learns to be aggressive and violent by observing and imitating the behavior of his or her abusive parents. Aggressive behavior by these abused children often masks underlying feelings of vulnerability and helplessness.

After the therapist acknowledges the child's need to feel powerful and important and his or her tendency to "identify with the aggressor," the therapist must limit direct manifestations of aggression such as hitting and destroying toys and playroom materials. The child should be taught to verbalize anger or express it symbolically through play. Limit setting must be clearly defined with respect to entering and leaving the playroom, removing toys and materials, and the length of the sessions. Control of aggression may be achieved through the introduction of sublimating activities and typical latency games.

> Juan, an 11-year-old boy, was referred to a child psychiatry clinic after he forced his 3-year-old half-brother to drink lye. Juan had returned to live

with his mother and her boyfriend 1 year before this incident, after having spent the previous 7 years with his father and stepmother in Puerto Rico. Juan had been subjected to chronic and severe physical abuse by his father during this period, which consisted of beatings on the head and burns on his body inflicted with a hot iron. Since returning to his mother, Juan became hyperactive and aggressive at home and in school and exhibited extreme jealousy toward his two half-brothers, whom he encountered for the first time. He hit both boys frequently before the lye incident. Juan confided to this therapist that he enjoyed catching mice, placing them in boiling water, and smashing their heads with a hammer, after which he would flush them down the toilet. When asked to explain this cruel behavior, Juan pointed to the scars and ridges on his scalp and the burn marks on his shoulder, exclaiming, "This is what my father did to me."

The therapist was able to interpret Juan's compulsion to repeat and reenact the abuse inflicted by his father with his half-brother, his schoolmates, and the mice. Juan's jealousy of his half-brother as a new sibling rival and his mother's favorite child was also explored with the therapist. This proved to be a turning point in the therapy. As Juan began to verbalize the feelings of rage, helplessness, and fear he experienced during the beatings inflicted by his father, he felt less compelled to reenact them. Through identification with the aggressor, the child displaces some of his or her original rage at the abusive parent onto a substitute. Identification with the aggressor may also serve as a tension-relieving device and as a pathological form of self-esteem regulation. The therapist's interpretations regarding the origins of Juan's rage were supplemented by strict limit setting during the therapy.

Hypersexual behavior in sexually abused children.   Sexually abused children also appear to be driven to reenact their victimization experiences, also using identification with the aggressor as a conspicuous defense mechanism. The traumatic memories of the molestation intrude into the child's dreams, fantasies, and play and are also likely to be reenacted with peers and even adults. These children often become sexually aroused in the treatment setting by routine physical or psychological closeness and have difficulty in differentiating between affectionate and sexual relationships. The therapist tries to set limits on the child's seductive behavior in the playroom and explains to the child how behaving like his or her molester makes the child feel less vulnerable and more in control.

Betty, the 6-year-old discussed in a previous case illustration, who had been forced to participate in sex orgies by her father, began to seduce her classmates by taking them into the school bathroom and fondling their genitals. This seductive behavior also appeared during the second month of play therapy. Betty began to polish her nails and apply her mother's lipstick and makeup. The therapist questioned the appropriateness of this behavior for a 6-year-old and prohibited it. However, Betty proceeded to improvise her makeup by using crayons and magic markers. She made herself a cardboard crown and called herself "the queen of Europe." She made a crown for her male therapist, invited him to be the "king," and tried to color his nails and eyebrows with the markers. Finally, she tried to sit on the therapist's lap and was gently restrained.

Careful questioning and exploration about her participation in the sexual parties revealed that Betty's father used to dress her up in seductive women's clothing and helped her apply lipstick and makeup as a prelude to their sexual activity. The therapist commented that Betty was repeating with him the same "makeup" game that her father played with her, and perhaps she wondered if the therapist was going to give her "bad touches" as her father had. Betty responded, "That's what people do when they like each other, and I wanted you to like me." The therapist was then able to discuss more appropriate, nonsexual ways of showing affection.

Countertransference Problems

The major countertransference problem confronting therapists who work with abused children is the tendency to overidentify with the victim, become enraged with the abuser, and develop exaggerated rescue fantasies. This situation may lead to an intolerance for the child's positive feelings toward the perpetrator or encourage the child to vent his or her own anger prematurely. These therapists easily become impatient with the progress of therapy and cannot tolerate the child's resistance and hostility, which threaten the rescue mission.

Working with physically abused children may elicit the therapist's feelings about his or her own aggression and views regarding discipline and child rearing. Working with sexually abused children may stir up the therapist's own incestuous feelings either as a child or as an adult. The therapist must become aware of his or her own feelings about sexual abuse and sexuality. If the therapist is uncomfortable about sexual matters or is sexually repressed, this discomfort might be communicated to the child, who might then be reluctant to talk about details of the molestation. Such a therapist might believe that the child's disclosure of incest is based on fantasy.

Some male therapists might overidentify with the father and blame the victim for the incest. Female therapists may overidentify with the mother and overlook the pathological mother-child relationship commonly encountered in incest families. Many therapists cannot tolerate the highly aggressive and provocative physically abused child because this behavior elicits their own aggression. In a similar vein, some therapists cannot tolerate the seductiveness and precocious sexuality of sexually abused children because they fear becoming sexually aroused.

Because working with abused children and their families can be a demanding and emotionally draining experience, therapists should have access to supervision and the ability to discuss their cases with peers. This support will result in greater awareness of the turbulent feelings evoked by the physical and sexual assault of children and should reduce the likelihood of major countertransference errors.

GROUP THERAPY

Group therapy has been recommended for physically abused (Kempe and Kempe 1978), sexually abused (Blick and Porter 1982; Sturkie 1983), and traumatized (Terr 1990) children. Group therapy may be used as the primary treatment modality, but it is often used in conjunction with individual treatment. Group therapy may be open ended and psychodynamic, with a focus on what the children introduce in each session (Steward et al. 1986), or it may be time limited with structured, preplanned formats. An example of the structured approach has been described by Sturkie (1983), who designed an eight-session format with each session devoted to a different theme. These themes were believability, guilt and responsibility, body integrity, secrecy and sharing, anger, powerlessness, other life crises, and court appearances. Groups are usually led by male and female cotherapists to re-create the parental dyad. In some cases, however, sexually abused girls might be more comfortable with a female therapist.

A group size of six to eight is optimal. Such a group is large enough to maintain continuity and group process in case of absences or dropouts, but not so large that the needs of the group members are overlooked.

The beneficial elements of group therapy are providing the abused child with a positive socialization experience designed to diminish his or her estrangement and sense of isolation from peers, reducing stigmatization and guilt by sharing of the abusive experiences, validating the child's reality, and correcting distorted perceptions induced by the abuser. The group also offers an opportunity for valuable learning experiences in areas such as sex education, prevention of further abuse, and preparation for court. The therapists also become positive role models for the group members.

INTERVENTION WITH THE ABUSIVE FAMILY

Because of the significant degree of psychopathology in individual family members and in the family system in cases of physical and sexual abuse, the treatment of the child victim should be supplemented by intervention with the parents and other family members.

In physically abusing families, the abuse is often inflicted on a background of poverty, neglect, and environmental stress. Individual treatment of the abusing parent is complemented by parenting education designed to help the parent develop nonabusive disciplinary and child-rearing techniques and to improve the overall parent-child relationship. Intervention should include a strong outreach component providing home visits, social services, and a crisis hot line, and the families should be assisted in obtaining medical care and legal assistance (Green 1980). Crisis or therapeutic nurseries may benefit physically abused preschool children and their mothers. Mothers of physically abused children also benefit from therapeutic and educational group therapy.

In families involved with sexual abuse and incest, the mother is a key figure and must be a focus for intervention. The major treatment goal with the mother is the establishment of a closer, empathic relationship with the incest victim. The most salient treatment issues are the mother's guilt at failing to prevent the incest, low self-esteem, anger at the husband, anger and depression about the breakup of the marriage, and the tendency to blame or disbelieve the victimized child. These mothers can benefit from individual and group therapy. Other types of intervention that have been helpful are conjoint mother-child individual and group therapy and mother-child groups working in parallel fashion, with ongoing communication between the therapists from each group (Damon and Waterman 1986).

Giarretto (1982) developed a family therapy approach to incestuous families. This approach includes the perpetrator (usually the father), the mother, and the child victim and is designed to change the pathological family system that created and maintained the incest. The family therapy is preceded by individual and dyadic treatment of the family members and is contingent on the prior admission of guilt by the offender.

Intervention with the offender, usually the father or father surrogate, commences with his removal from the home and denial of unsupervised access to the child. Behavior modification techniques that help the offenders control their deviant patterns of sexual arousal have been more successful than psychotherapy (Abel et al. 1985).

SUCCESS OF INTERVENTION

The results of a nationwide evaluation of federally funded treatment programs providing services to families involved in all types of abuse and neglect have been disappointing (Cohn and Daro 1987). Thirty percent of this population continued to abuse or neglect their children during their involvement with the program. At the termination of the treatment, only 42% of the parents were judged by their therapists to have a reduced potential for maltreatment of their children. The optimistic side of this evaluation revealed that the children exhibited the highest rates of improvement, in the range of 70%. Green et al. (1981a) reported a more successful treatment outcome in a multidisciplinary hospital-based program; two-thirds of the abusing parents demonstrated some improvement, with a recidivism rate of 16%.

Several group therapy outcome studies have been done using standardized instruments to measure posttreatment improvement. James (1977) and Verleur et al. (1986) found that sexually abused girls demonstrated more improvement in self-esteem after treatment than did untreated control groups. Nelki and Watters (1989) documented a significant decline in problematic behaviors exhibited by sexually abused children at the end of group therapy, according to parent rating scales.

There is an obvious need for treatment outcome studies using standardized instruments to determine the efficacy of intervention with abused children and their families. Follow-up studies should also be done with treated and untreated abused children to find out whether a diminution or reversal of symptoms and psychopathology attributed to the intervention persists over time.

CONCLUSION

The recent documentation of the high prevalence of child physical and sexual abuse in our society and the serious immediate and long-term psychological sequelae in the maltreated children highlight the urgent need for prevention and early intervention. The primary goals of intervention in cases of physical and sexual abuse are protection of the children from further maltreatment, amelioration or reversal of psychological impairment in the children, strengthening of parental functioning, and reduction in the environmental stressors associated with the abuse.

Treatment begins with crisis intervention and a careful psychiatric assessment of the child and the parents to determine their psychopathology and the dysfunctional family interaction. A wide variety of treatment modalities have been successfully utilized in cases of child abuse, such as individual and group therapy for children and parents, family therapy, parenting education, and the provision of concrete social services with outreach.

Validation of the victimization and the retrieval and integration of repressed and dissociated traumatic memories are crucial issues in the therapy of abused children. Other important treatment issues are betrayal and the establishment of trust, the use of primitive defenses, stigmatization and low self-esteem, emergence of repressed anger, the quest for control and mastery, role confusion, difficulty with impulse control, and countertransference problems.

Thus far, a handful of treatment outcome studies have demonstrated fair to moderate improvement when various types of intervention are used with abused children. However, more treatment outcome and follow-up studies are needed to determine the success of various types of intervention and the duration of their effects.

REFERENCES

Abel GG, Mittleman M, Becker JV: Sex offenders: results of assessment and recommendations for treatment, in Clinical Criminology: Current Concepts. Edited by Ben-Aron H, Hucker S, Webster C. Toronto, Canada, M & M Graphics, 1985, pp 191–205

Adams-Tucker C: The unmet needs of sexually abused youths: referrals from a child protection agency and clinical evaluation. Journal of the American Academy of Child Psychiatry 23:659–667, 1984

Aiosa-Karpas CJ, Karpas R, Pelcovitz D, et al: Gender identification and sex role attribution in sexually abused adolescent females. Journal of the American Academy of Child Psychiatry 30:266–271, 1991

Alfaro JD: Report on the relationship between child abuse and neglect and later socially deviant behavior. New York, New York State Assembly Select Committee on Child Abuse, 1977

Blick LC, Porter FS: Group therapy with female adolescent victims, in Handbook of Clinical Intervention in Child Sexual Abuse. Edited by Sgroi SM. Lexington, MA, Lexington Books, 1982, pp 147–175

Briere J: The long-term effects of childhood sexual abuse: defining a post-sexual abuse syndrome. Paper presented at the Third National Conference on Sexual Victimization of Children, Washington, DC, 1984

Briere J, Runtz M: Post sexual abuse trauma, in Lasting Effects of Child Sexual Abuse. Edited by Wyatt GE, Powell GJ. Newbury Park, CA, Sage, 1988, pp 85–99

Cohn AH, Daro D: Is treatment too late: what ten years of evaluative research tells us. Child Abuse Negl 11:433–442, 1987

Courtois C: The incest experience and its aftermath. Victimology: An International Journal 4:337–347, 1979

Damon L, Waterman J: Parallel group treatment of children and their mothers, in Sexual Abuse of Young Children. Edited by MacFarlane K, Waterman J. New York, Guilford, 1986, pp 244–298

Elmer E, Gregg CS: Developmental characteristics of abused children. Pediatrics 40:596–602, 1967

Finkelhor D: Child Sexual Abuse: New Theory and Research, New York, Free Press, 1984

Finkelhor D: Sourcebook on Child Sexual Abuse. Beverly Hills, CA, Sage, 1986

Friedrich WN, Reams R: Course of psychological symptoms in sexually abused young children. Psychotherapy 24:160–171, 1987

Gaensbauer T, Sands K: Regulation of emotional expression in infants from two contrasting environments. Journal of the American Academy of Child Psychiatry 21:167–171, 1979

Geller M, Ford-Somma L: Violent homes, violent children: a study of violence in the families of juvenile offenders (Division of Juvenile Services, New Jersey State Department of Corrections, Trenton). Report prepared for the National Center on Child Abuse and Neglect, Department of Health and Human Services, Washington, DC, 1984

George C, Main M: Social interactions and young abused children: approach, avoidance, and aggression. Child Dev 50:306–319, 1979

Giarretto H: Integrated Treatment of Child Sexual Abuse. Palo Alto, CA, Science & Behavior Books, 1982

Goodwin J: Post-traumatic symptoms in incest victims, in Post-Traumatic Stress Disorder in Children. Edited by Eth S, Pynoos RS. Washington, DC, American Psychiatric Press, 1985, pp 157–168

Green AH: Psychiatric treatment of abused children. Journal of the American Academy of Child Psychiatry 17:356–371, 1978

Green AH: Child Maltreatment: A Handbook for Mental Health and Child Care Professionals. New York, Jason Aronson, 1980

Green AH: Children traumatized by physical abuse, in Post-Traumatic Stress Disorder in Children. Edited by Eth S, Pynoos RS. Washington, DC, American Psychiatric Press, 1985, pp 135–154

Green AH, Power E, Steinbook B, et al: Factors associated with successful and unsuccessful intervention with child abusing families. Child Abuse Negl 5:45–52, 1981a

Green AH, Voeller K, Gaines R, et al: Neurological impairment in battered children. Child Abuse Negl 5:129–134, 1981b

Herman J: Father-Daughter Incest. Cambridge, MA, Harvard University Press, 1981

Herman J, Perry JC, van der Kolk B: Childhood trauma in borderline personality disorder. Am J Psychiatry 146:490–495, 1989

James K: Incest: the teenager's perspective. Psychotherapy: Theory, Research, and Practice 14:146–155, 1977

Kempe R, Kempe CH: Child Abuse. Cambridge, MA, Harvard University Press, 1978

Kluft R: Childhood Antecedents of Multiple Personality. Washington, DC, American Psychiatric Press, 1985

Lindberg F, Distad L: Post-traumatic stress disorder in women who experienced childhood incest. Child Abuse Negl 9:329–334, 1985

Martin HP: The child and his development, in Helping the Battered Child and His Family. Edited by Kempe CH, Helfer RE. Philadelphia, PA, Lippincott, 1972

McCarty L: Mother-child incest: characteristics of the offender. Child Welfare 65:447–458, 1986

Morrison J: Childhood sexual histories of women with somatization disorder. Am J Psychiatry 146:239–241, 1989

Nelki J, Watters J: A group for sexually abused young children. Child Abuse Negl 13:369–377, 1989

Oates K: Child Abuse and Neglect: What Happens Eventually? New York, Brunner/Mazel, 1986

Oppenheimer R, Howells K, Palmer L, et al: Adverse sexual experiences in childhood and clinical eating disorders: a preliminary description. J Psychosom Res 19:157–161, 1985

Putnam F: The psychophysiologic investigation of multiple personality disorder. Psychiatr Clin North Am 7:31–40, 1985

Sedney MA, Brooks B: Factors associated with a history of childhood sexual experience in a nonclinical female population. Journal of the American Academy of Child Psychiatry 23:215–218, 1984

Seghorn TK, Prentky RA, Boucher RJ: Child sexual abuse in the lives of sexually aggressive offenders. J Am Acad Child Adolesc Psychiatry 26:262–267, 1987

Sgroi S: Handbook of Clinical Intervention in Child Sexual Abuse. Lexington, MA, Lexington Books, 1982

Steele BF: The effect of abuse and neglect on psychological development, in Frontiers of Infant Psychiatry. Edited by Call JD, Galenson E, Tyson RL. New York, Basic Books, 1983, pp 235–244

Steward M, Farguhar L, Dicharry D, et al: Group therapy: a treatment choice for young victims of child abuse. Int J Group Psychother 36:261–277, 1986

Sturkie K: Structured group treatment for sexually abused children. Health Soc Work 8:299–308, 1983

Terr L: Too Scared to Cry: Psychic Trauma in Childhood. New York, Harper & Row, 1990

U.S. Department of Health and Human Services: Study findings: study of the national incidence and prevalence of child abuse and neglect. Washington, DC, U.S. Department of Health and Human Services, 1988, pp 5–8

Verleur D, Hughes R, De Rios M: Enhancement of self-esteem among female adolescent incest victims: a controlled study. Adolescence 21:843–854, 1986

Yates A: Children eroticized by incest. Am J Psychiatry 139:482–485, 1982

Afterword to Section IV

Clarice J. Kestenbaum, M.D., and Owen Lewis, M.D.,
Section Editors

In presenting these six chapters, we wanted to demonstrate several features of child and adolescent psychotherapy. The range of disorders treated with psychotherapy, either alone or in conjunction with other modalities of intervention, is broad. Classical principles evolved from the treatment of neurotic children. With appropriate adaptations, these principles may be used in the treatment of psychotic children. Disorders span the gamut from neuropsychiatric problems, in which there is a clear constitutional deficit, to the sequelae of child abuse, which arise from an environment insult.

Treatment relies on accurate diagnosis. Various components of treatment may include cognitive, behavioral, family, and pharmacological therapy, as well as psychodynamic therapy, which may serve as a principle component of treatment or be the organizing matrix. Even within psychodynamic psychotherapy, different aspects can be modified. From all these components, a treatment approach is forged that addresses both the developmental level of the child and the specific disorder.

The specific modalities required for each disorder in turn enhance our understanding of what makes therapy therapeutic. Often, well-timed focal behavioral work enables the working-through aspect of conflict resolution. Periodic or ongoing family work can further the dynamic inquiry. The limits of any specific intervention become clear as the integrative collaboration of therapies progresses.

As can be seen from each chapter, knowledge of each disorder is based on scientific research. We have included a chapter on psychotherapy research because our practice of therapy can only evolve if it is based on the scientific assessment of outcome.

In summary, then, several general principles apply to the practice of child and adolescent psychotherapy. It is not a generic modality of treatment. Rather, it is diagnosis specific. Diagnosis involves careful assessment of cognitive, familial, biological, and psychological factors. Child and adolescent psychotherapy is also essentially integrative, combining many modalities of treatment. Of the various disciplines of professionals who treat children, we feel that it is the child psychiatrist who can uniquely integrate these various approaches and affect both our concept of disease and its treatment.

V

Sleep Disorders

Section V

Sleep Disorders

Foreword

Charles F. Reynolds III, M.D., and David J. Kupfer, M.D.,
Section Editors

The recent publication of DSM-IV and the completion of the related American Psychiatric Association–National Institute of Mental Health field trials in insomnia represent advances that make it particularly appropriate to revisit the current state of knowledge about sleep disorders, from the dual perspectives of both psychiatric research and practice. During the past quarter-century, psychiatric researchers and clinicians have played a major role in the development of the new field of sleep disorders medicine. This is not too surprising when considering that disturbances in sleep and circadian rhythms of sleeping and waking function are among the most disabling and persistent features of psychiatric disorders and that many psychiatrists have long had an interest in sleep as a window on the inner lives of patients.

Further, as Donna E. Giles, Ph.D., Ronald E. Dahl, M.D., and Patricia A. Coble, R.N., discuss in Chapter 25, "Childbearing, Developmental, and Familial Aspects of Sleep," we now know that sleep is abnormal in individuals at risk for psychiatric disorders such as depression (even in the absence of a personal history of depression). Such an observation, which arises from recently completed family studies of sleep, is strongly convergent with other data from epidemiological studies indicating that disturbed sleep is a harbinger of future mental disorders, particularly depression and anxiety, as reviewed by Daniel J. Buysse, M.D., and Eric A. Nofzinger, M.D., in Chapter 26, "Sleep in Depression: Longitudinal Perspectives."

During the past decade, since the last appearance of a section devoted to sleep in 1985 in Volume 4 of *Review of Psychiatry*, the field of psychiatric sleep research has taken large strides forward. That progress is reflected abundantly in the chapters of this section and also informed our selection of the chapter authors, who are among the key contributors to progress in our field.

Several key themes are interwoven throughout the chapters:

1. Sleep and circadian rhythms provide a critical window into the functioning of the central nervous system.
2. Sleep and circadian rhythms change profoundly as a function of the continuum of aging (from successful aging to pathological aging).
3. The study of psychiatric sleep disorders has become integrated with other contemporary neuroscientific approaches, including genetics, imaging, neuropharmacology, and psychophysiology.
4. The study of psychiatric sleep disorders has also been integrated with epidemiological approaches, as illustrated particularly by the Epidemiologic Catchment Area studies.

Thus, the utility of sleep and circadian physiology as a window into normal and pathological aging is strongly underscored in reviews of work at opposite ends of the life cycle, in Chapter 25 by Giles and colleagues on childhood and adolescence and in Chapter 30, "Sleep in Dementing Illness," by Donald L. Bliwise, Ph.D., on old age. Progress in integrating psychiatric sleep research with other avenues of neuroscience is amply illustrated in the reviews of affective disorders in Chapter 26, by Buysse and Nofzinger, and of schizophrenia in Chapter 27, "Sleep Abnormalities in Schizophrenia and Other Psychotic Disorders," by Kathleen L. Benson, Ph.D., and Vincent P. Zarcone, Jr., M.D. Both reviews also highlight the value of integrating studies of sleep with different types and phases of treatment, including the acute and maintenance phases of psychotherapy and pharmacotherapy. Likewise, progress in the management of sleep disturbances and psychosocial sequelae of circadian rhythm disruption is richly detailed in Chapter 29, "Disorders Relating to Shift Work and Jet Lag," by Timothy H. Monk, Ph.D. Finally, the impact of daytime sleepiness on mood and performance as well as its differential diagnosis is an important topic for mental health professionals. Readers will find the discussion of these issues by Thomas Roth Ph.D., Timothy A. Roehrs, Ph.D., and Leon Rosenthal, M.D., in Chapter 28, "Normative and Pathological Aspects of Daytime Sleepiness," timely and useful.

We come to the ultimate justification for this *Review* section on psychiatric sleep disorders: namely, to help treat patients. The progress now being made on many fronts only underscores the practical utility for psychiatric clinicians of understanding sleep and its disorders, whether for early recognition and intervention to prevent the psychiatric complications of disordered sleep, or for using sleep to understand how central nervous system functioning changes across the life cycle and (in a related vein) to identify those factors that promote the vitality of healthy aging. We believe that the study of sleep and circadian rhythms will continue to be a vital component of understanding the factors that promote healthy aging.

Chapter 25

Childbearing, Developmental, and Familial Aspects of Sleep

Donna E. Giles, Ph.D., Ronald E. Dahl, M.D., and Patricia A. Coble, R.N.

The goals of this chapter are to provide brief overviews of 1) sleep during the course of pregnancy and the postpartum period; 2) sleep in normal childhood development, in primary sleep disorders, and in psychiatric disorders of children and adolescents; and 3) sleep as a familial and genetic entity. These three areas of interest will be considered in turn. Descriptions of sleep are based on terminology derived from electroencephalogram (EEG) studies of sleep. There are three broad categories of state: awake, rapid eye movement (REM) sleep, and non–rapid eye movement (NREM) sleep. NREM sleep is divided into four stages: 1, 2, 3, and 4. These stages represent progressive slowing of electrical activity in the brain. Stage 1 is light sleep or drowsiness. Stage 2 is of medium depth and is characterized by spindles and K complexes in the EEG. Stages 3 and 4 are called slow-wave or delta sleep because of the low-frequency and high-amplitude EEG waves.

SLEEP IN PREGNANT AND POSTPARTUM WOMEN

Although few would dispute that perturbations in sleep are common in childbearing women, the underlying causes of these disturbances are unknown. Hormonal factors as well as physical discomfort have been speculated to account for sleep disturbances during pregnancy, whereas sleep disruption after parturition has been associated primarily with nocturnal child care (American Sleep Disorders Association 1990; Mauri 1990). Published reports on the characteristics of sleep disturbances in pregnant and postpartum women have been sparse, however. Only eight reports describe EEG sleep characteristics in *healthy* women during pregnancy and postpartum (Branchey and Petre-Quadens 1968; Brownell et al. 1986; Driver and Shapiro 1992; Hertz et al. 1992; Karacan et al. 1968, 1969; Petre-Quadens et al. 1967; Roffwarg et al. 1968).

Taken together, these studies of sleep in childbearing women involved a total of only about 60 women. This number is reduced to just over 40 women if only those studies with a longitudinal design are considered. Most reports compared sleep measurements in the final trimester with those on a single follow-up recording obtained 3–6 months postpartum. Only two studies (Driver and Shapiro 1992; Karacan et al. 1968)—involving 3 and 5 women, respectively—examined sleep at time points earlier in pregnancy. Similarly, only those two studies presented postpartum data (for 13 and 5 women, respectively) obtained at points earlier than the third postpartum month. Studies have been performed in the sleep laboratory; however, only one study (Driver and Shapiro 1992) obtained postpartum measurements with infants present at night. Overall, sleep-continuity disturbances have been found most consistently in late pregnancy and the early postpartum period (Branchey and Petre-Quadens 1968; Driver and Shapiro 1992; Hertz et al. 1992; Karacan et al. 1968, 1969; Petre-Quadens et al. 1967), although the degree of disturbance has varied from study to study. Alterations in sleep staging have been less consistently reported, although they have been noted by some investigators (Driver and Shapiro 1992; Hertz et al. 1992; Karacan et al. 1968, 1969).

Clearly, our present capacity to distinguish normal from abnormal disturbances in sleep among childbearing women is limited by available data for this population. In light of this deficiency, we recently studied EEG sleep recordings for 34 women over the course of childbearing, using a home monitoring system (Coble et al., in press [a], in press [b]). To enter our study, all women were required to be less than 12 weeks pregnant, to have prenatal care, to be medically and obstetrically healthy, to have reported no sleep problems in the year before pregnancy, and to have been free of any current psychiatric disorders for at least 1 year before conception. Mean age was 28.8 years (range, 23–36 years). Social adjustment was good to excellent for all subjects, and all pregnancies were planned. Over a third (38.2%) were primigravidae, and most (85.3%) breast-fed their infants for at least 6 weeks postpartum. At study entry, 14 women (41.2%) had a history of affective disorder (minimum interval since the most recent episode: 2 years), whereas the remaining 20 women had no lifetime history of *any* psychiatric disorder. Only one woman, with a personal and family history of affective disorder, had an episode of psychiatric illness (nonpsychotic major depression) during the course of study.

EEG sleep recordings were obtained in subjects' homes using a remote monitoring system, the Telediagnostic System, for which reliability data had been established in our setting (Sewitch and Kupfer 1985). Two consecutive nights of sleep were recorded at 12, 24, and 36 weeks of gestation and at 1 and 8 months postpartum.

EEG sleep measurements were stable from 12 to 36 weeks of gestation. Although a modest increase in wakefulness after sleep onset and a slight decrease in sleep efficiency were observed at 36 weeks of gestation, the variability in these measures increased as well, and total sleep time remained unchanged. Values obtained for the pregnant women in our sample were not significantly different from those previously reported for healthy subjects ($n = 19$) evaluated by the same procedure (Sewitch and Kupfer 1985). Complaints of difficulty falling asleep were rarely endorsed. Restless sleep with one or more awakenings to use the bathroom *without* difficulty returning to sleep was endorsed by the majority of women at each assessment. Nocturnal awakenings associated *with* difficulty returning to sleep were reported by few women in our sample at 12 and 24 weeks of gestation, whereas a third reported such difficulty at 36 weeks of gestation.

The most pronounced effects of childbearing on EEG sleep were observed at 1 month postpartum. At this point, sleep continuity was clearly disrupted because these women experienced approximately an hour of nocturnal wakefulness associated with nighttime feeding of their infants. Comparison of EEG sleep at 1 month postpartum with EEG sleep at 36 weeks of gestation revealed a significant increase in awake time, decreased sleep efficiency, and increased slow-wave sleep. No significant differences were noted for any of the REM sleep measurements. In contrast, slow-wave sleep was not different in women at 1 month postpartum compared with nonchildbearing healthy subjects studied at home (Sewitch and Kupfer 1985), although sleep continuity was more impaired in postpartum women. REM sleep parameters were not different between the two groups. By 8 months postpartum, sleep continuity in childbearing women was markedly improved and EEG sleep did not differ significantly from that of control subjects. As in pregnancy, endorsement of midnocturnal awakenings was common in our subjects, and reports of difficulty returning to sleep after nocturnal awakenings were infrequent.

These findings add substantially to available data on EEG sleep in childbearing women, particularly regarding EEG sleep in the first and second trimesters. Sleep disturbances over the course of childbearing primarily involve sleep-continuity disruption, characterized by increased wakefulness after sleep onset. Some studies have noted increased slow-wave sleep after parturition (Driver and Shapiro 1992; Karacan et al. 1968, 1969), but these changes have generally been modest and have been accompanied by a high degree of individual variability. Earlier findings (Karacan et al. 1968, 1969) indicating increased sleep time in the first trimester, with normalization of sleep in the second trimester and increasing sleep disruption beginning in the third trimester, have not been confirmed by more recent longitudinal research (Driver and Shapiro 1992) nor by our data. Rather, sleep disturbances are actually quite modest: EEG sleep has shown little deviation from normal, and has shown remarkable stability from the first trimester to as late as 39 weeks of gestation. Also in contrast to the earlier findings (Karacan et al. 1968, 1969), more recent studies have indicated disturbances in sleep continuity at 1 month postpartum. This discrepancy is almost certainly due to the recording site. Earlier recordings were obtained for mothers who slept uninterrupted by the needs of their infants in the sleep laboratory; more recent data were obtained in the home with infants present and reflect disturbances associated with nocturnal child care. Despite interruptions in their sleep, however, few postpartum women subjectively report difficulty in returning to sleep.

To summarize, there is substantial stability of objective EEG sleep measures throughout pregnancy; however, child care requirements are associated with a clear decrease in sleep-continuity measures in the postpartum period. Subjective reports of sleep disturbance were largely related to midnocturnal awakenings, but women reported very little difficulty in returning to sleep. The third trimester was associated with greater variability in EEG sleep measures and a somewhat greater number of subjective sleep disturbances. Greater variability in sleep measures during the third trimester suggests that some individuals may suffer more than others from sleep loss, but that in general sleep architecture is preserved. When pregnant women in their third trimester were compared with matched nonpregnant control subjects, there were no objective differences in EEG sleep. Thus, on average, sleep is relatively robust during pregnancy and the *capacity* to sleep is retained postpartum, although demands of child care exert nightly effects on sleep.

SLEEP IN CHILD AND ADOLESCENT DEVELOPMENT

In this section, we provide a brief overview of sleep disorders relevant to child and adolescent psychiatry. Four essential topics are considered: 1) basic sleep physiology, 2) normal maturational changes in sleep across these ages, 3) primary sleep disorders in children and adolescents, and 4) sleep disturbances associated with child and adolescent psychiatric disorders. Expanded discussions of these topics are included in Dahl (1992) and Dahl (in press).

Sleep Physiology

Despite decades of basic and clinical research, the function of sleep has remained an elusive mystery. Whatever its purpose, sleep appears to be particularly important for the developing brain. Infants and young individuals require more sleep than mature individuals across species. Both the amount of sleep and the patterning of sleep stages undergo significant changes across early maturational development. Before considering these maturational sleep changes, a brief review of sleep physiology is warranted.

From a physiological perspective, it is helpful to contrast REM and delta sleep. REM sleep (or paradoxical sleep) has features of deep and light sleep. During REM sleep, muscle tone drops dramatically because of inhibition stemming from the pons. This relative muscle paralysis may prevent body movements during dreaming. Regulation of temperature, blood pressure, heart rate, and respiration has greater variability during REM sleep. Sympathetic nerve activity, cerebral metabolic activity, and brain oxygen consumption are high during REM sleep, comparable to what they are during wakefulness. The timing of REM sleep is linked to the circadian cycle of body temperature regulation, with most REM sleep occurring between 4 and 6 A.M., when body temperature is lowest in the 24-hour day.

When individuals are awakened from REM sleep, return to alertness is rapid and is associated with descriptions of dreams. In contrast, when individuals are awakened from delta sleep, they are often in a disoriented or "foggy" state and require a few minutes of transition before complete alertness. The amount and intensity of delta sleep are related to the length of prior wakefulness and to brain maturity. Children have a great deal of delta sleep and are very resistant to being awakened. Tones set just below the danger level for human hearing (123 decibels) delivered through bilateral earphones failed to result in behavioral or EEG arousal in children in delta sleep (Busby and Pivik 1983).

The patterning of sleep stages in a 10-year-old child is illustrated in Figure 25–1. REM sleep is shown at the same level as stage 1, but with hatched boxes, indicating the paradoxical nature of sleep depth. This child briefly enters stage 1, descends quickly to stage 2, and then descends to stages 3 and 4 (delta sleep). The first delta period lasted approximately 60 minutes, was followed by a brief return to stage 2 and an arousal, and then returned to a second delta period for another hour. An adult typically enters an REM period approximately 90 minutes into sleep. Children often "skip" this first REM period (Goetz et al. 1985) and return to a second delta sleep, possibly because of their increased depth of sleep and increased sleep needs. REM periods occur cyclically, approximately every 60–90 minutes for the rest of the night, with increasing duration of REM sleep toward morning. Three important points are illustrated by this sleep pattern in children:

1. The majority of delta sleep occurs in the first 1–3 hours. Concordantly, delta sleep–related problems are most likely early in the night.
2. Most REM sleep occurs in the second half of the night; thus, REM sleep–related disorders are more frequent in the early morning hours.

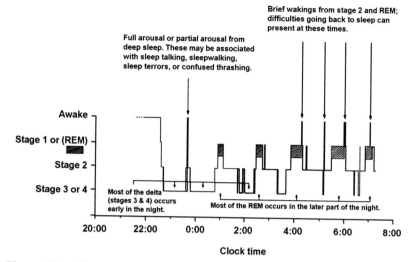

Figure 25–1. Sleep pattern in an early school-age child. *Hatched boxes* indicate rapid eye movement (REM) sleep. *Source.* Reprinted from Dahl RE: "Child and Adolescent Sleep Disorders," in *Child and Adolescent Neurology for Psychiatrists.* Edited by Kaufman DM, Solomon GE, Pfeffer CR. Baltimore, MD, Williams & Wilkins, 1992, p. 171. Used with permission.

3. Short periods of awakening normally occur five to seven times a night. Difficulties returning to sleep after these normal arousals can often appear to parents as though something is recurrently awakening the child.

Normal Development

The total amount of sleep, the patterning of stages, and the rate of cycling all change significantly through early development. Newborns usually sleep over 16 hours a day and begin each sleep cycle with REM sleep, called "active sleep" in newborns. REM–non-REM cycles occur every 50–60 minutes in infants. Short bouts of sleep equally distributed between night and daytime gradually give way to longer periods of daytime wakefulness. Although there is considerable individual variation, the typical 1-year-old child sleeps 11 hours at night with another 2.5 hours of sleep in two daytime naps. By age 3, an average nighttime sleep is 10.5 hours with one 60- to 90-minute nap during the day. Children in our culture typically cease to take naps by age 4 or 5 years.

There is a gradual decrease in total sleep time from age 5 (approximately 10.5 hours) to age 18 (adult level of approximately 8 hours a night). Changes in sleep architecture across childhood and adolescence include a gradual decrease in REM sleep and a significantly diminished amount and amplitude of delta sleep. Across all ages, sleep requirements and patterning are highly variable among individuals and are thought to be influenced by genetic, cultural, and situational factors.

Sleep efficiency also decreases during development. Young children spend almost all of their sleep time in stages 2, 3, 4, or REM sleep, with very little arousal, wakefulness, or light stage 1 sleep. With increasing age, children experience more frequent wakefulness and stage 1 sleep throughout sleep.

One of the most intriguing maturational changes in sleep is the increase in daytime sleepiness corresponding to puberty. Prepubertal children are remarkably alert throughout the daytime, but children at midadolescence show significant daytime sleepiness (Carskadon et al. 1987). Although some sleepiness may result from inadequate nighttime sleep, there is strong evidence that physiological changes in sleep regulation occurring with puberty account for increases in daytime sleepiness (Carskadon and Dement 1987).

Despite this apparent increase in the requirement for sleep during puberty, many adolescents in our society follow schedules resulting in markedly restricted sleep. Late-night social schedules and early morning school schedules frequently result in short sleep times in this age group. Although many high school students appear to get by on 6–7 hours of sleep during the school week, their sleep behaviors on weekends and vacations indicate that their true sleep needs are much greater. Many of these adolescents show significant sleepiness in the classroom. The effects of this relative sleep deprivation have implications for a wide range of issues, including school performance, mood changes, and substance use (Carskadon 1990). From a clinical perspective, many of these adolescents develop erratic sleep-wake schedules because of increasingly later bedtimes, erratic napping, and dramatically altered schedules on weekends. These issues are covered in the section on adolescent sleepiness.

Sleep Disorders in Children and Adolescents

Sleep disorders are highly relevant to the practice of child and adolescent psychiatry because sleep disorders can be mistaken for psychiatric disorders and psychiatric disorders are often associated with sleep problems and complaints. The connection between sleep and emotional and behavioral regulation appears to be complex and is probably bidirectional. Some of these interactions are straightforward: a sleep-deprived child becomes irritable and emotionally labile; an anxious child has difficulty falling asleep. Other interactions—such as sleep changes in children and adolescents with depressive disorders—may reflect more complex neurobiological connections between the regulation of sleep and the control of emotions and arousal.

Clinically, it is simplest to consider sleep disorders according to categories of the presenting complaints: 1) difficulty in falling (and staying) asleep, 2) excessive daytime sleepiness, 3) disorders of sleep-wake scheduling, and 4) unusual events during sleep.

Difficulties in Falling and Staying Asleep

Bedtime and middle-of-the-night difficulties surrounding sleep are frequent sources of considerable stress to both parents and children and may contribute to inadequate sleep for several family members. Among children ages 1–5 years, 20%–30% have sleeplessness that disturbs their parents (Beltramini and Hertzig 1983; Lozoff et al. 1985). Although medical problems (e.g., pain from an ear infection, cow-milk allergy, colic, or the itching of atopic dermatitis) can contribute significantly to this problem in some children, the majority of cases result from behavioral and learned factors. The single most critical factor in toddler sleep problems concerns the associations the child makes with falling asleep. Children who are able to sleep alone the entire night in their own beds ("good sleepers") have learned self-comforting behaviors, such as touching a favorite blanket, thumb sucking, body rocking, and so forth. These behaviors provide comfort at bedtime and are repeated after normal arousals between sleep cycles. Many "bad sleepers" simply have comforting behaviors that require parental involvement, such as being rocked, and subsequently require the same condition to return to sleep after night arousals. Treatment has been well reviewed elsewhere (Ferber 1987).

In school-age children and adolescents, anxieties and worries can contribute to difficulties in falling asleep in the same way that they do in adults. Lying down to go to sleep can be a time to reflect on sources of anxiety and conflicts of the day. In some children, anxiety and tension associated with bedtime can lead to severe, conditioned insomnia. There are many variations of this problem. Some children will lie quietly in bed, and parents are relatively unaware of the insomnia. Other children will be disruptive, repeatedly get out of bed, or require long intervals of intermittent parental involvement at bedtime.

One central theme in childhood insomnia is the issue of subjective feelings of safety. The process of going to sleep is essentially the process of letting go of vigilance—relinquishing the ability to respond to threats in the environment. The evolutionary biology of sleep is linked to restricting sleep to safe places. There is great survival value in preventing sleep in any situation where vigilance may be required. For humans—children in particular—a subjective sense of threat can severely disrupt sleep. Two examples are children with separation anxiety (who can be highly threatened by separating from a parent at bedtime) and abused children (who can have very threatening associations with bed or nighttime). In addition, regulation of vigilance and anxiety may be biologically controlled, with some individuals showing strong genetic or temperamental tendencies toward high vigilance and, hence, vulnerability to insomnia. It is essential to address sources of perceived threats for effective treatment of insomnia in children. Reasonable approaches include identifying sources of anxiety and worry, encouraging the child to express worries in appropriate ways during waking hours, and teaching age-appropriate relaxation techniques. Helping the child to learn to focus on positive images (which bring on relaxation) at bedtime can be essential. Limits that are consistently set, a regular sleep-wake schedule, and positive associations with bedtime (including a pleasant prebedtime ritual) can also be important factors.

Sleepiness

The child or adolescent with excessive sleepiness could have a problem in one of three areas: 1) inadequate amounts of sleep, 2) disturbed sleep, and 3) disorders associated with an increased need for sleep.

Inadequate amounts of sleep. The most common cause of mild to moderate sleepiness in adolescents is insufficient time in bed. A combination of late-night schedules and early morning school requirements effectively compresses the number of hours available for sleep. Part-time jobs, sports activities, hobbies, and active social lives can exacerbate this problem. The catch-up sleep of naps, weekends, and holidays further contributes to the problem by leading to erratic circadian schedules.

In taking a sleep history, it is important to obtain specific information concerning schedules. Retrospective estimates of "usual" bedtime are unlikely to be good sources of accurate information. A prospective, detailed, 2-week sleep diary verified by parents provides the most reliable information and often clarifies the inadequacy of the total number of sleep hours. Details about bedtime (with lights out and the child or adolescent attempting to fall asleep), estimates of sleep latency, nighttime arousals, rising time, difficulty getting up, and the frequency, timing, and duration of daytime naps should be assessed. It is essential to get details about sleep-wake schedules on weekends as well as during the school week.

When insufficient sleep is identified, the role of the clinician is often to help the family recognize the consequences of inadequate sleep. Sleep deprivation frequently contributes to falling asleep in school, oversleeping in the morning, fatigue, and irritability. When school or social functioning are impaired, a strict behavioral contract agreed on by the entire family can be essential. The contract should specify hours in bed with only small deviations on weekends and should target behaviors contributing to bad sleep habits, such as specific late-night activities, erratic napping, and oversleeping on school days. Choice of rewards and negative consequences, as well as accurate assessment of compliance, are essential components of the contract.

Disturbed nocturnal sleep.   A variety of factors can contribute to nocturnal disturbances in sleep. Two important sources include substance use and sleep apnea.

Use of substances.   Sources of disrupted sleep can be blatant or extremely subtle. Use of drugs or alcohol is an important consideration in youngsters with disturbed sleep. In addition to obvious effects of late-night stimulants such as cocaine, there are also more complex drug-sleep interactions. Alcohol, for example, can facilitate the onset of sleep but leads to sleep fragmentation and midnocturnal awakenings. Withdrawal from stimulants, alcohol, and marijuana can produce transient but severe sleep disruptions. Adolescents also commonly use caffeine in the form of caffeinated sodas, coffee, and tea. Elimination of caffeine can be an important step in treating difficulty in falling asleep. Medications such as β-adrenergic agonists for asthma or stimulants for attention-deficit disorder can also result in significant sleep disruptions.

Obstructive sleep apnea syndrome.   One source of disturbances leading to sleepiness is sleep-disordered breathing. During sleep, particularly in REM sleep, there is diminished muscle tone, including muscles maintaining the airway and assisting in respiration. In susceptible individuals, these physiological changes can lead to obstructive sleep apnea syndrome. Adults with obstructive sleep apnea syndrome are typically obese, hypersomnolent, lethargic individuals. Children with this disorder often are thin, have large tonsils or adenoids, and may appear more irritable than hypersomnic. Severe, prolonged apneic episodes during sleep can result in nocturnal hypoxemia and bradycardia and can lead to pulmonary hypertension with cor pulmonale.

Many children, however, present with subtle versions of obstructive sleep apnea syndrome. Actual apneic episodes may last less than 10 seconds, followed by a rapid, brief arousal, resumption of breathing, and quick return to sleep. When there is incomplete obstruction, the increased work of breathing through a very small airway can disturb sleep (Guilleminault et al. 1982). Although the actual number of minutes of wakefulness may be few, the chronic, brief disruptions in sleep can lead to significant daytime symptoms. The child is usually unaware of waking up. The parent often describes restless sleep but usually does not realize that the child is awakening repeatedly.

Symptoms include loud chronic snoring or noisy breathing, physically restless sleep, difficulties arousing the child in the morning, a history of problems with tonsils, adenoids, or ear infections, and signs of inadequate nighttime sleep. Signs of inadequate sleep can include irritability, difficulty concentrating, decreased school performance, and oppositional behavior. Many of these children paradoxically appear hyperactive as a result of inadequate nighttime sleep (Guilleminault and Winkle 1981). The diagnosis of obstructive sleep apnea syndrome can often be made clinically. Many pediatric otolaryngologists are experienced in assessing children with signs of snoring and disturbed sleep for evidence of adenoidal hypertrophy. Even moderate-size adenoids and tonsils that cause minimal problems in the awake examination may produce obstructive symptoms during sleep. In questionable cases, or when there are reasons to avoid tonsillectomy and adenoidectomy, polysomnographic studies can aid in the diagnosis. Clinical situations associated with high risk for sleep apnea include maxillofacial abnormalities, micrognathia, cleft palates (particularly with pharyngeal flap repairs), and Down's syndrome.

Disorders associated with increased need for sleep. Specific disorders associated with increased need for sleep include narcolepsy, idiopathic hypersomnolence, and Kleine-Levin syndrome. Each will be considered separately.

Narcolepsy. Narcolepsy is a chronic disorder characterized by excessive daytime sleepiness and intrusions of REM physiology on wakefulness, such as loss of muscle tone (cataplexy and sleep paralysis) and dream imagery (hypnagogic and hypnopompic hallucinations). The classic tetrad of symptoms include 1) sleep attacks, 2) cataplexy (the sudden loss of muscle tone without change of consciousness), 3) sleep paralysis (inability to move on awakening), and 4) hypnagogic hallucinations (dreamlike imagery before falling asleep). Not all symptoms are present in most cases of narcolepsy. Particularly in younger patients, signs of sleepiness may be the only initial symptom. Cataplexy is typically provoked by laughter, anger, or sudden emotional changes and may be as subtle as a slight weakness in the legs or as dramatic as a patient falling to the floor limp and unable to move. If cataplectic attacks last long enough, full sleep can occur.

Narcolepsy as it affects adults is discussed elsewhere (see Chapter 28). Issues relevant to narcolepsy in children and adolescents are described here. First, childhood narcolepsy is not nearly as rare as is generally believed. Although narcolepsy is rarely *diagnosed* in childhood, over 50% of adult narcoleptic patients report that their symptoms began during the school-age years (Navelet et al. 1976); only 4% of adult narcoleptic patients were diagnosed in childhood. Second, the clinical presentation of narcolepsy is highly variable in young patients. In our pediatric sleep center, only 1 of 15 patients with documented cases of narcolepsy had the full tetrad of symptoms. In nearly half the cases, excessive sleepiness was the only symptom for years. Further, cataplexy was often subtle and easy to miss on clinical history. A little weakness in the legs when a child laughs can easily escape notice. Similarly, it can be difficult to distinguish mild hypnagogic hallucinations from children's vivid imaginations at bedtime. Third, narcolepsy in young patients can easily be mistaken for psychiatric disorders (Allsopp and Zaiwalla 1992; Dahl et al., in press; Navelet et al. 1976).

Clinically, then, detection of early onset narcolepsy can be very difficult. Therefore, narcolepsy should be part of any differential diagnosis of unexplained daytime sleepiness or any history of cataplexy-like episodes. Diagnosis of narcolepsy requires evaluation in a sleep laboratory. Narcoleptic patients show REM periods near the onset of sleep, fragmented nighttime sleep, excessive daytime sleepiness in nap studies, and sleep-onset REM periods in naps. In prepubertal children, this diagnosis can be difficult to establish. Following the case clinically and repeating sleep studies may be necessary to reach a final diagnosis (Kotogol et al. 1990).

Idiopathic hypersomnolence. Some patients have significantly increased sleep needs without evidence of REM abnormalities seen in narcolepsy. This condition has been called idiopathic hypersomnolence. These individuals show objective sleepiness in nap studies despite adequate nighttime sleep. These disorders are treated with stimulant medication when the diagnosis is definitively established and daytime functioning is impaired.

Kleine-Levin syndrome. Symptoms of excessive somnolence, hypersexuality, and compulsive overeating were first described in adolescent boys by Kleine (1925) and Levin (1929). Mental disturbances (irritability, confusion, and occasional auditory or visual hallucinations) have also been reported in these cases. This syndrome is three times more likely to occur in males, may have a gradual or abrupt onset, and follows a flulike illness or injury with loss of consciousness in about half the cases. Frequently, symptoms are episodic with cycles lasting from 1–30 days. The syndrome often disappears spontaneously during late adolescence or early adulthood.

Laboratory tests, imaging studies, EEGs, and endocrine measures are not helpful in making the diagnosis of Kleine-Levin syndrome. Other organic causes of similar symptoms must be excluded, such as a hypothalamic tumor, localized central nervous system (CNS) infection, or vascular accident. Neurological signs, increased CNS pressure, abnormalities in temperature or water regulation, or other endocrine abnormalities indicate an organically based abnormality. A family history of bipolar illness or other signs suggesting bipolar illness should also be considered in the differential diagnosis. Although stimulant medication or use of lithium carbonate has been reported to be helpful in individual cases, there is no clear consensus on treatment.

Circadian and Scheduling Disorders

Our understanding of normal circadian physiology has advanced considerably over the past two decades and has contributed to the clinical management of a variety of sleep and schedule disorders (see Chapter 29). Among adolescents, the most common circadian problem is delayed sleep phase syndrome. The process often begins on weekends, holidays, or summer vacations. Many adolescents follow a 3:00 A.M. to noon sleep schedule during the summer and then abruptly try to shift to school schedules in the fall. On the night before the first day of school, the adolescent may try to go to bed early but is unable to fall asleep. For a few days, he or she manages to get up for school by overriding the system (despite inadequate sleep), but then takes a long nap after school. On the weekend, the late schedule is again followed, and the adolescent's biological clock is never reset.

This schedule can set up a chronic pattern of intermittent sleep deprivation, difficulties getting up for school, and disturbances of mood and concentration. These individuals have no trouble falling asleep with late bedtimes and no problems when following their usual late schedules, but they do not successfully adjust to the early school schedules. Although many adolescents follow this type of sleep pattern to some degree, certain individuals appear to develop severe problems and are unable to get up for school on time despite high motivation.

Treatment of delayed sleep phase syndrome in adolescents consists of two parts. The first is to align the sleep system *gradually* to the desired schedule. The second is to maintain that alignment. Treatment requires gradual, small, *consistent* advances in bedtime and wake-up time (15–30 minutes a day). It is often best to begin from the time the adolescent is usually able to go to sleep without difficulty. Naps must be avoided, and the schedule must be consistent across weekends and holidays.

In severe cases, some adolescents on very late schedules respond better to going around the clock with successive *delays* of bedtime, a process described as phase-delay "chronotherapy" (Czeisler et al. 1981). Because the biological clock tends to run on a 25-hour cycle, human physiology accommodates phase delays more easily than advances. Thus, schedule changes can proceed with longer delays (2–3 hours) per day. During chronotherapy, the adolescent must take no naps. Some activity and, if possible, exposure to bright light (e.g., by walking outside) should coincide with waking.

Although many adolescents do well with chronotherapy, the first weekend or vacation of returning to old habits can undo a lot of hard work. Particularly in the first 2–3 weeks after chronotherapy, rigid requirements should be set about wake-up time *7 days a week*. Later, if the adolescent wants to stay up late on an occasional weekend night, he or she may be able to do so but should *not* be permitted to sleep more than 1–2 hours later than his or her usual wake-up time for school. Strict behavioral contracts worked out with the parents, with specific rewards for success and serious consequences for failures, are essential in this type of intervention. Other treatments, including bright-light therapy, are addressed in Chapter 29.

Some adolescents may have the same sleep patterns but are not motivated to correct the problem, and they are not particularly troubled by recurrently being late for or missing school. These adolescents are *choosing* a late-night schedule. Unless the clinician is able to alter the larger realm of priorities and motivators, these adolescents are unlikely to respond to treatments for the sleep schedule problem.

Unusual Events During Sleep (Parasomnias)

Parasomnia is the term given to one of a group of unusual behaviors emerging from sleep. These behaviors include sleepwalking, sleep terrors, confused partial arousals, enuresis, and nightmares. Head banging and nocturnal seizures are also addressed in this section as other unusual sleep-related events in children.

Partial arousals.   Sleepwalking, sleep talking, sleep terrors, and confusional arousals are all variations of partial arousals from deep sleep. As discussed earlier, most children have a period of very deep slow-wave sleep during the first third of the night. At the end of this period, the transition to lighter sleep is often accompanied by unusual transition behaviors. If observed closely (such as in a sleep laboratory), many children will mumble, grimace, or demonstrate some awkward movements. These episodes can also consist of talking, calm or agitated sleepwalking, confused partial arousals, and at times, near paniclike behavior. The episodes can last from seconds to 30 minutes, with most events lasting 2–10 minutes.

Because many parents think the child is having a nightmare or dream, they often attempt to awaken and reassure the child. This attempt can be disturbing for the parent because the child often stares blankly, does not recognize parents, can appear incoherent, and may even thrash wildly, let out bloodcurdling screams, and bolt away. The event usually terminates spontaneously with the child returning to deep sleep. Attempts at waking the child are usually unsuccessful. He or she may have a vague image of what happened, but it is not as detailed as the imagery of dreaming or nightmares.

The cause of these events is unknown. It appears that an abnormal transition occurs: some neural components become activated, whereas other components remain dormant. The intensity of delta sleep may be integral to the occurrence of these events; they are most frequent in the age groups with the highest amount of delta sleep (ages 3–8 years). In addition, conditions that lead to increased delta sleep, such as sleep loss or being overly tired, are associated with increased partial arousals. As the pressure for delta sleep increases, the transition out of delta sleep appears to be more difficult. The history of children with frequent night terrors or partial arousals often indicates that these events occur in conjunction with chaotic sleep schedules, on the nights of recovery sleep after sleep loss, in conjunction with a change in schedule (such as beginning to wake earlier in the morning for school or day care), or after periods of stress.

The role played by psychological characteristics has also been extensively discussed. Unexpressed anxieties and conflicts may contribute to the occurrence of partial arousals (Klackenberg 1982). In our pediatric sleep center, children with frequent night terrors tend to be anxious and tense. These children are often well behaved, but are emotionally restricted. Although there appears to be some convergence of clinical impressions, at this time there is little empirical evidence to support these observations.

Partial arousals are quite common in younger children. Estimates vary, but approximately 5% of the children ages 3–12 years may sleepwalk regularly, and as many as 20% have had at least one episode of sleepwalking. Sleep terrors are less frequent, with estimates ranging from 1% to 6% in this age group. As delta sleep decreases in adolescence, so too does the frequency of these delta sleep–related events.

There are a number of considerations in evaluation and treatment of these problems. The first is to identify that the episode is a partial arousal. Differentiating sleep terrors from nightmares is important. Unlike nightmares, sleep terrors occur during the first third of the night, increase in frequency after sleep loss (or from being overly tired), and are associated with confusion and partial arousal, lack of memory of the event, and quick return to sleep. Once the episodes are identified as sleep terrors, one of the most important roles of the clinician is to provide meaningful explanations and reassurance. The next step should be to address the adequacy of the child's sleep schedule. Increasing the amount of sleep, introducing more consistency into the schedule, and removing causes of sleep disturbances (such as sleep-disordered breathing) can result in a dramatic decrease in the frequency of events. Finally, focusing on safe, relaxing thoughts at bedtime can be very helpful because tension or worry at bedtime makes these episodes more likely.

Medications such as diazepam or imipramine at bedtime significantly decrease delta sleep and the frequency of sleep terrors. Often when the medication is stopped, however, there is rebound of delta sleep and partial arousals. Nonetheless, medications can be an important temporary adjunct to treatment, particularly when partial arousals are extremely frequent, occur repeatedly within a night, or are severely disruptive to the family. In these situations, there is often such tension and fear surrounding bedtime that it is important to "break the cycle" of sleep deprivation, disturbed sleep, increased pressure for delta sleep, and night terrors. Short-term use of medication (such as 25–75 mg of imipramine at bedtime) can help create an opportunity for more lasting intervention.

Physical safety must also be considered. Although such events are rare, children can fall down stairs, walk through windows, or fall from upper bunks during partial arousals. Altering the sleep environment to minimize the risk of serious injuries is an essential aspect of dealing with these problems.

Nightmares.   Nightmares, in contrast to sleep terrors, are REM-sleep events—basically, dreams with sufficient anxiety to result in complete awakening. Many children have an occasional frightening dream. Frequent and recurrent nightmares, however, are not common. One of the first steps in assessing nightmares is distinguishing them from sleep terrors. Because nightmares usually occur during REM sleep, they are more likely in the second half of the night. Further, children awake fully from the nightmare, are usually alert, and can remember specific scenes or frightening images. In contrast to children with sleep terrors, children with nightmares have difficulty going back to sleep, often want to remain with parents, and remember nightmares in the morning. These distinctions, however, can be difficult in a younger child with limited verbal abilities.

Frightening daytime television programs, movies, videotapes, and threatening events can contribute to nightmares. In addition, traumatic events can lead to recurrent nightmares (Terr 1983). Commonsense approaches that address the sources of fears and anxieties are often sufficient. There is a wide range of clinical opinion, particularly in the psychoanalytic literature, on issues relating to dream content and nightmares.

Enuresis.   Nocturnal enuresis is a common sleep-related problem with a variety of causes. There is increasing understanding of a small functional bladder capacity, variance in the strength of the urethral sphincter, and variance in the neurological connections sensing and responding to bladder contractions and sphincter tone. There is also a subset of children for whom very deep sleep is an important component to nocturnal enuresis. In some cases, enuresis often occurs in the first third of the night. It is hard to imagine that bladder capacity or inadequate amounts of a hormone to concentrate urine are important factors in children who wet the bed 1–2 hours after going to sleep.

Many children with enuresis will respond to any of the traditional treatments: imipramine, nocturnal alarm, reinforcement techniques, or combinations of these. Other children, however, may have enuresis as a variant of a partial arousal from very deep sleep. The same factors contributing to partial arousals (sleep loss, obstructive sleep apnea, being overtired) are also associated with enuresis in these cases and should be treated with the same procedures, such as increasing total sleep, regularizing bedtime schedules, or treating sleep apnea.

Head banging, rocking, and variants.   Head banging (jactatio capitis nocturna) is the stereotypical, rhythmic movement of the head and upper body during sleep, drowsiness, or rest and has been named rhythmic movement disorder in the *International Classification of Sleep Disorders Diagnostic and Coding Manual* (American Sleep Disorders Association 1990). Estimates indicate that 3%–15% of normal healthy children evidence some head banging in the first year of life. The behavior usually disappears by age 4 but can persist through adolescence and into adulthood.

Most head banging occurs during the drowsiness before onset of sleep and may continue into stage 2 sleep. Children may also head bang to go back to sleep after waking up between sleep cycles. Often, head banging appears to be a self-comforting behavior even during awake rest periods during the day. Organic and psychopathological etiologies have been suspected on the basis of association with mental retardation, but head banging also occurs in normal children. Rhythmic movements may be learned behavior, reinforced by pleasurable sensations arising from the activity itself. Pleasurable sensations mediated by vestibular pathways can be a form of self-stimulation.

Behavior modification has been successful in many younger children. Psychiatric and neurological evaluations may be indicated when head banging persists beyond ages 3–6 years. Benzodiazepines and tricyclic antidepressant medications have also been reported to be helpful in some cases.

Sleep and seizures.   Normal behaviors associated with transitions out of stage 4 sleep and events during partial arousals can be quite bizarre in nature. Although many of these are easily typified as partial arousals, one complicating difficulty is that seizures occur predominantly during sleep or on arousal from sleep in up to 50%–80% of epileptic patients (Shouse 1989). The EEG synchronization during non-REM sleep appears to be conducive to the spread of abnormal electrical discharges. In addition, the transition into and out of sleep can activate seizures, one reason to perform diagnostic EEGs in the sleep-deprived state.

The relationship between sleep and seizures is not well understood. From a clinical perspective, it is important to note that 1) in rare cases, seizures can occur during sleep when a seizure disorder was not otherwise suspected, and 2) a standard sleep study is not the equivalent of a clinical EEG evaluation. The limited number of EEG electrodes and the slow paper speed (to permit all-night recording) do not permit the specific EEG information obtained in a full 10/20 EEG for a neurological evaluation. In complicated cases, it may be necessary to obtain input from a neurologist and sleep clinician working together to reach a diagnosis of unusual events occurring in sleep.

Sleep Changes Associated With Psychiatric Disorders

Disturbed sleep is a common symptom in many psychiatric disorders. In studies of adult psychiatric patients, these complaints are frequently accompanied by objective alterations in sleep and are potentially valuable as psychobiological markers, particularly of adult affective disorders (see Chapter 26). Although subjective sleep disturbances are prominent in child and adolescent psychiatric disorders, psychobiological studies have not yielded consistent findings of objective changes in sleep. There are numerous methodological and theoretical considerations regarding these discrepancies that are beyond the scope of this chapter. A brief overview of sleep studies addressing a few child psychiatric disorders follows.

Child and Adolescent Depression

Among adults with major depressive disorder, controlled sleep studies find altered EEG sleep, including short REM sleep latency, increased phasic activity, decreased delta sleep, and decreased sleep efficiency. Among eight well-controlled studies in children and adolescents, only three found reduced REM sleep latency and a few found evidence of decreased sleep efficiency. Most studies failed to find any evidence of increased phasic activity during REM sleep, and none of the controlled studies reported diminished delta sleep associated with depression (Dahl et al. 1990).

Our research group has found adult-pattern sleep changes in only a small subgroup of children with major depressive disorder (Dahl et al. 1991). One possibility is that normal maturational influences on sleep (intense delta sleep and high sleep efficiency) may mask sleep disturbances associated with depression. Researchers have also hypothesized that age and depression may interact in producing the sleep changes associated with depression. An interaction among genetic factors, age, and depression has also been postulated (Giles et al. 1992).

In contrast to the paucity of objective evidence of sleep disturbances, subjective complaints are common in children and adolescents with major depressive disorder. These symptoms include difficulty falling asleep, midnocturnal awakenings, early morning awakening, and restless sleep. In addition, many children and adolescents report hypersomnia during depression. In a recent review of the clinical picture of child and adolescent major depressive disorder (which included 187 subjects), 74% presented with complaints of disturbed sleep, whereas

25% reported hypersomnia (Ryan et al. 1987). Severe insomnia was reported in 38%, with many complaining they almost never sleep and always feel exhausted during the day. Again, it must be emphasized that in EEG sleep studies, including studies of subjects drawn from this sample, there were no objective sleep disturbances in the depressed children and adolescents complaining of insomnia.

When a child or an adolescent presents with significant sleep complaints, the possibility of depression should be considered and symptoms should be assessed in the context of other signs and symptoms of major depression. Likewise, a primary sleep disorder should be considered. There can be considerable overlap between sleep schedule disturbances and major depression. Depressed adolescents can develop difficulties in falling asleep, take naps, and develop late-night and erratic schedules. It may become necessary to address both sleep schedule issues and symptoms of depression.

Attention-Deficit Disorder

Sleep complaints in children with attention-deficit disorder (ADD) are frequent. Parents of children with ADD report more difficulties associated with their children falling asleep, waking in the night, waking early, and having restless sleep than parents of control children (Kaplan et al. 1987; Ross and Ross 1982). Despite subjective sleep disturbances, objective sleep studies have not revealed significant sleep disruption in children with ADD (Busby et al. 1981; Greenhill et al. 1983).

As with affective disorders, discrepancies between subjective and objective sleep complaints are a source of speculation and disagreement. It may be that only a small subgroup of children with ADD have sleep disturbances of clinical significance. We have seen children with ADD who show increased behavioral symptoms after sleep loss. As noted, inadequate sleep can cause behavioral symptoms in children that overlap with ADD (e.g., inattention, irritability, distractibility, and impulsivity). We recently reported the case of a 10-year-old girl with a clear diagnosis of ADD and long-standing sleep difficulties (delayed sleep phase insomnia) whose ADD and learning-disability symptoms improved significantly—as determined by blind raters in a controlled setting—after her sleep problem was treated (Dahl et al. 1991b).

Careful assessment and treatment of sleep problems in children with ADD are recommended. When sleep disturbances are identified, treatment should address both behavioral and physiological components. One clinical difficulty concerns defining adequate sleep. Because of the wide range of individual sleep needs, definitions of sleep requirements have traditionally been reported as the amount of sleep necessary for "optimal daytime functioning." In children with ADD, attempts at defining optimal daytime functioning can be difficult. When inadequate sleep or sleep disturbances are suspected, one prudent approach is to increase or improve sleep and evaluate for signs of improved daytime functioning.

Another important consideration in the relationship of sleep and ADD is the effects on sleep of stimulants used to treat the disorder. Late doses of stimulants or long-acting preparations can prolong sleep latency. Paradoxically, we also have seen *improvement* in sleep when a child is placed on stimulants and even further improvement when the child is given doses later in the day and placed on long-acting preparations. This improvement may result from better-organized behavior around bedtime and compliance with going to bed.

Control of arousal and attention, regulation of sleep, and the psychobiology of ADD are areas with probable, but little understood, overlap. More well-controlled studies are needed that address the relationship between ADD symptomatology and sleep regulation in children.

Tourette's Syndrome

Sleep disturbances are commonly reported in patients with Tourette's syndrome and tic disorders and occur more frequently in family members of patients with Tourette's syndrome. Patients with Tourette's syndrome have motor and vocal tics throughout all sleep stages (Burd and Kerbeshian 1988; Glaze et al. 1983) as well as increased rates of partial arousals out of deep sleep. Partial arousals can manifest as sleep terrors, sleepwalking, enuresis, or Tourette-like behaviors such as coprolalia or birdcalls. Both tics and partial arousals decrease with treatment of Tourette's syndrome. We recently treated a boy with Tourette's syndrome who had a significant decrease in partial arousals and tics during sleep after a change in his medication to a dose near bedtime. Parents of this boy reported not only an improvement in sleep-related symptoms, but also a decrease in daytime irritability and tiredness, side effects of chronic sleep disturbances.

GENETIC INFLUENCE ON SLEEP

Personal estimates of sleep duration and quality, objective sleep measures of normal sleep, and transmission of sleep disorders are substantially influenced by genetic factors. EEG sleep measures have also shed light on familial processes in some psychiatric disorders. Each of these areas will be considered briefly.

Genetics of Normal Sleep

Individual personal estimates of sleep duration are more correlated between monozygotic than between dizygotic twins and support a substantial heritable component in studies with adolescents (Gedda and

Brenci 1979) and adults ranging in age from 17 to 88 years (Gedda and Brenci 1979; Heath et al. 1990; Partinen et al. 1983). Younger individuals (ages 6–8 years) may also show a genetic influence, but the variability between monozygotic and dizygotic twins was so limited that genetic tests were not possible (Gedda and Brenci 1979). Reports of sleep quality have also shown significant genetic influence (Heath et al. 1990; Partinen et al. 1983).

When normal EEG sleep is assessed, genetic effects are also found in several components of non-REM sleep, including sleep duration, sleep structure, stages 2 and 4 sleep, and slow-wave sleep for children, older adolescents, and young adults (Linkowski et al. 1989; Webb and Campbell 1983; Zung and Wilson 1967). Time to onset of REM sleep, duration of REM sleep, and phasic activity during REM sleep have shown a genetic influence in some studies (Gould et al. 1978; Hori 1986; Webb and Campbell 1983), whereas other studies have argued that concordance in REM measures may be influenced as much by cohabitation (shared environment) as by shared genes (Linkowski et al. 1989, 1991). The cohabitation position has not been substantiated in animal studies (Valatx 1984) and is inconsistent with findings regarding human leukocyte antigen (HLA) typing in subjects with normal sleep patterns. For example, subjects who possessed the HLA-DR2 antigen reliably had a substantially shorter time to onset of the first REM period than subjects who were HLA-DR2 negative (Schulz et al. 1986), suggesting genetic control over the onset of REM sleep. In summary, both subjective and objective measures of normal sleep have a substantial heritable component.

Genetics of Sleep Disorders

Childhood-Onset Disorders
Sleep disorders with clear evidence of genetic involvement can be grouped using categories described in a previous section, "Sleep in Child and Adolescent Development." Disorders associated with increased need for sleep, including narcolepsy and idiopathic hypersomnolence, have been found to have a genetic component. Substantial heritability has also been determined in disorders of partial arousal, including sleepwalking, sleep terrors, and sleep enuresis.

Genetic mechanisms have been localized only in narcolepsy. The short arm of chromosome 6 (see Parkes and Lock 1989 for a review) has been identified in this disorder. HLA typing has demonstrated that the DR2 antigen is positive in almost 100% of narcoleptic patients with or without cataplexy, regardless of race. This finding in narcoleptic patients spurred the investigation of normal sleep described above (Schulz et al. 1986). REM mechanisms in subjects with normal sleep patterns did not appear to be pathological, yet even in unaffected individuals, the presence of HLA-DR2 was associated with a substantial decrease in time to the first REM period.

Idiopathic hypersomnia shares with narcolepsy the symptom of excessive daytime sleepiness, but patients do not manifest other signs or symptoms of narcolepsy. Almost 40% of the patients have a positive family history of hypersomnia (Roth 1980). Of interest, 60% of the patients *without* a positive history of hypersomnia in first-degree relatives have been found to be positive for the HLA-DR2 antigen (Honda et al. 1986). This condition has been described as monosymptomatic narcolepsy (Parkes and Lock 1989).

Sleepwalking and sleep terrors assort together in families even when the proband is identified as having only one disorder (Kales et al. 1980). When one parent is affected with sleepwalking, 45% of the offspring are also affected; this rate increases to 60% when both parents are affected. Of interest, unaffected family members tend to be deep sleepers, with higher-than-normal thresholds for arousal from sleep. Disorders of partial arousal are most likely expressions of a common genetic predisposition, although environmental factors, such as sleep deprivation and fever, influence their manifestation.

In some cases, sleep enuresis is also a disorder of partial arousal and has shown evidence of transmission by a single dominant gene (Bakwin 1970). If one parent has a history of sleep enuresis, the probability of enuresis in offspring is 44%. When both parents are affected, the risk for offspring is 77%.

Adult-Onset Disorders
Adult-onset sleep disorders with familial associations include familial sleep paralysis, obstructive sleep apnea, primary snoring, and restless leg syndrome.

Sleep paralysis, as described earlier, is a major symptom of narcolepsy but can exist alone. Sleep paralysis occurs on a single occasion in 40%–50% of the general population; more frequent occurrences indicate a familial disorder. Symptoms include brief paralysis of voluntary muscles in the trunk and limbs at either initiation or termination of sleep, extraocular muscle sparing, and often intense fear. The individual is fully cognizant of the inability to move. Mechanisms for muscle inhibition in REM sleep have been proposed also to induce sleep paralysis. The genetic variant of sleep paralysis is chronic, appears to be X chromosome–linked, and occurs more frequently in females.

Obstructive sleep apnea and primary snoring have shown familial aggregation. Apnea may be due to heritable neuromuscular, anatomical, or physiological defects (Redline et al. 1992). Snoring is heritable to the extent that weight and anatomy are heritable.

Restless leg syndrome, with or without myoclonus, is associated with an irresistible urge to move the legs and with unpleasant deep sensations in the legs. Family studies have indicated that the disorder is familial in 33% of cases and may be autosomal dominant in transmission (Ambrosetto et al. 1965).

Genetics of Sleep and Psychiatric Disorders

The genetic influence on sleep regulation and the sleep dysregulation observed in several major mental disorders imply that sleep may be a productive tool for further elucidating the genetics of these mental disorders. The genetic influence on several major mental disorders—including depression, schizophrenia, anxiety disorders, obsessive-compulsive disorder, and alcoholism—has been well described.

The proposition that EEG sleep measures may elucidate the genetic influence on psychiatric disorders is based on studies of sleep and the pathophysiology of major mental disorders (see Benca et al. 1992 for a meta-analysis and review). Patients with alcoholism (Adamson and Burdick 1973), schizophrenia (Ganguli et al. 1987; Zarcone et al. 1987), anxiety disorders (Insel et al. 1982; Reynolds et al. 1983), borderline personality disorder (Reynolds et al. 1985), eating disorders (Waller et al. 1989), and mood disorders (Reynolds and Kupfer 1987) have specific sleep disturbances. The relationship between sleep and mental disorders has been most extensively researched for schizophrenia and mood disorders.

EEG sleep abnormalities identified in patients with schizophrenia include fragmentation of sleep, decreased time asleep, abnormal REM sleep, and inability to mount an appropriate physiological response to REM sleep deprivation. Several EEG sleep abnormalities may arise out of circadian disorganization that occurs when patients are agitated or psychotic. Preliminary data suggest that schizophrenic patients with abnormal REM sleep have a higher prevalence of affective disorders among their first-degree relatives than schizophrenic patients without such abnormalities (M. Keshavan, personal communication, October 1989).

Ongoing work in our group has focused on EEG sleep abnormalities as a means of identifying familial and genetic transmission of unipolar depression. Our study paradigm involves high-risk families. In addition to a series of clinical criteria, index patients were selected based on the presence of abnormal sleep physiology. Two comparison groups were identified. One group included patients who had unipolar depression but who did *not* have abnormal sleep. The second group included healthy control families without any psychiatric disorder. These comparison groups provide information on transmission of abnormal sleep physiology as well as on cosegregation of abnormal sleep physiology and depression. Two parents and at least two siblings have been studied for each patient and healthy control subject.

Our findings to date indicate that sleep dysregulation has a familial association (Giles et al. 1988, 1989a), as well as a predictable relationship to lifetime prevalence of depression (Giles et al. 1988), and may increase the risk for new onset of depression (Giles et al. 1990). We also have evidence that rates of abnormal sleep are constant from generation to generation among families of depressed patients with abnormal sleep and that rates of depression tend to be slightly higher in siblings compared with parents. In contrast, the rates of depression in siblings of patients with *normal* sleep are substantially higher than the rates in their parents, yet remain lower than the rates in siblings of depressed patients from families with abnormal sleep (Giles et al. 1989b). Taken together, our findings suggest that EEG sleep abnormalities are familial, are associated with risk for depression, occur before the onset of depression, and may provide insight into the observed birth-cohort effect in depression, in which more recently born generations are at greater risk for depression.

This series of findings along with those of others (e.g., Mendlewicz et al. 1989) suggest that physiological measures of sleep have the potential to elucidate the genetic basis of unipolar depression in some cases. Not only are sleep abnormalities and depression transmitted together in families of depressed patients with abnormal sleep, but unaffected relatives with sleep abnormalities appear to be at increased risk for new onset of depression. Evidence that the onset of REM sleep is genetically controlled (as has been found in narcolepsy) suggests that HLA typing might be productive in patients with major depression. Research to examine this hypothesis did not find such an association, however (Staner et al. 1991). Nonetheless, EEG sleep measures may be useful in reducing the heterogeneity in unipolar depression and may increase the likelihood of determining the subtype that is genetically mediated.

SUMMARY

In this chapter, we summarized studies of sleep during the normal course of pregnancy and the postpartum period. Next, we reviewed developmental aspects of sleep from infancy through adolescence, including both the normal evolution of sleep and sleep disturbances as they occur in this age group. Sleep disturbances were considered in the context of primary sleep disorders and as symptoms in primary psychiatric disorders. Finally, evidence of genetic influences on normal sleep and on sleep disorders was reviewed briefly.

During the normal course of pregnancy, objective measures of sleep indicate that sleep is relatively unperturbed except for sleep continuity, when increased awakenings occur during the third trimester. In the postpartum period, infant care is associated with substantial mid-nocturnal awakenings. These objective findings mesh well with subjective reports of disrupted sleep continuity. Most pregnant women report mild problems with nocturnal wakefulness until the third trimester, when getting back to sleep becomes more difficult for a substantial subset of women. The reported postpartum sleep deficit is borne out by objective findings indicating compensatory increased slow-wave sleep for new mothers.

The course of sleep across the period from neonate to late adolescence is marked by consolidation of sleep to the nighttime period, increased stage 1 sleep, and decreased REM sleep. Slow-wave sleep reaches peak levels at age 3–5 years and then diminishes over time during school age and adolescence. Although adolescents and adults often get the same total amount of sleep, controlled studies indicate that the actual sleep needs of adolescents appear to be increased.

Difficulty in falling asleep and maintaining sleep are often related to scheduling disturbances, inconsistency of parental involvement in the sleep routine, or fears and anxieties in children. Causes for sleepiness during the day can range from scheduling problems to organic bases to apparently fundamental dysregulation of mechanisms related to sleep onset. Sleep in children and adolescents can also be punctuated by emergence of normal waking behaviors (such as walking, talking, and urinating) in the sleep period. Most of these behaviors, although worrisome and even potentially dangerous, can be modified with appropriate attention to sleep schedules and the sleep environment or with medication. Usually, these behaviors decrease markedly with maturation.

Symptoms of sleep disturbances are common in child psychopathology. Differentiating the range of normal minor sleep complaints in children and adolescents from the more significant complaints associated with pathology must be based on clinical judgment and experience. For the most part, objective physiological studies have not yet produced specific, clinically beneficial evidence of sleep disruptions in youngsters with psychiatric disorders. That may be because of technical limitations associated with measuring sleep or because of maturational factors that protect the sleep of children and mask disturbances. Because both the fields of sleep disorders and biological approaches to child psychopathology are relatively new areas, further research directed toward a better understanding of the interactions among the regulation of sleep, mood, behavior, and development remains promising.

Finally, studies support a genetic influence on normal sleep staging, duration and quality of sleep, and several sleep disorders. Despite this consensus, few genetic mechanisms involved in sleep processes—whether those processes foster normal sleep or disordered sleep—have been identified. Determinations of genetic influence have been based on the familial nature of identified sleep processes and on greater concordance for sleep measures in monozygotic twins than in dizygotic twins. Some work has been done to evaluate whether we can take advantage of both the familial nature of sleep and the familial nature of depression to identify those individuals who have a predisposing genetic vulnerability to the disorder. The results are promising, but comparable studies should be performed in patients with other psychiatric disorders. These studies could help elucidate whether a range of molecular-genetic probes could provide useful information in selected families with specified disorders.

REFERENCES

Adamson J, Burdick JA: Sleep of dry alcoholics. Arch Gen Psychiatry 28:146–149, 1973

Allsopp MR, Zaiwalla Z: Narcolepsy. Arch Dis Child 67:302–306, 1992

Ambrosetto C, Lugaresi E, Coccagna G, et al: Clinical and polygraphic remarks in the restless leg syndrome. Rivista Di Patologia Nervosa E Mentale 86:244–251, 1965

American Sleep Disorders Association: The International Classification of Sleep Disorders: Diagnostic and Coding Manual. Rochester, MN, American Sleep Disorders Association, 1990, pp 297–300

Bakwin H: Sleep walking in twins. Lancet 2:446–447, 1970

Beltramini AU, Hertzig E: Sleep and bedtime behavior in preschool-aged children. Pediatrics 71:153–158,1983

Benca RM, Obermeyer WH, Thisted RA, et al: Sleep and psychiatric disorders: a meta-analysis. Arch Gen Psychiatry 49:651–668, 1992

Branchey M, Petre-Quadens O: A comparative study of sleep parameters during pregnancy. Acta Neurol Belg 68:453–459, 1968

Brownell LG, West P, Kryger MH: Breathing during sleep in normal pregnant women. Am Rev Respir Dis 133:38–41, 1986

Burd L, Kerbeshian J: Nocturnal coprolalia and phonic tics (letter). Am J Psychiatry 145:132, 1988

Busby K, Pivik RT: Failure of high intensity auditory stimuli to affect behavioral arousal in children during the first sleep cycle. Pediatr Res 17:802–805, 1983

Busby K, Firestone P, Pivik RT: Sleep patterns in hyperkinetic and normal children. Pediatrics 4:366–383, 1981

Carskadon MA: Adolescent sleepiness: increased risk in a high-risk population. Alcohol, Drugs, and Driving 5/6:317–328, 1989/1990

Carskadon MA, Dement WC: Sleepiness in the normal adolescent, in Sleep and Its Disorders in Children. Edited by Guilleminault C. New York, Raven, 1987, pp 53–66

Carskadon MA, Orav EJ, Dement WC: Evolution of sleep and daytime sleepiness in adolescents, in Sleep and Its Disorders in Children. Edited by Guilleminault C. New York, Raven, 1987, pp 43–52

Coble PA, Reynolds CF III, Kupfer DJ, et al: Childbearing in women with and without a history of affective disorder, I: psychiatric symptomatology. Compr Psychiatry (in press [a])

Coble PA, Reynolds CF III, Kupfer DJ, et al: Childbearing in women with and without a history of affective disorder, II: electroencephalographic sleep. Compr Psychiatry (in press [b])

Czeisler CA, Richardson GS, Coleman RM, et al: Chronotherapy: resetting the circadian clocks of patients with delayed sleep phase insomnia. Sleep 4:1–2, 1981

Dahl RE: Child and adolescent sleep disorders, in Child and Adolescent Neurology for Psychiatrists. Edited by Kaufman DM, Solomon GE, Pfeffer CR. Baltimore, MD, Williams & Wilkins, 1992, pp 169–194

Dahl RE: Psychiatric disorders and sleep in the child, in Principles and Practice of Sleep Medicine, 2nd Edition. Edited by Kryger M, Roth T, Dement W. Philadelphia, PA, WB Saunders (in press)

Dahl RE, Puig-Antich J, Ryan ND, et al: EEG sleep in adolescents with major depression: the role of suicidality and inpatient status. J Affect Disord 19:63–75, 1990

Dahl RE, Ryan ND, Birmaher B, et al: EEG sleep measures in prepubertal depression. Psychiatry Res 38:201–214, 1991a

Dahl RE, Pelham WB, Wierson MC: The role of sleep disturbance in attention deficit disorder symptomatology: a case study. J Pediatr Psychol 16:229–239, 1991b

Dahl RE, Holttum J, Trubnick L: A clinical picture of early onset narcolepsy. J Am Acad Child Adolesc Psychiatry (in press)

Driver HS, Shapiro CM: A longitudinal study of sleep stages in young women during pregnancy and postpartum. Sleep 15:449–453, 1992

Ferber R: Sleeplessness, night awakening, and night crying in the infant and toddler. Pediatr Rev 9:69–82, 1987

Ganguli R, Reynolds CF III, Kupfer DJ: EEG sleep in young never-medicated schizophrenic patients: a comparison with delusional and nondelusional depressives and with healthy controls. Arch Gen Psychiatry 44:36–45, 1987

Gedda L, Brenci G: Sleep and dream characteristics in twins. Acta Genet Med Gemellol (Roma) 28:237–239, 1979

Giles DE, Biggs MM, Rush AJ, et al: Risk factors in families of unipolar depression, I: incidence of illness and reduced REM latency. J Affect Disord 14:51–59, 1988

Giles DE, Kupfer DJ, Roffwarg HP, et al: Polysomnographic parameters in first-degree relatives of unipolar probands. Psychiatry Res 27:127–136, 1989a

Giles DE, Roffwarg HP, Kupfer DJ, et al: Secular trend in unipolar depression: a hypothesis. J Affect Disord 16:71–75, 1989b

Giles DE, Kupfer DJ, Roffwarg HP: Abnormal EEG sleep antedates the onset of depression (abstract). Biol Psychiatry 27:93A, 1990

Giles DE, Roffwarg HP, Dahl RE, et al: EEG sleep abnormalities in depressed children: a hypothesis. Psychiatry Res 41:53–63, 1992

Glaze DG, Frost JD, Jankovic J: Sleep in Gilles de la Tourette's syndrome: disorder of arousal. Neurology 33:586–592, 1983

Goetz RR, Hanlon HS, Puig-Antich J, et al: Sign of REM prior to the first REM period in prepubertal children. Sleep 8:1–10, 1985

Gould J, Austin F, Cook P: A genetic analysis of sleep stage organisation in newborn twins (abstract). Sleep Research 7:132, 1978

Greenhill L, Puig-Antich J, Goetz R, et al: Sleep architecture and REM sleep measures in prepubertal children with attention deficit disorder with hyperactivity. Sleep 6:91–101, 1983

Guilleminault C, Winkle R: A review of 50 children with OSAS. Lung 159:275–287, 1981

Guilleminault C, Winkle R, Korobkin R, et al: Children and nocturnal snoring: evaluation of the effects of sleep-related respiratory resistive load and daytime functioning. Eur J Pediatr 139:165–171, 1982

Heath AC, Kendler KS, Eaves LJ, et al: Evidence for genetic influences on sleep disturbance and sleep pattern in twins. Sleep 13:318–335, 1990

Hertz G, Fast A, Feinsilver SH, et al: Sleep in normal late pregnancy. Sleep 15:246–251, 1992

Honda Y, Juji T, Matsuki K, et al: HLA-DR2 and Dw2 in narcolepsy and other disorders of excessive somnolence without cataplexy. Sleep 9:133–142, 1986

Hori A: Sleep characteristics in twins. Jpn J Psychiatry Neurol 40:35–46, 1986

Insel TR, Gillin JC, Moore A, et al: The sleep of patients with obsessive-compulsive disorder. Arch Gen Psychiatry 39:1372–1377, 1982

Kales A, Soldatos CR, Bixler EO, et al: Hereditary factors in sleep walking and night terrors. Br J Psychiatry 137:111–118, 1980

Kaplan BJ, McNicol J, Conte RA, et al: Sleep disturbance in preschool-aged hyperactive and nonhyperactive children. Pediatrics 80:839–844, 1987

Karacan I, Heine W, Agnew HW Jr, et al: Characteristics of sleep during late pregnancy and the postpartum periods. Am J Obstet Gynecol 101:579–586, 1968

Karacan I, Williams RL, Hursch CJ, et al: Some implications of the sleep patterns of pregnancy for postpartum emotional disturbances. Br J Psychiatry 115:929–935, 1969

Klackenberg G: Somnambulism in childhood: prevalence, course and behavioral correlation. Acta Paediatr Scand 71:495–499, 1982

Kleine W: Periodische Schlafsucht. Monatsschr Psychiatr Neurol 57:285–298, 1925

Kotogol S, Hartse KM, Walsh JK: Characteristics of narcolepsy in preteenaged children. Pediatrics 85:205– 209, 1990

Levin M: Narcolepsy and other varieties of morbid somnolence. Arch Neurol Psychiatry 22:1172–1200, 1929

Linkowski P, Kerkhofs M, Hauspie R, et al: EEG sleep patterns in man: a twin study. Electroencephalogr Clin Neurophysiol 73:279–284, 1989

Linkowski P, Kerkhofs M, Hauspie R, et al: Genetic determinants of EEG sleep: a study in twins living apart. Electroencephalogr Clin Neurophysiol 79:114–118, 1991

Lozoff B, Wolf AW, Davis NS: Sleep problems seen in pediatric practice. Pediatrics 75:477–483, 1985

Mauri M: Sleep and the reproductive cycle: a review. Health Care for Women International 11:409–421, 1990

Mendlewicz J, Sevy S, deMaertelaer V: REM sleep latency and morbidity risk of affective disorders in depressive illness. Neuropsychobiology 22:14–17, 1989

Navelet Y, Anders T, Guilleminault C: Narcolepsy in children, in Narcolepsy. Edited by Guilleminault C, Dement W, Passouant P. New York, Spectrum, 1976, pp 171–177

Parkes JD, Lock CB: Genetic factors in sleep disorders. J Neurol Neurosurg Psychiatry 52 (suppl):101–108, 1989

Partinen M, Kaprio J, Koskenvuo M, et al: Genetic and environmental determination of human sleep. Sleep 6:179–185, 1983

Petre-Quadens O, DeBarsey AM, Devos J, et al: Sleep in pregnancy: evidence of foetal-sleep characteristics. J Neurol Sci 4:600–605, 1967

Redline S, Tosteson T, Tishler PV, et al: Studies in the genetics of obstructive sleep apnea: familial aggregation of symptoms associated with sleep-related breathing disturbances. Am Rev Respir Dis 145:440–444, 1992

Reynolds CF III, Kupfer DJ: Sleep research in affective illness: state-of-the-art circa 1987. Sleep 10:199–215, 1987

Reynolds CF III, Shaw DH, Newton TF, et al: EEG sleep in outpatients with generalized anxiety: a preliminary comparison with depressed outpatients. Psychiatry Res 8:81–89, 1983

Reynolds CF III, Soloff PH, Kupfer DJ, et al: Depression in borderline patients: a prospective EEG sleep study. Psychiatry Res 14:1–15, 1985

Roffwarg HP, Frankel B, Pessah M: The nocturnal sleep patterns in pregnancy. Psychophysiology 5:227–228, 1968

Ross DM, Ross SA: Hyperactivity: Current Issues, Research and Theory, 2nd Edition. New York, Wiley, 1982

Roth B: Narcolepsy and Hypersomnia. Basel, Karger, 1980

Ryan ND, Puig-Antich J, Rabinovich H, et al: The clinical picture of major depression in children and adolescents. Arch Gen Psychiatry 44:854–861, 1987

Schulz H, Geisler P, Pollmaecher T, et al: HLA-DR2 correlates with rapid-eye-movement sleep latency in normal human subjects (letter). Lancet 2:803, 1986

Sewitch DE, Kupfer DJ: Polysomnographic telemetry using Telediagnostic and Oxford Medilog 9000 systems. Sleep 8:288–293, 1985

Shouse MN: Epilepsy and seizures during sleep, in Principles and Practices of Sleep Medicine. Edited by Kryger M, Roth T, Dement W. Philadelphia, PA, WB Saunders, 1989, pp 364–376

Staner L, Bouillon E, Andrien M, et al: Lack of association between HLA-DR antigens and sleep-onset REM periods in major depression. Biol Psychiatry 20:1199–1204, 1991

Terr L: Chowchilla revisited: the effects of psychic trauma four years after a school-bus kidnapping. Am J Psychiatry 140:1543–1550, 1983

Valatx JL: Genetic as a model for studying the sleep-waking cycle, in Sleep Mechanisms (Experimental Brain Research, Suppl 8). Edited by Borbely A, Valatx JL. Berlin, Springer, 1984, pp 135–145

Waller DA, Hardy BW, Pole R, et al: Sleep EEG in bulimic, depressed, and normal subjects. Biol Psychiatry 25:661–664, 1989

Webb W, Campbell SC: Relationships in sleep characteristics of identical and fraternal twins. Arch Gen Psychiatry 40:1093–1095, 1983

Zarcone VP, Benson KL, Berger PA: Abnormal rapid eye movement latencies in schizophrenia. Arch Gen Psychiatry 44:44–48, 1987

Zung WWK, Wilson WP: Sleep and dream patterns in twins: Markov analysis of a genetic trait, in Recent Advances in Biological Psychiatry. Edited by Wortis J. New York, Plenum, 1967, pp 119–130

Chapter 26

Sleep in Depression: Longitudinal Perspectives

Daniel J. Buysse, M.D., and Eric A. Nofzinger, M.D.

Approximately 20 years of focused research have established the subjective and electroencephalographic (EEG) sleep characteristics of patients with major depressive disorder. A number of recent review articles describe these findings and contrast them with the sleep characteristics of other psychiatric disorders (e.g., Benca et al. 1992; Nofzinger et al. 1993c).

Although debate continues regarding the sensitivity and specificity of particular EEG sleep findings in depression (Buysse and Kupfer 1990), it has become increasingly clear that no single sleep variable can be considered a robust biological marker of depression that differentiates this disorder from others (see Section II). Early hopes that rapid eye movement (REM) sleep latency could fit this role (Kupfer 1976) have yielded to recent examinations of published data, which also demonstrate this feature in at least some patients with other conditions, such as schizophrenia (Benca et al. 1992). However, these analyses also suggest that sleep disturbances (including shortening of REM sleep latency) tend to be more severe in depression than in other psychiatric disorders. Moreover, sleep in depressed patients appears to be characterized by a consistent group of EEG sleep findings that are not commonly seen in other disorders; these findings include sleep-continuity disturbance, reduced REM sleep latency, increased phasic REM activity, a "shift" in the amount and intensity of REM sleep toward the beginning of the sleep period, and reduced slow-wave sleep (e.g., stages 3 and 4 of non–rapid eye movement [NREM] or "delta" sleep) (Reynolds and Kupfer 1987).

Ideally, examination of these sleep patterns in depression will lead to insights regarding the neurobiological mechanisms of mood dysregulation. Several authors have recently considered the implications of sleep disturbances in depressed patients using circadian, neurochemical, and neurobiological theoretical frameworks (e.g., Buysse and Kupfer 1993; Wehr 1990).

In this chapter, we will not review in detail the sleep characteristics

Supported by National Institute of Mental Health Grants MH48891, MH16804, and MH30915.

of depression, its subtypes, or cross-sectional clinical correlates; the references above cover these topics. Rather, we will focus on a growing body of literature that examines sleep in depression from a longitudinal, rather than a cross-sectional, perspective.

Longitudinal studies are important for several reasons. First, they can help to determine whether the sleep characteristics of depressed patients are persistent biological traits, state-related changes, or even epiphenomena. In a similar way, these studies can begin to address whether an episode of depression leads to "scarring" of sleep or whether sleep features are stable, or even premorbid, biological features. Second, longitudinal studies can address the more direct relationships between sleep and mood and can help to untangle the direction of causality between sleep and mood changes. Finally, longitudinal studies may identify neurobiological and psychological correlates of the short-term treatment response and the long-term course of depression. Longitudinal studies clearly demonstrate that EEG sleep studies provide a valuable research tool beyond the question of diagnosis or biological markers.

We will review four basic types of sleep studies that address longitudinal questions in depression: 1) population and sample surveys of subjective sleep and mood states, 2) cross-sectional EEG sleep studies of patients during acute depression compared with patients in remission, 3) longitudinal within-subject EEG sleep and physiological studies, and 4) studies that examine associations between EEG sleep and clinical characteristics over time. We will conclude by considering some of the neurobiological implications of longitudinal studies.

POPULATION AND CLINICAL-SAMPLE SURVEYS OF SUBJECTIVE SLEEP AND MOOD DISTURBANCES

Studies that examine longitudinal relationships between subjective sleep disturbance and subjective mood disturbance provide the broadest context for examining longitudinal sleep-mood relationships. Such studies have the advantage of including large numbers of subjects and lengthy follow-up intervals.

Depressed patients frequently report disturbed sleep, including difficulties with sleep onset, sleep maintenance, and "early morning awakening." The interactions between insomnia complaints and mood disturbance have been assessed in several longitudinal studies of community-dwelling individuals. Rodin et al. (1988) examined self-ratings of depressed mood and sleep problems over 3 years in a community sample of 264 elderly adults. One-half of the subjects reported insomnia at five or more of the eight evaluation points, indicating the high prevalence of such complaints. Logistic regression models showed consistent positive associations between the presence of depressed mood over time and the severity and persistence of sleep disturbance, even when controlling for factors such as age, sex, physical health, and medication use. A decrease over time in depression was associated with decreased complaints of early morning awakening. This study is significant because it demonstrates not only that depression is related to sleep complaints, but that this association pertains as well to the occurrence of such symptoms over time. The study does not, however, demonstrate directional effects.

Does insomnia lead to depression? Ford and Kamerow (1989), as part of the National Institute of Mental Health Epidemiological Catchment Area study, questioned 7,954 adults about insomnia and psychiatric symptoms at two points 1 year apart. Robust associations between these symptoms were noted, but more importantly, persistent insomnia complaints were associated with a much higher risk of developing a new episode of depression in the 1-year follow-up interval (odds ratio, 39.8). These findings suggest that insomnia could be an early symptom of, or a marker of vulnerability to, depression. Dryman and Eaton (1991), using a subset of the same Epidemiological Catchment Area sample, verified the relationship between sleep disturbance and the subsequent onset of major depression during a 1-year follow-up, although the relationship held for women only.

Another epidemiological report focused on 1,577 elderly subjects followed up at 2 years (Kennedy et al. 1991). Rather than focusing on the onset of depression, this study focused on the persistence or remission of symptoms as assessed by the Center for Epidemiological Studies Depression Scale. Patients with persistent depression had worse subjective sleep disturbance at baseline and at 24 months than patients who experienced remission. Discriminant function analyses showed that health status, age, persistent sleep disturbance, and support services accounted for 31% of the variance between groups.

A Swiss cohort of young adults assessed at three points over 7 years also showed that chronic insomnia was associated with major depression and that recurrent or occasional insomnia correlated positively with life events and interpersonal conflicts (Vollrath et al. 1989). Furthermore, any type of insomnia was associated with an increased risk of subsequent depression. The authors also investigated the question of directionality: did patients with any type of insomnia at the first interview have an increased likelihood of depression 1 or 2 years later? Although the proportion of patients with chronic insomnia who developed an episode of depression was higher than the proportion with no insomnia (50% versus 29%), this difference was not statistically significant.

Other studies have evaluated longitudinal sleep-depression associations in clinical samples. A study of 242 patients with rheumatoid arthritis revealed that an interaction factor of high pain levels and high levels of sleep disturbance was associated with the development of depression 2 years later. However, sleep disturbance alone did not independently predict increased depression (Nicassio and Wallston 1992). In a different type of study, Fawcett et al. (1990) examined the prognostic significance of various clinical features in predicting suicide among patients with affective disorders. Global insomnia (rated based on items on the Schedule for Affective Disorders and Schizophrenia) was one of the clinical symptoms associated with suicide during the following year. The authors consider insomnia to be one of the "modifiable risks" for suicide.

Does treatment of subjective sleep problems diminish depression or the risk of a new depression? Unfortunately, little information is available regarding this question. Mosko et al. (1989) found that 67% of patients presenting to a sleep disorders center reported an episode of depression within the previous 5 years. Other investigators have noted similarly high rates of psychiatric disorders among samples of patients with clinical insomnia. However, Mosko and colleagues also found that treatment of certain types of sleep disturbances (sleep apnea and periodic limb movements) was followed by a reduction in Profile of Mood States scores, including scores on the depressive subscale (McNair et al. 1971), whereas treatment of other sleep problems (narcolepsy) or withdrawal of sleeping pills from patients with chronic insomnia was not followed by such a change. Obviously, conclusions from this study are limited by the particular types of sleep disturbances and treatments used.

Major findings from these studies are summarized in Table 26–1. Having considered subjective sleep and mood findings in longitudinal surveys, we will now turn to longitudinal studies of objective sleep measures in depression. These clinical studies further clarify the longitudinal relationships between sleep and depression.

EEG SLEEP STUDIES IN DEPRESSION: CROSS-SECTIONAL INVESTIGATIONS DURING DEPRESSION AND RECOVERY

Cross-sectional studies of EEG sleep in depressed patients during acute depression and remission begin to address the question of persistent ("trait") versus episode-related ("state") abnormalities. Although these studies technically are not longitudinal (in the sense of being repeated within subject assessments), they have been helpful as preliminary studies using objective measures of sleep disturbance. Viewed as exploratory rather than definitive investigations, these studies also

Table 26–1. Population and clinical-sample surveys of subjective sleep and mood disturbances

- Question addressed

    What is the association between subjective sleep disturbance and subjective mood disturbance over time?

- Major findings

    1. Depressive symptoms correlate with insomnia symptoms over time.
    2. The presence of continued insomnia is associated with the new onset of depression in some (but not all) studies.
    3. Continued insomnia is associated with poor response to treatment of depression.
    4. Treatment of sleep disturbances can improve depression in at least some patients.

- Unresolved issues

    1. What is the direction of causality between sleep and mood disturbance?
    2. Does early treatment of sleep disturbance prevent subsequent episodes of depression?

have the advantage of being relatively easy to conduct.

Hauri et al. (1974) reported one of the earliest investigations of EEG sleep in depressed patients who were in remission. A group of remitted unipolar patients, free of antidepressant medications for 2 weeks, differed from age-matched control subjects in having longer sleep latency, more stage 1 sleep, and less delta sleep. REM sleep latency and most other measures of REM sleep did not differ between the groups. Remitted depressed patients also showed greater night-to-night and between-subject variability in most sleep measures. Knowles et al. (1986) found that drug-free remitted bipolar patients also had greater between-subject variability than control subjects, but these investigators did not find reliable differences in the mean values for EEG sleep measures.

Cholinergic-challenge paradigms have also been used to investigate EEG sleep in cross-sectional studies of depression and remission. Such studies address the possibility that REM sleep dysregulation in depressed patients may reflect increased cholinergic sensitivity; infusion of cholinergic agents produces a more rapid onset of REM sleep in depressed patients than in control subjects (Gillin et al. 1991). The presence of an exaggerated response in remitted patients would argue for a persistent biological dysregulation. Sitaram et al. (1980) found that remitted, drug-free depressed patients (including both unipolar and bipolar patients, drug-free for ≥ 2 weeks) did not differ from control subjects with respect to baseline REM sleep latency. However, the remitted patients had significantly shorter REM sleep latency after the administration of the cholinergic agonist arecoline, suggesting increased cholinergic sensitivity in the remitted depressed patients. In contrast to these results, Berger et al. (1989) and Riemann and Berger (1989) found that the oral cholinergic agonist RS-86 did not lead to significant shortening of the REM sleep latency time in recovered depressed patients, as it did in symptomatic depressed patients. Differences between these studies may result from the difference in pharmacological probes or from the longer medication-free interval in the Berger et al. study.

Another very different type of cross-sectional study also addresses the question of the longitudinal sleep effects of depression. In this type of study, patients with single-episode depression or late age at onset are compared with those who have had repeated episodes or early age of onset. The finding of greater sleep disruption with recurrent illness would suggest either a progressive "scarring" of the sleep system caused by depressive episodes or an increased vulnerability to depressive episodes in these patients; on the other hand, an absence of differences would suggest that EEG sleep characteristics are stable findings or categorical vulnerability characteristics. Studies by Giles et al. (1990) and Buysse et al. (1988) support the latter hypothesis in middle-aged and elderly depressed patients. Single-episode and late-onset depressed patients did not differ in terms of REM sleep latency or other EEG sleep measures from patients with recurrent illness, even when controlling for the effects of current age and age at the first episode of depression.

Major findings from cross-sectional studies are summarized in Table 26–2. Inferences drawn from cross-sectional studies are limited by several factors, including sample bias, different treatment histories, different medication-free intervals, and different study methodologies. These studies do not yield consistent answers to the question of whether sleep findings in depression are more traitlike or are state related. True longitudinal, within-subject designs have proven more helpful in addressing this question.

LONGITUDINAL, WITHIN-SUBJECT STUDIES OF SLEEP IN DEPRESSION

Studies of this sort are better suited to address whether EEG sleep characteristics are episode related or whether they persist throughout the episode and into clinical recovery. The first question to resolve with longitudinal EEG sleep studies is whether sleep characteristics persist throughout an untreated depressive episode. An early study by Coble et al. (1979) indicated that the answer is *yes*. EEG sleep measures including REM sleep latency remained stable over a 35-day placebo treatment condition in a group of 12 depressed inpatients. Measures of phasic REM activity did show a small linear decrease over the same

Table 26–2. Cross-sectional EEG sleep studies during depressed episode and recovery

- Questions addressed
  1. Do EEG sleep findings in recovered depressed patients differ from those in healthy control subjects or in acutely depressed patients?
  2. Do EEG sleep findings in patients with single versus recurrent episodes of depression indicate progressive "scarring" of sleep?
- Major findings
  1. Recovered depressed patients have greater variability in sleep measures, less slow-wave sleep, and longer sleep latency than control subjects.
  2. Recovered depressed patients have increased cholinergic sensitivity in some (but not all) studies.
  3. EEG sleep findings in patients with recurrent versus single-episode depression do *not* suggest progressive sleep scarring over time.
- Unresolved issue
  Do EEG sleep findings in depressed patients change between the time of acute depression and the time of remission?

interval, suggesting that different sleep measures may actually show different longitudinal patterns during a depressive episode.

Treatment with antidepressant medications produces numerous acute changes from baseline EEG sleep patterns (e.g., Kupfer et al. 1981, 1989; Reynolds et al. 1991). Most tricyclics suppress REM sleep, increase REM sleep latency, and increase delta sleep in the first part of the night. However, studies of patients who are in clinical remission and still on medication cannot differentiate between the intrinsic effects of the medication on EEG sleep and changes that may occur as a function of the clinical state.

To address this problem, other studies have examined EEG sleep after recovery and after medication withdrawal. Several of these studies demonstrate stability of EEG sleep measures during depression and recovery in patients who have been off medication for a period of weeks or months. Rush et al. (1986) found no significant differences in any sleep measure, including REM sleep latency, between depression and recovery (after medication withdrawal) in 13 depressed patients; 10 of the 13 also maintained a stable categorical REM sleep latency classification. Giles et al. (1987) also reported stability of categorically defined REM sleep latency across clinical states after medication treatment and withdrawal. More recently, Steiger et al. (1989) found similar stability in most sleep measures, although early morning wakefulness decreased during clinical remission and (counterintuitively) stage 4 sleep decreased slightly and the number of awakenings increased. Early morning wakefulness also decreased in a study of elderly depressed patients after acute treatment and withdrawal from nortriptyline, whereas other variables showed no change (Lee et al. 1993). Further analysis of these data showed significant within-subject correlations between depression and recovery for REM measures, but not for sleep continuity and sleep stage architecture.

Other studies demonstrate a more notable trend toward normalization of sleep measures during drug-free clinical remission. Schulz et al. (1979), focusing on REM sleep latency, found sleep-onset REM periods in 31% of sleep records during depression but in only 5% during remission after drug treatment and withdrawal. Relative normalization in REM sleep latency was also noted by Reimann and Berger (1989) in eight depressed patients after successful treatment and withdrawal of medications. In addition, sleep latency, intermittent wakefulness, and phasic REM activity moved toward normal values (not statistically significant), but slow-wave sleep remained stable. Puig-Antich et al. (1983) also found improved sleep continuity during recovery in adolescent patients with depression; REM sleep latency was normal during the depressed state and actually became shorter during recovery but was still well within the normal range.

Although the above studies were conducted weeks to months after patients had been withdrawn from medications, one could legitimately question whether medications had long-lasting effects, particularly because most antidepressants have prominent effects on both REM sleep and sleep continuity. Two recent studies avoid this criticism by focusing on EEG sleep in patients treated with psychotherapy alone (Buysse et al. 1992b; Thase and Simons 1992). In each investigation, visually scored EEG sleep variables showed no significant changes from symptomatic depression to early recovery. Strong intraindividual correlations were noted for most sleep measures as well. Buysse et al. also found that automated period and amplitude measures of delta EEG activity and phasic REM showed subtle state-related differences, with delta activity increasing and REM activity decreasing during recovery. The major criticism of these studies is that patients treated with psychotherapy may have less severe depressive symptoms and EEG sleep disturbances compared with more ill inpatient and pharmacotherapy patient samples.

Yet another type of longitudinal study examines sleep at different points in the course of successive depressive episodes within individuals. With this strategy, patients are studied first during an index episode, which typically has lasted several weeks or months, and again in the course of a recurrence episode, which typically has lasted a much shorter length of time. Kupfer et al. (1988, 1991) reported that REM sleep latency, the percentage of REM sleep, and phasic REM activity all appear more abnormal early in the course of a recurrent episode compared with later in the course of the index episode. Slow-wave sleep and clinical measures of depression severity were not different at the two time points. EEG spectral power during REM episodes was also lower during the recurrence episode compared with the index episode. The exact significance of this last finding remains unclear, but it supports the notion that REM sleep regulation is more disturbed within the first few weeks of a depressive episode than several weeks or months later.

A final type of longitudinal EEG sleep study concerns patients with depressive *symptoms* but not necessarily a depressive *syndrome*. These studies address the possibility that sleep changes may be related to depression in a continuous (as opposed to a categorical) sense. The prototype of such investigations is the work of Cartwright and colleagues. Cartwright initially studied 29 women undergoing divorce and followed up on 13 of these women after 1–2 years. Among those subjects studied longitudinally, REM sleep latency lengthened significantly at follow-up (Cartwright 1983). In a subsequent investigation, however, Cartwright et al. (1991) found that REM latencies at baseline and 1-year follow-up were strongly correlated and not apparently different with respect to mean level. However, only 7 of 15 categorically depressed patients with short REM sleep latency at baseline continued to display this feature at follow-up when not depressed. Thus, Cartwright's data on patients with depressive symptoms contrast with studies of clinically depressed individuals in that they suggest that REM sleep latency may "normalize" during the resolution of mood-disturbing events.

Although most longitudinal sleep studies in depression have focused on the EEG abnormalities associated with depression, some longitudinal investigations have explored other physiological parameters during sleep as well. For instance, C. F. Reynolds, M. E. Thase, E. A. Nofzinger, and colleagues have studied nocturnal penile tumescence (NPT) over the longitudinal course of depression as a potential physiological correlate of altered sexual interest and function in depressed men. In healthy men, penile erections occur cyclically during sleep in close association with REM sleep (Fisher et al 1965). Penile tumescence precedes and follows the appearance of REM sleep by several minutes.

In an effort to determine whether depressed men's complaints of diminished sexual interest had a physiological correlate, Thase et al. (1987) reported that 10 depressed men had significantly reduced tumescence time, which was not attributable to alterations in REM sleep or sleep efficiency. They also presented preliminary information suggesting that alterations in NPT may be state related, because three patients who had abnormal NPT recordings while depressed had reversal of abnormal NPT after treatment with either cognitive-behavior therapy or antidepressant medication therapy. The initial finding of reduced penile tumescence during sleep was supported in both a larger sample ($n = 34$) of depressed men (Thase et al. 1988) and in a replication study of 51 different depressed men (Thase et al. 1992). Although these early studies indicated a state-dependent physiological change associated with alterations in daytime sexual function during the depressive episode, it remained unclear whether recovery from depression would reverse this change.

In a subsequent longitudinal study, self-report, behavioral, and NPT measures of sexual function were collected in 40 outpatient depressed men both before and after treatment with cognitive-behavior therapy (Nofzinger et al. 1993b). Overall, the results did not support the reversibility hypothesis. Rather, NPT measures were relatively stable from pretreatment to posttreatment despite clinical remission of depressive symptoms. NPT measures were reduced both before and after treatment compared with those in healthy control subjects. Although a subset of depressed men with reduced NPT measures before treatment did show improvement in NPT after recovery, this improvement may have represented a regression to the mean, given the considerable variability in some NPT measures on repeat assessment (Nofzinger et al. 1993a). Because changes in depression over the course of treatment did not correlate with alterations in NPT measures or with alterations in daytime sexual attitudes and behavior, the authors concluded that NPT profiles in depressed men reflect traitlike physiological alterations.

Major findings from longitudinal EEG sleep studies are summarized in Table 26–3. In the next section, we consider the longitudinal relationships between sleep and clinical measures in depressed patients.

Table 26–3.   Longitudinal within-subject studies of EEG sleep in depression

- Questions addressed
    1. Are EEG sleep findings stable during a depressive episode?
    2. Do EEG sleep findings or other sleep physiological measures change between the time of the acute episode and the time of recovery?
- Major findings
    1. Most EEG sleep characteristics remain stable during the acute episode of depression, but phasic REM sleep tends to "normalize."
    2. Sleep continuity, sleep-onset REM periods, and (in some studies) phasic REM sleep tend to normalize with recovery from depression.
    3. Categorically defined REM sleep latency and slow-wave sleep do not change between the time of acute depression and the time of recovery.
    4. Nocturnal penile tumescence does not change between the time of depression and the time of recovery.
    5. Strong intraindividual correlations exist for most sleep measures between the time of depression and the time of recovery.
- Unresolved issue
    Do more sophisticated measures of sleep (e.g., spectral analysis, period and amplitude analysis) show state-related changes?

CLINICAL CORRELATES OF LONGITUDINAL EEG SLEEP STUDIES

Investigators have long been interested in determining whether EEG sleep measures correlate with clinical features such as ratings of depression severity. Similarly, there has been a great deal of interest in knowing how baseline EEG sleep measures correlate with short- or longer-term clinical outcomes and how sleep and clinical measures relate to one another over time. We will consider four types of studies: 1) studies that examine associations between baseline EEG sleep and short-term pharmacotherapy outcome; 2) studies that examine the same associations for psychotherapy outcome; 3) studies that examine EEG sleep as a correlate of longer-term clinical outcome; and 4) studies that examine longitudinal associations among sleep, dreaming, and mood.

EEG Sleep and Short-Term Pharmacotherapy Outcome

A number of studies have found associations between EEG sleep features during depression and the acute response to pharmacotherapy. In particular, short REM sleep latency has been associated with a favorable response to medications such as desipramine or amitriptyline during acute treatment (Rush et al. 1985, 1989). Although mean REM sleep latency also tended to be shorter in amitriptyline responders (Mendlewicz et al. 1991) and in clomipramine responders (Riemann and Berger 1990), these differences did not reach statistical significance. In both studies, responders also tended to have more disturbed sleep continuity.

In other studies, investigators examined correlations between the *change* in sleep measures and the *change* in clinical ratings during drug administration. For example, Kupfer et al. (1981) found that the clinical antidepressant effect of amitriptyline (after 4 weeks) correlated more strongly with sleep latency and REM sleep latency during the first two nights of drug administration than it did with the same measures at drug-free baseline. Hochli et al. (1986) initially found that REM sleep suppression during the first night of clomipramine treatment correlated with the treatment response at day 19, but subsequent analyses did not bear out this observation (Riemann and Berger 1990). In a recent report on elderly depressed patients, Reynolds et al. (1991) reported very strong correlations between changes in clinical ratings and changes in EEG sleep during the first 5 weeks of nortriptyline treatment; the strongest sleep correlates included prolongation of REM sleep latency, improvement in sleep maintenance, and an increase in early night delta EEG activity. Mendlewicz et al. (1991) found no similar correlates in their group of younger depressed patients treated with amitriptyline. Looking at the other end of treatment, Gillin et al. (1978) found that REM sleep rebound on abrupt discontinuation of amitriptyline was significantly more robust in responders compared with non-responders.

Like antidepressant drugs, sleep deprivation has been used as both a physiological probe and a short-term treatment in depression. Baseline EEG sleep measures do not differentiate between responders and nonresponders to sleep deprivation (Duncan et al. 1980; Gerner et al. 1979; Riemann and Berger 1990), nor do the effects of sleep deprivation on EEG sleep measures strongly predict pharmacological treatment outcome (Kasper et al. 1990; Riemann and Berger 1990). Among older depressed patients, however, Reynolds et al. (1986a) found that the change in sleep continuity after one night of sleep deprivation correlated significantly with the end-of-treatment (after medication or electroconvulsive therapy) score on the Hamilton Rating Scale for Depression.

Finally, in a somewhat different vein, Greenhouse et al. (1987) examined whether baseline EEG sleep measures were associated with time to stabilization in depressed patients treated with imipramine and psychotherapy. None of four candidate variables (sleep latency, sleep efficiency, REM density, REM sleep latency) was significantly associated with time to clinical stabilization.

EEG Sleep and Psychotherapy Outcome

A growing number of studies have begun to focus on EEG sleep predictors of response to nonsomatic therapies, that is, psychotherapy. Such studies are attractive because they contest long-held notions regarding the distinctions between psychological and biological origins and treatments of depression, and because they may provide different predictors for different types of therapies (i.e., medication and psychotherapy). In one of the first studies of this sort, R. B. Jarrett et al. (1990) found that categorically defined REM sleep latency was *not* related to treatment outcome in 39 depressed outpatients treated with psychotherapy. Patients with reduced and nonreduced REM sleep latency did not have different posttreatment depression ratings, and patients in both groups were equally likely to be classified as responders. Although responders and nonresponders were not compared statistically, they did not appear to have systematic differences in any other baseline sleep measures, and selected baseline sleep measures did not relate significantly to posttreatment depression ratings.

In a similar study, Buysse et al. (1992a) found small differences in the baseline sleep of responders and nonresponders to interpersonal psychotherapy; nonresponders had longer sleep-onset latency, lower sleep efficiency, and altered temporal distribution of phasic REM activity. In addition, the groups showed different sleep adaptation patterns across two nights. However, baseline sleep measures did not correlate significantly with depression ratings after 4 weeks of treatment in the total sample.

Thase and Simons reported the most comprehensive analyses of EEG sleep during psychotherapy treatment. In the first of their reports (Thase and Simons 1992), the investigators found that several baseline sleep variables correlated with final Hamilton Rating Scale for Depression scores. The direction of the correlations showed that those with a greater percentage of delta sleep, longer sleep time, and more phasic and tonic REM had the highest posttreatment scores, suggesting that hypersomnia is associated with worse response to cognitive-behavior therapy. In a more detailed subsequent report, the investigators found that none of four key sleep variables were significantly related to end-of-treatment Hamilton Rating Scale for Depression scores (Simons and Thase 1992). Specifically, REM sleep latency, defined categorically or continuously, did not predict treatment response by most outcome definitions, and patients with reduced and nonreduced REM sleep latency did not show different temporal patterns of clinical response (using life-table analyses). In a set of exploratory analyses, the authors reported that greater night-to-night variability in REM sleep latency was associated with worse treatment response.

Relationships Between Sleep and Longer-Term Clinical Outcomes

The two previous sections deal with the use of EEG sleep measures as predictors of short-term treatment response. Several studies have also demonstrated that sleep measures may predict longer-term outcomes, such as recurrence of depression or even death.

Among elderly patients with concurrent symptoms of depression and dementia, poor sleep continuity, together with higher scores on cognitive measures and higher depression ratings, predicted favorable clinical outcome (in terms of cognitive and mood symptoms) at 2 years (Reynolds et al. 1986b). The authors interpret these data as suggesting that more "depressive" EEG sleep and clinical measures are associated with a better prognosis. However, during a 2-year follow-up of a more homogeneous group of elderly depressed patients, Reynolds and colleagues (1989) found that a baseline REM sleep latency of less than or equal to 20 minutes was associated with a relative risk of 3.7 for experiencing a recurrence during active nortriptyline maintenance therapy. The difference in these findings relates to differences in the definition of a positive outcome; the former study examined symptoms of dementia as well as depression, whereas the second study focused only on depression.

Both REM sleep latency and reduced "delta ratio" (a measure of the temporal pattern of EEG delta activity) have been associated with recurrence of depression (Figures 26–1 and 26–2). Giles et al. (1987) reported that categorically defined reduced REM sleep latency was significantly associated with recurrence in a group of drug-free patients followed for up to 24 months after successful pharmacotherapy and psychotherapy. Kupfer et al. (1990) found similar results using the delta ratio as a categorical variable; those with a reduced delta ratio (i.e., a more abnormal temporal pattern of delta EEG activity) had a shorter mean time to recurrence during a 3-year follow-up period than those

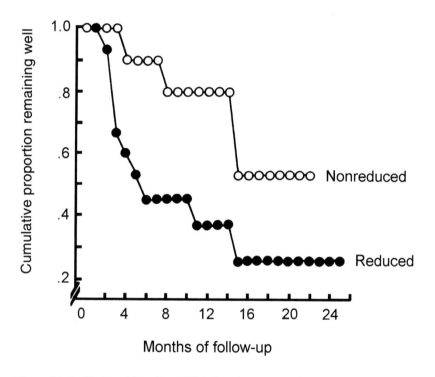

Figure 26–1. Reduced baseline REM sleep latency predicts shorter time to recurrence in depressed patients treated with combined pharmacotherapy and psychotherapy. ○ indicate 10 patients with an REM sleep latency of >65 minutes; ● indicate 15 patients with an REM sleep latency of ≤65 minutes. *Source.* Reprinted by permission of Elsevier Science Publishing Co., Inc., from Giles DE, Jarrett RB, Roffwarg HP, et al.: "Reduced Rapid Eye Movement Latency: A Predictor of Recurrence of Depression." *Neuropsychopharmacology* 1:33–39, 1987. Copyright 1987 by the American College of Neuropsychopharmacology.

with a higher delta ratio (47.1 versus 81.1 weeks). All patients had been treated acutely with imipramine, but were medication-free during follow-up. Interestingly, maintenance psychotherapy interacted with the delta ratio effects; in patients with a "normal" delta ratio, mean time to recurrence was twice as long in those treated with maintenance psychotherapy compared with those not treated with maintenance psychotherapy.

EEG sleep measures may also predict mortality. In a group of patients with concurrent symptoms of depression and dementia followed up for 2 years, Hoch et al. (1989) found that decedents had longer REM sleep latency, less REM sleep rebound after sleep deprivation, and greater amounts of sleep apnea (although still in the subclinical range for most subjects). Logistic regression showed that REM sleep latency and sleep apnea measures correctly identified 77% of the survivors and nonsurvivors, and parametric correlations showed survival time to be significantly related to REM sleep measures. Although the cause for these associations is not clear, the authors suggest that REM sleep reduction and apnea may be subtle indicators of early "brain failure" in these patients.

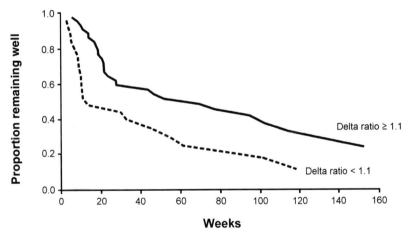

Figure 26–2. Low "delta ratio" at baseline predicts shorter time to recurrence in depressed patients after combined treatment with pharmacotherapy and psychotherapy. The delta ratio was obtained by dividing the delta EEG counts per minute in the first NREM period by the delta EEG counts per minute in the second NREM period. The *solid curve* indicates 45 patients with a delta ratio of ≥ 1.1; the *dashed curve* indicates 25 patients with a delta ratio of <1.1.

Source. Reprinted from Kupfer DJ, Frank E, McEachran AB, et al.: "Delta Sleep Ratio: A Biological Correlate of Early Recurrence in Unipolar Affective Disorder." *Arch Gen Psychiatry* 47:1100–1105, 1990. Used with permission. Copyright 1990, American Medical Association.

Longitudinal Associations Between Sleep, Dreaming, and Mood

In contrast to the lines of investigation previously described, other research has focused on the possibility that EEG sleep changes, especially changes in REM sleep or dreaming, may signal fundamental alterations in cognitive or affective processing among depressed patients. This research is based on the observation that storylike dreams occur predominantly during REM sleep and on theories that sleep and dreaming serve the psychological function of processing affective material aroused during wakefulness. These studies concentrate on the interrelations among daytime mood, EEG sleep variables, and dreaming sleep—either directly by collecting dream reports or indirectly by studying REM sleep variables.

After a series of investigations into the relations between daytime mood and sleep, especially dreaming sleep, Kramer (1993) theorized that dreaming serves a "selective mood regulatory function." Specifically, dreams may serve an adaptive function by problem-solving emotionally significant experiences from the preceding day. Across the night, mood intensity and variability decrease as the emotional preoccupations from the preceding day are altered by the dream process. The success of the dream experience in containing emotional surges and effectively resolving emotional problems from the preceding day is related subsequently to the mood on the following day. Breger (1967) suggested a similar function of dreaming, stating that "the dream [is] a unique place for the integration or mastery of psychological material related to a state of affective arousal" (p. 25).

Given the psychological theories suggesting that dreaming sleep has an affective-processing function and the EEG sleep studies citing abnormalities in REM sleep in depressed individuals, the hypothesis can be advanced that disturbances in affective processing may be reflected in disturbed dreaming of depressed individuals and subsequently in disturbed REM sleep. A review of research on the dreams of depressed patients suggests that the manifest dreams of depressed individuals do seem to differ from those of control subjects and of other patient populations. Although not all findings have been replicated among studies, data have been reported suggesting that acutely depressed individuals have shorter, more barren dreams (Hauri 1976; Kramer et al. 1966, 1968; Van de Castle and Holloway 1970), with more "masochistic" and depressive themes such as hopelessness and helplessness (Beck 1961; Hauri 1976; Kramer et al. 1966) and an excessive focus on the past (Cartwright et al. 1984; Hauri 1976), on family members, and on images of the self as wrong or unattractive (Van de Castle and Holloway 1970).

Longitudinal studies following patients into remission and cross-sectional studies of remitted patients have given variable reports as to the state-dependent and trait-dependent features of the dreams of depressed patients. Kramer et al. (1966, 1968) reported that some, but not all, of the characteristic features of dreams in depressed patients improve during remission while patients are on antidepressant treatment. Cartwright et al. (1984) also found that the dysfunctional themes manifest in dreams during acute depression appear to reverse on remission. However, Hauri (1976) reported that the dreams of patients remitted from depression remain disturbed, revealing persistent "allusions to a hostile environment, excessive focus on the past, labile affect and masochism" (p. 9). Although these studies should be replicated using standardized methods among laboratories, the existence of persistent abnormalities as well as state-dependent disturbances in the dreams of depressed patients would be consistent with the presence of both state-dependent and traitlike features in the EEG sleep disturbances of depressed patients.

It is less clear whether there is a relationship between the relatively specific REM sleep abnormalities seen in depressed individuals and their disturbed dream content. An indirect manner of approaching this question is to compare the EEG sleep alterations of depressed patients with emotional experiences during the daytime, which may be "worked through" in the dreaming process. Cartwright (1983) reported a study designed to test the hypothesis that "the REM sleep disturbance that accompanies depression is an indication of a difficulty in handling waking dysphoric states." In her study, REM sleep latency and REM density were found to relate to mood changes in persons undergoing divorce, that is, those predicted to be undergoing significant cognitive-affective reorganization. The implication was that dreaming may serve to "assimilate and/or accommodate new affective information." Thus, on resolution of the mood-disturbing event, both dreaming and REM sleep latency returned toward normal.

Greenberg and Pearlman (1975) reported significant correlations between a psychological state (defensive strain) and REM sleep latency and REM time in a patient in psychoanalysis. They also were working on a hypothesis that dreaming sleep serves an adaptive function to resolve or defend against emotional conflicts aroused during daytime experiences. Hauri and Hawkins (1971) showed that phasic REM sleep was one of the few EEG sleep variables that directly related to day-to-day fluctuations in psychological state in a sample of nine depressed inpatients treated with a variety of somatic treatments. Although they recognized that alterations in the content of dreams may result from depression and its treatment, they emphasized a neurobiological deficit rather than the primacy of dreaming for affective processing.

Nofzinger et al. (in press) further explored the relation between daytime affect and REM sleep in 45 depressed men before and after treatment with cognitive-behavior therapy and in a control group of

43 healthy subjects. The intensity of daytime affect (as measured by the sum of positive and negative affects) in depressed men correlated significantly and positively with phasic REM sleep measures both at pretreatment and posttreatment. This relationship was not found in healthy control subjects. In depressed men, both affect intensity and phasic REM sleep measures decreased over the course of treatment. In light of research on affect intensity and phasic REM sleep, they hypothesized that longitudinal alterations in phasic REM sleep seen in depressed patients may relate, in part, to fundamental features of their affective experience. In particular, the inability of depressed individuals to adequately process even normal levels of affect intensity may be associated with emotional instability, increased levels of physiological arousal, and ultimately a negative affective balance. They further hypothesized that the primary disturbance in affective processing and subsequent arousal may be reflected by elevations in phasic REM sleep, a physiological state of autonomic instability.

Successful treatment of depression may help depression-prone persons deal with limitations in processing affective information. Such individuals can be treated either by increasing their affective-processing capacity so that they can successfully manage a "normal" level of affect intensity or by reducing or dampening their level of affect intensity, which allows them to maintain a positive, stable state of mind, albeit at the cost of a reduced level of emotional experience. The persistence of the relationship between affect intensity and phasic REM sleep in depressed patients (but not in control subjects) may represent an underlying vulnerability in terms of affective-processing capability for some depressed persons.

Major findings from longitudinal studies of relationships between EEG sleep and clinical findings are summarized in Table 26–4.

IMPLICATIONS OF LONGITUDINAL SLEEP STUDIES IN DEPRESSION

Sleep disturbance is a frequent subjective correlate of depression, and insomnia complaints may represent early symptoms of, or risk factors for, new depressive episodes. Some particular aspects of EEG sleep and related physiological phenomena remain stable through the course of a depressed episode and into remission; examples include slow-wave sleep, REM sleep latency, and measurements of NPT. Other sleep measures—most notably, subjective estimates of sleep quality, objective sleep continuity, and phasic REM activity—improve as depressive symptoms remit. Sleep measures may help to predict both short-term and long-term clinical response to either pharmacotherapy or psychotherapy, and subjective dream experiences during the course

Table 26–4.   Clinical correlates of longitudinal EEG sleep studies

- Questions addressed
    1. Are EEG sleep studies helpful for predicting treatment outcome with medications or psychotherapy?
    2. Are EEG sleep studies helpful for predicting longer-term clinical outcome?
    3. What are the longitudinal associations among sleep, dreaming, and mood?
- Major findings
    1. Short REM sleep latency and disturbed sleep continuity during baseline EEG sleep studies—and prolongation of REM sleep latency with acute administration of tricyclic medication—predict a favorable short-term response to antidepressant medication.
    2. Baseline EEG sleep measures do not predict acute response to psychotherapy, but nonresponders show more night-to-night variability than responders.
    3. REM sleep latency and temporal distribution of slow-wave activity are associated with time to recurrence of depression.
    4. REM sleep characteristics are associated with the waking affective state over time in depressed patients.
- Unresolved issues
    1. Can EEG sleep measures predict differential response to specific antidepressants or general forms of treatment (e.g., pharmacotherapy versus psychotherapy)?
    2. Do EEG sleep measures indicate which patients require maintenance pharmacotherapy or psychotherapy?

of depression reflect not only the individual's affective state but also his or her affective-processing capacity.

What are the implications of these findings for understanding the neurobiology of depression? At this point, inferences must remain cautious and largely theoretical. The common findings in longitudinal studies to date may, however, point toward more definitive future areas of investigation.

Further investigation of the commonalities between sleep and endocrine regulation provides one way to further understand the longitudinal neurobiology of depression. A substantial body of literature exists to suggest that, as with sleep variables, different neuroendocrine measures show different patterns of dysregulation over the course of a depressive episode. For example, growth hormone secretion is often blunted in depressed patients and remains lower after recovery. This finding has been noted for both adult and adolescent depressed patients and in both basal and "challenge" paradigms (D. B. Jarrett et al. 1990b; Mitchell et al. 1988).

On the other hand, several studies of the hypothalamic-pituitary-adrenal axis suggest normalization of cortisol regulation as patients recover from their depressive symptoms (e.g., Greden et al. 1983; Holboer et al. 1982). Given that growth hormone is usually secreted in association with slow-wave sleep (D. B. Jarrett et al. 1990a), that the circadian pattern of cortisol secretion is temporally associated with REM sleep (Weitzman et al. 1974), and that common neurotransmitter systems affect sleep and endocrine regulation, simultaneous investigation of sleep and endocrine measures may elucidate underlying dysregulations more effectively than either type of study alone. Ehlers and Kupfer (1987) and Kupfer and Ehlers (1989) suggested a theoretical model for the link between sleep and endocrine regulation in depression, which includes both persistent (traitlike) and episodic (statelike) abnormalities. Future investigations and analyses may benefit from improved measurement and analytic tools, including more sophisticated EEG sleep measurements (e.g., period and amplitude analysis, spectral analysis, and measures of "dimensionality") and multivariate statistical models.

Linking sleep and other circadian-rhythm measurements may also clarify the neurobiological implications of longitudinal sleep studies in depression. Studies of core body temperature and cortisol suggest that decreased amplitude constitutes the major circadian dysregulation in depression (unipolar depression in particular) (Schulz and Lund 1985; Wehr 1990). Shortened REM sleep latency correlates with this "flattening" (Schulz and Lund 1985) during depression. Furthermore, treatment with antidepressants both prolongs REM sleep latency and "deepens" the temperature rhythm, and the changes in these two measures correlate significantly (Avery et al. 1982; Monk et al., submitted for publication; Souetre et al. 1988).

Further studies must clarify whether temperature and other circadian rhythms "normalize" with successful nonpharmacological treatments or after withdrawal of antidepressant agents. Preliminary data indicate that temperature-rhythm amplitude is not substantially altered at baseline in moderately depressed outpatients who respond to psychotherapy and that these rhythms do not change significantly after symptomatic remission. It may be that short REM sleep latency and decreased amplitude of core body temperature rhythm reflect a single underlying rhythm disturbance in a subgroup of depressed patients; the clinical and further neurobiological characterization of such a subgroup awaits further clarification.

Ultimately, one would like to understand the longitudinal relationships between sleep and depression from a neuropharmacological perspective. However, despite recent advances in the neuropharmacology of depression, we are still at a relatively early stage in our understanding of this area. Early cholinergic-monoaminergic models of depression still hold considerable interest for investigators studying sleep abnormalities in depression. McCarley (1982) and others have noted that both mood regulation and cyclic alternations in REM-NREM sleep involve interactions between cholinergic and monoaminergic neuronal systems. Tipping this balance in favor of cholinergic tone leads to depression-like symptoms, a more rapid occurrence of REM sleep (i.e., short REM sleep latency), and suppression of slow-wave sleep. Steriade and McCarley (1990) further argued, based on mathematical models of REM-NREM sleep interaction, that a relative lowering of monoaminergic tone most closely predicts the actual sleep changes seen in depressed patients.

Adapting the cholinergic-monoaminergic model to longitudinal studies proves somewhat more problematic, because some studies of cholinergic induction of REM sleep indicate a persistent (traitlike) vulnerability (e.g., Sitaram et al. 1980), whereas others show normalization of cholinergic supersensitivity (Berger et al. 1989). Discrepancies among studies may relate to the particular agents used (which may have different specificities for cholinergic systems), different capacities for suppressing monoaminergic activity, or both.

Building on the model proposed by Kupfer and Ehlers (1989), one might further hypothesize that sleep abnormalities in major depression include two sorts of defects: a persistent, traitlike weakening of monoaminergic tone, which leads to reduced slow-wave sleep and provides increased sensitivity to cholinergic agents; and an episodic, statelike heightening of cholinergic sensitivity, which leads to increased phasic REM activity, sleep-continuity disturbances, and disturbed dreaming during the episode. Both defects could contribute to short REM sleep latency, and the combination could make sleep-onset REM periods more likely during the acute episode. Either reduced monoaminergic tone or heightened cholinergic tone could result, at least in part, from instability in circadian rhythms of the neuronal systems. This model could be tested by longitudinal studies that examine a number of physiological systems (e.g., sleep, temperature, endocrine) simultaneously, using both basal and challenge conditions. A longitudinal perspective on these physiological changes would also benefit from increased attention to studies not only of depressed probands but also of at-risk family members (see Chapter 25). This strategy offers the best chance to determine whether EEG sleep measures and physiological dysregulation may actually precede an initial episode of depression.

Finally, longitudinal sleep studies in depression may benefit from more sensitive statistical techniques to maximize the informational value of the data collected. Dew et al. (in press) recently demonstrated the utility of such techniques in a longitudinal study of sleep and psychosocial measures in healthy elderly subjects. Using cluster analysis and discriminant function analysis, the investigators found three distinct sleep subgroups among the sample. More importantly, these subgroups differed not only in terms of concurrent and antecedent psychosocial variables, but also in terms of psychosocial measures—including depression ratings—obtained 1 year later. Adapting these techniques to apparently homogeneous groups of depressed patients may identify relevant subgroups in terms of longitudinal sleep and clinical patterns and may help to clarify the role of acute and chronic psychosocial stressors in the sleep patterns and clinical symptoms of these patients.

REFERENCES

Avery D, Gildschiodtz G, Rafaelsen O: REM latency and temperature in affective disorder before and after treatment. Biol Psychiatry 17:463–470, 1982

Beck AT, Ward CH: Dreams of depressed patients. Arch Gen Psychiatry 5:66–71, 1961

Benca RM, Obermeyer WH, Thisted RA, et al: Sleep and psychiatric disorders: a meta-analysis. Arch Gen Psychiatry 49:651–668, 1992

Berger M, Riemann D, Hochli D, et al: The cholinergic rapid eye movement sleep induction test with RS-86. Arch Gen Psychiatry 46:421–428, 1989

Breger L: Function of dreams. J Abnorm Psychol Monograph 72:1–28, 1967

Buysse DJ, Kupfer DJ: Diagnostic and research applications of electroencephalographic sleep studies in depression: conceptual and methodological issues. J Nerv Ment Dis 178:405–414, 1990

Buysse DJ, Kupfer DJ: Sleep disorders in depressives disorders, in The Biology of Depressive Disorders, Part A: A Systems Perspective. Edited by Mann JJ, Kupfer DJ. New York, Plenum, 1993, pp 123–154

Buysse DJ, Reynolds CF III, Houck PR, et al: Age of illness onset and sleep EEG variables in elderly depressives. Biol Psychiatry 24:355–359, 1988

Buysse DJ, Kupfer DJ, Frank E, et al: Electroencephalographic sleep studies in depressed patients treated with psychotherapy, I: baseline studies in responders and nonresponders. Psychiatry Res 40:13–26, 1992a

Buysse DJ, Kupfer DJ, Frank E, et al: Electroencephalographic sleep studies in depressed patients treated with psychotherapy, II: longitudinal studies at baseline and recovery. Psychiatry Res 40:27–40, 1992b

Cartwright RD: Rapid eye movement sleep characteristics during and after mood-disturbing events. Arch Gen Psychiatry 40:197–201, 1983

Cartwright RD, Lloyd S, Knight S, et al: Broken dreams: a study of the effects of divorce and depression on dream content. Psychiatry Res 47:251–259, 1984

Cartwright RD, Kravitz HM, Eastman CI, et al: REM latency and the recovery from depression: getting over divorce. Am J Psychiatry 148:1530–1535, 1991

Coble PA, Kupfer DJ, Spiker DG, et al: EEG sleep in primary depression: a longitudinal placebo study. J Affect Disord 1:131–138, 1979

Dew MA, Reynolds CF III, Monk TH, et al: Psychosocial correlates and sequelae of EEG sleep in healthy elders. J Gerontol (in press)

Dryman A, Eaton WW: Affective symptoms associated with the onset of major depression in the community: findings from the U.S. National Institute of Mental Health Epidemiologic Catchment Area Program. Acta Psychiatr Scand 84(1):1–5, 1991

Duncan WC, Gillin JC, Post RM, et al: Relationship between EEG sleep patterns and clinical improvement in depressed patients treated with sleep deprivation. Biol Psychiatry 15:879–889, 1980

Ehlers CL, Kupfer DJ: Hypothalamic peptide modulation of EEG sleep in depression: a further application of the S-process hypothesis. Biol Psychiatry 22:513–517, 1987

Fawcett J, Scheftner WA, Fogg L, et al: Time-related predictors of suicide in major affective disorder. Am J Psychiatry 147:1189–1194, 1990

Fisher C, Gross J, Zuch J: Cycle of penile erection synchronous with dreaming (REM) sleep: preliminary report. Arch Gen Psychiatry 12:29–45, 1965

Ford DE, Kamerow DB: Epidemiologic study of sleep disturbances and psychiatric disorders: an opportunity for prevention? JAMA 262:1479–1484, 1989

Gerner RH, Post RM, Gillin JC, et al: Biological and behavioral effects of one night's sleep deprivation in depressed patients and normals. J Psychiatr Res 15:21–40, 1979

Giles DE, Jarrett RB, Roffwarg HP, et al: Reduced rapid eye movement latency: a predictor of recurrence of depression. Neuropsychopharmacology 1:33–39, 1987

Giles DE, Roffwarg HP, Rush AJ: A cross-sectional study of the effects of depression on REM latency. Biol Psychiatry 28:697–704, 1990

Gillin JC, Wyatt RJ, Fram D: The relationship between changes in REM sleep and clinical improvement in depressed patients treated with amitriptyline. Psychopharmacology 59:267–272, 1978

Gillin JC, Sutton L, Ruiz C, et al: The cholinergic rapid eye movement induction test with arecoline in depression. Arch Gen Psychiatry 48:264–270, 1991

Greenberg R, Pearlman C: REM sleep and the analytic process: a psychoanalytic bridge. Psychoanal Q 44:391–403, 1975

Greenhouse JB, Kupfer DJ, Frank E, et al: Analysis of time to stabilization in the treatment of depression: biological and clinical correlates. J Affect Disord 13:259–266, 1987

Hauri P: Dreams in patients remitted from reactive depression. J Abnorm Psychol 85:1–10, 1976

Hauri P, Hawkins DR: Phasic REM, depression, and the relationship between sleeping and waking. Arch Gen Psychiatry 25:56–63, 1971

Hauri P, Chernik D, Hawkins D, et al: Sleep of depressed patients in remission. Arch Gen Psychiatry 31:386–391, 1974

Hoch CC, Reynolds CF III, Houck PR, et al: Predicting mortality in mixed depression and dementia using EEG sleep variables. J Neuropsychiatry Clin Neurosci 1:366–371, 1989

Hochli D, Riemann D, Zulley J, et al: Initial REM sleep suppression by clomipramine: a prognostic tool for treatment response in patients with a major depressive disorder. Biol Psychiatry 21:1217–1220, 1986

Jarrett DB, Greenhouse JB, Miewald JM, et al: A reexamination of the relationship between growth hormone secretion and slow wave sleep using delta wave analysis. Biol Psychiatry 27:497–509, 1990a

Jarrett DB, Miewald JM, Kupfer DJ: Recurrent depression is associated with a persistent reduction in sleep-related growth hormone secretion. Arch Gen Psychiatry 47:113–118, 1990b

Jarrett RB, Rush AJ, Khatami M, et al: Does the pretreatment polysomnogram predict response to cognitive therapy in depressed outpatients? a preliminary report. Psychiatry Res 33:285–299, 1990

Kasper S, Voll G, Vieira A, et al: Response to total sleep deprivation before and during treatment with fluvoxamine or maprotiline in patients with major depression—results of a double-blind study. Pharmacopsychiatry 23:135–142, 1990

Kennedy GJ, Kelman HR, Thomas C: Persistence and remission of depressive symptoms in late life. Am J Psychiatry 148:174–178, 1991

Knowles JB, Cairns J, MacLean AW, et al: The sleep of remitted bipolar depressives: comparison with sex and age-matched controls. Can J Psychiatry 31:295–298, 1986

Kramer M: The selective mood regulatory function of dreaming: an update and revision, in The Function of Dreaming. Edited by Moffitt AR, Kramer M, Hoffman RF. Albany, NY, State University of New York Press, 1993

Kramer M, Whitman RM, Baldridge W, et al: Dreaming in the depressed. Can J Psychiatry 11:178–192, 1966

Kramer M, Whitman RM, Baldridge B, et al: Drugs and dreams, III: the effects of imipramine on the dreams of depressed patients. Am J Psychiatry 124:1385–1392, 1968

Kupfer DJ: REM latency: a psychobiologic marker for primary depressive disease. Biol Psychiatry 11:159–174, 1976

Kupfer DJ, Ehlers CL: Two roads to rapid eye movement latency. Arch Gen Psychiatry 46:945–948, 1989

Kupfer DJ, Spiker DG, Coble PA, et al: Sleep and treatment prediction in endogenous depression. Am J Psychiatry 138:429–434, 1981

Kupfer DJ, Frank E, Grochocinski VJ, et al: Electroencephalographic sleep profiles in recurrent depression: a longitudinal investigation. Arch Gen Psychiatry 45:678–681, 1988

Kupfer DJ, Ehlers CL, Pollock BG, et al: Clomipramine and EEG sleep in depression. Psychiatry Res 30:165–180, 1989

Kupfer DJ, Frank E, McEachran AB, et al: Delta sleep ratio: a biological correlate of early recurrence in unipolar affective disorder. Arch Gen Psychiatry 47:1100–1105, 1990

Kupfer DJ, Ehlers CL, Frank E, et al: EEG sleep profiles and recurrent depression. Biol Psychiatry 30:641–655, 1991

Lee JH, Reynolds CF III, Hoch CC, et al: EEG sleep in recently remitted, elderly depressed patients in double-blind placebo-maintenance therapy. Neuropsychopharmacology 8:143–150, 1993

McCarley RW: REM sleep and depression: common neurobiological control mechanisms. Am J Psychiatry 139:565–570, 1982

McNair DM, Lorr M, Droppleman LF: EdITS Manual for the Profile of Mood States. San Diego, CA, Educational and Industrial Testing Service, 1971

Mendlewicz J, Kempenaers C, DeMaertelaer V: Sleep EEG and amitriptyline treatment in depressed inpatients. Biol Psychiatry 30:691–702, 1991

Mitchell PB, Bearn JA, Corn TH, et al: Growth hormone response to clonidine after recovery in patients with endogenous depression. Br J Psychiatry 152:34–38, 1988

Mosko S, Zetin M, Glen S, et al: Self-reported depressive symptomatology, mood ratings, and treatment outcome in sleep disorders patients. J Clin Psychol 45:51–60, 1989

Nicassio PM, Wallston KA: Longitudinal relationships among pain, sleep problems, and depression in rheumatoid arthritis. J Abnorm Psychol 101:514–520, 1992

Nofzinger EA, Fasiczka AL, Thase ME, et al: Are buckling force measurements reliable in nocturnal penile tumescence studies? Sleep 16:156–162, 1993a

Nofzinger EA, Thase ME, Reynolds CF III, et al: Sexual function in depressed men: assessment by self-report, behavioral, and nocturnal penile tumescence measures before and after treatment with cognitive behavior therapy. Arch Gen Psychiatry 50:24–30, 1993b

Nofzinger EA, Buysse DJ, Reynolds CF III, et al: Sleep disorders related to another mental disorder (non-substance/primary): a DSM-IV literature review. J Clin Psychiatry 54:244–255, 1993c

Nofzinger EA, Schwartz RM, Reynolds CF III, et al: Affect intensity and phasic REM sleep in depressed men before and after treatment with cognitive behavior therapy. J Consult Clin Psychol (in press)

Puig-Antich J, Goetz R, Hanlon C, et al: Sleep architecture and REM sleep measures in prepubertal major depressives. Arch Gen Psychiatry 40:187–192, 1983

Reynolds CF III, Kupfer DJ: Sleep research in affective illness: state of the art circa 1987. Sleep 10:199–215, 1987

Reynolds CF III, Kupfer DJ, Hoch CC, et al: Sleep deprivation effects in older endogenous depressed patients. Psychiatry Res 21:95–109, 1986a

Reynolds CF III, Kupfer DJ, Hoch CC, et al: Two-year follow up of elderly patients with mixed depression and dementia: clinical and EEG sleep findings. J Am Geriatr Soc 34:793–799, 1986b

Reynolds CF III, Perel JM, Frank E, et al: Open-trial maintenance nortriptyline in geriatric depression: survival analysis and preliminary data on the use of REM latency as a predictor of recurrence. Psychopharmacol Bull 25:129–132, 1989

Reynolds CF III, Hoch CC, Buysse DJ, et al: Sleep in late-life recurrent depression: changes during early continuation therapy with nortriptyline. Neuropsychopharmacology 5:85–96, 1991

Riemann D, Berger M: EEG sleep in depression and in remission and the REM sleep response to the cholinergic agonist RS 86. Neuropsychopharmacology 2:145–152, 1989

Riemann D, Berger M: The effects of total sleep deprivation and subsequent treatment with clomipramine on depressive symptoms and sleep electroencephalography in patients with a major depressive disorder. Acta Psychiatr Scand 81:24–31, 1990

Rodin J, McAvay G, Timko C: Depressed mood and sleep disturbances in the elderly: a longitudinal study. J Gerontol 43:45–52, 1988

Rush AJ, Erman MK, Schlesser MA, et al: Alprazolam vs amitriptyline in depressions with reduced REM latency. Arch Gen Psychiatry 42:1154–1159, 1985

Rush AJ, Erman MK, Giles DE, et al: Polysomnographic findings in recently drug-free and clinically remitted depressed patients. Arch Gen Psychiatry 43:878–884, 1986

Rush AJ, Giles DE, Jarrett RB, et al: Reduced REM latency predicts response to tricyclic medication in depressed outpatients. Biol Psychiatry 26:61–72, 1989

Schulz H, Lund R: On the origin of early REM episodes in the sleep of depressed patients: a comparison of three hypotheses. Psychiatry Res 16:65–77, 1985

Schulz H, Lund R, Cording C, et al: Bimodal distribution of REM sleep latencies in depression. Biol Psychiatry 14:595–600, 1979

Simons AD, Thase ME: Biological markers, treatment outcome, and one-year follow-up in endogenous depression: EEG sleep studies and response to cognitive therapy. J Consult Clin Psychol 60:392–401, 1992

Sitaram N, Nurnberger JI, Gershon ES, et al: Faster cholinergic REM sleep induction in euthymic patients with primary affective illness. Science 208:200–201, 1980

Souetre E, Salvati E, Wehr TA, et al: Twenty-four-hour profiles of body temperature and plasma TSH in bipolar patients during depression and during remission and in normal control subjects. Am J Psychiatry 145:1133–1137, 1988

Steiger A, Van Bardeleben V, Herth T, et al: Sleep EEG and nocturnal secretion of cortisol and growth hormone in male patients with endogenous depression before treatment and after recovery. J Affect Disord 16:189–195, 1989

Steriade M, McCarley RW: Brainstem mechanisms of dreaming and of disorders of sleep in man, in Brainstem Control of Wakefulness and Sleep. New York, Plenum, 1990, pp 395–482

Thase ME, Simons AD: The applied use of psychotherapy in the study of the psychobiology of depression. Journal of Psychotherapy Practice and Research 1:72–80, 1992

Thase ME, Reynolds CF III, Glanz LM, et al: Nocturnal penile tumescence in depressed men. Am J Psychiatry 144:89–92, 1987

Thase ME, Reynolds CF III, Glanz LN, et al: Diminished nocturnal penile tumescence in depressed men. Biol Psychiatry 24:33–46, 1988

Thase ME, Reynolds CF III, Jennings JR, et al: Diminished nocturnal penile tumescence in depression: a replication study. Biol Psychiatry 31:1136–1142, 1992

Van de Castle RL, Holloway J: Dreams of depressed patients, non-depressed patients, and normals. Psychophysiology 7:326–327, 1970

Vollrath M, Wicki W, Angst J: The Zurich study, VIII: insomnia: association with depression, anxiety, somatic syndromes, and course of insomnia. Eur Arch Psychiatr Neurol Sci 239:113–124, 1989

Wehr TA: Effects of wakefulness and sleep on depression and mania, in Sleep and Biological Rhythms: Basic Mechanisms and Applications to Psychiatry. Edited by Montplaisir J, Godbout R. New York, Oxford University Press, 1990, pp 42–86

Weitzman ED, Nogiere C, Perlow M, et al: Effects of a prolonged 3-hour sleep-wake cycle on sleep stages, plasma cortisol, growth hormone and body temperature in man. J Clin Endocrinol Metab 38:1018–1030, 1974

Chapter 27

Sleep Abnormalities in Schizophrenia and Other Psychotic Disorders

Kathleen L. Benson, Ph.D., and
Vincent P. Zarcone, Jr., M.D.

REVIEW OF SUBJECTIVE SLEEP COMPLAINTS AND POLYSOMNOGRAPHIC FINDINGS

As Bleuler pointed out over 90 years ago, "In schizophrenia, sleep is habitually disturbed" (1950, pp. 168–169). In the ensuing decades, there have been many similar descriptions. For example, Mark Vonnegut (1975) stated in *The Eden Express* that at the onset of his first schizophrenic episode, "I realized that this meant I could never sleep again" (p. 12). R. D. Laing (1960), in *The Divided Self*, observed that the patient, before the first episode, is "persecuted by his own insight and lucidity" and so lacks "the assurance" required for sleep (p. 119). That this "assurance" might have a biological basis is strongly suggested by the studies reviewed in this chapter.

Sleep disturbance, particularly at the onset of the first psychotic symptoms and with each subsequent relapse, can be marked. The patient can experience profoundly disturbing, terrifying hypnagogic hallucinations. Fairly frequently, sleeping and waking times are reversed, so that the patient sleeps in the daylight hours; the cause of this reversal has not yet been determined. Unfortunately, the patient may come to prefer a diurnal sleep period because some of the responsibility and anxiety associated with interacting with other people is reduced. Many schizophrenic patients have nightmares. Although there are no systematic studies, anecdotal clinical reports indicate that alcohol abuse and certainly psychedelic drug abuse can both disturb sleep and cause the patient to relapse. During psychotic episodes, hospitalization is almost always required so that antipsychotic medications can be administered

Portions of this chapter are reprinted with permission from Benson KL, Zarcone VP Jr.: "Sleep in Schizophrenia," in *Principles and Practice of Sleep Medicine*. Edited by Kryger MH, Roth T, Dement WC. Philadelphia, PA, WB Saunders, 1994. Used with permission.

and dosages adjusted. Although there is usually a marked improvement in sleep with adequate antipsychotic medications, schizophrenic patients have many enduring abnormalities of sleep structure.

Insomnia—Poor Sleep Efficiency

Schizophrenic patients in a state of psychotic agitation experience profoundly disturbed sleep, often characterized by prolonged periods of total sleeplessness documented by polysomnography. During less severe psychotic agitation, schizophrenic patients experience marked insomnia—long sleep-onset latencies, reduced total sleep time, and sleep fragmented by bouts of waking.

Empirical studies of sleep patterns in schizophrenia consistently report a marked increase in sleep-onset latency. Typically, sleep-onset latency in healthy control subjects is less than 20 minutes; in contrast, sleep-onset latency in schizophrenic patients typically exceeds 30 minutes. Kempenaers et al. (1988) report a mean sleep-onset latency of 104 minutes in schizophrenic patients compared to 28 minutes in depressed patients and 17 minutes in healthy control subjects. The wide divergence in the criteria used to define sleep onset warrants some caution in comparing statistics regarding sleep-onset latency across studies. Van Kammen et al. (1986) reported that severe insomnia is one of the prodromal symptoms associated with psychotic decompensation and that this insomnia may actually precede the occurrence of ratable symptoms of relapse.

REM Sleep and Psychosis

Studies of REM sleep time.   Dreaming has many similarities to psychosis. As Jackson (1958) and Wundt (1987) noted, everyone experiences temporary insanity during dreaming sleep. During rapid eye movement (REM) sleep, hallucinations, perceptual distortions, bizarre thinking, and temporary delusions occur intimately mixed with more normal thought and perceptual processes. This similarity between dreaming and psychosis led to the hypothesis that in schizophrenia the dream state intrudes into wakefulness or *at least* that REM sleep is abnormal in schizophrenic patients.

This spillover hypothesis implies that hallucinating patients have more abnormalities of REM sleep than nonhallucinating patients. Koresko et al. (1963) found that there was essentially little difference in total REM time when hallucinating patients were compared with nonhallucinating patients. Subsequent studies are in broad agreement that total REM time in schizophrenic patients does not significantly differ from normal standards (Caldwell and Domino 1967; Ganguli et al. 1987; Hiatt et al. 1985; Jus et al. 1968; Kempenaers et al. 1988; Stern et al. 1969; Traub 1972; Zarcone et al. 1987). However, total REM time in the acute, waxing phase of the illness may be markedly reduced (Kupfer et al. 1970). This observation may be secondary to the reduced total sleep time that also characterizes relapse. Because REM periods increase in length as total sleep time increases, reduced total sleep has an adverse impact on the development of REM sleep.

REM deprivation.   Research has shown abnormal REM rebound after REM sleep deprivation. Studies by Zarcone et al. (1975), Gillin et al. (1975), and Jus et al. (1977) showed an REM rebound failure in acutely symptomatic schizophrenic patients. Although two studies reported contradictory evidence of a normal REM rebound, the effects of another variable confounded the effects of the REM sleep deprivation by awakenings in both these studies. In one of these two studies, Vogel and Traub (1974) supplemented experimental awakenings with amphetamine administration because amphetamines reduce REM sleep. In the other study, DeBarros-Ferreira et al. (1973) did not control for age or total sleep time. Thus, the majority of studies indicate that REM rebound after REM sleep deprivation by awakenings is abnormally reduced or absent in patients with acute schizophrenia. The mechanism of this abnormality and its relation to the symptoms of schizophrenia remain unknown.

Phasic-event intrusion hypothesis.   The finding of REM rebound failure in acutely symptomatic schizophrenic patients led to the REM phasic-event intrusion hypothesis. Phasic events are those intermittent bursts of rapid eye movements and muscle twitches that occur during REM sleep. This hypothesis contends that the failure of REM rebound in patients with acute schizophrenia occurs because phasic REM events migrate from REM sleep into non–rapid eye movement (NREM) sleep and into wakefulness, thus decreasing phasic events during REM sleep. This decrease of phasic events, which presumably underlie the development of REM sleep, would reduce the duration of REM sleep and would account for the failure of REM rebound. The occurrence of phasic REM events in wakefulness could cause the thought disorders or attention deficits of schizophrenia.

Dement et al. (1969) developed an animal model of the REM phasic-event intrusion hypothesis. Cats depleted of serotonin (5-hydroxytryptamine; 5-HT) by chronic administration of parachlorophenylalanine developed pontine-geniculate-occipital (PGO) spikes not only in REM sleep but also in NREM sleep and wakefulness. In the animal model, the PGO spikes during wakefulness were associated with "hallucination-like" behavior, that is, orienting responses with no stimuli in the environment. When deprived of REM sleep, cats treated with parachlorophenylalanine showed an REM rebound failure with PGO spikes occurring in the waking state. Chlorpromazine reversed the rebound failure and decreased the hallucination-like orienting responses.

Investigators have attempted to test the REM phasic-event intrusion hypothesis in schizophrenic patients, but surface electrodes cannot directly record PGO spike–like activity in human subjects. As an alternative, research focused on possible indirect indicators of PGO spikes such as surface recordings during sleep of periorbital integrated potentials of the ocular muscles and middle-ear muscle activity. However, a comprehensive study of periorbital integrated potentials and middle-ear muscle activity failed to show any significant abnormality in the NREM to REM distribution in schizophrenia compared with schizoaffective disorder, major depressive disorder, and nonpsychiatric conditions (Benson and Zarcone 1985).

REM sleep eye movements.   Investigators have also studied phasic REM sleep eye-movement activity in patients with schizophrenia. In these studies, investigators used measures of eye-movement density to correct for differences in the amount of REM time. Eye-movement density is generally defined as the ratio of eye-movement frequency to the minutes spent in REM sleep, but investigators have used different visual and computer-based methods to define and count eye-movement frequency.

In an early study, Gulevich et al. (1967) reported a trend toward increased eye-movement density in schizophrenic patients compared with nonpsychiatric control subjects. However, Feinberg et al. (1965) found no difference in eye-movement density between schizophrenic patients and control subjects, although among the schizophrenic patients, eye-movement density was higher in the hallucinating patients than in the nonhallucinating patients. Moreover, Benson and Zarcone (1993) confirmed and extended Feinberg's observations using computerized measures to detect eye movement. This recent study found no difference in eye-movement density among schizophrenic patients, nonpsychiatric control subjects, and patients with major depressive disorder, although again, among schizophrenic patients, eye-movement density correlated positively with ratings of hallucinatory behavior on the Brief Psychiatric Rating Scale (BPRS).

REM sleep latency.   Although the studies described above have reported no global abnormality in REM sleep time or eye-movement density in schizophrenic patients, investigators have demonstrated an abnormality in REM sleep latency. During the past 30 years, many cross-sectional and longitudinal sleep studies have reported short REM sleep latencies in schizophrenic patients (Gulevich et al. 1967; Hiatt et al. 1985; Jus et al. 1973; Keshavan et al. 1991; Kupfer et al. 1970; Maggini et al. 1986; Stern et al. 1969; Tandon et al. 1992; Zarcone et al. 1987). Although some studies (Feinberg et al. 1965; Ganguli et al. 1987; Kempenaers et al.

1988) have not found short REM sleep latencies, their averaged group data included variability that suggested the presence of subgroups of schizophrenic patients with very short REM sleep latencies.

In general, we caution that studies of REM sleep latency are not directly comparable because the studies used patient samples differing in medication status, diagnostic subtypes (acute, chronic, schizoaffective), and symptom severity. The more recent studies have explicitly described and applied diagnostic criteria. Moreover, these studies did not necessarily use the same definition of REM sleep latency. The definition of REM sleep latency depends in large part on the definition of sleep onset, which can range from very liberal to very conservative. REM sleep latency can vary by as much as 20 minutes depending on the definition of sleep onset that is used.

Although many investigators have documented short REM sleep latencies in schizophrenic patients, they do not agree about the mechanism(s) that shorten the interval between sleep onset and the first REM period. Feinberg et al. (1969) suggested that a slow-wave sleep deficit in the first NREM period (the interval between sleep onset and the start of the first REM period) could permit the passive advance or early onset of the first REM period. Alternatively, short REM sleep latencies could represent an active or primary alteration of REM sleep mechanisms.

Slow-Wave Sleep

The slow-wave sleep deficit in schizophrenia is one of the most robust research findings. Investigators have observed slow-wave sleep abnormalities in patients with acute schizophrenia (Ganguli et al. 1987; Kupfer et al. 1970; Stern et al. 1969), patients with chronic schizophrenia (Benson et al. 1991a; Feinberg et al. 1969; Hiatt et al. 1985; Itil et al. 1972; Traub 1972), patients with remitted schizophrenia (Kupfer et al. 1970), and long-term-institutionalized schizophrenic patients (Caldwell and Domino 1967). Other investigators reported slow-wave sleep abnormalities in never-medicated patients (Ganguli et al. 1987; Jus et al. 1968), unmedicated patients (Benson et al. 1991a; Caldwell and Domino 1967; Feinberg et al. 1969; Hiatt et al. 1985; Itil et al. 1972; Kupfer et al. 1970; Stern et al. 1969; Vigneri et al. 1974), and phenothiazine-treated patients (Traub 1972). Four negative findings based on visually scored data have been reported, but they may reflect the confounds of advanced age (Jus et al. 1973), small sample size (Kempenaers et al. 1988), sampling bias (van Cauter et al. 1991), or slow-wave sleep deficits in control subjects (Tandon et al. 1992).

The strength of these observations warrants some discussion of the methods used to measure slow-wave sleep. Visually scored slow-wave sleep represents the summation of NREM stages 3 and 4. In an examination of slow-wave sleep deficits in schizophrenia, Benson and Zarcone (1989) showed that the amount of stage 3 sleep is relatively normal in schizophrenic patients and that the deficit in slow-wave sleep is largely confined to the stage 4 component. Furthermore, the night-to-night reliability is higher for stage 4 than for stage 3.

Several computer-based methods are commonly used to analyze slow EEG activity during NREM sleep. These include spectral analysis and combined period and amplitude analysis. Spectral analysis quantifies power density in a select EEG frequency range using the tool of fast Fourier transform; period and amplitude analysis provides baseline crossing counts (the waveform period), integrated amplitude, and first and second derivative measures in user-specified EEG frequency bands. The strength of period and amplitude analysis, in contrast to spectral analysis, lies in its ability to independently quantify both waveform incidence and waveform amplitude. In fact, the visual scoring of slow-wave sleep stages 3 and 4 is based on the confluence of both incidence and amplitude criteria. Stage 3 is scored when delta waves (0–2 Hz) that exceed 75 mV in peak-to-peak amplitude constitute 20%–50% of an epoch; stage 4 is scored when delta waves that exceed 75 mV occupy more than 50% of an epoch. Computer analysis of the sleep EEG is not only more accurate and reliable than human visual scoring, but it is more sensitive to delta activity 1) because, unlike visual scoring of stages 3 and 4, all delta activity is quantified, not just that in excess of 75 mV; and 2) because all NREM sleep epochs are analyzed, not just those visually scored as stages 3 and 4. Although there is as yet no consensus as to the empirical circumstances under which spectral analysis or period and amplitude analysis is preferable, period and amplitude analysis may be the more sensitive technique because of potential dissociations between waveform incidence and amplitude (e.g., benzodiazepines suppress delta wave amplitude while conserving incidence).

In 1974, Feinberg proposed a recovery model of sleep; according to this model, sleep reverses the consequences of plastic brain activity during waking and thus is sensitive to both the duration and intensity of prior waking. This reversal process would take place during NREM sleep and would be greatest during stage 4 sleep. Both spectral analysis and period and amplitude analysis sensitively capture the increased slow-wave activity that occurs during recovery from prior sleep deprivation in healthy young adults. Because slow-wave sleep processes respond homeostatically to the amount of prior waking, slow-wave sleep may serve an important restorative role in the central nervous system and thus may have important neuropsychiatric effects.

Two studies (Benson et al. 1993a; Luby and Caldwell 1967) have used total sleep deprivation as a naturalistic probe to determine whether schizophrenic patients can respond to sleep deprivation with an increase in slow-wave sleep on recovery nights. Luby and Caldwell (1967) deprived four schizophrenic patients of sleep for 85 hours; none showed an increase in visually scored slow-wave sleep during recovery sleep. Luby and Caldwell (1967) concluded that the lack of slow-wave sleep recovery suggested an irreversible brain defect in schizophrenia.

More recently, Benson et al. (1993a) deprived four schizophrenic patients of sleep for one night (40 hours of waking) and quantified recovery sleep using both visual scoring and period and amplitude analysis. On the first recovery night, Benson et al. (1993a) observed a decline in sleep-onset latency, minutes of waking after sleep onset, the number of awakenings, and the amount of stage 1 sleep. Total sleep time increased only modestly due in part to an imposed 8-hour recording period for both baseline and recovery nights. With regard to slow-wave sleep, the duration of the first NREM period (REM sleep latency) increased, as did the amount of stage 3 sleep. Virtually no stage 4 sleep was observed at baseline or on recovery nights, replicating Luby and Caldwell's finding. However, period and amplitude analysis of the delta (0–3 Hz) band EEG revealed an increase in slow-wave activity on the recovery night. Both average baseline crossing counts and average integrated amplitude increased during recovery sleep. These results suggest that the mechanism responsible for the functional relationship between slow-wave sleep and the amount of prior waking is impaired, but not lost, in schizophrenic patients. Finally, the reader is encouraged to entertain the possibility of a significant dissociation between the *function* of slow-wave sleep as a neurophysiological process and EEG indicators of that process. The presumptive *restorative process* may be preserved despite significantly reduced slow-wave activity.

DIFFERENTIAL DIAGNOSIS: ISSUES OF SPECIFICITY

In the preceding section, we reviewed the subjective complaints and polysomnographic findings associated with sleep abnormalities in schizophrenia; however, similar abnormalities can be found in other forms of psychiatric illness. Benson and Zarcone (1991) addressed this issue of specificity in a comprehensive study of sleep measures in four diagnostic groups: nonpsychiatric control subjects, schizophrenic patients, schizoaffective patients, and depressed patients meeting Research Diagnostic Criteria for major depressive disorder. As described by Benson and Zarcone (1991), both schizophrenic patients and schizoaffective patients had longer sleep-onset latencies than depressed patients or nonpsychiatric control subjects (see Figure 27–1, A). Benson and Zarcone (1991) also reported that the amount of waking after sleep onset could *not* differentiate among the three psychiatric disorders (see Figure 27–1, *B*), nor could it differentiate patients with these psychiatric disorders from nonpsychiatric control subjects after correcting for a very strong age effect. Compared with the nonpsychiatric control subjects, schizophrenic patients, schizoaffective patients, and depressed patients had less total sleep and poorer sleep efficiency (see Figure 27–1, *C*); moreover, schizophrenic patients and schizoaffective patients had significantly less total sleep and poorer sleep efficiency than depressed patients. Figure 27–1, *D*, shows that REM sleep latency was significantly shorter in schizophrenic patients, schizoaffective patients, and depressed patients compared with nonpsychiatric control subjects; these three psychiatric disorders did not differ from one another.

Because of significant differences in total sleep time across the four diagnostic groups, sleep stages as a percentage of total sleep are shown in Figure 27–2. These data are also derived from the work of Benson and Zarcone (1991). To summarize these data, the percentage of stage 2

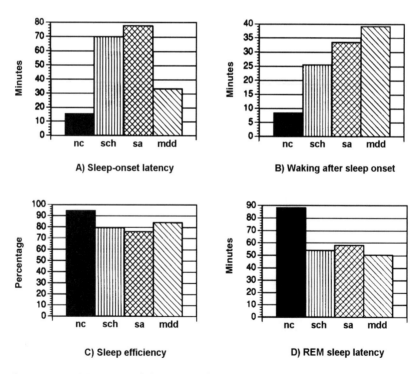

Figure 27–1. Measures of sleep-onset latency *(A)*, waking after sleep onset *(B)*, sleep efficiency *(C)*, and REM sleep latency *(D)* in four diagnostic groups: nonpsychiatric control subjects (nc), schizophrenic patients (sch), schizoaffective patients (sa), and patients with major depressive disorder (mdd).

sleep did not differentiate among the three groups with psychiatric disorders, nor did it differentiate the psychiatric patients from the non-psychiatric control subjects; the percentage of stage 2 sleep was not an age-related measure. The percentages of stage 3 and REM sleep also did not differentiate among the four diagnostic groups after correcting for a modest, but significant, age effect. The percentage of stage 1 sleep was significantly higher in the schizophrenic patients, schizoaffective patients, and depressed patients compared with the nonpsychiatric control subjects after correcting for a strong age effect, whereas the percentage of stage 4 sleep was significantly reduced in the psychiatric patients compared with the nonpsychiatric control subjects—also after

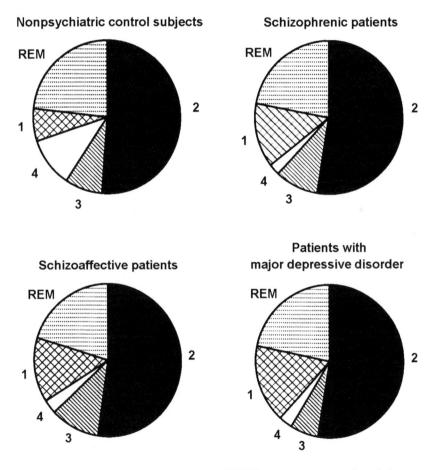

Figure 27–2. Sleep stages (1, 2, 3, 4, and REM) as a percentage of total sleep time in four diagnostic groups: nonpsychiatric control subjects, schizophrenic patients, schizoaffective patients, and patients with major depressive disorder.

correcting for a moderate, but significant, age effect. In conclusion, schizophrenic and schizoaffective patients had longer sleep latencies and poorer sleep efficiency than nonpsychiatric control subjects and depressed patients; furthermore, compared with the nonpsychiatric control subjects, the schizophrenic patients, schizoaffective patients, and depressed patients accrued more light sleep (stage 1) at the expense of a stage 4 deficit.

To date, there have been no systematic investigations comparing the sleep of nonpsychiatric control subjects with the sleep patterns of patients who have major psychotic disorders: schizophrenia, schizoaffective disorder, mania, and psychotic depression. However, various pairwise and three-way comparisons have been undertaken, resulting in the following conclusions: Even though a profound insomnia is a cardinal feature of the sleep of schizophrenic patients, long sleep latencies and poor sleep efficiency also characterize the sleep of schizoaffective patients (Benson and Zarcone 1991; Reich et al. 1975), manic patients (Hudson et al. 1988), and patients with psychotic depression (Ganguli et al. 1987; Thase et al. 1986). Slow-wave sleep deficits also are prominent features in the sleep of schizoaffective patients (Benson and Zarcone 1991; Reich et al. 1975) and patients with delusional depression (Ganguli et al. 1987; Thase et al. 1986), although the presence of slow-wave sleep deficits in manic patients is uncertain. Finally, short REM sleep latencies are clearly characteristic of the sleep of schizoaffective patients (Benson and Zarcone 1991; Reich et al. 1975), manic patients (Hudson et al. 1988), and patients with delusional depression (Ganguli et al. 1987; Thase et al. 1986). In particular, Thase et al. (1986) demonstrated a higher incidence of sleep-onset REM periods in patients with psychotic depression than in patients with nonpsychotic depression.

We turn now to other parameters of REM sleep. Because high levels of eye-movement activity have frequently been associated with depressive illness, the diagnostic specificity of this abnormality has also been investigated. Kupfer et al. (1979) reported that eye-movement densities were similar in psychotic depression and schizoaffective depression. Hudson et al. (1988) found significantly greater eye-movement activity in manic patients than in healthy control subjects. Consequently, high levels of REM sleep eye-movement activity are found not only in patients with depressive illness but also in patients with affective or mood disorders (broadly defined).

In a recent publication, Benson and Zarcone (1993) further explored the issue of specificity by studying the all-night total and the within-night evolution of REM sleep eye-movement density in unmedicated schizophrenic patients, depressed patients, and healthy nonpsychiatric control subjects. The all-night measures of eye-movement density could not distinguish the depressed patients from either the schizophrenic patients or the nonpsychiatric control subjects; all three groups demonstrated considerable within-group variance. However, the pattern of change in the evolution of eye-movement density and length of the REM period from the first through the third REM period differed with diagnosis. Compared with the steeper within-night increase in both eye-movement density and length of REM period shown by the schizophrenic patients and nonpsychiatric control subjects, the depressed patients showed less gain, or a flatter within-night pattern; this effect was associated with the older age of the depressed patients. Consequently, the increased eye-movement density in the first REM period and the increased length of the first REM period seen in depressed patients are largely age-related phenomena. The high levels of eye-movement density found in both psychiatric and nonpsychiatric populations raise questions about the narrow association of eye-movement density with mood disorder and suggest a broader interpretation based on a shared biochemical mechanism, increased central or autonomic arousal, or perhaps some stress-related factor.

BIOLOGICAL MECHANISMS AND CORRELATES OF SLEEP ABNORMALITIES

The pathophysiology and mechanism(s) underlying sleep abnormalities in psychotic disorders are unknown. There are, however, several factors known to modulate or covary with measures of sleep maintenance and sleep staging; these include age, brain structural concomitants, activity of select neurotransmitter systems, endogenous hypnogens, and abnormalities of the hypothalamic-pituitary-adrenal axis.

Brain Structure Correlates

In 1983, Feinberg proposed that an error occurs in the programmed decrease in synaptic density during the adolescence of some schizophrenic patients, resulting in decreased capability for synchronous delta band (0–3 Hz) EEG activity and thus revealing a deficit in slow-wave sleep. Certainly, structural abnormalities in schizophrenia have been implied by many brain-imaging studies (e.g., Suddath et al. 1990). For example, Pfefferbaum et al. (1988) showed that the ventricular system is larger in schizophrenic patients than in control subjects; in a related study, ventricular enlargement was associated with reduced cortical gray matter (Zipursky et al. 1992). Using computed tomography (CT) imaging, van Kammen et al. (1988) reported a significant negative correlation between stage 4 time and ventricular enlargement in schizophrenic patients. More recently, Benson and Zarcone (1992) replicated this finding using regression techniques to quantitatively correct ventricular system volume for variations in both age and head size. Van Kammen et al. (1988) also observed a negative correlation between total sleep time and the size of the third ventricle. Furthermore, Keshavan et al. (1991), using CT technology, reported a negative correlation between the size of the third ventricle and sleep efficiency. The third ventricle may be an important region to image because of its proximity to diencephalic structures (e.g., thalamus, preoptic area, hypothalamus) and the basal forebrain, which have been associated with sleep induction and maintenance (Mancia and Marini 1990).

These studies suggest that sleep abnormalities in schizophrenia may have underlying brain structural concomitants. Furthermore, given the observation by Zipursky et al. (1992) that enlarged ventricles in schizophrenic patients are related to diffuse differences in gray matter, these studies are consistent with Feinberg's model of reduced cortical synaptic density in schizophrenic patients as a potential mechanism underlying deficits in slow-wave sleep. Consequently, if deficits in slow-wave sleep in schizophrenic patients are associated with concomitant structural brain abnormalities, they may be more traitlike than statelike in character. In conclusion, the relationship of brain morphology to sleep abnormalities in schizophrenia should continue to be investigated systematically and should use more sensitive imaging (e.g., magnetic resonance imaging) and sleep quantification (e.g., period and amplitude analysis, power spectral analysis) technology.

Neurotransmitter Systems and Psychopharmacology

Serotonin. For decades, researchers (e.g., Koella 1985) have observed that 5-HT plays a key role in sleep regulation. Although older publications suggested that 5-HT might play a direct role as a hypnogenic neurotransmitter, more recent models (Jouvet 1984) define a more permissive or indirect role for 5-HT as a neuromodulator, possibly inducing the synthesis or release—or both—of hypothalamic hypnogens responsible for the development of slow-wave sleep. Reports (e.g., Idzikowski et al. 1986) that 5-HT_2 antagonists, like ritanserin, markedly increase slow-wave sleep in healthy subjects strengthen the hypothesis that 5-HT plays an important role in sleep regulation. However, these reports simultaneously suggest not a simple modulatory role for 5-HT, but rather a complex and possibly reciprocal interaction among 5-HT receptor subtypes, for example, excitatory 5-HT_2 receptors and inhibitory 5-HT_{1a} receptors.

Recent evidence has emerged to suggest that stage 4 deficits in schizophrenic patients are related to a serotonergic defect. Benson et al. (1991a) demonstrated that cerebrospinal fluid (CSF) levels of the 5-HT metabolite 5-hydroxyindoleacetic acid (5-HIAA) are positively correlated with total slow-wave sleep as well as with the stage 4 component in unmedicated schizophrenic patients. This was the first report of a direct correlation between measures of human slow-wave sleep and 5-HIAA in drug-free subjects. Because low amounts of 5-HIAA in CSF are found in patients with many psychiatric disorders and because deficits in slow-wave sleep are not specific to schizophrenia, low levels of 5-HIAA in CSF may be associated with deficits in slow-wave sleep across a broad spectrum of psychiatric disorders. Support for the nonspecificity of this relationship comes from a recent study showing that measures of slow-wave sleep are correlated with CSF 5-HIAA levels in patients with major depressive disorder (Benson et al. 1993b). Consequently, deficits in slow-wave sleep strongly characterize the sleep of schizophrenic as well as depressed patients, and serotonergic mechanisms significantly influence measures of slow-wave sleep in both diagnostic groups.

Although 5-HT antagonists such as ritanserin markedly increase slow-wave sleep in healthy control subjects (Idzikowski et al. 1986), Benson et al. (1991b) demonstrated that the 5-HT defect underlying stage 4 sleep deficits in some schizophrenic patients is markedly resistant to 5-HT$_2$ antagonists. This sample of 10 schizophrenic patients, in whom visually scored stage 4 sleep was virtually absent at baseline, did not show an increase in stage 4 sleep after the acute administration of 10 mg of ritanserin. (If the sample had included some schizophrenic patients with scorable amounts of stage 4 sleep at baseline, a threshold relationship between stage 4 and the effectiveness of ritanserin might have been observed.) Although ritanserin did not increase stage 4 sleep in these schizophrenic patients, it did promote sleep continuity; the amount of waking after sleep onset, the number of awakenings after sleep onset, and the amount of light stage 1 sleep were significantly reduced. These effects were correlated with plasma levels of ritanserin. In summary then, ritanserin proved to be a centrally active, sleep-promoting probe in schizophrenic patients, but it had no demonstrable effect on visually scored slow-wave sleep. These visually scored data might suggest that deficits in slow-wave sleep in schizophrenic patients are a seemingly permanent or irreversible defect, perhaps of serotonergic origin. However, a more sensitive computer analysis of the sleep EEG, using period and amplitude analysis, determined that ritanserin was at least partially successful in increasing slow-wave activity. Relative to baseline levels, the average number of delta band (0–3 Hz) baseline crossings in each 30-second epoch of NREM sleep increased 18.5% with ritanserin, whereas the average integrated amplitude of these delta band half-waves in each 30-second epoch of NREM increased 22.4% with ritanserin. Although these changes were statistically significant, their magnitude was not great enough to have an impact on the visual scoring of stages 3 and 4 sleep; they were, however, consistent with the demonstrated increase in sleep efficiency.

Clozapine, like ritanserin, is a potent 5-HT$_2$ antagonist, but unlike ritanserin, clozapine falls into the class of newer, atypical neuroleptics with established therapeutic efficacy as antipsychotics. In animal and human studies, clozapine promotes sleep and increases sleep efficiency (Blum and Girke 1973; Spierings et al. 1977; Touyz et al. 1978). Clozapine's effects on slow-wave sleep and REM sleep variables remain inconsistent and may in fact vary with dose, chronicity, and species. In chronic doses, clozapine may increase slow-wave sleep in schizophrenic patients, but it remains to be determined whether any clozapine-induced increases in slow-wave sleep will be associated with clinical improvement; alternatively, slow-wave sleep might not increase with clozapine in those patients with brain morphological changes and large deficits in slow-wave sleep. Finally, chlorpromazine's ability to modestly enhance visually scored slow-wave sleep in schizophrenic patients (Kaplan et al. 1974) might be explained by the relatively high level of 5-HT$_2$ antagonism associated with this conventional antipsychotic.

Norepinephrine. As we previously reported, van Kammen et al. (1986) demonstrated that severe insomnia is one of the prodromal symptoms associated with psychotic decompensation and that this severe insomnia may actually precede the occurrence of ratable symptoms of relapse. Van Kammen et al. (1986) also observed that increased CSF levels of norepinephrine and its primary metabolite, 3-methoxy-4-hydroxyphenylglycol (MHPG), are associated with this relapse-related insomnia.

Dopaminergic-cholinergic hypothesis of schizophrenia. Given the prominent role assigned to dopaminergic dysfunction in the pathophysiology of schizophrenia, there is surprisingly little information on the relationship of sleep abnormalities in schizophrenia to dopaminergic abnormalities. As reviewed above, CSF levels of the 5-HT metabolite 5-HIAA are correlated with slow-wave sleep in schizophrenia. In that study, Benson et al. (1991a) also observed a similar, but weaker, association with CSF amounts of homovanillic acid (HVA), the principal metabolite of dopamine. This association may derive from the fact that HVA and 5-HIAA are often highly intercorrelated in CSF analyses; however, the role of dopamine in sleep abnormalities in schizophrenia certainly warrants further attention. Such studies may likely be confounded by long-term exposure to the dopamine-antagonist properties of antipsychotics. Thaker et al. (1990) observed that patients with longer neuroleptic exposure as well as tardive dyskinesia have more abnormalities of REM sleep time and REM sleep latency during medication-free sleep recordings than do schizophrenic patients with a briefer history of neuroleptic exposure without tardive dyskinesia. There is a higher incidence of nocturnal periodic limb movements in schizophrenic patients than in nonpsychiatric control subjects (see Table 27–1). This observation might be related to an intrinsic dopaminergic abnormality or perhaps to lifetime exposure to antipsychotics.

One might infer that dopamine plays a role in sleep regulation in schizophrenia by observing the effects of antipsychotics on measures of sleep maintenance and sleep staging. In general, antipsychotics improve sleep maintenance by increasing total sleep time and by reducing sleep-onset latency, light stage 1 sleep, and intermittent wakefulness (Adam et al. 1976; Brannen and Jewett 1969; Hartmann and Cravens 1973; Kaplan et al. 1974; Kupfer et al. 1971). With one exception, these studies reported no significant changes in REM sleep time or slow-wave sleep. Kaplan et al. (1974) reported a modest increase in slow-wave sleep; slow-wave sleep as a percentage of total sleep increased from 4% to 6% with chronic chlorpromazine administration (approximately 400 mg daily). One should be cautious, however, when attributing these effects solely to dopaminergic blockade

Table 27–1. Sleep diagnostic studies ($n = 141$) classified according to psychiatric condition and percentage of sleep disorders per psychiatric condition

Psychiatric or control condition	No. reporting sleep disorders (%)
Healthy control subjects ($n = 33$)	
OSAS	5 (15)
Patients with schizophrenia ($n = 55$)	
OSAS	8 (14.5)
PLM	6 (10.9)
OSAS and PLM	1 (1.8)
Other psychiatric disorders ($n = 53$)	
OSAS	10 (18.9)
PLM	8 (15.1)
OSAS and PLM	2 (3.8)

Note. OSAS = obstructive sleep apnea syndrome. PLM = periodic limb movements.

because most antipsychotics are characterized by a profile of diverse receptor antagonism.

One might also infer that dopamine is involved in sleep regulation in schizophrenia by observing the effects of antipsychotic withdrawal. The time course of the acute effects on sleep of antipsychotic withdrawal has not been widely studied. Thaker et al. (1989) reported on sleep in a small sample of schizophrenic patients during chronic antipsychotic treatment and after abrupt antipsychotic withdrawal. The antipsychotics were relatively specific dopamine antagonists, and the administration of anticholinergic medication was continued during the period of antipsychotic withdrawal. During the initial withdrawal period, total sleep and REM sleep declined, REM sleep latency did not change, and slow-wave sleep increased but only in those patients with tardive dyskinesia. In the 2–4 weeks after withdrawal, sleep measures stabilized at a level between the levels observed during chronic treatment and during the first week of withdrawal. Thaker et al. (1989) attributed these changes to the possible unmasking of supersensitive dopamine receptors. Finally, the reader should be aware that most studies of unmedicated sleep in schizophrenic patients occur after 2–4 weeks of medication withdrawal and that antipsychotic withdrawal is often accompanied by the withdrawal of anticholinergic agents.

We turn now to the role of cholinergic mechanisms in the development of sleep abnormalities in schizophrenia. The effect of cholinergic mechanisms on total sleep architecture and REM sleep eye-movement activity has not been rigorously studied in healthy subjects or in patients with psychiatric disorders. Preliminary data suggest that cholinergic agonists decrease slow-wave sleep in depressed patients (Riemann and Berger 1989) and that anticholinergic agents reduce burst eye-movement activity in schizophrenic patients (Douglass et al. 1990).

In contrast, many studies have looked at the effect of cholinergic agents on REM sleep latency. Arecoline (a muscarinic receptor agonist) reduces REM sleep latency, whereas scopolamine (a muscarinic antagonist) prolongs REM sleep latency (Gillin et al. 1982). Given the fact that both schizophrenic patients and mood disorder patients can have short REM sleep latencies, abnormalities in the cholinergic regulation of REM sleep initiation may be present in schizophrenic patients as well. In fact, Riemann et al. (1991) recently demonstrated that schizophrenic patients and depressed patients respond similarly to the Cholinergic REM Induction Test (Gillin et al. 1983), suggesting that short REM sleep latencies in schizophrenic patients may also reflect some cholinergic supersensitivity.

Independent of sleep abnormalities, a link between cholinergic hyperactivity and schizophrenia has been proposed as part of a comprehensive model of cholinergic-dopaminergic interaction in schizophrenia. Tandon and Greden (1989) suggested that cholinergic hyperactivity is related to the development of negative symptoms in schizophrenia. According to their model, cholinergic activity increases as a protective mechanism in the face of elevated dopaminergic activity and psychotic exacerbation. Negative symptoms accompany this cholinergic hyperactivity. With effective treatment, dopamine activity may normalize, but some residual cholinergic hyperactivity may persist, accompanied by negative symptoms. Tandon et al. (1992) suggested that the underlying mechanism of short REM sleep latencies in schizophrenia may be cholinergic hyperactivity.

The Hypothalamic-Pituitary-Adrenal Axis and the Role of Endogenous Sleep and Waking Factors

Since 1980, our knowledge of endogenous hypnogenic factors has rapidly advanced. Some hypnogens enhance slow-wave sleep and, like factor S, were originally collected from sleep-deprived animals (Pappenheimer et al. 1975). The identification of factor S as a muramyl peptide, a component of bacterial cell walls, motivated numerous studies linking modulators of the immune response (e.g., interleukin-1, prostaglandins, interferon, and tumor necrosis factor) to enhancement of slow-wave sleep (Krueger and Karnovsky 1987). Prostaglandin D_2 is an endogenous CNS factor that has been shown to promote sleep in monkeys (Onoe et al. 1988). Alternatively, other endogenous factors may promote waking or arousal. For example, prostaglandin E_2 may be a wakefulness factor in hypothalamic regions known to be important in the regulation of sleep and waking (Matsumura et al. 1989). Because of the profound insomnia seen in schizophrenic patients, prostaglandin E_2 may be elevated in schizophrenic patients compared with nonpsychiatric control subjects; the relevant findings, however, disagree. Mathe et al. (1980) found increased CSF prostaglandin E_2 in schizophrenic patients compared with control subjects, whereas Gerner and Merrill (1983) did not. This discrepancy may be related to the fact that schizophrenic patients vary markedly in their degree of insomnia or sleep efficiency. Prostaglandin E_2 may be positively correlated with wakefulness variables such as sleep-onset latency, the amount of waking, and the number of arousals after sleep onset.

Endogenous factors associated with slow-wave sleep have also been collected during the sleep period. The most investigated substance of this type is delta sleep–inducing peptide. Delta sleep–inducing peptide levels in CSF and plasma are lower in schizophrenic patients than in healthy control subjects (Lindstrom et al. 1985), but their relationship to deficits in slow-wave sleep in schizophrenic patients has not yet been demonstrated.

Other hypothalamic substances, not necessarily identified as hypnogens or wake factors, may covary with or modulate sleep and waking behavior. One example is corticotropin-releasing factor. This factor has been associated with increased EEG arousal and decreased slow-wave sleep (Ehlers et al. 1986). More recently, it has been reported that corticotropin-releasing factor receptor antagonists can restore sleep time previously suppressed by restraint stress (Shibasaki et al. 1986). Corticotropin-releasing factor (like prostaglandin E_2) may be elevated in schizophrenic patients compared with nonpsychiatric control subjects (because of schizophrenic patients' poor sleep efficiency) and may be inversely correlated with measures of sleep efficiency.

Feinberg and March (1988) modeled the within-night distribution of slow-wave sleep as cyclic or pulsatile bursts in the amplitude of delta band (0–3 Hz) EEG possibly linked to the pulsatile release from the hypothalamus of some hypnogenic hormone or neuropeptide. In contrast to some of the previously described studies that sampled basal hypothalamic-pituitary-adrenal axis output at one point in the 24-hour cycle, this model strongly underscores the need for continuous, nocturnal plasma profiles of hormonal activity. Several studies have been attempted, but because few actively ill schizophrenic patients can tolerate the invasive nature of this type of protocol, the sample sizes are not large and any generalizations to be made are limited.

In healthy control subjects, the circadian rhythm of growth hormone and prolactin is characterized by a sleep-related peak. Meltzer et al. (1978) and Vigneri et al. (1974) reported impaired release of growth hormone during sleep in medicated and unmedicated schizophrenic patients, respectively. In contrast, Syvalahti and Pekkarinen (1977) and van Cauter et al. (1991) found a normal sleep-onset pulse of growth hormone. Concurrent EEG sleep recordings were conducted only in the Vigneri et al. (1974) and van Cauter et al. (1991) studies. Slow-wave sleep time was normal in the van Cauter et al. (1991) study, and stage 4 sleep was totally absent in all subjects in the Vigneri et al. (1974) study. The van Cauter et al. (1991) study reported three other findings: 1) no abnormalities in the levels or circadian distribution of corticotropin, 2) an absence of the normal inhibitory effect of the first few hours of sleep on cortisol secretion, and 3) an exaggerated increase in prolactin secretion after sleep onset.

This finding of supranormal sleep-related prolactin release in schizophrenic patients may be related to some underlying dopaminergic or serotonergic dysfunction, or both. Long sleep-onset latencies, deficits in slow-wave sleep in the first NREM period, short REM sleep latencies, exaggerated increase in prolactin secretion after sleep onset, and lack of cortisol inhibition during the early hours of the sleep period—taken together—indicated that the mechanism(s) leading to sleep onset and the elaboration of the first NREM period are impaired in schizophrenic patients.

CLINICAL CORRELATES OF SLEEP ABNORMALITIES IN SCHIZOPHRENIA

Both Ganguli et al. (1987) and van Kammen et al. (1988) reported an inverse correlation between slow-wave sleep and the negative symptoms of schizophrenia (e.g., affective flattening, inattentiveness, and motor retardation). Across these studies, measurement of slow-wave sleep as well as the assessment of negative symptoms differed, and both studies used a small sample of 10 or fewer subjects. Their observations are, however, consistent with the earlier work of Orzack et al. (1977), who reported normal amounts of slow-wave sleep in *good attenders* and low amounts of slow-wave sleep in *poor attenders* using the Continuous Performance Test. In contrast, Zarcone et al. (1990) and Tandon et al. (1992) found no association between negative symptoms and slow-wave sleep. However, Tandon et al. (1992) did note that REM sleep latency was inversely correlated with both negative and positive symptoms.

Also in regard to positive symptoms, recall that both Feinberg et al. (1965) and Benson and Zarcone (1993) found that REM sleep eye-movement density was higher in hallucinating than in nonhallucinating schizophrenic patients. Other studies have examined positive symptoms in relationship to sleep measures. Zarcone et al. (1990) observed no correlation between slow-wave sleep and the BPRS subfactor for positive symptoms (e.g., unusual thought content, conceptual disorganization, and hallucinatory behavior). They did, however, note a strong positive correlation between sleep-onset latency and the positive symptom subfactor of the BPRS, thus supporting the association of psychosis with insomnia.

Global measures of psychosis as well as total BPRS scores have also been investigated in relationship to sleep abnormalities in schizophrenic patients. Kempenaers et al. (1988) found that the BPRS was positively correlated with waking and inversely correlated with both REM sleep time and the amount of slow-wave sleep. Thaker et al. (1990) reported that REM sleep latency was inversely correlated with total BPRS scores. Finally, Neylan et al. (1992), using the Bunney-Hamburg Psychosis Scale (Bunney and Hamburg 1963), noted that in medication-free patients, the psychosis scale was negatively correlated with measures of sleep efficiency and slow-wave sleep; however, in patients who were clinically stabilized on haloperidol, the psychosis scale was positively correlated with REM sleep time and inversely correlated with REM sleep latency.

Across a broad spectrum of psychiatric disorders including schizophrenia, acts of aggression toward self and others have been associated with a defect in serotonergic mechanisms, often demonstrated by low levels of 5-HIAA in CSF. To summarize many studies, low amounts of 5-HIAA in CSF may define a biological indicator of *behavioral impulsivity* rather than violence or aggression per se. Because stage 4 sleep deficits in schizophrenia and depression have been associated with low CSF amounts of 5-HIAA (Benson et al. 1991a; Benson et al. 1993b), stage 4 sleep deficits may define a low 5-HT syndrome that, in turn, may mark a propensity for poor impulse control. When poor impulse control is added to dysphoria or delusional ideation, schizophrenic patients may be at serious risk for a suicide attempt.

CLINICAL APPLICATIONS

Therapeutic Intervention

To isolate themselves socially and avoid painful interactions with other people, many schizophrenic patients develop bad habits in relation to sleep initiation and sleep maintenance. These habits include sleep reversals and polyphasic sleep patterns sometimes complicated by heavy self-medication with alcohol or other psychoactive drugs. There are no systematic studies of the application of sleep hygiene to inpatient groups of schizophrenic patients; however, there is every reason to believe that patients would respond to sleep hygiene counseling and to relaxation training to help sleep initiation, sleep maintenance, and stress management. Ideally, most schizophrenic patients are seen for long-term follow-up in day hospitals and outpatient clinics; in these settings, the opportunity exists to work with patients on sleep hygiene to improve their overall level of functioning.

The chronic administration of antipsychotic medications typically improves sleep maintenance; there is, however, some question as to whether these changes in sleep architecture occur secondary to clinical improvement. As reviewed previously, antipsychotics uniformly produce some sedation (increased total sleep, reduced sleep-onset latency, reduced stage 1 sleep, and reduced intermittent awakenings), but they produce only modest changes in REM sleep time and slow-wave sleep. One study by Kaplan et al. (1974) demonstrated that chlorpromazine produced a statistically significant but rather minor increase in visually scored slow-wave sleep.

Although REM sleep deprivation has demonstrated therapeutic efficacy in patients with mood disorders, neither selective REM sleep deprivation nor total sleep deprivation has been used in the treatment of schizophrenic patients. From a research perspective, total sleep deprivation has been noted to increase the social interaction of schizophrenic patients (Luby and Caldwell 1967) and to decrease symptom severity after recovery sleep (Benson et al. 1993a). However, a large systematic study of the effects of total sleep deprivation on schizophrenic patients has not been performed.

Diagnostic Intervention

The sleep disorders specialist is not likely to be asked to assist in the differentiation of schizophrenia from other psychiatric disorders because there is as yet no consensus that abnormalities of sleep maintenance or architecture can differentiate among psychiatric disorders. Schizophrenic patients do, however, suffer from a variety of sleep disorders other than the sleep disruption associated with their psychosis. Some of the most common include sleep disorders associated with the abuse of, or dependence on, alcohol and illicit drugs. The incidence of intrinsic sleep disorders is also high in psychiatric populations. Sleep studies may assist in the differential diagnosis of excessive daytime somnolence in schizophrenic patients for whom overdosage with neuroleptics may be suspected. It is obvious that schizophrenic patients who are sleepy have to be assessed in the same manner as any other patients referred to the sleep disorders specialist. Given the higher prevalence of comorbidity of sleep disorders seen in schizophrenic patients, causes of excessive daytime somnolence in schizophrenic patients other than neuroleptic overdoses have to be strongly entertained. For example, schizophrenic patients can also meet criteria for narcolepsy, but the incidence of comorbidity of schizophrenia and narcolepsy is currently unknown.

Alternatively, the sleep clinic may be of value in differentiating narcolepsy *from* schizophrenia (Douglass et al. 1991). This distinction may be particularly important because a mistake in diagnosis can result in a very high risk-benefit ratio for the patients. Antipsychotics with their risk of causing tardive dyskinesia should not be prescribed to patients with narcolepsy; however, stimulants and anticataplexy medication may cure a narcoleptic patient misdiagnosed as schizophrenic. In addition to narcolepsy, psychiatric patients are often comorbid for obstructive sleep apnea syndrome or sleep-related periodic leg movements (see Table 27–1). These disorders can have a profound impact on sleep-onset latency, sleep fragmentation, sleep staging, and daytime somnolence. In particular, deficits of slow-wave sleep associated with these conditions can mask or confound *true* slow-wave sleep potential clearly demonstrated after treatment (e.g., with nasal continuous positive airway pressure).

THEORETICAL ISSUES AND DIRECTIONS FOR FUTURE INVESTIGATION

Longitudinal Studies

We turn now to proposing some general strategies and specific projects that might shape the future direction of sleep research in schizophrenia. The general strategy we most strongly advocate is the elucidation of state versus trait phenomena among the sleep abnormalities associated with schizophrenia. The central issue here is the stability of the sleep abnormalities when changes in clinical state or symptom severity occur.

To address this issue, a longitudinal study of sleep patterns in schizophrenic patients is required, with data collected from the same patients during different phases of their illness. Each patient would be observed during a period of clinical stability, during relapse when psychotic symptoms are seriously exacerbated, during the return to clinical stability, and, in some patients, during periods of clinical remission. The primary study variables should include sleep-onset latency, the amount of slow-wave sleep, and REM sleep latency. As a starting hypothesis, sleep-onset latency as well as REM sleep latency may vary with the phase of the illness or covary with the symptom severity, whereas deficits in slow-wave sleep may prove to be independent of clinical state.

A secondary issue that can be addressed by this type of longitudinal study is the prediction of future relapse. Here we would hypothesize that deficits in slow-wave sleep might predict a poorer prognosis. A recent publication of Kupfer et al. (1990) indicated that in depressive illness measures of slow-wave sleep predict relapse, whereas REM sleep latency does not correlate with relapse. Neylan et al. (1992) addressed the issue of relapse by observing patients who were clinically stable on haloperidol and observing them again after antipsychotic withdrawal. Sleep recordings were conducted during relapse or after a 6-week medication-free period if the patient remained clinically stable. Sleep measures during haloperidol treatment could not predict relapse; however, slow-wave sleep declined between haloperidol treatment and the medication-free period only in those schizophrenic patients who relapsed.

This strategy of longitudinal study is confounded by the effect of medication (either chronic administration or withdrawal) on clinical symptoms as well as on sleep architecture. Whenever possible, medication-free studies are desirable, but unfortunately these are not feasible for a majority of patients. Consequently, the effects of antipsychotics and other adjunct medication on sleep parameters also need careful study and control. Indeed, another way to assess the state-trait issue and the stability of sleep abnormalities is to use a pharmacological probe or medication.

This general approach gives rise to several more specific questions. First, does the administration of an antipsychotic alter sleep architecture in a rational, dose-dependent manner, and are the effects of chronic treatment sustained? Second, which components of sleep architecture are affected by pharmacological probes? For example, the sedating properties of most antipsychotics should reduce sleep-onset latency and stage 1 sleep while increasing total sleep time, but their ability to promote sustained increases in both REM sleep latency and slow-wave sleep is unresolved. Third, can the sustained use of antipsychotics *normalize* sleep architecture? It is well known that conventional sleeping pills, which fall into the benzodiazepine class of medication, reduce sleep-onset latency and promote total sleep time, but they markedly *reduce* slow-wave sleep. Atypical antipsychotics (e.g., clozapine) may actually increase slow-wave sleep. Fourth, are changes in sleep maintenance and sleep staging independent of changes in clinical symptoms? We highly recommend longitudinal studies of the newer antipsychotics, like clozapine, to answer these last two questions. For example, do these agents produce sustained increases in slow-wave sleep, and do changes in slow-wave sleep correlate with therapeutic response?

Investigators can also examine the relationship between a naturalistic probe such as total sleep deprivation and the stability of deficits in slow-wave sleep in schizophrenic patients. Specifically, do schizophrenic patients respond to sleep deprivation with a homeostatic increase in slow-wave sleep, or are their deficits in slow-wave sleep essentially intractable? Recall that Luby and Caldwell (1967) as well as Benson et al. (1993a) found no homeostatic recovery of visually scored stage 4 sleep after total sleep deprivation in four schizophrenic patients. Benson et al. (1993a) did report a significant but modest increase in stage 3 sleep, as well as an increase in the integrated amplitude of delta band EEG of about 25%. This study warrants replication in a larger sample of schizophrenic patients.

The sleep deprivation paradigm directly examines the stability of sleep architecture and offers two other advantages. First, investigators can conduct sleep deprivation experiments over a brief interval to minimize the confound of changes in clinical state. Second, investigators can use sophisticated computer analyses of the human EEG to examine what brain wave changes occur in schizophrenic patients during recovery sleep. Specifically, will the recovery sleep of schizophrenic patients produce an increase in select EEG frequencies (e.g., 1–2 Hz), as occurs in healthy control subjects during recovery sleep? Such detailed quantification of the sleep EEG can distinguish between global slowing of EEG frequencies more characteristically associated with some pharmaceutical agents and frequency-specific increases (e.g., 1–2 Hz) characteristic of natural slow-wave sleep recovery. This distinction becomes particularly important in analyzing the frequency-specific changes in EEG in response to specific pharmacological probes or medication regimens.

If research can establish the stability of sleep abnormalities in schizophrenic patients, then we would recommend extending the longitudinal strategy to include the onset of schizophrenia in adolescence. If adolescents genetically at risk for schizophrenia develop abnormalities of sleep architecture, particularly deficits in slow-wave sleep, before the explicit onset of the first psychotic episode, then the deficit in slow-wave sleep could provide a marker for greater susceptibility and permit early intervention. Moreover, the longitudinal strategy could also examine the relationship between deficits in slow-wave sleep and an abnormal process of brain development—particularly in those adolescents genetically at risk or those in the early stage of schizophrenia.

Finally, if investigators can establish stability of sleep abnormalities between and across episodes, then such traitlike abnormalities would suggest some permanent or irreversible alteration in the underlying sleep mechanism(s). However, large sample studies of the families of schizophrenic patients with short REM sleep latencies and slow-wave sleep abnormalities may be premature until we confirm the stability of sleep abnormalities. We also note that stability in sleep abnormalities does not necessarily imply a genetic origin; for example, deficits in slow-wave sleep could be associated with perinatal brain damage, which is also linked to the development of schizophrenia. As another example, short REM sleep latencies might reflect a kind of "scar" that marks repeated responses to environmentally determined psychological stress.

Cross-Sectional Studies

The second general strategy we advocate is the cross-sectional study of the biological correlates of sleep disorders in schizophrenia. Studies of biological correlates assume greater importance when we recognize that abnormalities of sleep maintenance, REM sleep latency, and slow-wave sleep are present in patients with a variety of psychiatric conditions, including schizophrenia. The presence of sleep abnormalities in patients with many psychiatric disorders could reflect the global effects of chronic stress or central or autonomic arousal, but the psychophysiological impact of these factors on sleep continuity, REM sleep latency, and slow-wave sleep has not been adequately investigated. On the other hand, the mechanism(s) underlying these abnormalities might vary with diagnosis and thus map in some unique way to the pathophysiology or even the genetic defect associated with schizophrenia as opposed to mood disorder.

We previously alluded to the possible relationship between deficits in slow-wave sleep and brain structural concomitants. This model strongly suggests that future studies should jointly examine sleep architecture and brain morphology both in schizophrenic patients and in psychiatric control subjects. In particular, studies should use magnetic resonance imaging to examine both the morphology of brain structures implicated in the etiology of schizophrenia (e.g., cortical gray matter volume, left temporal cortex, hippocampi) and the brain regions associated with sleep *centers* (e.g., thalamus, hypothalamus, basal forebrain, preoptic area). This area of research could also benefit from the use of functional (as opposed to structural) imaging such as positron-emission tomography. Because the mechanisms of slow-wave sleep in schizophrenic patients appear to be associated with a serotonergic defect, functional imaging could examine the relationship of deficits in slow-wave sleep to the binding of ligands to the various serotonergic receptor subtypes.

Cross-sectional studies can further extend the rapid growth in our knowledge of the body's endogenous sleep-wake factors. Many of these endogenous hypnogens, like delta sleep–inducing peptide and prostaglandin D_2, enhance slow-wave sleep. On the other hand, prostaglandin E_2 and corticotropin-releasing factor, which have been associated with waking, may be elevated in schizophrenic patients compared with control subjects. More research could systematically investigate these endogenous factors in schizophrenic patients as a possible way to understand both the insomnia and the deficits in slow-wave sleep seen in these patients. Other cross-sectional studies could examine the relationship of sleep abnormalities to hypothalamic mechanisms. In particular, the pulsatile profile of slow-wave sleep clearly suggests the need for substantive investigation of continuous, nocturnal hypothalamic and pituitary output.

Finally, cross-sectional studies could evaluate the relationship between abnormalities in slow-wave sleep and abnormal temperature regulation in schizophrenic patients. Research has shown a strong link between sleep and temperature regulation. Normally, the body's thermostat is turned down during sleep and the body (as well as the brain) cools. Some research has suggested that there is a brain-specific *restorative* function associated with the cooling during slow-wave sleep. If sleep-related cooling is absent in schizophrenic patients with deficits in slow-wave sleep, one might speculate that the brain-specific restorative function is defective and that deficits in slow-wave sleep might be risk factors for the development of thought disorders in schizophrenia.

REFERENCES

Adam K, Allen S, Carruthers-Jones I, et al: Mesoridazine and human sleep. Br J Clin Pharmacol 3:157–163, 1976

Benson KL, Zarcone VP: Testing the REM sleep phasic event intrusion hypothesis of schizophrenia. Psychiatry Res 15:163–173, 1985

Benson KL, Zarcone VP: Slow wave sleep deficits: their magnitude, distribution and reliability (abstract). Sleep Research 18:165, 1989

Benson KL, Zarcone VP: REM latency, eye movement density and slow wave sleep in schizophrenia and depression, in Biological Psychiatry, Vol 1. Edited by Racagni G, Brunello N, Fukuda T. Amsterdam, Elsevier Science Publishers BV, 1991, pp 811–813

Benson KL, Zarcone VP: Slow wave sleep and brain structural imaging in schizophrenia (abstract). Sleep Research 21:149, 1992

Benson KL, Zarcone VP: REM sleep eye movement activity in schizophrenia and depression. Arch Gen Psychiatry 50:474–482, 1993

Benson KL, Faull KF, Zarcone VP: Evidence for the role of serotonin in the regulation of slow wave sleep in schizophrenia. Sleep 14:133–139, 1991a

Benson KL, Csernansky JG, Zarcone VP: The effect of ritanserin in slow wave sleep deficits and sleep continuity in schizophrenia (abstract). Sleep Research 20:170, 1991b

Benson KL, Sullivan EV, Lim KO, et al: The effect of total sleep deprivation on slow wave sleep recovery in schizophrenia. Sleep Research 22, 1993a

Benson KL, Faull K, Zarcone VP: The effects of age and serotonergic activity on slow wave sleep in depressive illness. Biol Psychiatry 33:842–844, 1993b

Bleuler E: Dementia Praecox. New York, International University Press, 1950

Blum A, Girke W: Marked increase in REM sleep produced by a new antipsychotic compound. Clin Electroencephalogr 4:80–84, 1973

Brannen JO, Jewett RE: Effects of selected phenothiazines on REM sleep in schizophrenics. Arch Gen Psychiatry 21:284–290, 1969

Bunney WE, Hamburg D: Methods for reliable longitudinal observations of behavior. Arch Gen Psychiatry 9:280–294, 1963

Caldwell DF, Domino EF: Electroencephalographic and eye movement patterns during sleep in chronic schizophrenic patients. Electroencephalogr Clin Neurophysiol 22:414–420, 1967

DeBarros-Ferreira M, Goldsteinas L, Lairy G: REM sleep deprivation in chronic schizophrenics: effects on dynamics of fast sleep. Electroencephalogr Clin Neurophysiol 34:561–569, 1973

Dement W, Zarcone V, Ferguson J, et al: Some parallel findings in schizophrenic patients and serotonin-depleted cats, in Schizophrenia: Current Concepts and Research. Edited by Sankar D. Hicksville, NY, PJD Publications, 1969, pp 775–811

Douglass AB, Tandon R, Shipley JE, et al: REM density changes in schizophrenia due to biperiden. Biol Psychiatry 27:108A, 1990

Douglass AB, Hays P, Pazderka F, et al: Florid refractory schizophrenias that turn out to be treatable variants of HLA-associated narcolepsy. J Nerv Ment Dis 179:12–18, 1991

Ehlers CL, Reed TK, Henriksen SJ: Effects of corticotropin-releasing factor and growth hormone-releasing factor on sleep and activity in rats. Neuroendocrinology 42:467–474, 1986

Feinberg I: Changes in sleep cycle patterns with age. J Psychiatry Res 10:283–306, 1974

Feinberg I: Schizophrenia: caused by a fault in programmed synaptic elimination during adolescence? J Psychiatr Res 17:319–334, 1983

Feinberg I, March JD: Cyclic delta peaks during sleep: result of a pulsatile endocrine process? Arch Gen Psychiatry 45:1141–1142, 1988

Feinberg I, Koresko RL, Gottlieb F: Further observations on electrophysiological sleep patterns in schizophrenia. Compr Psychiatry 6:21–24, 1965

Feinberg I, Braum N, Koresko RL, et al: Stage 4 sleep in schizophrenia. Arch Gen Psychiatry 21:262–266, 1969

Ganguli R, Reynolds CF III, Kupfer DJ: EEG sleep in young, never medicated, schizophrenic patients: a comparison with delusional and nondelusional depressives and with healthy controls. Arch Gen Psychiatry 44:36–45, 1987

Gerner R, Merrill J: Cerebrospinal fluid prostaglandin E in depression, mania and schizophrenia compared to normals. Biol Psychiatry 18:565–569, 1983

Gillin JC, Buchsbaum MS, Jacobs LS: Partial sleep deprivation, schizophrenia and field articulation. Arch Gen Psychiatry 32:1431–1436, 1975

Gillin JC, Sitaram N, Mendelson WB: Acetylcholine, sleep, and depression. Human Neurobiol 1:211–219, 1982

Gillin JC, Sitaram N, Nurnberger JI, et al: The Cholinergic REM Induction Test. Psychopharmacol Bull 19:668–670, 1983

Gulevich GD, Dement WC, Zarcone VP: All-night sleep recordings of chronic schizophrenics in remission. Compr Psychiatry 8:141–149, 1967

Hartmann E, Cravens J: The effects of long term administration of psychotrophic drugs on human sleep, IV: the effects of chlorpromazine. Psychopharmacologia (Berl) 33:203–218, 1973

Hiatt JF, Floyd TC, Katz PH, et al: Further evidence of abnormal NREM sleep in schizophrenia. Arch Gen Psychiatry 42:797–802, 1985

Hudson JI, Lipinski JF, Frankenburg FR, et al: Electroencephalographic sleep in mania. Arch Gen Psychiatry 45:267–273, 1988

Idzikowski C, Mills F, Glennard R: 5-hydroxytryptamine-2 antagonist increases human slow wave sleep. Brain Res 378:164–168, 1986

Itil TM, Hsu W, Klingenberg H, et al: Digital computer analyzed all-night sleep EEG patterns (sleep prints) in schizophrenics. Biol Psychiatry 4:3–16, 1972

Jackson JH: Selected writings of John Hughlings Jackson, Vol 2. Edited by Taylor J, Holmes G, Walshe FMR. New York, Basic Books, 1958

Jouvet M: Indolamines and sleep-inducing factors, in Sleep Mechanisms. Edited by Borbely A, Valatx JL. Berlin, Springer-Verlag, 1984, pp 81–94

Jus K, Kiljan A, Wilczak H, et al: Etude polygraphique du sommeil de nuit dans la schizophrenie. Ann Med Psychol (Paris) 1:713–725, 1968

Jus K, Bouchard M, Jus AK, et al: Sleep EEG studies in untreated long-term schizophrenic patients. Arch Gen Psychiatry 29:386–390, 1973

Jus K, Gagnon-Binette M, Desjardins D, et al: Effets de la deprivation du sommeil rapide pendant la premiere et la seconde partie de la nuit chez les schizophrenes chroniques. La Vie Medicale au Canada Francais 6:1234–1242, 1977

Kaplan J, Dawson S, Vaughn T, et al: Effect of prolonged chlorpromazine administration on the sleep of chronic schizophrenics. Arch Gen Psychiatry 31:62–66, 1974

Kempenaers C, Kerkhofs M, Linkowski P, et al: Sleep EEG variables in young schizophrenic and depressive patients. Biol Psychiatry 24:833–838, 1988

Keshavan MS, Reynolds CF III, Ganguli R, et al: Electroencephalographic sleep and cerebral morphology in functional psychosis: a preliminary study with computed tomography. Psychiatry Res 39:293–301, 1991

Koella WP: Serotonin and sleep, in Sleep: Neurotransmitters and Neuromodulators. Edited by Wauquier A, Gaillard JM, Monti JM, et al. New York, Raven, 1985, pp 185–196

Koresko R, Snyder F, Feinberg I: "Dream time" in hallucinating and non-hallucinating schizophrenic patients. Nature 199:1118–1119, 1963

Krueger JM, Karnovsky ML: Sleep and the immune response. Ann N Y Acad Sci 496:510–516, 1987

Kupfer DJ, Ehlers CL: Two roads to rapid eye movement latency. Arch Gen Psychiatry 46:945–948, 1987

Kupfer DJ, Wyatt RJ, Scott J, et al: Sleep disturbance in acute schizophrenic patients. Am J Psychiatry 126:1213–1223, 1970

Kupfer DJ, Wyatt RJ, Snyder F, et al: Chlorpromazine and sleep in psychiatric patients. Arch Gen Psychiatry 24:185–189, 1971

Kupfer DJ, Broudy D, Spiker DG, et al: EEG sleep and affective psychoses, I: schizoaffective disorders. Psychiatry Res 1:173–178, 1979

Kupfer DJ, Frank E, McEachran AB, et al: Delta sleep ratio: a biological correlate of early recurrence in unipolar affective disorder. Arch Gen Psychiatry 47:1100–1105, 1990

Laing RD: The Divided Self. Baltimore, MD, Penguin Books, 1960

Lindstrom LH, Ekman R, Walleus H, et al: Delta-sleep-inducing-peptide in cerebrospinal fluid from schizophrenics, depressives and healthy volunteers. Prog Neuropsychopharmacol Biol Psychiatry 9:83–90, 1985

Luby ED, Caldwell DF: Sleep deprivation and EEG slow wave activity in chronic schizophrenia. Arch Gen Psychiatry 17:361–364, 1967

Maggini C, Guazzelli M, Pieri M, et al: REM latency in psychiatric disorders, polygraphic study on major depression, bipolar disorder manic and schizophrenic disorder. New Trends in Experimental and Clinical Psychiatry 2:93–101, 1986

Mancia M, Marini G (eds): The Diencephalon and Sleep. New York, Raven, 1990

Mathe A, Wiesel F, Sedvall G, et al: Increased content of immunoreactive prostaglandin E in cerebrospinal fluid of patients with schizophrenia. Lancet 1:16–17, 1980

Matsumura H, Honda K, Goh Y, et al: Awakening effect of prostaglandin E2 in freely moving rats. Brain Res 481:242–249, 1989

Meltzer HY, Goode DJ, Fang VS: The effect of psychotropic drugs on endocrine function, I: neuroleptics, precursors, and agonists, in Psychopharmacology—A Generation of Progress. Edited by Lipton MA, DiMascio A, Killam KF. New York, Raven, 1978, pp 522–523

Neylan TC, van Kammen DP, Kelley ME, et al: Sleep in schizophrenic patients on and off haloperidol therapy. Arch Gen Psychiatry 49:643–649, 1992

Onoe H, Ueno R, Fugita I, et al: Prostaglandin D2, a cerebral sleep-inducing substance in monkeys. Proc Natl Acad Sci U S A 85:4082–4086, 1988

Orzack MH, Hartmann EL, Kornetsky C: The relationship between attention and slow-wave sleep in chronic schizophrenia. Psychopharmacol Bull 13:59–61, 1977

Pappenheimer JR, Koski G, Fencl V, et al: Extraction of sleep-promoting factor S from cerebrospinal fluid and from brains of sleep deprived animals. J Neurophysiol 38:1299–1311, 1975

Pfefferbaum A, Zipursky RB, Lim KO, et al: Computed tomographic evidence for generalized sulcal and ventricular enlargement in schizophrenia. Arch Gen Psychiatry 45:633–640, 1988

Reich L, Weiss BL, Coble P, et al: Sleep disturbance in schizophrenia. Arch Gen Psychiatry 32:51–55, 1975

Riemann D, Berger M: EEG sleep in depression and in remission and the REM sleep response to the cholinergic agonist RS86. Neuropsychopharmacology 2:145–152, 1989

Riemann D, Gann H, Hohagen F, et al: Cholinergic stimulation with RS 86 and REM sleep in healthy controls, primary MDD and schizophrenia (abstract). Biol Psychiatry 29:99A, 1991

Shibasaki T, Yamauchi N, Hotta M, et al: Brain corticotropin-releasing hormone increases arousal in stress. Brain Res 554:352–354, 1986

Spierings ELH, Dzoljic MR, Godschalk M: Effect of clozapine on the sleep pattern in the rat. Pharmacology 15:551–556, 1977

Stern M, Fram D, Wyatt R, et al: All night sleep studies of acute schizophrenics. Arch Gen Psychiatry 20:470–477, 1969

Suddath RL, Christison GW, Torrey EF, et al: Anatomical abnormalities in the brains of monozygotic twins discordant for schizophrenia. N Engl J Med 322:789–794, 1990

Syvalahti E, Pekkarinen A: Serum growth hormone levels in schizophrenic patients during sleep. J Neural Transm 40:221–226, 1977

Tandon R, Greden JF: Cholinergic hyperactivity and negative schizophrenia symptoms. Arch Gen Psychiatry 46:745–753, 1989

Tandon R, Shipley JE, Taylor S, et al: Electroencephalographic sleep abnormalities in schizophrenia. Arch Gen Psychiatry 49:185–194, 1992

Thaker GK, Wagman AM, Kirkpatrick B, et al: Alterations in sleep polygraphy after neuroleptic withdrawal: a putative supersensitive dopaminergic mechanism. Biol Psychiatry 25:75–86, 1989

Thaker GK, Wagman AMI, Tamminga CA: Sleep polygraphy in schizophrenia: methodological issues. Biol Psychiatry 28:240–246, 1990

Thase ME, Kupfer DJ, Ulrich RF: Electroencephalographic sleep in psychotic depression. Arch Gen Psychiatry 43:886–893, 1986

Touyz SW, Saayman GS, Zabow T: A psychophysiological investigation of the long-term effects of clozapine upon sleep patterns of normal young adults. Psychopharmacology 56:69–73, 1978

Traub AC: Sleep stage deficits in chronic schizophrenia. Psychol Rep 31:815–820, 1972

van Cauter E, Linkowski P, Kerkhofs M, et al: Circadian and sleep-related endocrine rhythms in schizophrenia. Arch Gen Psychiatry 48:348–356, 1991

van Kammen DP, van Kammen WB, Peters JL, et al: CSF MHPG, sleep and psychosis in schizophrenia. Clin Neuropharmacol 9 (suppl 4):575–577, 1986

van Kammen DP, van Kammen WB, Peters J, et al: Decreased slow-wave sleep and enlarged lateral ventricles in schizophrenia. Neuropsychopharmacology 1:265–271, 1988

Vigneri R, Pezzino V, Squatrito S, et al: Sleep-associated growth hormone (GH) release in schizophrenia. Neuroendocrinology 14:356–361, 1974

Vogel GW, Traub A: REM deprivation, I: the effect on schizophrenic patients. Arch Gen Psychiatry 30:653–662, 1974

Vonnegut M: Eden Express. New York, Praeger, 1975

Wundt W: Outlines of Psychology. East St Clair Shores, MI, Scholarly Publication, 1987

Zarcone VP, Azumi K, Dement W, et al: REM phase deprivation and schizophrenia, II. Arch Gen Psychiatry 32:1431–1436, 1975

Zarcone VP, Benson KL, Berger PA: Abnormal rapid eye movement latencies in schizophrenia. Arch Gen Psychiatry 44:45–48, 1987

Zarcone VP, Benson KL, Csernansky JG: BPRS symptom factors and sleep variables in schizophrenia, in Treatment of Negative Symptoms in Schizophrenia—Proceedings of a Symposium Held at the VIIIth World Congress of Psychiatry in October 1989. Oxford, Oxford Clinical Communications, 1990, pp 18–20

Zipursky RB, Lim KO, Sullivan EV, et al: Widespread cerebral gray matter volume deficits in schizophrenia. Arch Gen Psychiatry 49:195–205, 1992

Chapter 28

Normative and Pathological Aspects of Daytime Sleepiness

Thomas Roth, Ph.D., Timothy A. Roehrs, Ph.D., and Leon Rosenthal, M.D.

EPIDEMIOLOGY AND MORBIDITY OF SLEEPINESS

Sleepiness in Various Populations

Surveys have found that between 0.5% and 12% of the population complain of excessive sleepiness. Variations in prevalence depend on the particular subpopulation sampled and the specific question asked. Many of the surveys have asked about "hypersomnia" or "too much sleep" and not specifically about daytime sleepiness or unintended sleep episodes during the daytime. Those surveys that focused specifically on daytime sleepiness generally found rates of 5% and higher.

A 1962 survey (McGhie and Russell 1962) of 2,466 Scottish people found that 0.5% reported "too much sleep," as did a 1976 random sample of people in rural Florida (Karacan et al. 1976). Of 1,006 representative households in the Los Angeles area, 4.2% of the respondents reported hypersomnia (Bixler et al. 1979). In the National Institute of Mental Health Epidemiologic Catchment Area study of sleep disturbances and psychiatric disorders, 3.2% of the respondents experienced "a two-week or longer period of sleeping too much" (Ford and Kamerow 1989). Two surveys of Israeli industrial workers found that 4.4% and 4.9% of those queried reported excessive daytime sleepiness (EDS) (Lavie 1981; Lavie et al. 1979). A random, stratified sample of the white, non–Mexican-American population of Tucson, Arizona, found that 12% of those surveyed reported EDS (Klink and Quan 1987). Moderate daytime sleepiness was reported by 16.7% of a random sample of Swedish people, and 5.7% thought that their sleepiness was a major problem (Gislason and Almqvist 1987). Among Finnish army recruits, 9.5% rated themselves "more sleepy than their peers"; among French army recruits, 5% reported "daytime sleep episodes which disrupted their function" (Billiard et al. 1987; Partinen 1982). A survey of the citizens of the Republic of San Marino went even further to distinguish between postprandial, or midday, sleepiness and sleepiness at other times of the day; the researchers found that 8.7% of the subjects experienced excessive sleepiness at some time during the day (Lugaresi et al. 1983).

Several subgroups have been identified as having higher rates of EDS. In several surveys, younger adults reported higher rates of sleepiness. In the Swedish and San Marino studies, excessive sleepiness was more common in the younger (≤ 30 years) age groups (Gislason and Almqvist 1987; Lugaresi et al. 1983). Similarly, in the Los Angeles and the Epidemiologic Catchment Area studies, young people were more likely to report increased sleepiness (Bixler et al. 1979; Ford and Kamerow 1989). An objective, polysomnographic study (using the Multiple Sleep Latency Test [MSLT]) showed young (ages 21–30 years) adults to be sleepier than a comparison group of middle-aged (ages 31–50 years) adults (Levine et al. 1988). Elderly people as a subgroup also appear to be sleepier than other age groups. Questionnaire studies have found that elderly persons report more daytime napping than middle-aged people, independent of employment status (Dement and Carskadon 1981). Studies using the MSLT have found elderly persons to be sleepier than other age groups (Dement and Carskadon 1981). Among the nearly 25% of the work force engaged in shift work, the rate of excessive sleepiness complaints during waking hours is very high (Akerstedt and Frober 1976).

Morbidity of Sleepiness

The morbidity of sleepiness falls into three general classes: enhanced risk of life-threatening accidents, diminished cognitive and job performance, and impaired psychosocial function. Histories of patients seen at sleep disorders centers point to the life-threatening impact of excessive sleepiness. Nearly half of the patients with excessive sleepiness report automobile accidents, and more than half report occupational accidents, some life threatening (Guilleminault and Carskadon 1977). Also, information regarding traffic and industrial accidents in the general population suggests a link between sleepiness and life-threatening events. For example, the highest rate of automobile accidents occurs in the early hours of the morning, when the fewest automobiles are on the road (Mitler et al. 1988). During these early morning hours, sleepiness reaches its circadian maxima (Richardson et al. 1982). Long-haul truck drivers experience accidents most frequently (even when corrected for the number of hours driving previous to the accident) during the early morning hours, again when sleepiness is maximal (Mackie and Miller 1978).

Shift workers, who were identified above as a particularly sleepy subpopulation, have the highest rate of industrial accidents (Folkard 1981). Sleepiness has also been suspected as playing a primary role in a number of accidents with dire consequences (i.e., the Three Mile Island nuclear accident and the Bhopal chemical accident).

Cognitive and job function are impaired by sleepiness. Many patients with sleep disorders report losing jobs because of their sleepiness (Guilleminault and Carskadon 1977). In industrial efficiency assessments, the poorest job performance consistently occurs on the night shift (Folkard 1981). In children, excessive sleepiness has been associated with learning disabilities (Navelet et al. 1976). A recent study of neuropsychological function showed impaired memory and cognitive function in patients with excessive sleepiness (Bedard et al. 1991). Laboratory studies in healthy, sleep-deprived control subjects have clearly shown a link between sleepiness and reduced cognitive function (Webb 1972).

The impact of sleepiness on psychosocial function is considerable. Patients with disorders of excessive sleepiness report that their family life is disrupted. Also, patients with excessive sleepiness sometimes present at psychiatric clinics with symptoms of anxiety and depression (Roth et al. 1988). Systematic evaluations of patients with various disorders of excessive sleepiness using the Minnesota Multiphasic Personality Inventory have found that these patients have higher scores than healthy control subjects, particularly on the hypochondriasis and depression scales (Beutler et al. 1981). When assessed with the Research Diagnostic Criteria for psychiatric diagnoses, a percentage of sleepy patients meet criteria for an affective disorder or alcohol abuse (Reynolds et al. 1984).

At the clinical level, patients report significant changes in their lives. They experience significant distress and, on many occasions, secondary depression. The impact may be so severe that patients with significant EDS are portrayed as having undergone a change in their personality (when their behavior is compared with their premorbid personality). At the systemic level, the impact on family life is considerable. Because the pathologies that cause significant EDS typically affect individuals during their most productive years, the manifestations of EDS are likely to be reflected in job performance. Sleepy patients are unable to engage in social intercourse without finding themselves awakened by a spouse or friend. This situation may result in an increased level of distress. Other symptoms frequently complicate the patient's life. For example, the effect of sleepiness during the day in conjunction with snoring during sleep or cataplexy during sexual activity can result in a serious challenge to intimacy.

MEASUREMENT OF SLEEPINESS

Self-Report Measures

Many of the various mood scales have factors reflecting sleepiness, fatigue, vigor, or alertness. The Clyde Mood Scale has a sleepy factor, and earlier sleep studies showed that diurnal changes in the sleepy factor relate to the quantity of nocturnal sleep (Kramer et al. 1976). The Profile of Mood States has a vigor and a fatigue factor, and this scale is regularly used in psychopharmacology research to assess the sedative effects of drugs (McNair et al. 1971). A unidimensional scale of sleepiness, the Stanford Sleepiness Scale, is a well-validated and frequently used scale within the sleep field (Hoddes et al. 1973). Visual analog scales of sleepiness and alertness also have been used successfully to assess level of sleepiness (Roth et al. 1982).

All of the previously described scales assess sleepiness at a specific point in time, as opposed to assessing the general level of sleepiness. A recently developed unidimensional scale attempts to measure a person's general level of daytime sleepiness (Johns 1991). The Epworth Sleepiness Scale inquires about the likelihood of falling asleep in eight different situations commonly encountered in daily life. Total scores on the Epworth Sleepiness Scale correlated with MSLT scores and with the nocturnal indices of respiratory disturbance in apnea patients (Johns 1991).

However, in clinical populations, sleepiness often is confused with fatigue, tiredness, and lassitude. In addition, some patients will respond in a socially desirable manner, denying any sleepiness. Thus, patients have rated themselves as alert while showing objective levels of sleepiness (Dement et al. 1978). In an attempt to overcome these problems, a multidimensional self-report scale—that includes psychic distress, social desirability, and behavioral activation factors in addition to the sleepiness factor—has been developed (Rosenthal et al. 1991a). The Sleep-Wake Activity Inventory has been shown to reliably predict MSLT scores, to differentiate sleepy, healthy control subjects without sleep complaints from patients with complaints, and to detect changes in daytime sleepiness after effective treatment of patients with apnea (Rosenthal et al. 1991a).

Electrophysiological Measures

A number of electrophysiological measures have been employed to assess daytime sleepiness. Auditory evoked potentials have been used to assess daytime sleepiness with some success (Broughton et al. 1986). The amplitude of the P300 wave is reduced in patients with narcolepsy compared with healthy control subjects. But compared with the MSLT, evoked potentials lack sensitivity. To a degree, this measure suffers from its state characteristics; that is, it may be a highly labile measure that changes from moment to moment.

The MSLT has gained wide acceptance within the field of sleep and sleep disorders as the standard method of quantifying sleepiness (Carskadon et al. 1986). Using standard polysomnographic methods (including the electroencephalogram [EEG], electrooculogram, and electromyogram), this test measures the latency until sleep onset while the subject lies in a quiet, dark bedroom on repeated opportunities at 2-hour intervals throughout the day. The MSLT is based on the assumption that sleepiness is a state of physiological need that leads to an increased tendency to fall asleep. The reliability and validity of this measure have been documented in a variety of experimental and clinical situations (Roehrs and Roth 1992). A mean sleep latency (i.e., the time to the first epoch scored as sleep) of less than 5 minutes on the MSLT has been viewed as evidence of pathological sleepiness. Mean latencies of 5–10 minutes are seen as a gray zone, and latencies of more than 10 minutes are considered normal.

Alternatives to the MSLT have been developed by some clinical investigators; one such alternative is the Maintenance of Wakefulness Test. This test requires that the subject sit in a chair in a darkened room and remain awake for 40 minutes (Mitler et al. 1982). Another test, the Modified Assessment of Sleepiness Test, alternates maintenance of wakefulness testing with sleep latency testing (Erman et al. 1987). None of these alternatives has produced improved sensitivity.

Behavioral Measures

Given that the MSLT is a valid and reliable measure of sleepiness, the question arises as to how this measure relates to an individual's capacity to function. Direct correlations of the MSLT with other measures of performance under normal conditions have not been very robust (Nicholson and Stone 1986). However, several studies have found that when sleepiness is at maximal levels, correlations with performance are high. For example, MSLT scores after sleep deprivation (Carskadon and Dement 1982), after administration of sedating antihistamines (Nicholson and Stone 1986), or after benzodiazepine administration (Roth and Roehrs 1985) correlate with measures of performance and even prove to be the most sensitive measure (Roehrs et al. 1986). Such findings suggest that significant sleepiness is the necessary basis, or background, to detect performance decrements. Another reason that correlations between performance and MSLT measures of normal or moderate sleepiness are not robust is that laboratory performance and MSLT measures are differentially affected by variables such as age, education, and motivation.

DETERMINANTS OF SLEEPINESS

Although individuals attribute the subjective experience of sleepiness to a variety of factors (e.g., boredom, heavy meals, dark rooms), the level of sleepiness is determined by four variables: sleep at night, circadian phase, drugs, and central nervous system (CNS) pathology. Other factors that are cited by individuals as causes of EDS do not determine the level of sleepiness as much as they modulate the expression of sleepiness. Thus, fully alert individuals (e.g., preadolescents) do not fall asleep in boring situations, whereas individuals who are sleepy because of a chronic sleep debt (e.g., college students) report falling asleep when bored.

The modulators of sleepiness are primarily environment and motivation. Environmental factors such as level of stimulation and posture can affect the expression of sleepiness. For example, sleep-deprived individuals are less likely to fall asleep, even briefly, if they are standing in a crowded room talking to someone compared with when they are lying down in a room alone, reading a book. Clearly, a distinction must be made between what causes an individual to be sleepy versus what facilitates or inhibits the behavioral expression of his or her physiological state.

Sleep at Night

For most individuals, the most important determinant of the degree of daytime sleepiness is nocturnal sleep. Nocturnal sleep both in terms of its duration and its continuity is directly related to daytime sleepiness. Studies in healthy volunteers have shown that total and partial sleep deprivation is followed by increased daytime sleepiness the next day (Rosenthal et al. 1993). The highly consistent and systematic nature of this relation is illustrated in Figure 28–1. Aside from the next-day effects of sleep deprivation, the sleepiness-promoting effect of sleep restriction accumulates over days. As little as 1 hour of sleep lost per night will result in progressive increases in daytime sleepiness (Carskadon and Dement 1981). Conversely, extending sleep beyond the usual 7–8 hours per night produces increases in alertness (Roehrs et al. 1989).

Sleep restriction accounts for the sleepiness of both symptomatic and asymptomatic individuals. Among patients presenting with EDS at a sleep clinic, a subgroup of patients have been identified in whom EDS can be attributed to chronic insufficient sleep (Roehrs et al. 1983). The effects of insufficient sleep have also been evaluated in asymptomatic individuals. In an MSLT study evaluating the level of sleepiness in a young, healthy, asymptomatic population, the sleepiest 20% of the population showed a mean sleep latency of less than 6 minutes (Levine et al. 1988). This level of sleepiness is consistent with that seen in EDS patient populations. The sleepiness seen in these sleepy, but otherwise healthy, individuals can be attributed to chronic insufficient sleep. This conclusion is based on the fact that these sleepy, but otherwise healthy, individuals, like sleep-deprived healthy control subjects, show high nocturnal sleep efficiencies (Roehrs et al. 1990), blunted nocturnal awakening threshold (Rosenthal et al. 1992), and impaired performance on daytime testing (Roehrs et al. 1990). Most importantly, extending nocturnal sleep by increasing nocturnal time in bed from 8 to 10 hours for 5 days leads to these individuals' sleepiness being reduced to levels seen in the general population (Roehrs et al. 1989).

Daytime sleepiness is related not only to the duration of sleep but also to the quality of sleep. Two approaches have been undertaken to evaluate the quality of sleep. The first approach looked at sleep-stage distribution. To date, no one has been able to successfully relate the quality of sleep or the refreshing nature of sleep to sleep stages. The other approach to sleep quality has been to look at sleep continuity. Sleep in patients with a variety of sleep disorders is fragmented by transient arousals that last 3–15 seconds. These arousals are characterized by EEG speeding and a transient increase in skeletal muscle tone. These arousals do not meet the Rechtschaffen and Kales criteria for an awakening, and thus do not affect the scoring of traditional sleep

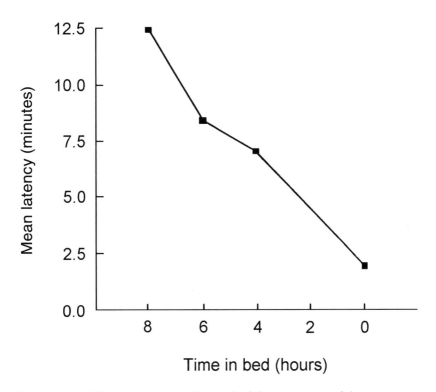

Figure 28–1. Effects of sleep loss (time in bed the previous night) on mean sleep-onset latency, as measured by the Multiple Sleep Latency Test the following day.

stages. Behaviorally, subjects are not aware of these arousals and do not report frequent awakenings during the night even when these arousals occur 60 times per hour. Correlational evidence suggests a relation between sleep fragmentation and daytime sleepiness (Carskadon et al. 1982). Fragmentation, as indexed by the number of brief EEG arousals, correlates with EDS in various patient groups (Stepanski et al. 1984b). Treatment studies also link sleep fragmentation and excessive sleepiness. Patients with sleep apnea syndrome who are successfully treated (i.e., apneas are reduced) by surgery or continuous positive airway pressure show fewer arousals from sleep as well as less sleepiness (Lamphere et al. 1989; Zorick et al. 1983).

Experimental fragmentation of the sleep of healthy persons has been produced by inducing arousals with auditory stimuli. Several studies have shown that subjects awakened at various intervals during the night demonstrate performance decrements and increased sleepiness on the following day (Bonnet 1985, 1986). In recent studies, sleep has been fragmented without awakening subjects by terminating the stimulus on EEG signs of arousal rather than on the appearance of a behavioral response. Increased daytime sleepiness resulted from nocturnal sleep fragmentation in one study (Stepanski et al. 1984a). In a second study, the recuperative effects of a nap after sleep deprivation were compromised by fragmenting the sleep during the nap (Levine et al. 1987).

One population in which sleep fragmentation is an important determinant of excessive sleepiness is elderly persons. Studies have shown that elderly people without sleep complaints show an increased number of apneas and periodic leg movements during sleep (Ancoli-Israel et al. 1981; Carskadon and Dement 1981). As noted previously, elderly people as a group are sleepier than other age groups. Furthermore, there is a significant correlation between the rates of transient arousal and the degree of daytime sleepiness (Carskadon et al. 1982).

Circadian Rhythms

A biphasic, objective pattern of sleep tendencies was clearly observed when healthy young adult and elderly subjects were tested every 2 hours over a complete 24-hour day (Richardson et al. 1982). Two troughs of alertness—one during the nocturnal hours (about 0200–0600 hours) and another during the daytime hours (about 1400–1800 hours)—were observed.

Other research protocols yielded similar results. In constant routine studies (in which external environmental stimulation is minimized and subjects remain awake), Froberg et al. (1972) noted a biphasic circadian rhythmicity of self-rated fatigue—similar to that seen for sleepiness—superimposed on the expected increase in self-rated fatigue resulting from sleep deprivation. In another constant routine study, in which the EEG was continuously monitored, a biphasic pattern of "unintentional sleep" was observed (Carskadon 1985). In studies with sleep scheduled at unusual times, the duration of the sleep periods has been used as an index of the level of sleepiness. A pronounced circadian variation in sleep duration was found, with the termination of sleep periods closely related to the biphasic pattern of sleep latency observed in the studies cited above (Akerstedt and Gillberg 1981; Strogatz 1986).

Earlier it was noted that shift workers are unusually sleepy, and that travelers experience sleepiness acutely in a new time zone. The sleepiness in these two groups of people results from the placement of sleep and wakefulness at times that are out of phase with the existing circadian rhythm. Thus, not only is nocturnal sleep shortened and fragmented, but also wakefulness occurs at the trough of alertness. Several studies have shown that pharmacological extension and consolidation of out-of-phase sleep can reduce daytime sleepiness (Seidel et al. 1984).

Drugs

Drugs also alter the levels of sleepiness and alertness. All of the sedative-hypnotic drugs increase sleepiness, which is their desired therapeutic effect. Benzodiazepines, barbiturates, and ethanol reduce sleep-onset latency as measured polysomnographically on either nighttime or MSLT studies (Gaillard 1989). The probable mechanism for this effect is facilitation of the function of γ-aminobutyric acid (GABA), a major inhibitory transmitter system of the CNS. Each of these drug classes has been shown to be a GABA agonist.

Sedating effects also are seen with some of the neuroleptic and antidepressant drugs. Depending on the patient, sedation may or may not be desirable. Most of the information regarding the sedating effects of these drugs is derived from clinical experience and subjective ratings. There have been few systematic studies using objective measures that compare drugs and doses with respect to their hypnotic properties. The mechanism of the sedation is not clear and may in fact be multiple. Many of these agents have histaminergic effects (see discussion below), but they also affect other neurotransmitter systems (e.g., acetylcholine, serotonin) that have been implicated in the control of sleep and wakefulness.

Many other drug classes produce sedation, but it is clearly an undesired side effect. A commonly reported side effect of the H_1 antihistamines is daytime sleepiness. The antihistaminic side effect has been confirmed in objective studies using the MSLT (Nicholson and Stone 1986). Any differences among the sedating effects of the H_1 antihistamines can be related to the differential liposolubility and CNS penetrance of the specific drugs (Nicholson and Stone 1986). Histamine is now recognized as a CNS active substance, and it is thought to have a role in the central control of wakefulness.

Among antihypertensives, particularly β-adrenoreceptor blockers, there are differences in liposolubility and reported CNS side effects. Several studies have documented the sedating effects of some of the β-blockers by using both performance and polysomnographic measures (Conway et al. 1978). These effects may be due to antagonism of the diffuse forebrain noradrenergic system, which maintains cortical activation.

As expected, stimulant drugs clearly reduce sleepiness and increase alertness. Amphetamine, methylphenidate, and pemoline are used in the symptomatic treatment of the EDS of narcolepsy and have been found to objectively reduce sleepiness (Mitler et al. 1986). These drugs facilitate catecholaminergic activity and thereby enhance and prolong wakefulness. A commonly used stimulant found widely in beverages and foods is caffeine. Caffeine has been shown to increase alertness as measured by MSLT and to improve performance degraded by sleep restriction (Lumley et al. 1987; Rosenthal et al. 1991b).

DIFFERENTIAL DIAGNOSIS

Sleep-wake behavior is inherently within the scope of the psychiatric evaluation. The majority of patients affected with a psychiatric disorder complain of sleep disturbances. Before the introduction of the systematic study of sleep and its pathologies, abnormal manifestations of sleepiness were frequently attributed to depression or personality disorders. With the development of the discipline of sleep disorders medicine, we are better able to recognize, diagnose, and treat sleep-wake symptoms (American Sleep Disorders Association 1990). Psychiatrists are likely to continue to play an important role in the accurate diagnosis of these pathologies, because many patients with sleep disorders experience significant behavioral morbidity and often present to a psychiatrist. As a result, the psychiatrist must be familiar with EDS and its differential diagnosis. In this regard, it is important to realize that it is not unusual for patients to misrepresent the experience of sleepiness as fatigue, decreased ability to concentrate, decreased interest in daily activities, and even depression (Reynolds et al. 1984). The ability to assess sleepiness and its manifestations should enable a more accurate clinical evaluation, earlier intervention, or adequate referral.

The clinical evaluation of a patient should always include an assessment of sleep-wake behavior. The patient should be questioned about his or her sleep-wake habits and about possible abnormal manifestations of sleep and their consequences during the wake period. The clinician must bear in mind that transient daytime sleepiness is a common experience. For most adults, it is the inevitable consequence of inadequate or insufficient sleep. This symptom is reversed by the return to a regular sleep schedule once the acute stressor or environmental disturbance is resolved. Thus, it is important to determine the chronicity and reversibility of the symptom. In general, patients or their families do not complain of EDS until it becomes disruptive. By then, the problem is a chronic one and in most instances warrants evaluation.

The manifestations of EDS should be conceptualized as occurring within a spectrum of severity. Feeling sleepy in the midafternoon can be considered as a mild manifestation of sleepiness (although still within the range of normality because of the known biphasic circadian rhythm of sleepiness). However, falling asleep while waiting for a red light to turn green, at any time of the day, is a clear sign of an abnormal manifestation of sleepiness. Within the spectrum of possible manifestations, patients might become accustomed to falling asleep at times that are undesirable, such as when listening to a lecture, sitting in a warm room, or waiting in a reception area (indicative of clinically significant sleepiness)—yet still interpret these events as "normal." The common denominator to these manifestations is that the individual is sedentary. As the severity of sleepiness increases, the time required for sleep to occur decreases, and the circumstances in which it occurs broaden. Further increments in sleepiness lead to involuntary sleep episodes that are manifested at increasingly inappropriate times, such as while visiting with friends, eating, or driving. A description of the most common disorders of EDS follows.

Obstructive Sleep Apnea Syndrome

Obstructive sleep apnea syndrome (OSAS) is the single most common diagnosis of EDS patients in sleep disorders centers in the United States (Coleman et al. 1982). Patients with OSAS tend to be middle-aged, obese men. Patients with OSAS usually present with a variety of symptoms, including snoring, EDS, difficulty concentrating, memory lapses, morning headaches, and irritability (Roth et al. 1988). Less frequently, patients may complain of depression, anxiety, loss of libido, impotence, falling out of bed, enuresis, or sleepwalking.

Affected individuals typically have normal breathing during the wake state but experience repetitive episodes of upper-airway occlusion during sleep. These episodes lead to numerous arousals and awakenings (i.e., sleep fragmentation) that result in a disruption of the normal sleep architecture. Patients with OSAS spend a high percentage of their sleep in stage 1 non–rapid eye movement (NREM) sleep and decreased time in stages 3 and 4 NREM sleep and rapid eye movement (REM) sleep. The sleep fragmentation that these patients experience is believed to be the primary etiology of their most significant symptom:

EDS. In fact, among OSAS patients the prevalence of EDS is surpassed only by the complaint of snoring. The latter symptom is usually elicited from a bed partner, who frequently describes the affected individual as having restless sleep and snoring punctuated by periods of silence or episodes during which breathing stops. This characteristic snoring is of utmost importance because the prevalence of snoring approaches 30% in the general population, whereas estimates of the prevalence of OSAS are less than 10%.

The upper-airway occlusion takes place at the level of the pharynx in the majority of patients. However, the site can vary, having been described as high as the nasopharynx or as low as the larynx. The pathophysiology of the upper-airway closure has been the subject of numerous investigations. Anatomical and functional factors have been identified as possible culprits in the occurrence of the upper-airway occlusion (Remmers 1989). The most common anatomical risk factor is obesity.

The apneas that are characteristic of OSAS are associated with episodes of hypoxia and hypercapnia, which in turn lead to arousals, enabling the resumption of breathing. Arousals per se are associated with a number of important sequelae, the most clinically relevant being daytime sleepiness. Daytime sleepiness is a well-documented cause of cognitive impairment in patients with OSAS and other sleep disorders. It is also believed that at least a proportion of the observed cognitive deterioration in these patients is secondary to hypoxia (Bedard et al. 1991). Other consequences of hypoxia include changes in both the pulmonary and systemic vasculature, which have been implicated in the high prevalence of pulmonary and systemic hypertension observed in OSAS patients (Shepard et al. 1985).

A variety of medical treatments are available for patients with OSAS. These include weight loss, use of medications (e.g., protriptyline, fluoxetine), and nasal continuous positive airway pressure. Nasal continuous positive airway pressure, the most commonly used medical treatment for OSAS, has its effect by pneumatically splinting the upper airway and thereby preventing obstruction. The treatment should be based on a thorough evaluation of the patient's symptoms and signs, as well as the severity of the OSAS episodes. Severity is determined by a polysomnographic evaluation that provides information about the frequency of apnea, its relation to sleep stage and sleep position, the degree of oxygen desaturation, abnormalities of heart rate, sleep fragmentation, and objective level of daytime sleepiness.

Surgical treatments are also available for OSAS. The most common include uvulopalatopharyngoplasty and mandibular and maxillary advancement. Surgical treatments are usually reserved for patients in whom significant anatomical abnormalities of the upper airway are documented. Regardless of the treatment modality selected, the success of treatment is measured by the normalization of sleep-disordered breathing, which leads to improved sleep continuity and reversal of EDS (Lamphere et al. 1989).

Narcolepsy

Narcolepsy is a CNS disorder of unknown etiology that is characterized by EDS. When narcolepsy is fully expressed, patients also experience periods of cataplexy, sleep paralysis, and hypnagogic hallucinations (Rosenthal et al. 1990). A variety of other symptoms are also frequently encountered. These may include memory lapses, difficulty concentrating, automatic behaviors, and secondary depression. The latter group of symptoms are not specific to narcolepsy and are relatively common in patients affected by EDS. The age at onset is adolescence and young adulthood (ages 15–35 years), and EDS is usually the initial symptom to be manifested.

Cataplexy is reported by 70%–80% of narcolepsy patients. The occurrence of cataplexy is considered as pathognomonic for the disorder, and many consider its occurrence essential for the diagnosis of narcolepsy. Cataplexy consists of a sudden muscle weakness (a partial loss of muscle tone or total atonia), which is most frequently triggered by affect-laden situations. Hypnagogic hallucinations (reported by 50%–70% of patients) are vivid perceptual experiences occurring at the onset of sleep and may be concomitant with sleep paralysis. The latter condition is reported by 40%–65% of patients. Sleep paralysis consists of a temporary loss of muscle tone during the transition between wakefulness and sleep. Because of the inability to move or speak in the presence of a clear sensorium, these episodes can be very frightening.

The full narcoleptic tetrad (i.e., EDS, cataplexy, hypnagogic hallucinations, and sleep paralysis) is seen in only 20%–30% of narcolepsy patients. Although the entire narcolepsy tetrad was described over 100 years ago, clinical experience has unmasked other symptoms in these patients. The majority of patients (> 80%) report disturbed nocturnal sleep. Many complain of vivid dreams, which are most likely the result of idiopathic awakenings from REM sleep. Automatic behaviors are also frequently reported and occur during monotonous or repetitive activities. They are semipurposeful activities of which the patient has no memory. These episodes are believed to be caused by microsleeps, which result in poor performance and amnesia. These abnormalities represent a challenge to the patient, and their consequences may frequently be reflected in the patient's personality, interpersonal relationships, education, and job performance. Symptoms of depression, marital and family problems, and loss of employment are reported by the majority of patients.

The high incidence of narcolepsy in families has been recognized.

However, cases with no genetic predisposition are also found. Monozygotic twins may be concordant or discordant for the disorder, which suggests that genetic factors may be necessary but not sufficient to manifest the disease. Thus, it is believed that the disease has a multifactorial model of heritability (Honda and Juji 1988). The finding that more than 90% of these patients carry the HLA-DR2 haplotype is remarkable compared with the 25%–30% frequency encountered in the general population (Honda and Juji 1988). Despite this association, the exact location of the narcolepsy susceptibility gene has not been determined.

Polysomnographic studies are essential for the accurate diagnosis of narcolepsy. Patients require overnight polysomnography and an MSLT on the following day. Patients need to be withdrawn from all psychoactive medications before the laboratory evaluation. Although a 2-week withdrawal period is typically recommended, longer periods may be required in patients receiving long-acting drugs (e.g., fluoxetine). The recognized polysomnographic criteria for the diagnosis of the disorder require confirmation of pathological sleepiness (mean sleep latency as measured by MSLT of ≤ 5 minutes), two or more sleep-onset REM periods, and the absence of other potential causes of EDS (e.g., sleep apnea, insufficient sleep). The unique polysomnographic feature of narcolepsy is the occurrence of multiple sleep-onset REM periods, which are rarely encountered in other pathologies. Infrequently, one might encounter multiple sleep-onset REM periods in OSAS. In the presence of OSAS, one should not make the diagnosis of narcolepsy until sleep-disordered breathing has been normalized. This diagnosis usually requires follow-up polysomnography after treatment of OSAS.

The intrusion of REM sleep into wakefulness is considered the defining characteristic of narcolepsy. In fact, the symptoms of cataplexy, hypnagogic hallucinations, and sleep paralysis are considered REM-related phenomena that intrude into wakefulness. REM intrusions into wakefulness must be differentiated from increased REM pressure. Short REM sleep latency, long first REM periods, high REM density, and an elevated percentage of REM sleep—all of which are indicative of increased REM pressure—are not found in narcolepsy patients. Conversely, these indices of heightened REM pressure, but not multiple sleep-onset REM periods, are encountered in psychiatric populations.

Other medical disorders can manifest themselves concurrent with the symptoms of narcolepsy. When psychiatric diseases coexist with narcolepsy, they present a challenge to the clinician. First, schizophrenic hallucinations need to be differentiated from the hypnagogic hallucinations of narcolepsy. Second, because many psychotropic drugs are sedating, the pharmacological management of narcolepsy concurrent with psychosis is problematic. Finally, a few cases are reported in the literature in which a brain lesion (e.g., craniopharyngioma, sarcoid granuloma), usually in the region of the third ventricle, has been associated with narcolepsy, cataplexy, or both (Aldrich and Naylor 1989). These cases suggest that diencephalic lesions can be associated with signs and symptoms of narcolepsy that are clinically indistinguishable from those of idiopathic narcolepsy.

The treatment of narcolepsy is mainly symptomatic. It is also essential to counsel patients about the importance of adequate sleep hygiene, including the use of prophylactic naps. However, naps only result in brief relief of sleepiness. This alerting effect of naps is a distinguishing characteristic of narcolepsy patients. EDS is generally treated with CNS stimulants (methylphenidate and pemoline being the most widely used). When cataplexy and the other auxiliary symptoms are present, their treatment usually includes nonsedating tricyclic antidepressants (e.g., protriptyline). All of the medications used in the treatment of the auxiliary symptoms have REM-suppressing properties. Other medications reported as being useful in the treatment of narcolepsy include fluoxetine and the monoamine oxidase inhibitors.

Chronic Insufficient Sleep

Individuals affected with chronic insufficient sleep fail to accrue as much sleep as they need. These patients have no difficulty with sleep initiation or sleep maintenance but rather voluntarily or unwittingly restrict their time in bed. When this behavior persists, it results in chronic sleep deprivation and EDS. These patients have no overt evidence of psychopathology, no auxiliary symptoms, and no other medical explanation for their sleepiness (Roehrs et al. 1983).

It has been found that chronic insufficient sleepers become symptomatic during the third decade of life. It should be recognized that many people with comparable sleep schedules do not become symptomatic with EDS. Although what precipitates the symptoms of EDS is not well understood, it is likely that individual differences in sleep need and in the amount and chronicity of sleep restriction are key issues in the development of symptoms.

No gender differences are known to exist regarding the prevalence of this disorder. Patients frequently complain of snoring and marked difficulty in arising in the morning. They may report sleeping through the alarm clock and usually use the snooze alarm on several occasions before being able to get their day started. Polysomnographic evaluation reveals a short latency to sleep onset at night, long sleep periods when patients are allowed to sleep ad libitum, and a high sleep efficiency. The MSLT reveals pathological sleepiness (mean sleep latency of ≤ 5 minutes) but no evidence of multiple sleep-onset REM periods (Roehrs et al. 1983).

A relevant characteristic of the sleepiness observed in patients who are chronic insufficient sleepers is its reversibility. Clinical experience indicates that extending the amount of time that these individuals spend in bed reverses their sleepiness. Not infrequently, however, it is difficult to convince these patients to change their sleep-wake behavior.

A subset of patients with sleepiness and comparable polysomnographic features do not respond to extension of sleep. These patients receive the diagnosis of idiopathic CNS hypersomnia. Clearly, idiopathic CNS hypersomnolence is a diagnosis made by exclusion, and this condition can only be differentiated from chronic insufficient sleep syndrome by a trial of sleep extension. Idiopathic CNS hypersomnolence is symptomatically managed with stimulant medications. Typically, stimulating antidepressants are the drugs of choice.

Mood Disorders

Sleep disturbance is a core symptom in various psychiatric conditions. In a study by the Epidemiologic Catchment Area project, it was found that 40.4% of those who reported insomnia (for 2 weeks or longer) and 46.5% of those with hypersomnia (defined as sleeping too much) had a psychiatric disorder (Ford and Kamerow 1989). These frequencies are substantially higher than the 16.4% observed in participants who reported no sleep disturbance but were found to have a psychiatric condition. The most common psychiatric disorders in patients with hypersomnia were anxiety disorders (phobias, obsessive-compulsive disorder, and panic disorder), mood disorders, and alcohol and drug use disorders. In the Epidemiologic Catchment Area study, the complaint of hypersomnia had a particularly strong association with depressive disorders (especially with major depression). Data from other studies suggest that hypersomnia might be more prevalent during the depressive phase of bipolar illness and in young depressed patients (Hawkins et al. 1985; Thase et al. 1989).

Most of the research done on sleep and psychiatric diseases has been focused on the abnormalities encountered in the nocturnal sleep of populations affected with various mood disorders. These abnormalities include decreased sleep continuity, diminished delta wave production, shortened REM sleep latency, and temporal redistribution of REM sleep. It has been said that a relatively low percentage of depressed patients (10%–20%) report spending more time in bed and show high sleep efficiencies on nocturnal sleep recordings (Thase et al. 1989). A majority of these patients also complain of anergia and psychomotor slowing. High rates of daytime drowsiness (30%–85%) have also been reported in patients with the diagnosis of seasonal affective disorder.

It is difficult to ascertain the prevalence of hypersomnia and daytime sleepiness in psychiatric populations. This difficulty can be partially explained by the lack of operational definitions of hypersomnia and daytime sleepiness for these populations. On many occasions, these terms are used interchangeably. The results of studies quantifying sleepiness indicate that these patients do not suffer from pathological levels of daytime sleepiness. In fact, their scores on the MSLT are comparable to those reported among populations with no history of EDS (Nofzinger et al. 1991). Thus, these findings have failed to confirm the symptom of hypersomnia or sleepiness with the use of electrophysiological measures. The existing evidence indicates that although patients are likely to report anergia and a higher need for sleep, this does not necessarily imply that they suffer from an increased propensity to fall asleep or an increased need for sleep.

Circadian-Rhythm Disorders

Sleep-wake behavior, like other physiological processes, is characterized by a temporal structure that matches the 24-hour day-night cycle. Other physiological processes that function with circadian rhythms include endocrine secretions, body temperature, sensory processing, cardiac and renal function, and cognitive performance. All of these rhythms are maintained in the correct phase relative to the environment because of the effect of light (virtually the universal zeitgeber). The entrainment effects of light are mediated via the retinohypothalamic tract. Under normal conditions, light entrains the circadian rest-activity rhythms in such a way that spontaneous sleep duration varies with the phase of the body temperature cycle.

When the external zeitgebers fall out of synchrony with the internal circadian rhythms, a significant deterioration in sleep quality is likely to result. Perhaps the most frequent form of desynchronization is precipitated by rapid travel across time zones (jet lag). Until the external zeitgebers and the internal rhythms fall back into synchrony, it is not unusual for people to complain of sleep disturbance and daytime fatigue, gastrointestinal distress, tired muscles, headaches, reduced cognitive skills, poor psychomotor coordination, and moodiness (Klein et al. 1972). It has been suggested that a small dose of a short-acting benzodiazepine (taken for the first few days) is helpful in alleviating the symptoms of insomnia (Seidel et al. 1984). More recently, exposure to bright light to reentrain the internal rhythms has been advocated (Czeisler et al. 1989).

Sleep-wake pathologies associated with circadian-rhythm disorders include the delayed sleep phase syndrome, the advanced sleep phase syndrome, the non–24-hour sleep-wake schedule, and the irregular sleep-wake pattern. All of these pathologies share a misalignment between the internal circadian rhythms and the desired (or required) sleep schedule. Such a misalignment frequently results in complaints of sleepiness secondary to sleep loss. Treatment of these conditions is usually complicated by societal demands and the difficulties in changing sleep-wake behavior. Fortunately, for most individuals, the circadian system has sufficient resetting capacity to accomplish the required reentrainment. Exposure to light at appropriate times usually results in successful realignment of the internal and external rhythms (Czeisler et al. 1989). However, if entrainment is not preserved, recurrence of the symptoms is a distinct possibility.

Other Pathologies

Restless leg syndrome and periodic leg movements during sleep can result in insomnia or EDS. It has been shown that patients initially suffer from insomnia (caused by sleep loss, sleep fragmentation, or both), which after several years might evolve to EDS. Thus, these patients may present with symptoms of insomnia or EDS (Rosenthal et al. 1984).

On some occasions, patients may complain of significant sleepiness; however, when they are tested in the laboratory, no objective evidence for their complaint is found. In these cases patients require reassurance and careful differential diagnosis to rule out other behavioral disorders.

SUMMARY

Daytime sleepiness is a rather common experience. It is usually determined by the amount of sleep at night, circadian phase, and drugs. For most people, it is a temporary state that is reversed by sleep, realignment of the internal and external rhythms, or elimination of a drug with CNS effects. However, for a subset of the population, daytime sleepiness is a chronic experience. It is for this latter population that referral to a sleep disorders center is indicated. Regardless of its chronicity, the manifestations of EDS have serious consequences because these individuals are at risk for having accidents, suffer from decreased performance, and, in general, experience significant distress. Thus, it is important to educate the general population about the potential impact of EDS on a person's life. In addition, it is important for the psychiatrist to become familiar with the concept of EDS because its manifestations are, to a great extent, behavioral in nature.

REFERENCES

Akerstedt T, Frober JE: Shift work and health: interdisciplinary aspects, in Shift Work and Health—A Symposium. Washington, DC, National Institute of Occupational Safety and Health, 1976, pp 179–197

Akerstedt T, Gillberg M: The circadian variation of experimentally displaced sleep. Sleep 4:159–169, 1981

Aldrich MS, Naylor MW: Narcolepsy associated with lesions of the diencephalon. Neurology 39:1505–1508, 1989

American Sleep Disorders Association: The International Classification of Sleep Disorders: Diagnostic and Coding Manual. Rochester, MN, American Sleep Disorders Association, 1990

Ancoli-Israel S, Kripke D, Mason W, et al: Sleep apnea and nocturnal myoclonus in a senior population. Sleep 4:349–358, 1981

Bedard M-A, Montplaisir J, Richer F, et al: Obstructive sleep apnea syndrome: pathogenesis of neuropsychological deficits. J Clin Exp Neuropsychol 13:950–964, 1991

Beutler LE, Ware JC, Karacan I, et al: Differentiating psychological characteristics of patients with sleep apnea and narcolepsy. Sleep 4:39–47, 1981

Billiard M, Alperovitch A, Perot C, et al: Excessive daytime somnolence in young men: prevalence and contributing factors. Sleep 10:297–305, 1987

Bixler ED, Kales A, Soldatos CR, et al: Prevalence of sleep disorders in the Los Angeles metropolitan area. Am J Psychiatry 136:1257–1262, 1979

Bonnet MH: The effect of sleep disruption on performance, sleep and mood. Sleep 8:11–19, 1985

Bonnet MH: Performance and sleepiness as a function of the frequency and placement of sleep disruption. Psychophysiology 23:263–271, 1986

Broughton R, Valley V, Aguirre M, et al: Excessive daytime sleepiness and the pathophysiology of narcolepsy-cataplexy: a laboratory perspective. Sleep 9:205–215, 1986

Carskadon MA: Sleep tendency on a constant routine (abstract). Sleep Research 14:292, 1985

Carskadon MA, Dement WC: Respiration during sleep in the aged human. J Gerontol 36:420–423, 1981

Carskadon MA, Dement WC: Nocturnal determinants of daytime sleepiness. Sleep 5:S73–S81, 1982

Carskadon MA, Brown E, Dement WC: Sleep fragmentation in the elderly: relationship to daytime sleep tendency. Neurobiol Aging 3:321–327, 1982

Carskadon MA, Dement WC, Mitler MM, et al: Guidelines for the Multiple Sleep Latency Test (MSLT): a standard measure of sleepiness. Sleep 9:519–524, 1986

Coleman M, Roffwarg H, Kennedy S, et al: Sleep-wake disorders based on a polysomnographic diagnosis—a national cooperative study. JAMA 247:997–1003, 1982

Conway J, Greenwood DT, Middlemiss DN: Central nervous actions of beta-adrenoreceptor antagonists. Clin Sci Mol Med 54:119–124, 1978

Czeisler CA, Kronauer RE, Allan JS, et al: Bright light induction of strong (type 0) resetting of the human circadian pacemaker. Science 244:1328–1333, 1989

Dement WC, Carskadon MA: An essay on sleepiness, in Actualites en Medecine Experimentale. Montpellier, France, Euromed, 1981, pp 47–71

Dement WC, Carskadon MA, Richardson GS: Excessive daytime sleepiness in the sleep apnea syndrome, in Sleep Apnea Syndromes. Edited by Guilleminault C, Dement WC. New York, Alan R Liss, 1978, pp 23–46

Erman MK, Beckham B, Gardner DA, et al: The Modified Assessment of Sleepiness Test (MAST) (abstract). Sleep Research 16:550, 1987

Folkard S: Shiftwork and performance, in The Twenty-Four Hour Workday: Proceedings of a Symposium on Variations in Work-Sleep Schedules (DHHS Publ No [NIOSH] 81-1270). Edited by Johnson LC, Tepas DI, Colquhoun WJ, et al. Washington, DC, U.S. Government Printing Office, 1981, pp 347–373

Ford DE, Kamerow DB: Epidemiologic study of sleep disturbances and psychiatric disorders: an opportunity for prevention? JAMA 262:1479–1484, 1989

Froberg J, Karlsson CG, Levi L, et al: Circadian variations in performance, psychological ratings, catecholamine excretion and diuresis during prolonged sleep deprivation. Int J Psychobiol 2:23–36, 1972

Gaillard JM: Neurotransmission and receptor pharmacology, in Principles and Practice of Sleep Medicine. Edited by Kryger MH, Roth T, Dement WC. Philadelphia, PA, WB Saunders, 1989, pp 198–201

Gislason T, Almqvist M: Somatic diseases and sleep complaints. Acta Medica Scandinavia 221:475–481, 1987

Guilleminault C, Carskadon M: Relationship between sleep disorders and daytime complaints. Sleep 6:95–100, 1977

Hawkins DR, Taub JM, Van de Castle RL: Extended sleep (hypersomnia) in young depressed patients. Am J Psychiatry 142:905–910, 1985

Honda Y, Juji T (eds): HLA in Narcolepsy. Heidelberg, Springer-Verlag, 1988

Hoddes E, Zarcone VP, Smythe H, et al: Quantification of sleepiness: a new approach. Psychophysiology 10:431–436, 1973

Johns MW: A new method for measuring daytime sleepiness: the Epworth Sleepiness Scale. Sleep 14:540–545, 1991

Karacan I, Thornby JI, Anch M, et al: Prevalence of sleep disturbance in a primarily urban Florida county. Soc Sci Med 10:239–244, 1976

Klein KE, Wegmann HM, Hunt BI: Desynchronization as a function of body temperature circadian rhythm as a result of outgoing and homecoming transmeridian flights. Aerospace Medicine 43:119–132, 1972

Klink M, Quan SF: Prevalence of reported sleep disturbances in a general adult population and their relationship to obstructive airways diseases. Chest 91:540–546, 1987

Kramer M, Roehrs T, Roth T: Mood change and the physiology of sleep. Compr Psychiatry 17:161–165, 1976

Lamphere J, Roehrs T, Wittig R, et al: Recovery of alertness after CPAP in apnea. Chest 96:1364–1367, 1989

Lavie P: Sleep habits and sleep disturbances in industrial workers in Israel: main findings and some characteristics of workers complaining of excessive daytime sleepiness. Sleep 4:147–158, 1981

Lavie P, Adam N, Nave N, et al: Prevalence of sleep complaints in Israel (abstract). Sleep Research 8:198, 1979

Levine B, Roehrs T, Stepanski E, et al: Fragmenting sleep diminishes its recuperative value. Sleep 10:590–599, 1987

Levine B, Roehrs T, Zorick F, et al: Daytime sleepiness in young adults. Sleep 11:39–46, 1988

Lugaresi E, Cirignotta F, Zucconi M, et al: Good and poor sleepers: an epidemiological survey of the San Marino population, in Sleep-Wake Disorders: Natural History, Epidemiology, and Long-Term Evolution. Edited by Guilleminault C, Lugaresi E. New York, Raven, 1983, pp 1–12

Lumley M, Roehrs T, Asker D, et al: Ethanol and caffeine effects on daytime sleepiness/alertness. Sleep 10:306–312, 1987

Mackie RR, Miller JC: Effects of hours of service, regularity of schedules, and cargo loading on truck and bus driver fatigue (technical report 1765-F DOT-HS-5-01142). Washington, DC, U.S. Government Printing Office, 1978

McGhie A, Russell SM. The subjective assessment of normal sleep patterns. Journal of Mental Science 108:642–654, 1962

McNair DM, Lorr M, Droppleman LF: EdITS Manual for the Profile of Mood States. San Diego, CA, Educational and Industrial Testing Service, 1971

Mitler MM, Gujavarty KS, Browman CP: Maintenance of wakefulness test: a polysomnographic technique for evaluating treatment efficacy in patients with excessive somnolence. Electroencephalogr Clin Neurophysiol 53:658–661, 1982

Mitler MM, Shafor R, Hajdukovich R, et al: Treatment of narcolepsy: objective studies on methylphenidate, pemoline and protriptyline. Sleep 9:260–264, 1986

Mitler MM, Carskadon MA, Czeisler CA, et al: Catastrophes, sleep, and public policy: consensus report. Sleep 11:100–109, 1988

Navelet Y, Anders T, Guilleminault C: Narcolepsy in children, in Narcolepsy. Edited by Guilleminault C, Dement WC, Passouant P. New York, Spectrum, 1976, pp 171–177

Nicholson AN, Stone BM: Antihistamines: impaired performance and the tendency to sleep. Eur J Clin Pharmacol 30:27–32, 1986

Nofzinger EA, Thase ME, Reynolds CF III, et al: Hypersomnia in bipolar depression: a comparison with narcolepsy using the Multiple Sleep Latency Test. Am J Psychiatry 148:1177–1181, 1991

Partinen M: Sleeping habits and sleep disorders of Finnish men before, during, and after military service (abstract). Annales Medicinae Militaris Fenniae 57 (suppl 1):96, 1982

Remmers JE: Anatomy and physiology of upper airway obstruction, in Principles and Practice of Sleep Medicine. Edited by Kryger MH, Roth T, Dement WC. Philadelphia, PA, WB Saunders, 1989, pp 525–536

Reynolds CF III, Kupfer DJ, McEachran AB: Depressive psychopathology in male sleep apneics. J Clin Psychiatry 45:287–290, 1984

Richardson GS, Carskadon MA, Orav EJ, et al: Circadian variation of sleep tendency in elderly and young adult subjects. Sleep 5:S82–S94, 1982

Roehrs T, Roth T: Multiple Sleep Latency Test: technical aspects and normal values. J Clin Neurophysiol 9:63–67, 1992

Roehrs T, Zorick F, Sicklesteel J, et al: Excessive sleepiness associated with insufficient sleep. Sleep 6:319–325, 1983

Roehrs T, Kribbs N, Zorick F, et al: Hypnotic residual effects of benzodiazepines with repeated administration. Sleep 9:309–316, 1986

Roehrs T, Timms V, Zwyghuizen-Doorenbos A, et al: Sleep extension in sleepy and alert normals. Sleep 12:449–457, 1989

Roehrs TA, Timms V, Zwyghuizen-Doorenbos A, et al: Polysomnographic, performance, and personality differences of sleepy and alert normals. Sleep 13:395–402, 1990

Rosenthal LD, Roehrs T, Sicklesteel J, et al: Periodic movements during sleep, sleep fragmentation, and sleep-wake complaints. Sleep 7:326–330, 1984

Rosenthal LD, Merlotti L, Young DK, et al: Subjective and polysomnographic characteristics of patients diagnosed with narcolepsy. Gen Hosp Psychiatry 12:191–197, 1990

Rosenthal LD, Rosen A, Wittig RM, et al: A sleep-wake activity inventory to measure daytime sleepiness (abstract). Sleep Research 20:130, 1991a

Rosenthal LD, Roehrs TA, Zwyghuizen-Doorenbos A, et al: Alerting effects of caffeine after normal and restricted sleep. Neuropsychopharmacology 4:103–108, 1991b

Rosenthal LD, Roehrs TA, Krstevska S, et al: Auditory awakening thresholds in sleepy, alert, and sleep deprived subjects (abstract). Sleep Research 21:111, 1992

Rosenthal L, Roehrs TA, Rosen A, et al: Level of sleepiness and total sleep time following various time in bed conditions. Sleep 16:226–232, 1993

Roth T, Roehrs TA: Determinants of residual effects of hypnotics. Accid Anal Prev 17:291–296, 1985

Roth T, Roehrs TA, Zorick F: Sleepiness: its measurement and determinants. Sleep 5:S128–S134, 1982

Roth T, Roehrs TA, Conway WA: Behavioral morbidity of apnea. Seminars in Respiratory Medicine 9:554–559, 1988

Seidel WF, Roth T, Roehrs TA, et al: Treatment of a 12-hour shift of sleep schedule with benzodiazepines. Science 224:1262–1264, 1984

Shepard JW Jr, Garrison M, Grither D, et al: Hemodynamic responses to O_2 desaturation in obstructive sleep apnea (abstract). Am Rev Respir Dis 131:A106, 1985

Stepanski E, Salava W, Lamphere J, et al: Experimental sleep fragmentation and sleepiness in normal subjects: a preliminary report (abstract). Sleep Research 13:193, 1984a

Stepanski E, Lamphere J, Badia P, et al: Sleep fragmentation and daytime sleepiness. Sleep 7:18–26, 1984b

Strogatz SH: The Mathematical Structure of the Human Sleep-Wake Cycle. New York, Springer-Verlag, 1986

Thase ME, Himmelhoch JM, Mallinger AG, et al: Sleep EEG and DST findings in anergic bipolar depression. Am J Psychiatry 146:329–333, 1989

Webb WB: Sleep deprivation: total, partial and selective, in The Sleeping Brain. Edited by Chase MH. Los Angeles, CA, BIS/BRS, 1972, pp 323–362

Zorick F, Roehrs T, Conway W, et al: Effects of uvulopalatopharyngoplasty on the day-time sleepiness associated with sleep apnea syndrome. Bulletin Europeen de Physiopathologie Respiratoire 19:600–603, 1983

Chapter 29

Disorders Relating to Shift Work and Jet Lag

Timothy H. Monk, Ph.D.

To be lost in time may be as disconcerting to a patient as it is to be lost in space. Just as a familiarity with the spatial domain of one's life is important to healthy functioning, so too is an equivalent familiarity with the temporal domain. Even the simple time structure associated with daytime employment can be important to well-being; Feather and Bond (1983) found that for both employed and unemployed persons, "structured and purposeful use of time was positively associated with self-esteem and negatively associated with depressive symptoms" (p. 241). One could argue that the "when" and "with whom" components of daily events are often just as important as the "where." Regular daily social rhythms enable people to make sense of the stream of activities they experience and to plan and predict their immediate future.

This chapter is concerned with patients who can be characterized as being "lost in time" because of the unusual routines required of them by their occupation. These patients are suffering either because their jobs involve shift work with nonstandard duty hours or because their jobs carry them to different geographical time zones on a frequent basis, causing them to suffer from chronic jet lag. Both groups are well represented in the population, the former because of the increased demand for around-the-clock services and the reluctance of manufacturing employers to hire new personnel, and the latter because of the increasingly multinational stance of most major commercial enterprises. Managers and supervisors from the home office must often travel abroad to visit and evaluate their company's overseas operations.

Typically, patients who are lost in time present with a whole package of complaints. Many of these complaints are specific to the individual patient, the precipitating agent, or both. However, it is safe to predict that in most cases the symptom list will include trouble sleeping at night, daytime sleepiness and irritability, impaired performance, and gastrointestinal distress. Very often, the patient's relationships with spouse and children are problematic, as are interpersonal processes in general. A feeling of general and pervasive malaise might lead to symptoms of clinical depression.

The aim of this chapter is to educate the clinician in the etiology of such disorders. Recent research findings in the area of human circadian rhythms are described, as well as more specific research related to shift work and jet lag. The chapter then gives separate consideration to the disorders of shift work and of chronic jet lag, with a discussion of the points specific to each area and the presentation of possible treatment strategies.

THE HUMAN CIRCADIAN SYSTEM

Homo sapiens is a diurnal species, endowed with a physiology that is oriented toward active wakefulness during the daylight hours and restful sleep at night. A central timekeeping process in the brain, located in the suprachiasmatic nucleus (SCN) of the hypothalamus (Moore 1982), generates signals with a period of about 24 hours (hence the term "circadian," from the Latin *circa dies*). This rhythmic signal is endogenous and self-sustaining. Indeed, the SCN of lower mammals has been shown to continue to generate rhythmic signals even when removed from the brain and studied in vitro. For humans, the consequences of this characteristic of the SCN are that circadian rhythms are self-sustaining and appear to have a momentum of their own (Aschoff 1981).

The *advantage* of the endogenous, self-sustaining nature of circadian rhythms is that they continue to run, even when the individual is kept awake and is unaware of the time of day. Thus, the circadian system is robust to transient changes in the activity-rest cycle or the exposure to time cues. The *disadvantage* is that the circadian timekeeping system is very slow to adjust to the abrupt changes in schedule required by shift-work and transmeridian travel (Aschoff et al. 1975). Indeed, some experts question whether, under normal conditions, night workers ever completely adjust the timing of their biological clocks (Knauth and Rutenfranz 1976). Likewise, for many people, the symptoms of jet lag can last for more than a week after travel to a different time zone (Winget et al. 1984).

Just as animal circadian rhythms are typically studied using measures of wheel-running activity, those of humans are usually studied using measures of body temperature (Wever 1979). The most frequently used measure is rectal temperature, which can be measured very easily on a minute-by-minute basis around the clock using a thermistor attached to a recording device. When rectal temperatures are plotted as a function of time (Figure 29–1), a clear rhythm emerges with a trough in the early hours of the morning and a peak in the mid-evening.

Although about one-half of the observed rhythm can be attributed to changes in posture, activity, or both, the remainder is generated more directly from signals emanating from the SCN. The latter can be seen in "constant conditions" or "unmasking" studies in which the patient is kept in wakeful bed rest (and unaware of time of day) for 36 hours or more at a time (Mills et al. 1978). As can be seen in our own data (Figure 29–2), reliable circadian rhythms in rectal temperature continue to emerge under these conditions, with approximately the same timing of peak and trough as is seen under normal sleep-wake regimens.

Although this chapter uses temperature rhythms quite extensively in discussing shift work and jet-lag effects, the reader should remember that body temperature is just one of many different circadian rhythms observed in human physiology. Indeed, one could argue that if the rhythms of plasma cortisol or plasma melatonin were as easy and inexpensive to measure as the rhythm of rectal temperature, then these neuroendocrine rhythms would instead be the rhythms of choice. Specifically, the onset of melatonin excretion by the pineal gland (which typically occurs in the evening hours) has been suggested as a particularly useful marker of circadian phase because of the relative absence

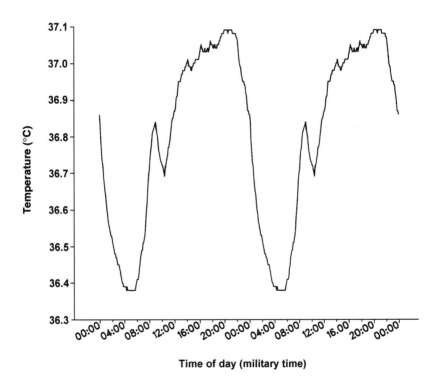

Figure 29–1. Double-plotted circadian rectal temperature rhythm averaged from 23 healthy young men. Mean temperature is plotted as a function of time of day, with each time plotted twice to highlight the rhythm.

of masking (interference) from sleep-wake patterns (Lewy et al. 1984).

The study of the response of the human circadian system to even one single abrupt shift in routine has revealed quite dramatic effects in both field and laboratory conditions. These effects are illustrated by Figure 29–3, which shows the response of the circadian temperature rhythm (measured in eight healthy middle-aged men) to one 6-hour phase advance in routine (accomplished by truncating night 6 of the 15-night protocol). The experiment was conducted in time isolation, and the subjects were unaware of the timing or extent of the phase shift. Indeed, most of them were unaware of what had happened and could not understand why they felt so sleepy. Nevertheless, the amplitude reduction consequent on the phase shift can be seen quite clearly. Quantifying the effects of the phase shift on rhythm amplitude and timing (phase) revealed that recovery of rhythm amplitude back to baseline values took well over a week and that the timing of the rhythm never

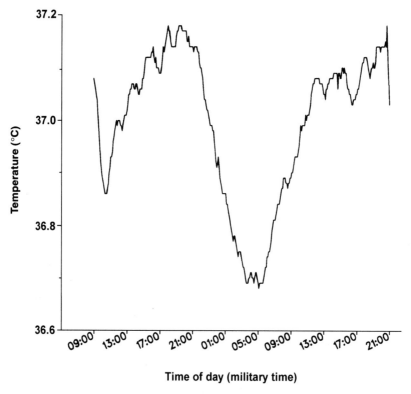

Figure 29–2. Mean rectal temperature plotted as a function of time of day, averaged from 15 healthy young adults experiencing 36 hours of wakeful bed rest ("constant conditions" or "unmasking"—see text). Each point is plotted once only.

completely achieved the new phase position (Figure 29–4). This result echoes those from previous studies involving phase shifts, which usually confirm that 1 day of recovery (at least) is required for each time zone crossed (Aschoff et al. 1975).

Two major problems arise when the circadian system is still in the slow process of realignment to a new routine. The first major problem is that the signals from the SCN, and thus the resulting endogenous circadian rhythms, are inappropriate for the particular schedule that the patient wants to live. Processes appropriate to sleep are present when wakefulness is desired and vice versa. The second major problem is that a disharmony of the circadian system is induced. One can use the analogy of a symphony orchestra, with the component processes that make up the circadian system likened to the individual instruments. When the patient commences night work or flies across time zones, it is as if a new conductor climbs the rostrum, beating at a different rhythm. Until all of the individual instruments switch to the new conductor, there is a cacophony of noise. In the circadian domain, this

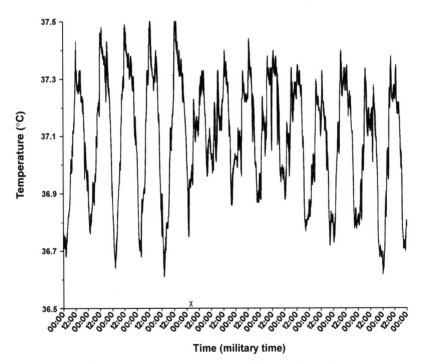

Figure 29–3. Mean rectal temperature from eight middle-aged men in a 15-day time-isolation laboratory protocol. A single acute 6-hour phase advance in routine (accomplished by truncating sleep period 6) occurred at the time point marked by X.

Source. Data from Monk et al. 1988.

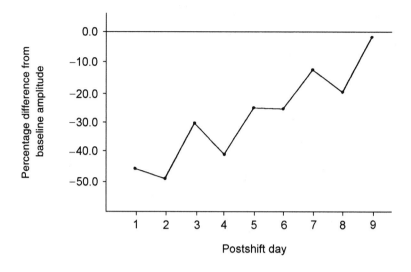

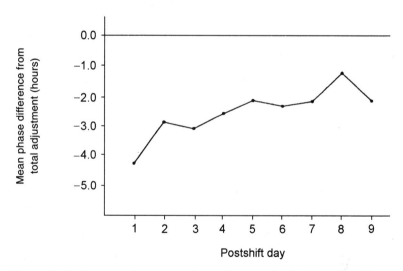

Figure 29–4. Recovery functions of circadian amplitude (size of oscillation; *upper panel*) and acrophase (timing of fitted peak; *lower panel*) from eight middle-aged men experiencing a 6-hour phase advance in routine. Estimates were derived from individual sinusoidal fits to each subject's daily rhythms and indicate the process of temporal alignment of the circadian system as it relates to the size (or strength) of the circadian rhythm (*upper panel*) and to the appropriateness of its timing or phase (*lower panel*).
Source. Data from Monk et al. 1988.

disharmony is referred to as "internal dissociation" (Wever 1975), and it presents in the patient as malaise, fatigue, irritability, and loss of appetite.

Although rhythmic changes in the patient's environment (e.g., daylight and darkness) are not needed for rhythm generation itself, these changes are needed to keep the SCN running exactly according to a 24-hour schedule and with the correct temporal orientation (i.e., with sleep at night and wakefulness during the day). These time cues are referred to as *zeitgebers* (from the German "time giver"). Zeitgebers are the agents of change when a patient works a night shift or flies across time zones.

Through the 1960s and 1970s, it was believed that the light-dark cycle did not represent the most potent zeitgeber for the human circadian system, as it does for lower animals. Instead, it was believed that the *social* zeitgebers of social communication and knowledge of clock time predominated (Wever 1979). However, in the early 1980s, this assumption was dramatically reversed when levels of illumination approaching those of daylight were employed. This reversal was heralded by the finding by Lewy et al. (1980) that only when *daylight* levels (> 2,000 lux) of artificial illumination were experienced could the normal nocturnal excretion of the hormone melatonin into the bloodstream be suppressed. Because melatonin was known to play an important role in the circadian system, this finding suggested that previous research had been misguided in using comparatively low levels of artificial illumination in human circadian studies. When such studies were repeated using bright illumination, it was found that light could be a very powerful zeitgeber in humans (Wever et al. 1983).

Through the 1980s to the present, much of the human circadian research reported has been concerned with light as a zeitgeber, and attention to nonphotic zeitgebers has been minimal. The few researchers (including myself) who believe that nonphotic zeitgebers do have significant effects in humans are, in the United States at least, regarded as slightly eccentric. We do, however, take heart from similar conclusions regarding nonphotic zeitgebers now drawn by researchers investigating animal circadian rhythms (Rusak et al. 1988). However, whether or not nonphotic zeitgebers are important in humans, it is undoubtedly true that daylight is a powerful circadian zeitgeber. Unfortunately, daylight is what very often makes life so difficult for the shift-worker patient.

SLEEP AND THE CIRCADIAN SYSTEM

Because one of the major duties of the circadian system is to prepare us for a restful period of sleep during the night, it is hardly surprising that when the circadian system fails, the sleep of the individual patient is disrupted. It is, after all, very unusual (except during a night's sleep) for a person to spend 7 or 8 hours without eating, drinking, voiding, or talking. Clearly, the circadian system must do some "shutting down" in anticipation of sleep, in terms of both the physical and the mental life of the individual. Without that shutting-down process, the desire to eat, drink, void, and talk will intrude into the "night," and the patient will be unable to sleep.

Several authors (e.g., Weitzman and Kripke 1981; Wever 1979) have objectively studied sleep in persons who were phase-shifted. In our own studies of phase-shifted subjects (Monk et al. 1988), we found that the disrupted circadian rhythms illustrated in Figures 29–3 and 29–4 were associated with quite profound changes in the various parameters of sleep (Figure 29–5). Specifically, in the "nights" after the phase shift, some measures (e.g., the percentage of rapid eye movement [REM] sleep) recovered to baseline levels in a monotonic manner, paralleling the phase adjustment of the circadian temperature rhythm; whereas others (e.g, actual sleep duration) recovered in a zig-zag manner. This difference was explained by dominance of SCN-generated rhythms in determining the amount of REM sleep obtained, whereas the other measures represented the output of a "tug of war" between rhythmic processes (from the misaligned circadian system) and homeostatic processes mediated by fatigue from truncated and disrupted "nights" of sleep.

This finding has an important practical message: very often, nights of comparatively good sleep can intrude into a pattern of otherwise-disrupted sleep in a patient doing shift work or experiencing chronic jet lag. These events, however, may only be a function of particularly high levels of fatigue "breaking through" to produce a consolidated sleep episode and may have nothing to do with a resolution of the underlying circadian dysfunction.

SHIFT WORK

Definition and Prevalence

The term "shift work" means different things to different people. For some, shift work means that the individual works at night; others use the term to label any system of work that requires regular attendance outside the normal 7 A.M. to 6 P.M. "window" (Monk and Folkard 1992). In this chapter the latter, less restrictive definition is used. Justification for that choice comes from the fact that many "evening only" or "morning-evening rotating" shift workers have significant coping problems. As shall be discussed later, these problems occur mainly in

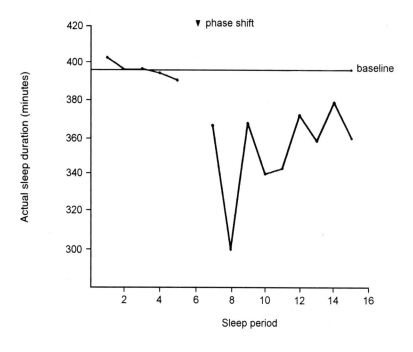

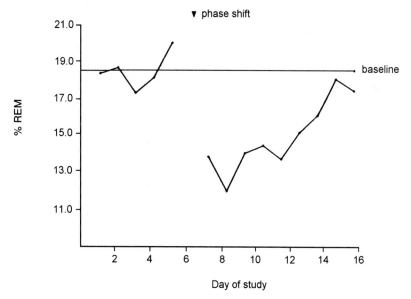

Figure 29–5. Mean actual sleep duration (time spent asleep; *upper panel*) and the percentage of REM sleep (*lower panel*) in eight middle-aged men experiencing a 6-hour phase advance in routine. The night of the phase shift (night 6) was truncated by 6 hours and is not plotted (see text).
Source. Data from Monk et al. 1988.

the social and domestic arenas rather than in the sleep or circadian ones, but they are nevertheless very real and troubling to the individuals involved.

According to the more inclusive definition of the prevalence of shift work, 20 million Americans are potentially affected, representing about 22% of the work force (16% of full-time and 47% of part-time employees) (Mellor 1986). This number can be expected to grow because of the demand for around-the-clock services; the high capital cost of machinery, which requires it to be operated around the clock to secure an acceptable return on the investment; and the *increase* rather than decrease in the total hours per week worked by the average U.S. employee (Schor 1991). Moreover, the proportional incidence of problems associated with shift work can be expected to rise because most workers do not nowadays have a full-time homemaker to help with child rearing, shopping, cooking, and household maintenance. The time pressures are becoming less and less tolerable (Schor 1991).

DSM-IV (American Psychiatric Association 1994) recognizes "shift work type" as a specific type of circadian rhythm sleep disorder (sleep-wake schedule disorder; 307.45). The description reads: "Insomnia during major sleep period or excessive sleepiness during major wake period associated with night work or frequently changing shift work."

A Triad of Factors

Because of the attention paid to circadian rhythms in the early part of this chapter, it may be tempting to assume that the problems of shift work are exclusively those of circadian adjustment. That assumption would, however, be mistaken. Sleep problems unrelated to circadian alignment, social problems, and domestic problems undeniably contribute in a major way to the distress of the shift-worker patient and may, indeed, precipitate the seeking of professional help.

Essentially, three domains must be functioning well for the individual to cope successfully with shift work. As shown in Figure 29–6, these can be represented by a triad: circadian rhythms, sleep, and social-domestic factors (Monk 1988). All three are interrelated, and problems with any one of them can negate gains that might otherwise be made by the other two. For example, without the social support of the patient's household, he or she might be totally unable to follow the routines and activities that good sleep hygiene and circadian zeitgeber management might dictate. Conversely, a shift worker's family life will undoubtedly suffer if a failure in the sleep and circadian domains leads to chronic fatigue and irritability. In this section, each component of the triad is considered in turn, concluding with a list of treatment recommendations for each area.

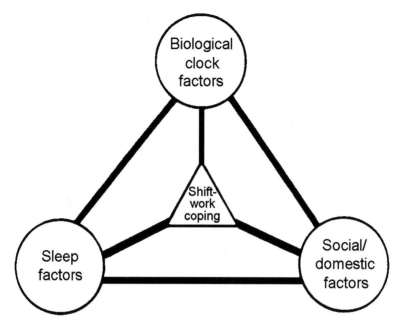

Figure 29–6. The triad of factors determining a shift worker's ability to cope.
Source. Adapted from Monk 1988.

Circadian Rhythms

As has been shown quite convincingly in a study by Knauth and Rutenfranz (1976), and recently confirmed in an experimental study by Czeisler et al. (1990), night workers' circadian rhythms do not, under normal circumstances, ever completely phase-adjust to be appropriate to a nocturnal routine. Although some authors (e.g., Wilkinson 1992a) still assert that permanent night-work schedules are preferable, others (e.g., Folkard 1992; Monk 1986) point out that retention of a nocturnal circadian orientation is infeasible in a real world of domestic commitments and unavoidable daylight exposure. As Van Loon (1963) has demonstrated, it only takes one weekend-style break for reversion to a diurnal (day-active) circadian orientation to occur.

Obtaining a nocturnal orientation can be likened to a salmon leaping up a waterfall, with the top of the waterfall representing a nocturnal circadian orientation and the bottom of the waterfall representing a diurnal one. It is very difficult to reach the top of the waterfall—and all too easy to drop back down. Just a few days on a day-oriented routine are enough to lose one's nocturnal circadian orientation. Shift workers who rotate through different shift timings on a regular (or an irregular) basis are even less likely to obtain the circadian alignment appropriate to their work schedule, and they often find themselves in a permanent state of flux or circadian desynchrony (Knauth and Rutenfranz 1976).

Not surprisingly, Gordon et al. (1986) found an increased incidence of alcohol use, tranquilizer use, and nervousness in rotating shift workers.

Bright artificial lights. Recently, there has been considerable interest in the development of bright-light strategies as a countermeasure against maladaptation to shift work. This trend started in the 1980s with the discovery that, contrary to the prevailing view of the 1970s, daylight levels of ambient illumination could be a potent zeitgeber for the human circadian system (see above). In the late 1980s, Eastman (1990) performed a careful series of studies with actual shift workers, using a combination of banks of bright lights ("light boxes") to simulate daylight and welders' goggles together with strict lightproofing in the bedroom to attenuate daylight. The aim was to entrain shift workers to a circadian cycle appropriate to their shift cycle. Although the approach had some success, the procedures required of the individual are rigorous, and Eastman (1991) has suggested caution in putting them forward as a panacea for disorders related to shift work.

Eastman's strategy was based on light exposure and darkness maintenance *outside* working hours. A rather different approach was adopted by Czeisler et al. (1990), who created a simulated workplace with extremely bright levels of illumination for the duration of the entire night shift. When combined with strict control of bedtimes (0900 hours) and wake times (1700 hours) and absolute darkening of the bedroom, this approach did lead (after a week) to successful complete phase shifts in a small group of young volunteer subjects (who were not real shift workers). Similar success (although less well verified objectively) was reported in NASA astronauts whose crew quarters were modified to allow extremely bright artificial levels of illumination. It is important to note here that we are not talking about putting in a few extra light bulbs. To acquire the appropriate levels of illumination in the room in question at NASA, the entire ceiling had to be filled with light fittings, and tables and floor coverings had to be lightened. The cost ran into tens of thousands of dollars. A special regimen of bright-light exposure was also used, and the astronauts were very enthusiastic about the results (Czeisler et al. 1991).

It is hard to dispute that Czeisler et al.'s package of manipulations involving extremely bright artificial light at work during the night shift and absolute darkening and rigid bedtime control at home can very adequately phase-shift ("reset") the timing of the circadian system. What is easy to dispute is whether this package of manipulations is at all realistic in general shift-work situations. Few workplaces have the particular facilities and resources of NASA—and few workers have the motivation levels of those volunteering for a Harvard study lasting a few weeks or a once-in-a-lifetime space mission. There are indeed some situations in which such strategies are feasible and appropriate.

Whether they have any general bearing whatsoever on the problems of the average shift worker remains questionable.

Shift schedules.   The other way in which researchers have attempted to ease the problems of shift workers is to manipulate the shift schedule. Many shift workers experience what is called a "rotating" shift schedule, in which several days or weeks on one shift timing is followed by an equivalent spell on a different shift timing. An example of this type of schedule is the "southern swing," in which a week of night shifts is followed by a week of evening shifts and then a week of morning shifts.

From the results presented earlier in this chapter, it is clear that weekly shift rotation such as the southern swing is likely to be a disaster with respect to adjustment of the worker's circadian rhythms. Because the circadian pacemaker is slow to adjust to a new timing, the worker is likely to be in a permanent state of flux, never fully adjusting to the hours he or she is being asked to work. Probably the only system worse than weekly rotation is the irregular, almost entirely unpredictable work hours suffered, for example, by locomotive drivers.

Thus, there is plenty of room for improvement regarding the direction and speed of shift rotation. Most experts agree that weekly rotation should be avoided, but the question of what should replace it has become a source of contention (Folkard 1992; Monk 1986; Wilkinson 1992a, 1992b). Some favor changing to permanent or extremely slowly rotating systems, whereas others favor the rapidly rotating shift systems—increasingly popular in Europe—where no more than two or three different shifts are worked before a change in timing. The advantages of rapid rotation are that the circadian system remains resolutely day oriented, lessening some of the "jet-lag" type symptoms, and that there are few enough night shifts in a row that a significant sleep debt can be avoided. However, both rapid rotation and slow rotation have their disadvantages. Workers on rapid rotation suffer particularly from low levels of alertness on the night shift and poor daytime sleep. Workers on slow rotation and fixed shifts suffer from the all-too-easy loss of nocturnal circadian orientation that can occur on weekend-type breaks.

The issue is a complicated one. Because the clinician is unlikely to be able to change the shift schedule worked by his or her patient, but rather will be forced to work within the constraints of the schedule imposed by the employer, this point will not be discussed further.

Sleep
Sleep loss is the most likely symptom to be presented to the clinician by the shift-worker patient. Surveys of problems related to shift work inevitably find sleep to be at or near the top of the list, and some authors put the prevalence rate of sleep disorders in shift workers at 60% (Rutenfranz et al. 1977, 1985). What the patient is probably not aware

of is that there are both endogenous and exogenous reasons why his or her sleep is disrupted. Endogenous reasons stem from misalignment of the circadian system; exogenous reasons stem from the noise and demands of a day-oriented society. Clearly, a misaligned circadian system is unable to "set the stage" for sleep. Thus, hunger and bathroom needs are not suppressed during the sleep episode, and alerting mechanisms (e.g., the cortisol surge, temperature rise) occur at the "wrong" times, making a prolonged period of restful sleep either difficult or impossible.

These endogenous effects have been quantified in both laboratory and field studies. In the laboratory, Akerstedt and Gillberg (1982) studied healthy volunteers whose sleep was delayed by various amounts of time. Figure 29–7 shows how the amount of sleep obtained varied as a function of the time of day at which the sleep was started. Thus, the average duration of morning sleeps was only 60% of the normal length, even though they followed a night of complete sleep deprivation. Analysis of urine volumes, rectal temperatures, and hormone excretion rates confirmed that the sleep interruptions could be attributable directly to the outputs of the circadian system (Akerstedt and Gillberg 1982).

In field studies, Foret and Lantin (1972) found a similar effect in a survey of French train drivers, a result confirmed in both West German and Japanese shift workers (Kogi 1985) (Figure 29–7). It should be remembered, however, that workers whose sleep is studied in the field may have additionally experienced *exogenous* interruptions in sleep. The most obvious of the exogenous factors are the noises coming from a day-active society (traffic, ringing telephones, children playing), which can be particularly disruptive for patients living in poor housing conditions (Rutenfranz et al. 1985). However, just as important are those interruptions resulting from the general attitude that a family may have toward the patient's day sleeps, regarding them as fair game for disruption to a much greater extent than is the case for the night sleep of day workers. Thus, for example, a day sleep might be interrupted to meet children off the school bus or for a dental appointment, whereas the equivalent disruption of day worker's night sleep would be unthinkable (Tepas and Monk 1987; Walsh et al. 1981).

It should be borne in mind that exogenous distractions can sometimes be used as scapegoats for a sleep disruption that is basically *endogenous* in origin. Thus, Folkard et al. (1979), when comparing responses of two night-working subgroups to a questionnaire, found that "rigid sleepers" reported more days of sleep disruption by noise than did "flexible sleepers." On examination, the sleeping accommodations of the two subgroups were entirely comparable; it was just that flexible sleepers had a better-adjusted circadian system and were thus less disturbed than rigid sleepers by any given noise. As is well known

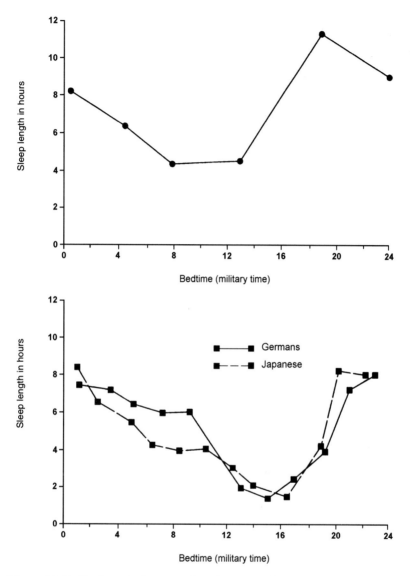

Figure 29–7. Replotted laboratory data *(upper panel)* and survey data on several thousand German *(solid line)* and Japanese *(dashed line)* shift workers *(lower panel)* relating hours of sleep obtained to the bedtime at which sleep was attempted. Morning bedtimes followed a night of total sleep loss.
Source. Adapted from Akerstedt and Gillberg 1982 (upper panel) and Kogi 1985 (lower panel).

from experience, if the body and mind are not ready for sleep, even the quiet dripping of a faucet can keep one awake.

Whether because of endogenous or exogenous processes (or a mixture of the two), day sleeps are undoubtedly shorter than equivalent night sleeps, and night workers will inevitably build up a deficit of 7 hours or more over their week of duty, usually dissipating it to some extent with long sleep-ins on the weekend (Knauth et al. 1980).

This buildup of a sleep debt is important in two respects. First is the obvious finding that partially sleep-deprived individuals perform less well than fully rested ones, particularly when doing monotonous tasks such as driving and quality control (Froberg 1985; Wilkinson 1972). Limiting one's night sleep to 3 hours, for example, results in performance decrements comparable to those observed in persons ingesting the British "legal limit" of alcohol (Folkard et al. 1977). Often these decrements result from "gaps" or "blocks" in performance when response times are considerably slower than normal. This slower response time may adversely affect the patient's safety while driving vehicles or operating dangerous machinery. Equally important, however, are the malaise and irritability that result from a chronic sleep debt. These effects can severely impair a patient's ability to interact well with workmates and family, and they may precipitate further problems in his or her life.

Social and Domestic Problems

It is important for clinicians (and, indeed, for researchers) to remember that the social and domestic problems of the shift-worker patient are as important as the problems associated with circadian rhythms and sleep. Not only can social and domestic problems be more salient and intractable than those related to the other two factors, but they can severely limit the application of strategies designed to enhance circadian adjustment and to improve sleep. Thus, a rocky marriage, a second job, or an unreasonable domestic load inevitably reduces the amount of sleep time available and renders an appropriate circadian routine infeasible. These social and domestic problems then result in sleep deprivation, jet-lag symptoms, or both for the patient, who will also be preoccupied with the problems themselves.

Marital problems, second jobs, and an excessive domestic load have all been documented as a source (or a result) of failure to cope with shift work. In a survey of 1,490 hourly workers, Tepas et al. (1985) found an almost 50% increase in divorces and separations for those on (fixed) night shifts compared with those on morning and evening shifts. When asked whether they were satisfied with the amount of time they had to spend with family and friends, workers on both night and evening shifts were about half as likely to respond "yes" as were their morning-shift colleagues (Tepas and Monk 1987).

Problems of access to spouse and children are particularly frequent in those persons working evening shifts, for whom circadian and sleep loss difficulties are often largely absent. Thus, for example, patients report that they can spend a whole week at a time without ever interacting with their day-working spouse or school-age children (Monk and Folkard 1992). The family becomes inert mounds under the bedsheets to the evening worker returning home after midnight; and the shift worker becomes a sleeping ogre to the family, who must tiptoe around the house as they get ready for school or work in the morning.

Excessive domestic load represents a major source of difficulties in coping with shift work and accounts for most, it not all, of the differences between the sexes in coping ability. Married women are often expected by their husbands to continue to run the household, raise the children, and do domestic chores in addition to their shift-work burden (Gadbois 1981). For these people, there is usually insufficient "leisure" time available for such duties, and time is therefore "borrowed" from the sleep period. Thus, Gadbois (1981) found that female night-shift workers with two children slept about 9 hours less per week than their unmarried female colleagues. Brown and Charles (cited in Walker 1985) concluded that women's night working "takes place *without* any fundamental transformation of the sexual division of labor and at considerable cost to the women themselves" (p. 225).

Societal problems are also encountered by shift workers. As mentioned at the beginning of this chapter, society expects a Monday-to-Friday day-work schedule. Several authors (reviewed by Walker 1985) have determined that shift workers feel alienated from the community because they are unable to attend evening educational, sports, or religious meetings, or weekend recreational events. Team or society membership becomes difficult because of irregularity of attendance, and few shift workers hold office in such clubs and societies. Shift workers can feel themselves to be "marginal," losing out on community benefits and prestige. Such a perception can be felt particularly keenly in reference to the company, where company picnics, sports events, and clubs are effectively closed to the shift worker. These feelings of alienation may further reduce shift-worker patients' self-esteem, which may already be battered by the perception (or, rather, misperception) that they have lost the love and respect of their families and have failed to show the strength needed to cope with the abnormal work hours.

Health Consequences

Because current shift workers represent a "survivor sample," it has not been easy to demonstrate the adverse health consequences of shift work—even with respect to gastrointestinal disorders (for which there is the best evidence). For example, it has proved to be *former* shift workers who show the increased incidence of peptic ulcers (Rutenfranz et al. 1977). Cardiovascular risk has also been implicated in some Swedish studies (Knutsson et al. 1986). Moreover, factors associated with cardiovascular risk have been shown to be lessened by improving the shift schedule (Orth-Gomer 1983). More longitudinal follow-up studies of shift workers are needed to make these finding more definitive.

Age and Experience

It is a nasty surprise to many shift workers to discover that, with regard to coping with shift work, age and experience weigh in as *negative* factors rather positive ones. Many who coped well with shift work in their 20s and 30s suddenly experience significant problems as they enter their late 40s and 50s. These problems may be associated with increased fragility of sleep, a change in the workers' circadian rhythms, or both (Monk and Folkard 1985). Moreover, even when age is controlled for in the analysis, years of shift-work experience correlate negatively with coping ability (Foret et al. 1981). Thus, long-term adjustment to shift work over one's life appears to be an unachievable goal.

SOLUTIONS FOR SHIFT WORK

Although it is easy to document the problems associated with shift work, it is more difficult to put forward solutions. A list of recommendations follows (Monk 1988). Although the recommendations make sense based on what we currently know, it should be recognized that much more research needs to be done in this area before these treatments can be considered to be properly validated.

Solutions for the Circadian System

Unless the shift-worker patient is on either a totally irregular routine (which is often encountered in the transportation sector) or a rapidly rotating one (which is used by many European companies and certain U.S. air traffic controllers), the aim of the coping strategy will be 1) to acquire as rapidly as possible the circadian temporal orientation that is most appropriate to the work shift and 2) to maintain that orientation throughout the patient's spell of duty on that shift (Monk 1986).

Studies of jet lag and laboratory phase shifts have suggested that phase delays are more easily accomplished by the biological clock than are phase advances (Aschoff et al. 1975; Klein et al. 1972). Thus, night workers should take their sleep straight after work, rather than waiting until the afternoon. This change corresponds to a delay of about 9 hours, which is easier for the biological clock to achieve than the advance of about 9 hours required by an afternoon bedtime. Because excessive napping can interfere with the quality of the major sleep episode, afternoon naps should be used only as a "topping off" device and should be limited to 2 hours or less.

Night workers should identify the time cues that are pulling their biological clock toward a nocturnal orientation and strengthen them and should identify those cues that are working against a nocturnal orientation and attenuate them. Time cues working in their favor are a regular morning bedtime; three meals per "day," with a proper lunch halfway through the working night; and physical activity and social interaction through the night. Time cues working against them will be daylight on the journey home from work (perhaps warranting the use of sunglasses), sleep during the night shift, and social or work commitments during the first half of the day (8 A.M. to 4 P.M.).

Not everyone's biological clock properties are the same, and certain characteristics will influence how easy or difficult an individual finds it to cope with shift work. In particular, "morning types" with an early phasing biological clock who like to get up with the dawn seem to experience extra problems in coping with shift work (Hildebrandt and Stratmann 1979). Also at risk are those in their late 40s or 50s, whose biological clocks have become earlier phasing and less robust with age (see above). For such individuals, the change from successful coping with shift work to significant sleep and well-being problems can be precipitated.

Sleep Coping Strategies
Shift workers should jealously guard the time set aside for their sleep. This time should be regular, predictable, and free from social or other commitments. During that time, telephones, doorbells, and domestic appliances should be silenced. Heavy curtains and thick carpets should be used to help make the bedroom as quiet and as dark as possible. The bedroom should be used only for sleep and lovemaking. Caffeine should be avoided within 5 hours of bedtime, and alcohol should not be used as a sedative because subsequent sleep would then be light and disrupted. Because of problems of tolerance and withdrawal, hypnotics should not be regularly used as sleeping aids. Hypnotics with a long half-life should be avoided because of possible intrusions of sleepiness into the work shift at a time (the night shift) when the patient is particularly vulnerable to such effects.

People who naturally need a lot of sleep to function well can find shift work particularly hard to cope with. Often, such individuals report that all they do is work and sleep, missing out on recreation and social interaction. This situation can become so problematic that a switch to day work is called for.

Social and Domestic Coping Strategies
Few of the coping strategies outlined for the other two factors in the triad will work unless the social and domestic milieu is supportive.

Shift workers should seek to gain their family's understanding of their predicament and to rally their family's support in coping with it. Relationships should be forged with other shift-work families, who are more likely than day-working friends to be supportive and understanding.

Particularly at risk from a domestic point of view are those shift workers who are still expected to run a household and look after children (Gadbois 1981). These shift workers are often "working wives," and husbands should realize that domestic chores can severely cut into the sleep time of the shift worker, thus increasing irritability and family tensions.

Spousal and parenting roles may also be compromised, particularly on the evening shift, which has little impact on sleep or biological clock factors. Efforts should be made to ensure that other times are specifically set aside for the shift worker to spend time with his or her spouse and children. In general, the presence of a shift worker in the household can either strengthen the family by drawing it closer together against the difficulties or destroy the family with strain and disharmony. The clinician should be aware of the need to involve the patient's family in the development of any shift-work coping strategy. Depending on the individual case, this involvement might range from a simple interview with the spouse to a course of marital therapy. Table 29–1 presents a simple checklist of strategies that shift-worker patients might find useful.

CHRONIC JET LAG

Like the term "shift work," the term "jet lag" can be confusing because it means different things to different people. To some, jet lag includes the short-term discomfort and somatic symptoms resulting from the air sickness, stress, fatigue, aching muscles, and dehydration that result from the flight itself (Graeber 1989). These symptoms occur even on North-South flights where no time zones are crossed. They are usually dissipated during the first day after arrival, however, and because of this are unlikely to result in the sufferer seeking professional help.

A more standard use of the term *jet lag* is to describe symptoms lasting several days after the flight itself, which result from a need to reset the circadian system to the timing appropriate to a new time zone. Like the symptoms of shift work (which have a similar etiology), those of jet lag include sleep disruption, daytime sleepiness, malaise, irritability, and gastrointestinal distress. Their severity depends on both the individual involved and the direction and extent of the difference in time zone between home and destination (Klein et al. 1972).

In the present age of relatively inexpensive air travel, many millions

Table 29–1. Summary of coping strategies for patients doing shift work

- Sleep immediately after a night shift, rather than before it.
- Keep to a regular schedule of three meals per day, avoiding excessive snacks.
- Keep a regular bedtime on each spell of duty.
- Avoid exposure to bright sunshine on the way home from a night shift (wear sunglasses).
- Jealously guard your sleep time, silencing telephones, doorbells, and domestic appliances.
- Keep the bedroom quiet and dark.
- Only use the bedroom for sleep and lovemaking.
- Avoid caffeine within 5 hours before sleep.
- Avoid the habitual use of alcohol or sleeping pills.
- Rally the support of your family in helping you to cope.
- Keep the channels of family communication open.
- Set aside special times to be with spouse and children.
- Forge links with other shift-working families.

Source. Adapted from Monk TH: "Coping With the Stress of Shift Work." *Work and Stress* 2:169–172, 1988. Used with permission.

of Americans have experienced jet lag at least once in their lives. For most people, the jet lag was, at worst, a transient inconvenience that marred the early part of a vacation or a visit to a grandchild. I agree with the recent international sleep disorders nosology in concluding that treatment in such situations is not warranted (American Sleep Disorders Association 1990). This chapter instead deals with a jet-lag problem that causes many people significant distress for months at a time. For such people, the crossing of time zones is not something that occurs once or twice per year, but several times a month, and the time zones involved often are radically different from that of home base.

DSM-IV recognizes "jet-lag type" as a specific type of circadian rhythm sleep disorder (sleep-wake schedule disorder; 307.45). The description reads: "Sleepiness and alertness that occur at inappropriate times of day relative to local time, occurring after repeated travel across more than one time zone."

Jet-Lag Findings

Properly controlled studies of jet lag, either in the field or in the laboratory, are very difficult and expensive to carry out. As a consequence, few are reported in the literature (see reviews by Aschoff et al. 1975; Graeber 1989; and Winget et al. 1984). Fortunately, however, a carefully conducted, definitive series of studies by Klein, Wegmann, and associates are available. These researchers concentrated primarily on the effects of the 6-hour time change involved in crossing the Atlantic Ocean, using groups of healthy young men as subjects (Klein and Wegmann 1975; Klein et al. 1972). Among their many findings, Klein and Wegmann concluded that circadian temperature rhythms took about 50% longer to adjust to eastbound flights than to westbound ones, that the homeward versus outward distinction was unimportant, and that jet-lag effects could be prolonged by requiring that subjects remain within their destination hotel for several days after arrival.

As one would expect, the circadian disruptions of jet lag are manifest in quite significant effects on sleep. These effects are reviewed extensively by Graeber (1989). As with the circadian dysfunction that underlies it, the extent of the sleep disruption depends on the number of time zones crossed and the direction of travel. Reported effects include reductions in sleep efficiency, decreased REM sleep latencies, increased REM sleep in the first part of the night, and in some cases a reduction in slow-wave sleep. In his review, Graeber noted that these effects were still present 7 days after the flight, a finding that is corroborated by our own laboratory studies simulating jet lag (Monk et al. 1988—see Figures 29–4 and 29–5).

The negative symptoms of jet lag are not restricted to sleep disruption, however. Daytime functioning is also impaired, with increases in sleepiness, malaise, and irritability and impairments in performance ability (Klein et al. 1972). Somatic symptoms also include gastrointestinal problems and headaches.

Chronic Jet-Lag Syndrome

This syndrome has not been properly studied before; thus, there are no literature results to be reported. Indeed, a major purpose of this chapter is to draw clinicians' attention to chronic jet-lag syndrome, so that patients suffering from the disorder can be properly diagnosed and treated. Its reality as a disorder became apparent to me at a seminar given for senior executives at a large multinational company. Somewhat surprisingly, *all* those present reported significant problems with the disorder, which stemmed from an occupational life-style that involved spending up to 2 weeks every month in a time zone radically different from that of the executive's home base. Trips were often to the Middle East or Far East and involved stressful and important negotiations and decisions.

The executives who had suffered from the syndrome reported all of the somatic, emotional, sleep-related, and performance-related decrements characteristic of jet lag, together with the health and marital disharmonies discussed earlier with regard to shift work. Interestingly, though, these executives only realized the extent of their impairment when they returned to a prolonged spell of duty at the home-base office. Only after several weeks of recovery did they remember what it was like to have a normal, stable affect again, to interact well with family and co-workers, and to perform at optimal levels of efficiency. Thus, one of the first cognitive effects of chronic jet-lag syndrome appears to be loss of awareness of the level of impairment one is experiencing. This loss is clearly insidious for those who must make crucial decisions in large-scale multinational companies.

Age effects are also involved in the etiology of chronic jet-lag syndrome. As noted above for shift work, late middle age and beyond is a vulnerable time of life for circadian-rhythm and sleep disorders related to work schedules. With some exceptions, many senior executives do not reach their level of seniority until the fifth or sixth decade of life. Thus, they are at a dangerous age, both for the syndrome itself and for the cardiovascular, psychiatric, and gastrointestinal disorders that are likely to be associated with it.

TREATMENT OF CHRONIC JET-LAG SYNDROME

The first point to recognize is that the comfort level of the travel (e.g., going first class, being met by limousines, staying in luxury hotels) may increase the comfort level of the individual but can never eliminate the basic cause of the disorder, which stems from the difference in time zone between the home base and the destination. Even supersonic travel will help only if it allows the patient to remain on home-base time by enabling the transatlantic meeting to take place within a single day. That is not to argue that such luxuries should not be afforded to the traveler, only that they can never comprise a full solution to the problem of chronic jet-lag syndrome.

The most useful approach for the person who has chronic jet-lag syndrome involves 1) minimizing the number of time zones crossed per month, 2) scheduling postflight recovery days, and 3) scheduling meetings at times that are appropriate to the *traveler's* biological clock (i.e., at a sensible time of day relative to the home-base time zone). This strategy is similar to the one adopted by Henry Kissinger in his "shuttle diplomacy" missions, who allegedly kept as much as possible to a U.S. time zone–based schedule and regarded every meal as breakfast.

On an individual-trip basis, the patient also needs concrete advice about how to lessen the symptoms of jet lag. This list of countermeasures is taken from a previous publication of mine (Monk 1987) and follows many of the guidelines suggested by Ehret and Scanlon (1983). Importantly, though, like many other researchers in this field (e.g., Graeber 1989), I am not convinced of the value of the widely publicized

Ehret jet-lag diet, particularly in regard to the feasting and fasting components. Indeed, in a recent objective laboratory test (Moline et al. 1990), the diet failed to lessen jet-lag symptoms at all (actually, it made some of them worse).

Like the night worker, the air traveler should first think carefully about the desired orientation of his or her circadian system. It may well be that the patient will decide to remain on home-based time. In that case, he or she should schedule meetings and avoid destination time cues accordingly, remaining indoors wherever possible.

Should such a strategy prove infeasible, then a rapid phase change of the circadian system is desirable, and the following coping procedures should be undertaken. Before the flight, if it is possible to do so without losing sleep, the patient should consider a gradual change in bedtime (1 hour or less per day) toward the new routine. For example, before a flight from New York to Paris, he or she could start going to bed progressively earlier than usual each night for a few days before the flight; in anticipation of a flight from New York to Honolulu, he or she could go to bed progressively later. It is very important, though, that the time of waking is also changed and that the patient avoids accumulating a sleep debt; otherwise, any potentially beneficial effects may be lost. This process might be helped by judicious use of bright lights from a light box or by timed daylight exposure in the evening to delay the routine or in the early morning to advance it (Daan and Lewy 1984).

On boarding the plane, the patient should immediately reset his or her wristwatch to the new time zone and attempt to follow activities appropriate to the new time (for example, sleeping if it is nighttime and staying awake if it is daytime). Food can sometimes help in this adjustment. For some people, carbohydrates induce sleepiness and proteins induce alertness, and judicious choices of menu or lunch box items may have the desired effect. If the flight is long and a (new time zone) daytime sleep becomes irresistible, the sleep should be short (less than 2 hours) and taken during the siesta (1 P.M.–4 P.M.) interval. If necessary, the patient should ask someone to wake him or her up; otherwise, it may turn into a long sleep, interfering with the subsequent night's sleep.

On arrival, the patient should immerse himself or herself in the society and activity patterns of the destination. He or she should *not* remain within the confines of the hotel, because studies have shown that this significantly impedes the process of adjustment (Klein and Wegmann 1975). Outdoor activities are recommended, because daylight levels assist in the adjustment of circadian rhythms. The patient should stay awake until standard bedtime in the new time zone. Again, if sleep is irresistible, a short siesta is permissible, but with an alarm clock to prevent it from becoming as long as a normal sleep. Meal choices can help in this process, and the patient should keep a snack at bedside (not chocolate) in case of hunger in the middle of the night. In general, sleep after the flight will be more fragile (easily disrupted) than usual, and earplugs may be needed to mask out sounds (e.g., an air conditioner) that would not normally be considered a problem.

There may be a second-night effect (particularly after eastward flights) wherein the second night is worse than the first. This reaction is quite normal and does not indicate particularly that the patient is doing anything wrong.

The same process should be done in reverse when the patient returns to home base. There is no evidence that adjustment is any more rapid in the homeward direction than in the outward one (Klein et al. 1972), so the patient should be careful in scheduling events and meetings during the week after return.

Scheduling of flight times can also help in the adjustment process. Wherever possible, the patient should seek to arrive at his or her destination in the evening. This schedule allows time for the patient to unwind, have a light meal (avoiding caffeine and alcohol), and retire to bed at an appropriate time. The direction of the flight can also be considered. Because phase delays are more easy to cope with than phase advances, around-the-world itineraries should always go in the westbound direction. Table 29–2 gives a list of hints and strategies that might be useful for the patient.

As was the case for the shift worker, the circadian aspects of chronic jet-lag syndrome do not represent the whole picture. Advice regarding sleep coping strategies and social and domestic coping strategies would still apply, and the reader is referred to those sections in the "Solutions for Shift Work" part of the chapter. Just as coping with shift work should include both home-based and work-based strategies, so too should coping with jet-lag syndrome involve both home-based and

Table 29–2.   Summary of advice for patients coping with jet lag

- Be well rested before the flights.
- Reset your wristwatch to the new time zone on boarding the plane.
- Avoid caffeine, alcohol, and smoking.
- Drink plenty of fluids.
- Get out and about in the daylight.
- Stay up until the normal destination bedtime.
- Keep a midnight snack and earplugs handy.
- Allow time to recover from jet lag on your return.
- Consider staying on home-based time.

Source. Adapted from Monk TH: "Coping With the Stress of Jet-Lag." *Work and Stress* 1:163–166, 1987. Used with permission.

away-based strategies. The social and domestic issues comprise a vitally important aspect of the treatment of chronic jet-lag disorder and should not be neglected.

CONCLUSIONS

A patient's occupation can, either through abnormal work hours or through transmeridian travel, destroy the orderly rhythms of life that are so important for the smooth functioning of his or her circadian system. Such disruptions can compromise sleep, waking function, mood, health, and interpersonal relationships. Like the problem itself, treatment should be multifaceted and should aim both to reduce the stresses and strains impinging on the patient and to bolster his or her ability to cope with the stresses and strains that are unavoidable.

REFERENCES

Akerstedt T, Gillberg M: Displacement of the sleep period and sleep deprivation: implications for shift work. Human Neurobiology 1:163–171, 1982

American Psychiatric Association: Diagnostic and Statistical Manual of Mental Disorders, 4th Edition. Washington, DC, American Psychiatric Association, 1994

American Sleep Disorders Association: The International Classification of Sleep Disorders: Diagnostic and Coding Manual. Rochester, MN, American Sleep Disorders Association, 1990

Aschoff J (ed): Handbook of Behavioral Neurobiology, Vol 4. New York, Plenum, 1981

Aschoff J, Hoffman K, Pohl H, et al: Re-entrainment of circadian rhythms after phase-shifts of the zeitgeber. Chronobiologia 2:23–78, 1975

Czeisler CA, Johnson MP, Duffy JF, et al: Exposure to bright light and darkness to treat physiologic maladaptation to night work. N Engl J Med 322:1253–1259, 1990

Czeisler CA, Chiasera AJ, Duffy JF: Research on sleep, circadian rhythms and aging: applications to manned spaceflight. Exp Gerontol 26:217–232, 1991

Daan S, Lewy AJ: Scheduled exposure to daylight: a potential strategy to reduce "jet-lag" following transmeridian flight. Psychopharmacol Bull 20:566–568, 1984

Eastman CI: Circadian rhythms and bright light: recommendations for shift work. Work and Stress 4:245–260, 1990

Eastman CI: Squashing versus nudging circadian rhythms with artificial bright light: solutions for shift work? Perspect Biol Med 34:181–195, 1991

Ehret CF, Scanlon LW: Overcoming Jet Lag. New York, Berkley, 1983

Feather NT, Bond J: Time structure and purposeful activity among employed and unemployed university graduates. Journal of Occupational Psychology 56:241–254, 1983

Folkard S: Is there a "best compromise" shift system? Ergonomics 35:1453–1463, 1992

Folkard S, Monk TH, Bradbury R, et al: Time of day effects in school children's immediate and delayed recall of meaningful material. Br J Psychol 68:45–50, 1977

Folkard S, Monk TH, Lobban MC: Towards a predictive test of adjustment to shiftwork. Ergonomics 22:79–91, 1979

Foret J, Lantin G: The sleep of train drivers: an example of the effects of irregular work schedules on sleep, in Aspects of Human Efficiency. Edited by Colquhoun WP. London, English Universities Press, 1972, pp 273–282

Foret J, Bensimon G, Benoit O, et al: Quality of sleep as a function of age and shift work, in Night and Shift Work: Biological and Social Aspects. Edited by Reinberg A, Vieux N, Andlauer P. Oxford, Pergamon, 1981, pp 149–160

Froberg JE: Sleep deprivation and prolonged work hours, in Hours of Work—Temporal Factors in Work Scheduling. Edited by Folkard S, Monk TH. New York, Wiley, 1985, pp 67–75

Gadbois C: Women on night shift: interdependence of sleep and off-the-job activities, in Night and Shift Work: Biological and Social Aspects. Edited by Reinberg A, Vieux N, Andlauer P. Oxford, Pergamon, 1981, pp 223–227

Gordon NP, Cleary PD, Parker CE, et al: The prevalence and health impact of shiftwork. Am J Public Health 76:1225–1228, 1986

Graeber RC: Jet lag and sleep disruption, in Principles and Practice of Sleep Medicine. Edited by Kryger MH, Roth T, Dement WC. Philadelphia, PA, WB Saunders, 1989, pp 324–331

Hildebrandt G, Stratmann I: Circadian system response to night work in relation to the individual circadian phase position. Int Arch Occup Environ Health 43:73–83, 1979

Klein KE, Wegmann HM: The resynchronization of human circadian rhythms after transmeridian flights as a result of flight direction and mode of activity, in Chronobiology. Edited by Scheving LE, Halberg F, Pauly JE. Tokyo, Igaku Shoin, 1975, pp 564–570

Klein KE, Wegmann HM, Hunt BI: Desynchronization of body temperature and performance circadian rhythms as a results of out-going and homegoing transmeridian flights. Aerospace Medicine 43:119–132, 1972

Knauth P, Rutenfranz J: Experimental shift work studies of permanent night, and rapidly rotating, shift systems, I: circadian rhythm of body temperature and re-entrainment at shift change. Int Arch Occup Environ Health 37:125–137, 1976

Knauth P, Landau K, Droge C, et al: Duration of sleep depending on the type of shift work. Int Arch Occup Environ Health 46:167–177, 1980

Knutsson A, Akerstedt T, Orth-Gomer K, et al: Increased risk of ischaemic heart disease in shift workers. Lancet 2:89–92, 1986

Kogi K: Introduction to the problems of shift work, in Hours of Work—Temporal Factors in Work Scheduling. Edited by Folkard S, Monk TH. New York, Wiley, 1985, pp 165–184

Lewy AJ, Wehr TA, Goodwin FK, et al: Light suppresses melatonin secretion in humans. Science 210:1267–1269, 1980

Lewy AJ, Sack RA, Singer CL: Assessment and treatment of chronobiologic disorders using plasma melatonin levels and bright light exposure: the clock-gate model and the phase response curve. Psychopharmacol Bull 20:561–565, 1984

Mellor EF: Shift work and flexitime: how prevalent are they? Monthly Labor Review 109:14–21, 1986

Mills JN, Minors DS, Waterhouse JM: The effects of sleep upon human circadian rhythms. Chronobiologia 5:14–27, 1978

Moline ML, Pollak CP, Wagner DR, et al: Effects of the "jet-lag" diet on the adjustment to a phase advance. Paper presented at the second annual meeting of the Society for Research Into Biological Rhythms, Amelia Island, FL, May 1990

Monk TH: Advantages and disadvantages of rapidly rotating shift schedules—a circadian viewpoint. Hum Factors 28:553–557, 1986

Monk TH: Coping with the stress of jet-lag. Work and Stress 1:163–166, 1987

Monk TH: Coping with the stress of shift work. Work and Stress 2:169–172, 1988

Monk TH, Folkard S: Individual differences in shiftwork adjustment, in Hours of Work—Temporal Factors in Work Scheduling. Edited by Folkard S, Monk TH. New York, Wiley, 1985, pp 227–237

Monk TH, Folkard S: Making Shift Work Tolerable. London, Taylor & Frances, 1992

Monk TH, Moline ML, Graeber RC: Inducing jet lag in the laboratory: patterns of adjustment to an acute shift in routine. Aviation, Space and Environmental Medicine 59:703–710, 1988

Moore RY: The suprachiasmatic nucleus and the organization of a circadian system. Trends Neurosci 5:404–407, 1982

Orth-Gomer K: Intervention on coronary risk factors by adapting a shift work schedule to biologic rhythmicity. Psychosom Med 45:407–415, 1983

Rusak B, Mistlberger RE, Losier B, et al: Daily hoarding opportunity entrains the pacemaker for hamster activity rhythms. J Comp Physiol [A] 164:165–171, 1988

Rutenfranz J, Colquhoun WP, Knauth P, et al: Biomedical and psychosocial aspects of shift work: a review. Scand J Work Environ Health 3:165–182, 1977

Rutenfranz J, Haider M, Koller M: Occupational health measures for nightworkers and shiftworkers, in Hours of Work—Temporal Factors in Work Scheduling. Edited by Folkard S, Monk TH. New York, Wiley, 1985, pp 199–210

Schor JB: The Overworked American. New York, Basic Books, 1991

Tepas DI, Monk TH: Work schedules, in Handbook of Human Factors. Edited by Salvendy G. New York, Wiley, 1987, pp 819–843

Tepas DI, Armstrong DR, Carlson ML, et al: Changing industry to continuous operations: different strokes for different plants. Behavior Research Methods, Instruments and Computers 17:670–676, 1985

Van Loon JH: Diurnal body temperature curves in shift workers. Ergonomics 6:267–272, 1963

Walker JM: Social problems of shift work, in Hours of Work—Temporal Factors in Work Scheduling. Edited by Folkard S, Monk TH. New York, Wiley, 1985, pp 211–225

Walsh JK, Tepas DI, Moss PD: The EEG sleep of night and rotating shift workers, in The Twenty-Four Hour Workday: Proceedings of a Symposium on Variations in Work-Sleep Schedules. Edited by Johnson LC, Tepas DI, Colquhoun WP, et al. Cincinnati, OH, Department of Health and Human Services (NIOSH), 1981, pp 451–465

Weitzman ED, Kripke DF: Experimental 12-hour shift of the sleep-wake cycle in man: effects on sleep and physiologic rhythms, in Variations in Work-Sleep Schedules: Effects on Health and Performance (Advances in Sleep Research, Vol 7). Edited by Johnson LC, Tepas DI, Colquhoun WP, et al. New York, Spectrum Publications, 1981, pp 125–149

Wever RA: The circadian multi-oscillator system of man. International Journal of Chronobiology 3:19–55, 1975

Wever RA: The Circadian System of Man: Results of Experiments Under Temporal Isolation. New York, Springer-Verlag, 1979

Wever RA, Poiasek J, Wildgruber CM: Bright light affects human circadian rhythms. Pflugers Arch 396:85–87, 1983

Wilkinson RT: Sleep deprivation—eight questions, in Aspects of Human Efficiency. Edited by Colquhoun WP. London, English Universities Press, 1972, pp 25–30

Wilkinson RT: How fast should the night shift rotate? Ergonomics 35:1425–1446, 1992a

Wilkinson RT: Reply to Folkard. Ergonomics 35:1465–1466, 1992b

Winget CM, DeRoshia CW, Markley CL, et al: A review of human physiological and performance changes associated with desynchronosis of biological rhythms. Aviation, Space and Environmental Medicine 55:1085–1096, 1984

Chapter 30

Sleep in Dementing Illness

Donald L. Bliwise, Ph.D.

In this chapter, I review sleep in patients with dementing illness. The initial focus will be on the clinical picture of sleep disturbance in patients with dementia. Second, I review polysomnographic and physiological studies of sleep and rhythms in some specific types of dementia. Finally, I end with a brief section on treatment and amelioration of sleep-related symptoms in these patients.

CLINICAL PICTURE OF SLEEP DISTURBANCE IN DEMENTIA

Familiar to most clinicians is the typical presentation of a family member with dementia by the spouse or other caregiver with the complaint that the identified patient becomes "difficult" or agitated at night. Caregivers tend to report this phenomenon in a variety of ways, sometimes describing the patient as "aggressive," "combative," or "confused." Occasionally, overt wandering is the presenting symptom, and there have been cases of the patient eloping outside the home during the night. More typically, the patient with dementia will go into the kitchen at night, open the refrigerator, turn on the stove, or turn on the radio and disturb other family members attempting to sleep. A number of investigators (e.g., Pollak et al. 1990) have noted that such nocturnal confusion is a major cause of institutionalization in patients with dementia, even more so than the stressors of physical incapacity and incontinence. Such behavioral disturbance, often referred to as "sundowning," has also been shown to relate to measures of caregiver burden more strongly than the rate of decline in mental function (Gallagher-Thompson et al. 1992).

To date, sundowning itself has been the subject of relatively few systematic studies. Some early investigators contended that a delirious state could be induced in patients with dementia merely by bringing them into a dark room during the daytime hours. Although attributed to the effects of darkness, this finding has never been replicated, and the putative mechanisms of the effect have never been understood.

Supported by Grant AG-10643 from the National Institute on Aging.

More recently, Evans (1987) compared 11 nursing home patients labeled as sundowners and 78 patients labeled as nonsundowners on a variety of demographic and medical variables. Variables such as incontinence and recent room transfer discriminated the groups, whereas variables such as use of psychoactive medication and differences in morning and afternoon body temperature did not. Although this study was valuable in generating empirical data related to this phenomenon, it is important to keep in mind that patients were classified into the sundowning and nonsundowning groups based on data collected over only 2 days, during which observations were made for only two 10-minute periods in the morning and afternoon. Patients were not observed during most of the day; hence, the validity of these data for discussing behavior patterns over the entire 24-hour period must be considered quite limited. Other work by Cohen-Mansfield et al. (1989), who attempted to document sundowning as a "trait" characteristic of nursing home patients, reported that two of eight patients showed such a pattern. Martino-Saltzman et al. (1991) investigated wandering in nursing home patients and reported that the time period from 7 to 10 P.M. appeared to be the most common time for such behavior to occur.

Finally, in a series of studies using systematic behavioral observations in nursing home patients, Bliwise et al. (1990; in press) noted that although sleep was less likely to occur during the period close to sunset, there was not a significant increase in agitation occurring at that time. Thus, the notion of sundowning proved difficult to validate using reliable observations of agitation and disturbed behavior. Curiously, however, detectable trends did occur in the seasonal variation of agitation: disruptive behaviors were worse in the winter months than in autumn. These trends were noted only during the period near sundown, defined as the actual time of sunset plus or minus 2 hours. No apparent seasonal variation was noted in agitation that occurred in the presunset or postsunset period.

Apart from these descriptive studies, typically made in institutionalized populations (which were probably heterogeneous insofar as the type of dementia was concerned), few data exist on the prevalence of sundowning behavior in patients with dementia. Several studies examining behavioral problems in patients with Alzheimer's disease have reported on "sleep disturbance" prevalence in their patient populations. The figures generally agree and suggest that about 40% of Alzheimer's disease patients show such problems with sleep (see Bliwise 1993). It is important to realize that these figures may be misleading in that a dementia patient's inability to sleep through the night may not be at all equivalent to sundowning.

Our own approach to this problem has been to ask caregivers to indicate the typical time of day when disruptive behaviors (e.g., agitation, wandering, combativeness) are likely to occur; then, we estimate the sundowning prevalence on that basis (Bliwise et al. 1992). Our data suggest that, over a 1-month reporting period, the apparent prevalence of sundowning was about 28%. Interestingly, some caregivers reported a pattern of morning disruptive behavior. This pattern was much less common, however, and did not relate to any assessments of mental function. By contrast, patients who displayed sundowning behavior showed a steeper rate of decline in mental abilities related to ideo-kinetic praxis (dysfunction of the ability to respond to commands). This decline suggested that patients' inability to respond appropriately to cues involving day versus those involving night might reflect a more general inability to respond nonlinguistically (i.e., behaviorally) to environmental cues.

SLEEP IN SPECIFIC DEMENTING CONDITIONS

The knowledge base of empirical research for Alzheimer's disease far outweighs that of other dementing conditions because 1) Alzheimer's disease is the most prevalent type of dementia (with estimates as high as 70% of all patients presenting with dementia), and 2) many other conditions (e.g., degenerative conditions involving the basal ganglia) do not invariably involve dementia until perhaps their most advanced stage. Far fewer patients with conditions like Huntington's disease or progressive supranuclear palsy have undergone sleep or rhythm studies. Hence, review of existing literature involving those diseases often relies on single groups, uncontrolled designs, or anecdotal reports.

Alzheimer's Disease

Sleep architecture. Studies of sleep architecture have generally shown higher amounts of stage 1 sleep and lower sleep efficiency in patients with Alzheimer's disease compared with age-matched control subjects. Studies from the Seattle group have shown that measures of general sleep disturbance such as reduced sleep efficiency actually parallel the extent of dementia (Prinz et al. 1982; Vitiello et al. 1990). Decreases in stages 3 and 4 sleep have been noted as well, but comparisons with control subjects may be limited because of floor effects (i.e., healthy elderly subjects also have decreased amounts of stages 3 and 4 sleep).

Rapid eye movement (REM) sleep parameters have shown inconsistent alterations in Alzheimer's disease. Because of the widespread cholinergic deterioration in patients with Alzheimer's disease and the dependence of REM sleep on intact cholinergic systems, a clear directional hypothesis can be formulated: measures of REM sleep quantity, duration, and intensity should be reduced in patients with Alzheimer's disease. Additionally, the time it takes to enter REM sleep at the beginning of the night (REM sleep latency) should be increased, although the latter effect might be posited additionally to reflect the decrease in stages 3 and 4 sleep typically occupying the first non–rapid eye movement (NREM) cycle. Despite the clarity in the direction of the predictions, evidence has been mixed as to whether REM sleep is unambiguously altered in patients with Alzheimer's disease. (For a more thorough review, see Bliwise 1993).

In addition to these studies employing visually scored polysomnography, several new studies examining sleep electroencephalographic (EEG) patterns in Alzheimer's disease patients have been reported recently. Petit et al. (1992) reported that asymmetry of temporal regions in REM sleep was a more powerful discriminator of Alzheimer's disease patients and elderly control subjects than was EEG asymmetry in the waking state. Prinz et al. (1992) also reported that increases in theta power in tonic REM sleep were able to distinguish a large group of patients with very mild Alzheimer's disease from control subjects without dementia.

It is of considerable import to place the findings regarding sleep architecture in Alzheimer's disease in the context of the differential diagnosis of depression in late life. The clinical presentations of the geriatric patient with depressive illness who complains about memory impairment, the dementia patient who denies any loss of mental capacities, and the mixed-syndrome patient who has features of both conditions are well recognized by those working in the field. The possibility that polysomnography might aid in the establishment of a diagnosis has been evaluated in great detail by the Pittsburgh group (Reynolds et al. 1988), who have shown that at baseline, affective disorder may be more strongly associated with measures of disturbed sleep (e.g., early morning awakening and shorter REM sleep latency) compared with early dementia.

Under conditions of experimentally induced sleep deprivation, alterations in REM sleep recovery functions (geriatric depressed patients showing an absence of REM sleep rebound, but early Alzheimer's disease patients showing REM sleep increases in the first REM period of the night) and in sleep continuity (depressed patients demonstrating poorer sleep continuity both before and after sleep deprivation compared with dementia patients) also suggest the utility of sleep studies in discriminating these diagnostic groups (Reynolds et al. 1987). Finally, in patients presenting with a mixed picture, sleep recordings have been shown to provide impressive discriminant validity in predicting which patients will later show deterioration versus improvement. The results of these studies suggested that higher amounts of stage 1 sleep and lower sleep efficiency were associated with clinical improvement on 2-year follow-up (Reynolds et al. 1986).

Respiration in sleep.   Data conflict as to whether patients with Alzheimer's disease have higher rates of sleep apnea than age-matched and gender-matched control subjects. Some studies have shown significantly higher, but nonetheless small, differences in rates of sleep-disordered breathing in Alzheimer's disease patients (see Bliwise 1989 for a review). This observation is consistent with some degeneration in the brain stem centers controlling ventilation in Alzheimer's disease patients; the differences between Alzheimer's disease patients and control subjects presumably are more manifest during a condition of altered chemoresponsivity. Other studies have not reported differences between Alzheimer's disease patients and control subjects and suggest that few of the Alzheimer's disease patients show marked oxyhemoglobin desaturation in sleep (Bliwise et al. 1989). Marked hypoxemia would be expected if the dementia of Alzheimer's disease were a consequence of sleep apnea (Bliwise 1989). Hence, the most prudent interpretation of the small possible differences in sleep apnea between Alzheimer's disease patients and age-matched, sex-matched control subjects is that such differences represent subtle deficiencies in ventilatory control mechanisms.

Although the evidence regarding sleep apnea in Alzheimer's disease is equivocal, there may be somewhat more compelling evidence that impaired respiration in sleep could be related to other forms of dementia (see "Vascular Dementia" section later in this chapter). Also of note are several reports that suggest that patients with Alzheimer's disease who have sleep apnea may be more confused and disoriented on awakening than those who do not (see Bliwise 1989). However, at least one group of researchers (Hoch et al. 1989) could not replicate the finding.

Movements in sleep.   There are several reasons to suspect that movements during sleep may be more pronounced in patients with Alzheimer's disease than in age-matched control subjects. First, myoclonus in wakefulness has long been noted to occur in some Alzheimer's disease patients with a prevalence of about 25%, particularly in later stages of the disease. Waking myoclonus in Alzheimer's disease is neither generalized nor stimulus sensitive (as it is in other dementias such as Creutzfeldt-Jakob disease) and typically involves only distal muscle jerks without paroxysmal EEG activity. As such, it bears some resemblance to periodic leg movements (PLMs) in sleep. Additionally, Alzheimer's disease may involve disruption of the dopaminergic system as well as the aforementioned cholinergic deficit. Because PLMs are often treated with L-dopa, such projected dopamine deficiencies in Alzheimer's disease would predict higher-than-normal rates of PLMs in patients with Alzheimer's disease. Few data are available to address this issue; however, three research groups reported no significant differences in PLMs between Alzheimer's disease patients and control subjects (Bliwise et al. 1986; Prinz et al. 1986; Reynolds et al. 1984).

Circadian rhythms.   Based on the clinical presentation of sundowning noted above, many investigators have attempted to document aberrations in the circadian timing systems of patients with Alzheimer's disease. Reductions in amplitude might be predicted on the basis of the higher levels of spontaneous daytime sleep observed in these patients (Allen et al. 1987; Prinz et al. 1982). Alterations in phase might be predicted in Alzheimer's disease patients as well, based on animal studies suggesting that phase advances in the temperature and rest-activity cycles in animals correspond to partial ablation of the suprachiasmatic nucleus. Swaab et al. (1985) noted that Alzheimer's disease patients show degeneration of this region of the hypothalamus, and patients with tumors of the third ventricle have long been known to present with daytime hypersomnolence.

In addition to the putative changes in amplitude and phase that are assumed to occur, there may well be alterations within the entrainment mechanism itself. These might occur anywhere in the retinohypothalamic tract and could prevent adequate signal transduction. For example, patients with Alzheimer's disease have been shown to incur degeneration of the optic nerve (Hinton et al. 1986).

Attempts to examine the circadian timing systems of patients with Alzheimer's disease have not provided convincing evidence that these patients have deficits in such functions. Several studies of body temperature rhythm and diurnal variation in a variety of hormones and blood constituents consistently failed to find significant differences between Alzheimer's disease patients and control subjects (see Bliwise 1993 for a review). Speculation concerning the basis for the absence of such differences has focused on selection bias operating in the inclusion of Alzheimer's disease patients capable of undergoing rectal temperature monitoring or tolerating indwelling catheters (Bliwise 1993).

Several studies of rest-activity rhythms in patients with Alzheimer's disease have suggested wide intraindividual and day-to-day variation in activity (Witting et al. 1990), but measures more closely related to the core oscillator (e.g., temperature) have not. A recent report by Okawa et al. (1991), however, is one of the few that suggests aberrations in the circadian timing of a physiological function in Alzheimer's disease patients. In this study, grossly demented nursing home patients were studied intermittently with oral temperatures taken at selected points around the 24-hour day over successive days. Results suggested "disorganized" and highly variable temperature rhythms in these institutionalized patients.

Vascular Dementia

Sleep architecture.   Very little is known about changes in sleep architecture specific to vascular dementia. Allen et al. (1987) reported minimal differences between patients with Alzheimer's disease and patients with multi-infarct dementia on waking after sleep onset or other sleep-stage measures. More recently Aharon-Peretz et al. (1991) reported that, based on wrist actigraphic measurements (activity "counts" using arbitrary units of movement), patients with multi-infarct dementia showed more nocturnal sleep fragmentation than patients with Alzheimer's disease. A brief report using polysomnography (Gilley et al. 1988) noted similar results. In contrast to patients with Alzheimer's disease, there appeared to be no correlation between the severity of the dementia and the extent of sleep fragmentation in patients with multi-infarct dementia.

Respiration in sleep.   Several studies have shown that patients with multi-infarct dementia have more sleep-disordered breathing relative to patients with Alzheimer's disease (Erkinjuntti et al. 1987; Manni et al. 1991). Because of the association of sleep apnea with cardiovascular disease in general, the possibility that sleep apnea may be causally related to cerebrovascular disease has been proposed. For example, snoring has been implicated as a risk factor for stroke (Palomaki et al. 1989). The possibility exists that some of the reported associations could represent disturbances in respiration subsequent to the stroke or retrospective reporting bias. However, the role of sleep apnea in the development of cardiovascular disease in general would suggest that this form of dementia may well be related to untreated, severe sleep apnea.

Movements in sleep.   Except for the brief report by Gilley et al. (1988), which suggested no differences in PLMs between patients with multi-infarct dementia and patients with Alzheimer's disease, there appear to be no studies addressing this issue. Inami et al. (1987) reported that PLMs were apparently common in patients with hemiplegic stroke on the affected side.

Circadian rhythms.   Of historical interest are the clinical observations of Hachinski et al. (1975), who reported that nocturnal confusion was mildly pathognomonic of multi-infarct dementia relative to Alzheimer's disease. More recently, Aharon-Peretz et al. (1991), using actigraphy, reported greater disruption in the 24-hour sleep-wake cycle in patients with multi-infarct dementia compared with patients with Alzheimer's disease. However, in a 24-hour polysomnographic study, Allen et al. (1987) reported no differences between the two patient populations on any daytime sleep parameters. Tarquini et al. (1978) reported absence of diurnal variation in thyroid-stimulating hormone in elderly atherosclerotic patients compared with elderly control subjects, although again this finding might be secondary to the disease rather than representing an underlying causal mechanism.

Parkinson's Disease

An examination of sleep patterns in Parkinson's disease, more than in any other type of dementia, requires a consideration of sleep both in the medicated and unmedicated states. Because such a large proportion of patients with Parkinson's disease are treated pharmacologically and because clinical evidence suggests that more than 90% of patients with Parkinson's disease experience sleep disturbance (Lees et al. 1988), it is considerably more common to encounter sleep problems in treated rather than untreated patients. Additionally, pharmacotherapy for Parkinson's disease involves manipulation of dopaminergic and, to a lesser extent, cholinergic systems, which are the same functional systems that are most impaired in patients with the disease. Hence, interpretation of drug effects must be made in the context of dopamine depletion—already presumed to be as high as 70% before clinical presentation of the disorder.

Movement in sleep is an apparent final confound in the interpretation of potential alterations in sleep architecture in patients with Parkinson's disease. Because Parkinson's disease patients often show persistence of their waking movement disorder into the state of sleep, such events could represent an immediate cause of sleep disruption in these patients. Although an increasing number of studies have examined characteristics of sleep-related movement in Parkinson's disease (see "Movements in Sleep" within this section), these studies have seldom addressed whether alterations in sleep-stage measures in such patients might not reflect these disruptive events.

Sleep architecture.   In early studies of unmedicated Parkinson's disease patients or Parkinson's disease patients withdrawn from medication, Mouret (1975) reported few, if any, differences between a subgroup of Parkinson's disease patients characterized by excessive eye blinking and blepharospasm and control subjects referenced in the literature. Another subgroup of Parkinson's disease patients, characterized by absence of atonia in REM sleep, showed considerably more sleep disturbance, with reduction in slow-wave and REM sleep. Kales et al. (1971) reported no differences in REM sleep between unmedicated patients and control subjects, but noted that the patients had less slow-wave sleep and increased sleep fragmentation. Decreases in both slow-wave and REM sleep under baseline conditions were noted by Bergonzi et al.

(1974), using control subjects from prior studies.

More recently, Askenasy and Yahr (1985) noted that in 5 patients with Parkinson's disease withdrawn from all medications for a 5-day period, sleep efficiency averaged 66% and the percentages of both slow-wave sleep and REM sleep were very low. This report essentially replicated an earlier report on 10 (presumably untreated) patients with Parkinson's disease (Askenasy 1981). Pronounced deficits in slow-wave sleep in unmedicated Parkinson's disease patients were specifically noted by Myslobodsky et al. (1982). Despite this previous literature, a recent report by Ferini-Strambi et al. (1991) is of interest. This group reported on 26 de novo, mild-stage (mean Hoehn-Yahr score = 2; Hoehn and Yahr 1967) Parkinson's disease patients compared with 15 age-matched, gender-matched control subjects. Measures of sleep maintenance and sleep stages failed to distinguish the two groups.

Because depression is not an uncommon symptom in patients with Parkinson's disease, several studies have attempted to study its role in sleep disruption in these patients. Depressed Parkinson's disease patients have comparatively worse sleep relative to nondepressed Parkinson's disease patients. Reduced REM sleep latencies were observed in depressed Parkinson's disease patients even after controlling for the duration of antiparkinsonian medication use (Kostic et al. 1989).

A summary of the effects of medication on sleep in patients with Parkinson's disease is complicated by the facts that 1) different doses and types of medications are often reported; 2) the patients studied may be in different stages of the disease or have different medication histories that would affect the integrity of the existing dopaminergic systems, or both; and 3) studies differ in the extent of medication withdrawal (if any) used before polysomnography. Given these factors, it is not surprising that there is considerable disagreement over not only the polysomnographic but even the clinical effects on sleep of various antiparkinsonian medications. Regarding the latter, some clinicians have noted that although L-dopa has mild stimulant properties in healthy subjects, in Parkinson's disease patients it can often induce profound and disabling hypersomnolence within 30–60 minutes after ingestion (Nausieda 1990).

Overnight polysomnographic studies suggest that L-dopa administered at low doses improves sleep quality, whereas at high doses it disturbs sleep (Bergonzi et al. 1974). Kales et al. (1971) reported decreases in REM sleep with L-dopa with no change in sleep fragmentation or slow-wave sleep, whereas others reported changes in the timing of REM sleep, with greater amounts occurring later in the night (Aldrich 1989). Lavie et al. (1980b) noted increased REM density in Parkinson's disease patients with chronic L-dopa administration. Emser et al. (1988) noted that even with combined administration of L-dopa and amantadine, Parkinson's disease patients showed relatively low amounts of slow-wave and REM sleep. The increase in REM density noted by Lavie et al. may be related to the troubling dream experiences and nightmares experienced by 30%–50% of Parkinson's disease patients (Lees et al. 1988; Sharf et al. 1978).

Recently, Cipolli et al. (1991) reported that age was a major covariate in examining the potentially disruptive effects of L-dopa on sleep. Regarding other antiparkinsonian medication effects, Stern et al. (1968) reported that amantadine had varying effects on REM sleep; some patients showed increases and some showed decreases with this medication. Vardi et al. (1979) compared sleep of the same Parkinson's disease patients on bromocriptine and on L-dopa and found no differences. In a more recent study that examined the effects of combined pergolide and carbidopa–L-dopa (Sinemet) and used clinical efficacy as an end point, Askenasy and Yahr (1985) reported that improvement was associated with increases in polysomnographically defined sleep efficiency. No changes in REM or slow-wave sleep were seen. Pronounced effects on muscle activity during sleep were also observed (see "Movements in Sleep" within this section).

A consistent feature of the sleep of patients with Parkinson's disease is a relative paucity of sleep-spindle activity. This effect is seen both in unmedicated patients compared with control subjects (Emser et al. 1987) and in treated patients, in whom an increase in spindle density has been noted (Emser et al. 1988; Puca et al. 1973). In patients with unilateral Parkinson's symptoms, administration of L-dopa differentially increased spindle activity of the afflicted (contralateral) hemisphere (Myslobodsky et al. 1982).

Respiration in sleep. During wakefulness, patients with Parkinson's disease have been shown to incur obstructive ventilatory deficits. For example, on the flow volume loop (ratio of expiratory flow to inspiratory flow), Parkinson's disease patients are likely to show a "flutter" pattern or a tendency for collapse on inspiration (Vincken et al. 1984). Alterations in upper-airway function such as those might be expected to predispose Parkinson's disease patients to have more sleep apnea than control subjects. Few polysomnographic studies have reported on respiratory patterns in patients with Parkinson's disease, but available data conflict. Some studies suggest higher amounts of sleep apnea (Emser et al. 1987; Hardie et al. 1986), whereas others do not (Apps et al. 1985; Ferini-Strambi et al. 1991). Patients with Parkinson's disease accompanied by autonomic nervous system dysfunction (Shy-Drager syndrome) have been reported to have more sleep apnea than patients with idiopathic Parkinson's disease (Apps et al. 1985). Recently, however, Ferini-Strambi et al. (1992) reported autonomic dysregulation of heart rate during sleep in patients with idiopathic Parkinson's disease, although rates of sleep-disordered breathing and oxygen saturation were no higher than those in control subjects.

Movements in sleep. Movements during sleep in patients with Parkinson's disease are of particular interest for several reasons. First, because Parkinson's disease is characterized by tremor, rigidity, and bradykinesia in the waking state, an obvious question arises regarding the occurrence of these disorders during sleep. Second, there is considerable evidence that movement disorders occurring primarily in sleep (i.e., nocturnal myoclonus) may be partially under dopaminergic control, because medications such as L-dopa can reduce their presence in sleep disorder patients without Parkinson's disease. Patterns of movement during sleep in Parkinson's disease patients (under both unmedicated and medicated conditions) may thus offer considerable promise for understanding sleep-related modulation in the motor system.

In Parkinson's early description of the disease that bears his name, he noted a cessation of tremor during sleep; however, he also noted anecdotally that in a few severe cases tremor appeared to commence within sleep (Askenasy 1981; Stern et al. 1968). With the advent of polysomnography, numerous researchers have attempted to examine physiologically measured tremor during sleep. Among the initial studies to examine this phenomenon, Stern et al. (1968) reported that tremor was occasionally seen during the sleep period, but that its presence was invariably preceded by evidence of awakening or arousal in NREM sleep or a burst of eye movement during REM sleep. April (1966) also noted the presence of tremor in sleep but suggested that preceding activation was not a necessary component to its elicitation.

It should be stressed that all investigators have noted that tremor occurring during wakefulness typically subsides during the onset of sleep and then later reappears. When tremor reappears, its amplitude is usually diminished, although its frequency is unchanged from the waking state (Stern et al. 1968). Also, it seldom occurs in stages 3 and 4 sleep. The extent of tremor in tonic REM sleep has been a matter of debate. More recently, Fish et al. (1991) examined 1) polysomnographic patterns in 2.0-second mini-epochs immediately before movement and 2) frequency of movements as a function of traditional sleep staging. As in the earlier studies, movement was usually associated with lightening of the existing sleep stage. Of particular note was the analysis using the short 2.0-second mini-epochs, which demonstrated that during REM bursts Parkinson's disease patients were over twice as likely to show associated movement compared with patients who had other movement disorders such as Huntington's disease. Most of the Parkinson's disease patients in this study were receiving antiparkinsonian medication, which raises the issue of whether such medications might partially suspend the motor inhibition characteristic of REM sleep.

Askenasy (1981) proposed that the high prevalence of PLMs in the sleep of patients with Parkinson's disease actually represents the sleep-related modulation of the same basal ganglia dysfunction manifested by the waking motor symptoms of Parkinson's disease. Critical to this hypothesis is the fact that the stage-related prevalence of such movements follows a pattern similar to that seen for tremor during sleep. Additionally, the movements may occur not only in the anterior tibialis but also in muscle groups such as the medial gastrocnemius, extensor digitorum, and flexor carpi.

Unlike Fish et al. (1991), Askenasy and Yahr (1990) contend that the conversion of tremor into repetitive muscle contractions is a subclinical event insofar as EEG activation is concerned and that such events are rare in REM sleep. One difference between the two data sets is that Fish et al. focused on movement per se in afflicted muscle groups, whereas Askenasy and Yahr defined muscle activity on the basis of bursts of at least six periodic events.

Although the issues of definition and characterization of movements during sleep in patients with Parkinson's disease remain somewhat controversial, it would appear that the continued occurrence of movement during sleep in these patients represents a major issue in the management of such cases (see "Treatment Considerations" later in this chapter).

Circadian rhythms.   Few studies have explicitly assessed circadian rhythms in patients with Parkinson's disease. In a preliminary report, elderly women with Parkinson's disease were more likely to report daytime napping, to have reduced amplitudes in their body temperature rhythm, and to have an earlier acrophase (peak temperature) compared with elderly female control subjects (Dowling 1992). Medication effects were not significant in these patients. Another brief report noted that 62% of Parkinson's disease patients treated with L-dopa showed aperiodic or otherwise "flat" rhythms of plasma cortisol (Nausieda et al. 1982a). Patients with normal rhythms had fewer psychiatric symptoms and sleep disturbances than did the patients with apparently aberrant rhythms.

Apart from these studies, some data exist suggesting that motor symptoms such as tremor and dystonia may be worse nocturnally (Aldrich 1989) and improve after sleep; however, other questionnaire data have suggested that this trend may not be apparent for most Parkinson's disease patients (Lees et al. 1988).

Huntington's Disease

Sleep architecture.   Huntington's disease, a progressive dementia involving degeneration of the motor system, primarily involves neuronal loss in the caudate and putamen. Several studies of sleep architecture in these patients have been reported, often with conflicting results. Hansotia et al. (1985) noted minimal differences between patients with mild Huntington's disease and control subjects but found that moderately afflicted patients showed abnormalities such as reduced sleep times, reduced sleep efficiency, and reduced slow-wave sleep. Emser et al. (1988) reported no differences between their Huntington's disease patients and age-matched control subjects, whereas their Parkinson's disease patients showed predictable patterns of sleep disruption and sleep architecture. The only variable differentiating the Huntington's disease patients from control subjects was stage 2 sleep-spindle density, with *higher* density observed in the Huntington's disease patients. Because the presence of sleep spindles is usually associated with movement inhibition, Emser et al. interpreted this result to reflect a weakening of a dopaminergic inhibitory system via intrastriatal neurons within the corpus striatum.

More recent work by Wiegand et al. (1991) confirmed the increased density of sleep spindles in patients with Huntington's disease, but they also reported polysomnographic findings more typical of other dementing illnesses—including decreased sleep efficiency, prolonged sleep latency, and reduced slow-wave sleep. Computed tomography–measured atrophy in the caudate, but not in the cortex, was associated with less slow-wave sleep and lower sleep efficiency (Emser et al. 1988; Wiegand et al. 1991). Many of these changes in sleep architecture in Huntington's disease patients might reflect either direct effects of neuronal degeneration on nuclei critical to sleep regulation or the disruptive effects of movements during sleep.

Because of possible abnormalities in extraocular motility in patients with Huntington's disease, effects on REM sleep have long been of interest in this condition. In an early report, Starr (1967) reported a virtual absence of phasic eye-movement activity during REM sleep in a small group of Huntington's disease patients. Later work showed either a normal (Emser et al. 1988; Wiegand et al. 1991) or a slightly reduced (Hansotia et al. 1985) percentage of REM sleep in patients with Huntington's disease, but nothing like the virtual absence of eye-movement activity originally reported by Starr (1967).

Respiration in sleep. Most polysomnographic studies in patients with Huntington's disease have focused on sleep architecture or movements in sleep. Hence, few have reported on, or apparently even recorded, breathing during sleep in this form of dementia. Bollen et al. (1988) reported no differences between Huntington's disease patients and control subjects in measures of sleep apnea, and Emser et al. (1987) noted a very low prevalence (10%) of significant sleep apnea in their Huntington's disease patients.

Movements in sleep. The dyskinetic movements of Huntington's disease have been shown to occur during sleep, although they were more likely during transitional sleep such as stage 1 or in a lightening of sleep stage (Fish et al. 1991). Such movements were rare in slow-wave sleep (stages 3 and 4) and in REM sleep. Huntington's disease patients typically showed a greater number of movements within the entire sleep period than did Parkinson's disease patients. Movements typically occurred within several seconds after arousal rather than being a cause of arousal per se (Fish et al. 1991). By contrast, PLMs often occur before or simultaneously with signs of EEG arousal. There are no reports regarding the presence of PLMs in Huntington's disease patients.

Circadian rhythms. There are few studies of circadian rhythms in patients with Huntington's disease, although Durso et al. (1983) noted that diurnal variation in growth hormone was preserved in Huntington's disease patients. Despite this preservation, mean growth hormone levels were higher in Huntington's disease patients compared with age-matched control subjects, consistent with dysregulation of hypothalamic control over the anterior pituitary.

Progressive Supranuclear Palsy

Progressive supranuclear palsy is a degenerative disease characterized by dementia, dysarthria, and impaired voluntary gaze. Disturbed sleep architecture is quite pronounced in these patients, with reduced sleep efficiency and considerable time awake after sleep onset (Aldrich et al. 1989). Despite this marked disturbance of nocturnal sleep, polysomnographic recordings indicate that there is little compensatory daytime sleep in these patients (Gross et al. 1978). As in the case of Alzheimer's disease, substantial correlations exist between measures of sleep disturbance and the level of dementia (Aldrich et al. 1989). REM sleep appears particularly diminished in patients with progressive supranuclear palsy (Aldrich et al. 1989; Gross et al. 1978), perhaps owing to selective deterioration in the pontine tegmentum and pedunculopontine nucleus. Curiously, however, REM sleep latency was very short in several patients. In the small number of cases evaluated to date, the prevalence of sleep apnea and PLMs appeared no higher than that in age-matched control subjects.

Creutzfeldt-Jakob Disease

This swiftly progressive dementia is characterized by extrapyramidal signs and periodic, generalized paroxysmal EEG activity. Discrimination of sleep stages and other sleep-related waveforms typically is not possible because spike-and-wave activity precludes identification of such features (Calleja et al. 1985). REM sleep is usually not discernible. Early in the disease, a distinct sleep-wake cycle can be detected, but this cycle disappears typically within several months. Episodes of sleep apnea, concurrent with diminution of spike-and-wave complexes, have been described (Mamdani et al. 1983). Diffuse myoclonus is seen in all limbs and is apparent throughout sleep and wakefulness.

TREATMENT CONSIDERATIONS

Regardless of the cause of dementia, some basic issues regarding treatment remain salient. Treatment for the sleep disturbance accompanying dementia can involve pharmacological and nonpharmacological approaches. The two should not be considered mutually exclusive because often use of a combined approach can result in additive effects not seen with either approach separately. However, it is important to keep in mind that, depending on the individual patient, combining pharmacotherapy and behavioral therapy may introduce new elements of risk. For example, the increased risk of hip fracture in elderly patients receiving psychoactive medications dictates good judgment when medications are combined with a nondrug approach requiring the patient to increase ambulation and avoid prolonged periods of sedentary activity.

Pharmacological Treatments

Typical benzodiazepine hypnotics, although effective in many cases of geriatric insomnia, are seldom helpful in the management of disruptive nocturnal behavior. With the exception of Parkinson's disease, which requires separate pharmacological considerations (see below), the medication of choice to treat sundowning and disruptive nocturnal behavior usually is haloperidol or thioridazine. Haloperidol and thioridazine have marked extrapyramidal and anticholinergic side effects, respectively. Current thinking generally concedes that all antipsychotic medications have similar efficacy; however, periodic withdrawal may be used to reestablish the necessity of treatment with such medications. Some anecdotal reports indicate that less commonly used medications have been successful in treating these types of agitation syndromes, including β-blockers such as propranolol and anticonvulsants such as valproic acid. There is no question that in the past many psychoactive medications were overused, particularly in the nursing home setting. It is of interest to note that new federal guidelines in the United States appear to be resulting in decreased use of such medications.

Pharmacological management of sleep disturbance in patients with Parkinson's disease represents an important exception to the principles of pharmacotherapy outlined in the preceding paragraph. Askenasy and Yahr (1985) demonstrated that appropriate clinical management of waking motor symptoms (whether with Sinemet alone or combined with pergolide or trihexyphenidyl) results in a reduction of motor activity during sleep and higher sleep efficiency as recorded polysomnographically. Although amelioration of waking motor symptoms is always the desired outcome, the fact that anywhere from 74% to 98% of medicated Parkinson's disease patients complain of sleep disturbance (Lees et al. 1988; Nausieda et al. 1982b) suggests that suboptimal management may well be the rule rather than the exception.

Clinical experience usually dictates that early in the course of treatment with Sinemet, daytime administration improves motor symptoms and may not disrupt sleep. As Parkinson's disease progresses and Sinemet use becomes long term, patients may experience "off" phenomena during the night. Not only dyskinesia but also immobility with subsequent inability to rise to use the bathroom (Lees et al. 1988) may be troubling for the patient. Nocturnal administration of Sinemet, particularly in sustained-release form, may be helpful in getting patients through the night. Additional use of selegiline has been shown to improve sleep in patients with Parkinson's disease even when L-dopa has minimal effect (Lavie et al. 1980a), and pergolide, a dopamine receptor agonist, may remaximize the beneficial effects of Sinemet.

It is possible that some of the nocturnal problems experienced by patients with Parkinson's disease are a function of frequent awakenings, which are complicated by the type of motor symptoms described above. Excessive daytime somnolence (either representing an acute effect of daytime L-dopa administration or possibly an alteration in intrinsic circadian rhythms) may reduce these patients' homeostatic drive to sleep nocturnally, thus indirectly causing many of their nocturnal symptoms. Nausieda (1990) suggested that alternate-day dosing of Sinemet may avoid the hypersomnolence that leads to disturbed nocturnal sleep, whereas others feel that such drug "holidays" may precipitate sudden freeze attacks and akinesia (Aldrich 1989). Nocturnal administration of clozapine has been reported to have sedative effects in patients with Parkinson's disease who experience dopaminomimetic-induced sleep disturbance (Wolters et al. 1990), and sedating tricyclic antidepressants such as amitriptyline may have beneficial effects as well.

Nonpharmacological Treatments

Nonpharmacological treatments for sleep disturbance in dementia should be considered because they may work well and thus obviate the need for medication. Enlistment of the caregiver's cooperation is a prerequisite for successful implementation of almost any intervention.

For example, simple avoidance of daytime napping and, more generally, avoidance of prolonged periods of daytime sedentary activity should be stressed. The homeostatic response to sleep deprivation appears to be preserved in patients with dementia, as evidenced in both experimental and descriptive studies (see Bliwise 1993 for a review). Helping the caregiver understand that the docile, afternoon drowsiness of a family member with dementia must be avoided may be the greatest challenge in using this type of intervention. Many caregivers deny the overt signs of daytime drowsiness in dementia patients and may prefer to use the quiet of those daytime hours for their own tasks and household chores.

In recent years, use of bright light for the treatment of sleep disturbance in patients with dementia has become increasingly recognized as a potentially important avenue of treatment (e.g., Satlin et al. 1992). Although issues remain regarding the cumulative amount of illumination required as well as the optimal time of day for exposure, bright light may be effective both in maintaining daytime alertness and in manipulating the putative underlying core oscillator, perhaps by increasing the amplitude or delaying the phase of the underlying body temperature rhythm. Although light may be a very good and simple treatment to attempt, many elderly individuals, particularly those with macular degeneration, may find the glare to be a noxious stimulus and be intolerant of it. Additionally, even if the illumination is tolerated, there can be no guarantee that sufficient light reaches the retina to induce biological effects. Nonetheless, exposure to bright light is an important innovation in attempting to improve sleep in the patient with dementia.

As a last resort, significant environmental management should be considered. In England, the "night watchers" system, in which a caregiver comes to the home only at night, has proved successful. In the institutional setting, specific assignment of sundowning patients to a nocturnal activities hour has been successfully implemented in a number of nursing homes. Approaches like these, in which patients with dementia are allowed to dictate their own sleep-wake schedule rather than conform to that of the surrounding milieu, may represent a final attempt at managing the elderly dementia patient with otherwise intractable sleep disturbance at the end of life.

REFERENCES

Aharon-Peretz J, Masiah A, Pillar T: Sleep-wake cycles in multi-infarct dementia and dementia of the Alzheimer type. Neurology 41:1616–1619, 1991

Aldrich MS: Parkinsonism, in Principles and Practice of Sleep Medicine. Edited by Kryger MH, Roth TS, Dement WC. Philadelphia, PA, WB Saunders, 1989, pp 351–357

Aldrich MS, Foster NL, White RF, et al: Sleep abnormalities in progressive supranuclear palsy. Ann Neurol 25:577–581, 1989

Allen SR, Seiler WO, Stahelin HB, et al: Seventy-two hour polygraphic and behavioral recordings of wakefulness and sleep in a hospital geriatric unit: comparison between demented and nondemented patients. Sleep 10:143–159, 1987

Apps MCP, Sheaff PC, Ingram DA, et al. Respiration and sleep in Parkinson's disease. J Neurol Neurosurg Psychiatry 48:1240–1245, 1985

April RS: Observations on parkinsonian tremor in all-night sleep. Neurology 16:720–724, 1966

Askenasy J: Sleep patterns in extrapyramidal disorders: Int J Neurol 15:62–76, 1981

Askenasy J, Yahr M: Reversal of sleep disturbance in Parkinson's disease by anti-parkinsonian therapy: a preliminary study. Neurology 35:527–532, 1985

Askenasy J, Yahr M: Parkinsonian tremor loses its alternating aspect during non-REM sleep and is inhibited by REM sleep. J Neurol Neurosurg Psychiatry 53:749–753, 1990

Bergonzi P, Chiurulla C, Cianchetti C, et al: Clinical pharmacology as an approach to the study of biochemical sleep mechanisms: the action of L-dopa. Confin Neurol 36:5–22, 1974

Bliwise DL: Neuropsychological function and sleep. Clin Geriatr Med 5:381–394, 1989

Bliwise DL: Sleep in normal aging and dementia. Sleep 16:40–81, 1993

Bliwise DL, Tinklenberg J, Davies H, et al: Sleep patterns in Alzheimer's disease (AD) (abstract). Sleep Research 15:49, 1986

Bliwise DL, Yesavage JA, Tinklenberg JR, et al: Sleep apnea in Alzheimer's disease. Neurobiol Aging 10:343–346, 1989

Bliwise DL, Bevier WC, Bliwise NG, et al: Systematic 24-hr behavioral observations of sleep and wakefulness in a skilled-care nursing facility. Psychology and Aging 5:16–24, 1990

Bliwise DL, Yesavage JA, Tinklenberg JR: Sundowning and rate of decline in mental function in Alzheimer's disease. Dementia 3:335–341, 1992

Bliwise DL, Carroll JC, Lee KA, et al: Sleep and sundowning in nursing home patients with dementia. Psychiatry Res (in press)

Bollen EL, Den Heijer JC, Ponsioen C, et al: Respiration during sleep in Huntington's chorea. J Neurol Sci 84:63–68, 1988

Calleja J, Carpizo R, Berciano J, et al: Serial waking-sleep EEGs and evolution of somatosensory potentials in Creutzfeldt-Jakob disease. Electroencephalogr Clin Neurophysiol 60:504–508, 1985

Cipolli C, Bolzani R, Massetani R, et al: Age-related modifications in sleep of Parkinson patients, in Sleep and Ageing. Edited by Smirne S, Franceschi M, Ferini-Strambi L. Milano, Italy, Masson SpA, 1991, pp 93–96

Cohen-Mansfield J, Watson V, Meade W, et al: Does sundowning occur in residents of an Alzheimer's unit? International Journal of Geriatric Psychiatry 4:293–298, 1989

Dowling GA: Circadian functioning in older women with Parkinson's disease (abstract). Gerontologist 32:10, 1992

Durso R, Tamminga CA, Ruggeri S, et al: Twenty-four hour plasma levels of growth hormone and prolactin in Huntington's disease. J Neurol Neurosurg Psychiatry 46:1134–1137, 1983

Emser W, Hoffmann K, Stolz T, et al: Sleep disorders in diseases of the basal ganglia. Interdisciplinary Topics in Gerontology 22:144–157, 1987

Emser W, Brenner M, Stober T, et al: Changes in nocturnal sleep in Huntington's and Parkinson's disease. J Neurol 235:177–179, 1988

Erkinjuntti T, Partinen M, Sulkava R, et al: Sleep apnea in multiinfarct dementia and Alzheimer's disease. Sleep 10:419–425, 1987

Evans LK: Sundown syndrome in institutionalized elderly. J Am Geriatr Soc 35:101–108, 1987

Ferini-Strambi L, Smirne S, Pinto P, et al: Parkinson's disease: sleep and respiration in de novo patients, in Sleep and Ageing. Edited by Smirne S, Franceschi M, Ferini-Strambi L. Milano, Italy, Masson SpA, 1991, pp 97–101

Ferini-Strambi L, Franceschi M, Pinto P, et al: Respiration and heart rate variability during sleep in untreated Parkinson patients. Gerontology 38:92–98, 1992

Fish DR, Sawyers D, Allen PJ, et al: The effect of sleep on the dyskinetic movements of Parkinson's disease, Gilles de la Tourette syndrome, Huntington's disease, and torsion dystonia. Arch Neurol 48:210–214, 1991

Gallagher-Thompson D, Brooks JO III, Bliwise D, et al: The relations among caregiver stress, "sundowning" symptoms, and cognitive decline in Alzheimer's disease. J Am Geriatr Soc 40:807–810, 1992

Gilley DW, Wilson RS, Ristanovic RK, et al: Sleep disturbance in subcortical multiinfarct dementia and Alzheimer's disease (abstract). Ann Neurol 24:134, 1988

Gross RA, Spehlmann R, Daniels JC: Sleep disturbances in progressive supranuclear palsy. Electroencephalogr Clin Neurophysiol 45:16–25, 1978

Hachinski VC, Iliff LD, Zilkha E, et al: Cerebral blood flow in dementia. Arch Neurol 32:632–637, 1975

Hansotia P, Wall R, Berendes J, et al: Sleep disturbances and severity of Huntington's disease. Neurology 35:1672–1674, 1985

Hardie RJ, Efthimiou J, Stern GM: Respiration and sleep in Parkinson's disease (letter). J Neurol Neurosurg Psychiatry 49:1326, 1986

Hinton DR, Sadun AA, Blanks JC, et al: Optic-nerve degeneration in Alzheimer's disease. N Engl J Med 315:485–487, 1986

Hoch CC, Reynolds CF III, Nebes RD, et al: Clinical significance of sleep-disordered breathing in Alzheimer's disease: preliminary data. J Am Geriatr Soc 37:138–144, 1989

Hoehn MM, Yahr MD: Parkinsonism: onset, progression, and mortality. Neurology 17:427–442, 1967

Inami Y, Shimizu T, Iijima S, et al: Nocturnal myoclonus syndrome in patients with hemiplegia due to cerebrovascular disease (abstract). Sleep Research 16:480, 1987

Kales A, Ansel R, Markham C, et al: Sleep in patients with Parkinson's disease and normal subjects prior to and following levodopa administration. Clin Pharmacol Ther 12:397–406, 1971

Kostic VS, Susie V, Covickovic-Sternic N, et al: Reduced rapid eye movement sleep latency in patients with Parkinson's disease. J Neurol 236:421–423, 1989

Lavie P, Wajsbort J, Youdim MBH: Deprenyl does not cause insomnia in parkinsonian patients. Communications in Psychopharmacology 4:303–307, 1980a

Lavie P, Bental E, Goshen H, et al: REM ocular activity in Parkinsonian patients chronically treated with levodopa. J Neural Transm 47:61–67, 1980b

Lees AJ, Blackburn NA, Campbell VL: The nighttime problems of Parkinson's disease. Clin Neuropharmacol 11:512–519, 1988

Mamdani MB, Masdeu J, Ross E, et al: Sleep apnea with unusual EEG changes in Jakob-Creutzfeldt disease. Electroencephalogr Clin Neurophysiol 55:411–416, 1983

Manni R, Romani A, Galimberti CA, et al: Sleep-disordered breathing in dementia: its relationship with dementia severity and outcome, in Sleep and Ageing. Edited by Smirne S, Franceschi M, Ferini-Strambi L. Milano, Italy, Masson SpA, 1991, pp 75–81

Martino-Saltzman D, Blasch BB, Morris RD, et al: Travel behavior of nursing home residents perceived as wanderers and nonwanderers. Gerontologist 31:666–672, 1991

Mouret J: Differences in sleep patients with Parkinson's disease. Electroencephalogr Clin Neurophysiol 38:653–657, 1975

Myslobodsky M, Mintz M, Ben-Mayor V, et al: Unilateral dopamine deficit and lateral EEG asymmetry: sleep abnormalities in hemi-Parkinson's patients. Electroencephalogr Clin Neurophysiol 54:227–231, 1982

Nausieda PA: Sleep in Parkinson disease, in Handbook of Sleep Disorders. Edited by Thorpy MJ. New York, Marcel Dekker, 1990, pp 719–733

Nausieda PA, Baum RA, Weiner WJ: Cortisol rhythm disruption as a side effect of chronic levodopa therapy (abstract). Neurology 32:180, 1982a

Nausieda PA, Weiner WJ, Kaplan LR: Sleep disruption in the course of chronic levodopa therapy: an early feature of the levodopa psychosis. Clin Neuropharmacol 5:183–194, 1982b

Okawa M, Mishima K, Hishikawa Y, et al: Circadian rhythm disorders in sleep-waking and body temperature in elderly patients with dementia and their treatment. Sleep 14:478–485, 1991

Palomaki H, Partinen M, Juvela S, et al: Snoring as a risk factor for sleep-related brain infarction. Stroke 20:1311–1315, 1989

Petit D, Montplaisir J, Lorrain D, et al: Spectral analysis of the rapid eye movement sleep electroencephalogram in right and left temporal regions: a biological marker of Alzheimer's disease. Ann Neurol 32:172–176, 1992

Pollak CP, Perlick D, Linsner JP, et al: Sleep problems in the community elderly as predictors of death and nursing home placement. J Community Health 15:123–135, 1990

Prinz PN, Vitaliano PP, Vitiello MV, et al: Sleep, EEG and mental function changes in senile dementia of the Alzheimer type. Neurobiol Aging 3:361–370, 1982

Prinz P, Frommlet M, Vitiello MV, et al: Periodic leg movements are unaffected by mild Alzheimer's disease (abstract). Sleep Research 15:200, 1986

Prinz PN, Larsen LH, Moe KE, et al: EEG markers of early Alzheimer's disease in computer selected tonic REM sleep. Electroencephalogr Clin Neurophysiol 83:36–43, 1992

Puca FM, Bricolo A, Rurella G: Effect of L-dopa or amantadine therapy on sleep spindles in parkinsonism. Electroencephalogr Clin Neurophysiol 35:327–330, 1973

Reynolds CF III, Kupfer DJ, Taska LS, et al: Comparative frequency of sleep apnea and nocturnal myoclonus among elderly depressives, dementing patients, and healthy controls (abstract). Sleep Research 13:159, 1984

Reynolds CF III, Kupfer DJ, Hoch CC, et al: Two-year follow-up of elderly patients with mixed depression and dementia: clinical and EEG sleep findings. J Am Geriatr Soc 34:793–799, 1986

Reynolds CF III, Kupfer DJ, Hoch CC, et al: Sleep deprivation as a probe in the elderly. Arch Gen Psychiatry 44:982–990, 1987

Reynolds CF III, Kupfer DJ, Houck PR, et al: Reliable discrimination of elderly depressed and demented patients by electroencephalographic sleep data. Arch Gen Psychiatry 45:258–264, 1988

Satlin A, Volicer L, Ross V, et al: Bright light treatment of behavioral and sleep disturbances in patients with Alzheimer's disease. Am J Psychiatry 149:1028–1032, 1992

Sharf B, Moskovitz Ch, Lupton MD, et al: Dream phenomena induced by chronic levodopa therapy. J Neural Transm 43:143–151, 1978

Starr A: A disorder of rapid eye movements in Huntington's chorea. Brain 90:545–564, 1967

Stern M, Roffwarg H, Duvoisin R: The parkinsonian tremor in sleep. J Nerv Ment Dis 147:202–210, 1968

Swaab DF, Fliers E, Partiman TS. The suprachiasmatic nucleus of the human brain in relation to sex, age and senile dementia. Brain Research 342:37–44, 1985

Tarquini B, Gheri R, Fanfani S, et al: Neuroendocrinological functionality and atherosclerosis: the tiretropo hormone. Giornale Di Gerontologia 26:661–662, 1978

Vardi J, Glaubman H, Rabey J, et al: EEG sleep patterns in parkinsonian patients treated with bromocriptine and L-dopa: a comparative study. J Neural Transm 45:307–316, 1979

Vincken WG, Gauthier SG, Dollfuss RE, et al: Involvement of upper-airway muscles in extrapyramidal disorders. N Engl J Med 311:438–442, 1984

Vitiello MV, Prinz PN, Williams DE, et al: Sleep disturbances in patients with mild-stage Alzheimer's disease. J Gerontol 45:M131–M138, 1990

Wiegand M, Moller A, Lauer C, et al: Nocturnal sleep in Huntington's disease. J Neurol 238:203–208, 1991

Witting W, Mirmiran M, Eikelenboom P, et al: Alterations in the circadian rest-activity rhythm in aging and Alzheimer's disease. Biol Psychiatry 27:563–572, 1990

Wolters ECh, Hurwitz TA, Mak E, et al: Clozapine in the treatment of parkinsonian patients with dopaminomimetic psychosis. Neurology 40:832–834, 1990

Afterword to Section V

Charles F. Reynolds III, M.D., and David J. Kupfer, M.D.,
Section Editors

The chapters composing this section on sleep disorders illustrate the pivotal importance of sleep changes in the pathogenesis, diagnosis, management, and prognosis of many psychiatric disorders, including mood disorders, psychotic disorders, and neurodegenerative disorders. This fact is not surprising when one considers that rapid eye movement sleep and non–rapid eye movement sleep constitute two of three known operating states of the central nervous system (the third state being wakefulness). Hence, as illustrated by the chapters in this section, study of these states has elucidated many potential mechanisms and useful correlates of psychiatric disorders.

Although we still have not defined the basic functions of sleep, there is much reason to believe that sleep subserves the basic information-processing functions of the brain, in both cognitive and affective spheres. In various psychopathological syndromes, we see a disturbance in the basic relationship of sleep to the affective and cognitive information-processing activities of the brain. As psychiatric clinicians, we try to restore this relationship to proper balance in focusing on states of the mind-brain and the rest-activity cycle. As investigators, we attempt to understand vulnerabilities to psychopathology (as well as mechanisms of treatment response) in terms of shifts in affect balance and information processing to more or less adaptive modes, together with the role of sleep in these processes.

The other challenges facing us pertain to further working out how homeostatic and circadian influences affect the timing and quality of sleep in health and in psychiatric disorders, together with elucidating the neurophysiological and biochemical mechanisms that generate observed sleep-wake changes in various psychopathological states. The substantial progress toward these goals is illustrated by the chapters in this section.

Afterword to Volume 13

John M. Oldham, M.D., and Michelle B. Riba, M.D.

Although historians like to tell us that there is nothing new under the sun, it is difficult to agree with this proposal when one observes the enormous progress in our field, as exemplified by several of the sections in this volume. History *is*, however, a great teacher, and the lessons learned from early wisdom, as well as the constant self-corrective process that occurs as we *make* history by building on our successes and "righting" ourselves from our mistakes, orient us toward a future that holds great promise for our patients. We hope that the selections presented in this volume bring home just that message—that we must constantly revisit our heritage as we look to the future.

And, speaking of looking to the future, Volume 14 of the *Review of Psychiatry* is already well under way. The first section of the volume, edited by Herbert Kleber, M.D., will focus on substance abuse. The second section is on psychiatric disorders in women and women's health care, edited by Myrna Weissman, Ph.D., and Michelle B. Riba, M.D. The third section, edited by Elliott Gershon, M.D., will bring us up to date in the area of psychiatric genetics; this is followed by a section on cross-cultural psychiatry, edited by Pedro Ruiz, M.D. And, finally, the volume will be completed by the last section, on sexual disorders, edited by Judith Becker, Ph.D., and Taylor Segraves, M.D. As in previous volumes, our effort has been to provide a mixture of clinically relevant and applicable up-to-date information, along with a chance to zero in on a few areas at the forefront of research.

Index

Page numbers printed in **boldface** *type refer to tables or figures.*

Accidents, excessive daytime
    sleepiness and, 708
Action for Mental Health (Mental
    Health Study Act of 1955),
    103–104
Addiction, as psychiatric
    subspecialty, 16
Adenylate cyclase system, 181, 214
Adjustment disorder, 488
Adolescents. *See also* Child
    psychiatry/psychotherapy
    developmental issues in Tourette's
        syndrome, obsessive-
        compulsive disorder, and
        attention-deficit
        hyperactivity disorder,
        529–531
    eating disorders in, 556–566
    prevalence of obsessive-
        compulsive disorder in,
        521–522
    puberty and daytime sleepiness,
        627
Adrenergic receptors, 173–174, 198
Adrenocorticotropic hormone
    (ACTH), 177–179
Affective disorders
    catecholamine hypothesis for, 172
    children at risk for, 580–581
Affective/impulsive personality
    disorders, biological markers
    for, 263–275
Affective instability, 263
Aftercare, development of, 94
Aggression
    in physically abused children,
        601–602
    serotonergic activity and, 272, 273,
        274, 696
Alcohol abuse
    in adult survivors of child abuse,
        591
    sleep disorders and, 630
Alcoholism
    biological markers for
        drug challenges, 218–220
        electrophysiology, 215–216

enzymes as, 212–215
    measures of cognitive
        impairment, 216–217
    methodological considerations
        in study of, 208–212
    family studies of, 207–208
    personality characteristics and,
        217
Alcohol-metabolizing enzymes,
    212–213
Aldehyde dehydrogenase (ALDH),
    212–213, 215
Alexander, F., 44
Alprazolam, 173, 181
Alzheimer's disease, sleep
    disturbances in, 759–762
Amenorrhea, in eating disorders,
    234
American Academy of Psychiatry
    and the Law (AAPL), 365, 366,
    377, 379, 382–385
American Association for Marriage
    and Family Therapy, 445
American Board of Psychiatry and
    Neurology, 15
American Medical Association,
    ethical standards, 319, 368, 371,
    380, 394, 433
American Psychiatric Association
    ethical principles relevant to
        treatment boundaries,
        419–421
    ethical standards of, 352, 356, 378,
        394
    formal charges of breach of
        confidentiality against
        members of, 343
    official positions of organized
        psychiatry on ethics, 319
    relevance of ethical annotations
        and opinions for forensic
        psychiatry, 379–381
    on sexual misconduct, 433,
        444–445
American Psychological
    Association, 352
Amitriptyline, 661, 662, 772

Bartering, in financial arrangements for psychiatric treatment, 424
Basal ganglia, biological markers of Tourette's syndrome, 302
Bassett, A., 45
Bayle, A. L., 27
Beard, George Miller, 36
Beers, Clifford W., 47, 102
Behavioral sciences
    ethical abuses in research, 323
    psychiatric education in, 10
Behaviorism, 467–468
Behavior therapy, history of psychotherapy, 58
Bender-Gestalt psychological examination, 574
Bennett, A. E., 32
Benzodiazepine
    biological markers in panic disorder, 191
    sleep disorders and dementia, 771
    sleep disorders and schizophrenia, 699
    sleepiness and alertness, 715
    treatment of social phobia, 278
Berne, Eric, 61
Bill of rights, patient's, 329
Billings, John Shav, 47
Biochemistry, biological markers
    for generalized anxiety disorder, 197
    for social phobia, 191–192
Biological markers, for psychiatric disease
    for alcoholism
        drug challenges, 218–220
        electrophysiology, 215–216
        enzymes, 212–215
        measures of cognitive impairment, 216–217
        methodological considerations in studies of, 208–212
        state markers for heavy drinking, 207
    for affective/impulsive personality disorders, 263–275
    for anxiety disorders
        generalized anxiety disorder, 196–199

obsessive-compulsive disorder, 192–194
        panic disorders, 188–191
        posttraumatic stress disorder, 194–196
        research on, 187–188
        simple phobia, 199
        social phobia, 191–192
        summary of, **200–201**
    in child psychiatry, 293–305
    definition of, 292–293
    depression and sleep abnormalities, 643–644, 651
    development of, 293–294
    diagnosis and, 129
    for eating disorders
        bone mineral density, 245–246
        energy regulation, 228–230
        growth hormone and somatomedins, 235–236
        hypothalamic-pituitary-adrenal axis, 232–233
        hypothalamic-pituitary-ovarian axis, 233–235
        metabolic abnormalities, 231–232
        neuroimaging studies, 245
        neuropeptides, 241–245
        neurotransmitters, 236–241
    for mood disorders
        neuroendocrinology, 176–180
        neurotransmitters and receptors, 172–176
        pineal function and circadian rhythm, 182
        potential state-dependent markers in, **183**
        research on, 171
        second-messenger systems, 180–182
    for personality disorders
        anxiety-related personality disorders, 275–278
        schizophrenia-related personality disorders, 255–262
    for schizophrenia
        neurochemistry, 146–154
        neuroendocrinology, 143–146
        neuroimaging, 154–161

Biological markers, for
    schizophrenia *(continued)*
        neuroimmunology, 142–143
        psychophysiology and, 133,
            138–142
        research on, 161–162
        summary of, **134–137**
Bipolar disorder
    children at risk for, 580–581
    diagnosis of in children, 571
    psychotherapy of children and
        adolescents with, 581–584
Blanket release-of-information
    forms, 395
Block grants, 110–111
Blood and injury phobia, 199
Borderline personality disorder
    in adult survivors of child abuse,
        591
    genetic factors for, 264
Boundary crossings, 416–417
Boundary violations, nonsexual,
    415–431. *See also* Sexual
    misconduct
Brain imaging
    affective/impulsive personality
        disorder and, 265, 267
    functional and pathophysiology
        of schizophrenia, 157–161
    generalized anxiety disorder and,
        198–199
    obsessive-compulsive disorder
        and, 194
    studies of in panic disorder, 191
Brain physiology
    history of psychiatric research, 42
    lesions and narcolepsy, 721
    sleep abnormalities and structure
        correlates in schizophrenia,
        687–688
Breach of confidentiality, definition
    of, 345
Broca, P., 28
Brodie, B. B., 43
Bromocriptine, 766
Bulimia nervosa
    in adolescents, 562–566
    cholecystokinin and, 243
    corticotropin-releasing hormone
        and, 233

description of, 227
energy regulation abnormalities
    in, 230
growth hormones in, 236
hypothalamic-pituitary-ovarian
    axis and, 234
metabolic abnormalities in,
    231–232
neuropeptide Y and peptide YY,
    244
noradrenergic system
    abnormalities in, 240–241
opioid activity in, 242–243
serotonin activity in, 238–239
Bunney-Hamburg Psychosis Scale,
    695–696
Buss-Durkee Hostility Inventory, 271

Caffeine, 199, 716
Calcium, regulation of neuronal
    processes, 181–182
Canada, development of psychiatric
    research in, 39
Cannon, W. B., 43
Caplan, Gerald, 103
Carbidopa-L-dopa, 766
Cataplexy, 631, 719
Catecholamine
    alprazolam and output of, 173
    hypothesis for affective disorders,
        172
Census, epidemiological studies, 47,
    48
Center for Epidemiological Studies
    Depression Scale, 653
Cerebral laterality, 160
Chapman Psychosis-Proneness
    Scale, 260
Child abuse. *See also* Physical abuse;
    Sexual abuse
    comparisons between physical
        and sexual abuse, 589–590
    confidentiality and mandatory
        reporting of, 352–356
    definitions and incidence of, 589
    group therapy for, 604, 606
    intervention in cases of, 592–595
    intervention with abusive family,
        604–605

long-term effects in adult
survivors of, 591
major treatment issues in
individual psychotherapy,
595–604
psychological impairment in
abused children, 590–591
success of intervention in,
605–606
Childbearing, sleep disturbances,
621–624
Child Global Assessment Scale
(CGAS), 483–484
Child psychiatry/psychotherapy.
See also Attention-deficit
hyperactivity disorder; Child
abuse; Obsessive-compulsive
disorder; Tourette's syndrome
beginning of with neurotic
children, 498–500
biological markers in
for specific disorders, 294–305
research on, 293–294, 305
for bipolar disorder, 581–584
concept of psychoneurosis,
494–496
conduct disorders and personality
disorders in, 496–497,
501–515
development of paradigms,
467–468
diagnosis of schizophrenia and
bipolar disorder, 571
for early-onset schizophrenia,
575–579
eating disorders in infants,
toddlers, and children,
541–556
efficacy of interventions with
psychotic children, 584–585
history of concepts of childhood
psychosis, 572–573
research on
methodological flaws in
studies, **474**
neurobiological and molecular,
291–292
reviews of, 475–490
schizophrenia and affective
disorders, 585–586

and risk for affective disorders,
580–581
role of in management of
childhood neuropsychiatric
disorders, 519
sleep disorders and, 627–640
thought processes and risk of
schizophrenia, 573–575
Children With Attention Deficit
Disorder (C.H.A.D.D.), 532
Chlordiazepoxide, 34
Chlorphenylpiperazine, 151–152
Chlorpromazine, 33, 99, 690
Cholecystokinin, 243
Cholinergic REM Induction Test,
692
Cholinergic system, affective/
impulsive personality disorder,
270
Chronotherapy, for sleep disorders,
633
Circadian rhythm
in Alzheimer's disease, 762
biological markers for mood
disorders, 182
excessive daytime sleepiness and,
714–715, 723–724
human system of, 730–735
in Huntington's disease, 770
neurobiological implications of
longitudinal sleep studies in
depression, 670
in Parkinson's disease, 768
scheduling disorders and sleep
disturbance in children and
adolescents, 632–634
shift work and, 739–745
sleep physiology and, 735–736
in vascular dementia, 763–764
Class, studies of mental illness and
socioeconomic, 74
Client-centered therapy, 65
Clinical care, ethics of, 326–328
Clinical neurophysiology, as
psychiatric subspecialty, 16
Clomipramine, 523, 661
Clonidine, 174, 521, 524
Clozapine, 148, 690, 699, 772
Clyde Mood Scale, 709–710
Cognitive-behavior therapy, 66, 468

Cognitive impairment
  alcoholism and measures of,
    216–217
  excessive daytime sleepiness and,
    709
Community mental health centers
  concepts of, **106**
  criticism of in 1970s, 109–111
  development of, 98, 107
  history of psychotherapy, 61
  program elements in, **105**
  transition to, 1955–1964, 98–105
Community Mental Health Center
  Amendment of 1975, 109
Comorbidity, research on in child
  psychotherapy, 487
Competitive bidding, 114
Conduct disorders, in children and
  adolescents, 496–497, 501–515
Confidentiality
  basis of, 346–347
  boundary violations involving, 430
  definitions of, 344–346
  duty to protect third parties,
    356–360
  empirical aspects of, 347–352
  managed care and, 394–397
  mandatory child abuse reporting
    and, 352–356
  value of in psychiatry and ethical
    dilemmas, 360–361
Conners Teacher Rating Scale, 532
Consumer movements, 111–112
Contingency fees, forensic
  psychiatry and, 383
Continuous Performance Task,
  257–258, 695
Contracted services, and boundary
  violations, 421–424
Control, child abuse victims and
  quest for, 600
Corporations, medical services, 114
Corticotropin-releasing hormone
  (CRH)
  biological markers for eating
    disorders, 232–233
  biological markers for mood
    disorders, 177–178
  sleep and waking behavior and,
    694

Cortisol
  in sleep disorders and depression,
    669–670
  suppression of plasma as
    biological marker of
    schizophrenia, 144
Countertransference
  child psychotherapy and, 506
  and treatment of abused children,
    603–604
  treatment of victims of sexually
    exploitative therapists, 448
Creutzfeldt-Jakob disease, 770–771
Cullen, William, 35
Culture, studies of influences on
  behavior, 74
Cushing's disease, 178–179
Cyclic adenosine, 214
Cyproheptadine, 238

Dayton, Neil A., 48
Death penalty, forensic psychiatry
  and, 371–372, 373
Decisional capacity, informed
  consent in psychiatric research,
  333–336
Defense mechanisms, 597–598
Deinstitutionalization
  attempts to reform from 1975 to
    1984, 109–112
  impact of from 1965 to 1974, 105–108
  transition to from 1955 to 1964,
    98–105
Delayed sleep phase syndrome, 633
Delta sleep–inducing peptide,
  693–694
Dementia, sleep disturbances in,
  757–773
Dental phobias, 199
Depression. *See also* Mood disorders
  average duration of disorders in
    school children, 488
  gender differences in studies of, 75
  noradrenergic system in, 271
  sleep
    abnormalities as biological
      markers of, 643–644, 651
    changes in children and
      adolescents, 638–639

differential diagnosis of
abnormalities of, 683–687
EEG studies of, 654–668
longitudinal studies of,
656–660, 668–672
Parkinson's disease and, 765
population and clinical-sample
surveys of, 652–654
and women's roles in society,
77–78
Deutsch, Albert, 11
Dexamethasone suppression test
(DST), 176–177, 233
Diagnosis. *See also* Nosology
of attention-deficit hyperactivity
disorder, obsessive-
compulsive disorder, and
Tourette's syndrome, 525–527
child psychopathology and
physical or sexual
victimization, 593
of narcolepsy in children, 632
and research on biological
markers, 129
of schizophrenia and bipolar
disorder in children, 571
sleep studies according to
psychiatric condition, **691**
thought disorders in young
children, 573–574
Diagnostic Interview Schedule, 49
Diagnosis-related groups (DRGs),
390
*Diagnostic and Statistical Manual of
Mental Disorders* (DSM) system,
129
Diazepam, 220, 635
Diet-induced thermogenesis, 230
Dix, Dorothea, 94, 408
L-Dopa, 765–766, 767, 768, 772
Dopamine
biological markers
for eating disorders, 241
for obsessive-compulsive
disorder, 194
for schizophrenia, 146–147
gender differences in response to
receptors, 79
sleep abnormalities in
schizophrenia, 690–692

social phobia and decreased,
277–278
stress-induced psychosis in
posttraumatic stress
disorder, 196
Double agentry, and managed care,
401–402
Dreams and dreaming, 666–668, 678
Drug abuse
in adult survivors of child abuse, 591
and sleep disorders, 630
Drug companies, 324
DSM-III
history of psychiatric research, 38,
49
history of psychotherapy and, 63
DSM-III-R
autism, 297–298
classification of conduct disorders,
497
classification of feeding disorders,
541
formal thought disorder, 574
gender-related disorders, 82–83
personality disorders, 255
schizophrenia and bipolar
disorder in children and
adults, 571
DSM-IV
diagnostic categories related to
women, 73, 84–85
jet lag as type of circadian rhythm
sleep disorder, 749
personality disorders, 255
schizophrenia and bipolar
disorder in children and
adults, 571
shift work as type of circadian
rhythm sleep disorder, 738
Dunbar, F., 44
Dunham, H. W., 48
Dunlap, C. B., 40
Dysthymic disorder, 488

Earle, Pliny, 9
Eating disorders
in adolescents, 556–566
in adult survivors of child abuse,
591

Eating disorders *(continued)*
  biological markers for
    bone mineral density, 245–246
    energy regulation, 228–230
    growth hormone and
      somatomedins, 235–236
    hypothalamic-pituitary-adrenal
      axis, 232–233
    hypothalamic-pituitary-ovarian
      axis, 233–235
    metabolic abnormalities,
      231–232
    neuroimaging studies, 245
    neuropeptides, 241–245
    neurotransmitters, 236–241
  in infants, toddlers, and children,
    541–556
  social etiology of, 83–84
Economics. *See also* Managed care
  high costs of medical care, 389
  impact of costs on patient care,
    407–410
  managed care and delivery of
    psychiatric services, 389–391
  present status of care for
    chronically mentally ill,
    113–14
Education
  psychiatric
    ethical issues in, 337–340
    gender differences in mental
      disorders and, 86
    history of, 9–24
    psychotherapeutic management
      of attention-deficit
      hyperactivity disorder,
      obsessive-compulsive
      disorder, and Tourette's
      syndrome, 526
Egeland, J. A., 45–46
Ehret jet-lag diet, 752
Electroconvulsive therapy (ECT),
  history of psychiatric research,
  31–32
Electrodermal response studies, 268
Electrophysiology, biological
  markers for alcoholism, 215–216
Empathy, in child psychotherapy, 506
Enabling, as boundary violation, 426
Enuresis, 636–637, 642

Enzymes, as biological markers for
  alcoholism, 212–215
Epidemiologic Catchment Area
  (ECA) studies, 75–76
Epidemiology, history of psychiatric
  research, 46–49
Epworth Sleepiness Scale, 710
Erikson, E. H., 44
Erlenmeyer-Kimling, N., 45
Eroticism, as type of nonsexual
  exploitation, 425
Esquirol, Jean Etienne, 27
Ethanol, 715
Ethics
  boundary violations and, 415–431
  confidentiality
    basis of, 346–347
    definitions of, 344–346
    duty to protect third parties,
      356–360
    empirical aspects of, 347–352
    managed care and, 394–397
    mandatory child abuse
      reporting and, 352–356
    value of in psychiatry and
      ethical dilemmas
      regarding, 360–361
  in education of psychiatrists,
    337–340, 431
  forensic psychiatry
    absence of traditional
      physician-patient
      relationship in, 367–369
    conflicting responsibilities in,
      369–370
    conflicts between values of
      medicine and law, 375–377
    ethical dilemmas in, 372–375
    ethical guidelines for practice
      of, 366, 382–386
    ethical surveys of, 375
    impartiality, honesty, and
      objectivity in, 377–378
    and legal adversary system,
      366–367
    philosophical underpinnings
      of, 370–372
  fundamental principles of, 319–320
  future roles of psychiatrists and,
    22

gender and public perception of
psychiatrists, 85–86
managed care
and changing role of
psychiatrists, 391–394
confidentiality in, 394–397
conflicts of interest in, 397–399
double agentry in, 401–402
honesty and, 402–403
impact of costs on patient care,
407–410
informed consent and, 399–401
interference in doctor-patient
relationship, 403–405
relationships with other mental
health professionals,
405–407
official positions of organized
psychiatry on, 319
research issues, 323–337
sexual misconduct
posttermination relationships,
445–446
prevalence of, 434–437
prevention of, 451–453
profile and psychodynamics of
therapists in, 438–443
profile of vulnerable patients,
437–438
sanctions against accused
therapists, 443–445
Ethics committees, and sexual
misconduct, 444–445
Ethological paradigm, 468
Eugenics movement, 47
Event-related brain potentials
(ERPs), 139–142, 267–268
Evoked potential studies, 258
Excessive daytime sleepiness (EDS)
determinants of, 711–716
differential diagnosis and, 716–724
epidemiology and morbidity of,
707–708
measurement of, 709–711
Excitatory amino acids, 152–153
Experimental therapies, ethical
issues, 331
Experiments, in mental health
services, 114–115
Exploitation Index, 417, **418–419**

Expressive therapy, 577
Eye-movement impairment, 257,
680, 686

Failure to thrive (FTT), 542
Falret, J. P., 28
Family. *See also* Family therapy;
Parents
evaluation of in child abuse cases,
593–594
interventions with abusive,
604–605
shift work and sleep disorders,
744–745, 748
Family studies and familiality. *See
also* Genetics
alcoholism and, 207–208
eye-movement dysfunction and
schizophrenia, 139
generalized anxiety disorder and,
197
simple phobias and, 199
Family therapy. *See also* Family;
Parents
conduct disorders in children,
501–502
eating disorders in adolescents,
560–561, 565
in attention-deficit hyperactivity
disorder, obsessive-
compulsive disorder, and
Tourette's syndrome, 531
research on efficacy of in child
psychotherapy, 477, 479–480
Farris, R. E. L., 48
Fear conditioning, 268
Feeding disorder
of attachment, 545–547
of homeostasis, 543–544
of separation, 547–551
use of term, 542
Fees, boundary violations and,
423–424
Feighner criteria, 63
Feminism, gender differences in
mental illness, 77, 80
Fenfluramine, 273
Ferguson v. Wilson (1986), 368
Fetal alcohol syndrome, 209

Glucose, eating disorders and metabolic abnormalities, 231, 232
Goldhamer, H., 48
Golga, G., 28
Gonadal hormone function, 144–145
Gonadotropin-releasing hormone (GnRH), 234
Greediness, as boundary violation, 426
Griesinger, Wilhelm, 27–28
Group for the Advancement of Psychiatry, 96
Group psychotherapy
    eating disorders in adolescents, 565
    for physically and sexually abused children, 604, 606
Growth hormone (GH)
    biological markers
        for eating disorders, 235–236
        for mood disorders, 173–174
        for schizophrenia, 143–144
    sleep abnormalities in schizophrenic patients, 694
    sleep disorders and depression, 669, 670
Growth-hormone releasing factor (GHRF), biological markers for schizophrenia, 144
Guided affective imagery, 57, 65
Gusella, J. F., 45

Hallucinations
    clinical significance of in preadolescent children, 575
    narcolepsy and, 719, 720
Haloperidol, 521, 771
Hamilton Rating Scale for Depression scores, 663
Harlow, H. F., 44
Hartmann, H., 44
Harvard Community Health Plan, 404
Head banging, as sleep disorder, 637
Health maintenance organizations (HMOs), 390, 391
Heath, R. G., 41

Hebb, D. O., 44
Hecker, E., 28
Heinroth, Johann Christian, 28
Hill, Joseph A., 47
Hill-Burton Program, 11
Himwich, H. E., 41
Hippocratic oath, 319, 343, 371, 392
History, of psychiatry
    concepts of childhood psychosis, 572–573
    education and, 9–24
    ethical abuses in research, 323
    gender differences in mental disorders, 74–80
    gender-related disorders, 80–84
    mental hospitals
        changes from 1945 to 1954, 96–98
        deinstitutionalization and community mental health centers, 1955–1964, 98–105
        early history of, 93–96
        impact of deinstitutionalization from 1965 to 1974, 105–108
        reform of deinstitutionalization from 1975 to 1984, 109–112
    psychotherapy
        background information, 56
        brief therapy and, 58–60
        changes in 1950s, 56–58
        changes in 1960s and 1970s, 60–62
        consolidation and methods of, 62–64
        present status of, 64–67
    research in
        beginnings of, 27–28
        changing attitudes toward, 29
        epidemiology and, 46–49
        nosology and, 35–38
        pathology and, 38–46
        therapy and, 30–35
    value of, 779
Hoffer, A., 41
Homeless, mentally ill, 109, 112
Homicides, third-party warnings and, 359–360
Homosexuality, cases of sexual misconduct, 437

Homovanillic acid, as biological
marker
for personality disorders, 260–261
for schizophrenia, 146–147
Honesty, and boundary violations,
428–430
Horney, K., 44
Hospitalization, eating disorders in
adolescents, 560. *See also* Mental
hospitals
Human leukocyte antigen (HLA), 641
Huntington's disease, sleep
disturbances and, 767, 768–770
5-Hydroxyindoleacetic acid
(5-HIAA), 148–149, 174
Hypercortisolemia, 178–179, 232–233
Hyperserotonemia, 299–300
Hypersomnia, 638–639, 642, 707, 722
Hyperventilation, in panic disorder,
190
Hypofrontality, 159–160
Hypothalamic-pituitary-adrenal axis
(HPA)
biological markers
eating disorders, 232–233
mood disorders, 176–177
panic disorder, 190–191
posttraumatic stress disorder,
196
endogenous sleep and waking
factors and, 693–695
sleep disorders and depression,
669–670
Hypothalamic-pituitary-ovarian
axis, biological markers of
eating disorders, 233–235
Hypothalamic-pituitary-thyroid
axis, biological markers for
mood disorders, 179–180
Hypothyroidism, 179
Hysteria, 77, 78
Hysteroid dysphoria, 271

Idiopathic hypersomnolence, 632
Imipramine, 34
Impulsivity
in affective/impulsive personality
disorders, 263
serotonin mechanisms and, 696

Identity, in psychotherapy for
attention-deficit hyperactivity
disorder, obsessive-compulsive
disorder, and Tourette's
syndrome, 530–531
Idiopathic hypersomnolence, 641,
642
Imipramine, 635, 662
Incest. *See also* Sexual abuse
interventions with abusive family,
605
role reversals in cases of, 601
Infantile anorexia nervosa, 547–551
Infantile neurosis, 494–495
Information processing,
affective/impulsive personality
disorder, 265, 267–269
Informed consent
as ethical issue in psychiatric
research, 333–337
managed care and, 399–401
patient's right of, 327–328
Insomnia
and depression, 639, 653
and mood disturbance, 652
and risk of suicide, 654
safety as central theme in
childhood, 628–629
in schizophrenic patients, 678
Institute of Medicine, 115
Insulin, bulimia nervosa and
metabolic abnormalities, 232
Insulin coma therapy, 31, 32
Insurance companies. *See also*
Managed care
boundary violations in financial
matters, 430
research on effectiveness of
psychotherapy, 64, 69
International Pilot Study of
Schizophrenia, 49
Internships, psychiatric education, 15
Interpersonal therapy, 66, 468
Irritability, noradrenergic system
and, 271–272

Jarvis, Edward, 46, 47
Jet lag, sleep disturbances and,
748–754

Jewish Chronic Disease Hospital
cancer research, 334
Job performance, daytime sleepiness
and, 709. *See also* Shift work
Journals, ethical standards in
research, 325
Juvenile offenders/delinquents
psychological subtypes of, 497–498
research on efficacy of treatments
by nonprofessionals, 481

Kahlbaum, K. L., 28
Kallmann, F. J., 45
Ketamine, 152
Klein, Melanie, 467
Kleine-Levin syndrome, 632
Korean War, 97
Korsakoff, S., 28
Kraepelin, Emil, 28

Lactate sensitivity, 189
Language
processing and affective/
impulsive personality
disorder, 265
use of as boundary violation, 427
Late luteal phase dysphoric
disorder, 73, 84
Lautebur, P. C., 41
Learning disabilities, excessive
sleepiness in children, 709
Learning Disabilities Association, 532
Legal issues. *See also* Forensic
psychiatry
duty to protect third parties and
confidentiality, 356–360
ethical obligations of psychiatrists,
345–346
mandatory child abuse reporting
and confidentiality, 352–356
sexual misconduct and, 443–444
value conflicts in forensic
psychiatry, 375–377
Leighton, Alexander, 48
Licensure boards, and sexual
misconduct, 444
Light, exposure to and
circadian-rhythm disorders,
723–724, 735, 740–741, 773

Lithium
bipolar disorder in children, 582
bipolar disorder and guanine
nucleotide–binding proteins,
180
eye-movement disorder and,
138–139
history of psychiatric research
and, 34
and phosphoinositide turnover,
181
Living wills, 336
Locus coeruleus,
affective/impulsive personality
disorder, 270–271
Lovesickness, sexual misconduct
and, 441–442
LSD, 323
Luteinizing hormone, 145, 234
Lynd, Robert and Helen, 48
Lysergic acid diethylamide (LSD),
323
Lysophosphatidylcholine, 153–154

Malpractice litigation, 443
Malzberg, Benjamin, 48
Managed care
changing role of psychiatrists in
context of, 391–394
and confidentiality, 394–397
conflicts of interest in, 397–399
as cost-control initiative, 114
double agentry and, 401–402
and honesty, 402–403
impact of costs on patient care,
407–410
informed consent in, 399–401
interference in doctor-patient
relationship, 403–405
prospective payment system,
389–391
relationships with other mental
health professionals,
405–407
research on efficacy of child
psychotherapy, 488–489
Mania
episodes of and alcohol abuse, 210
eye-movement activity in, 686

Marriage
shift work and sleep disorders, 744–745, 748
social roles of women and mental illness, 76, 82
therapists and former patients, 445–446
Marshall, A. W., 48
Masochistic surrender, 442–443
Massachusetts, Commission on Lunacy, 46
Medical Superintendents of American Institutions for the Insane, 9
Medicine
ethics in clinical, 325–326
value conflicts in forensic psychiatry, 375–377
Melatonin
circadian rhythm and, 731
output of in depressed patients, 182
Mental Health Act of 1946, 96–97
Mental Health Study Act of 1955, 103
Mental Health Systems Act of 1980, 110
Mental hospitals
alternatives to state, **95**
deinstitutionalization and populations of state, **100**
distribution of patients by type of institution, **108**
for-profit and inappropriate hospitalizations, 408
history of
changes in from 1945 to 1954, 96–98
early years of from 1492 to 1945, 93–96
evolution of psychiatric education, 12
patient statistics for state, **101**
Mental hygiene movement, 12, 29
Meprobamate, 33–34
Metabolism, eating disorders and abnormalities of, 231–232
3-Methoxy-4-hydroxyphenylglycol (MHPG)
biological markers for mood disorders, 172–173

biological markers for schizophrenia, 148
Methylphenidate, 150, 524, 716
Meyer, Adolf, 9–10, 29, 39, 44, 47, 102
Midtown Manhattan Study, 49
Minnesota Multiphasic Personality Inventory, 709
Mismatch negativity, 141–142
Missouri Board of Registration for the Healing Arts v. Levine (1991), 369
Mitchell, Weir, 29, 31, 36
Mobile treatment unit, 113
Modified Assessment of Sleepiness Test, 711
Molecular biology, biology of personality disorders, 279
Monoamine oxidase (MAO), as biological marker
for affective/impulsive personality disorder, 269
for alcoholism, 213–214
for mood disorders, 179
for personality disorders, 260–262
Monoamine oxidase inhibitors (MAOIs)
history of psychiatric research and introduction of, 34
treatment of social phobia, 277–278
Mood disorders
biological markers for
neuroendocrinology, 176–180
neurotransmitters and receptors, 172–176
pineal function and circadian rhythm, 182
research on, 171
second-messenger systems, 180–182
summary of, **183**
excessive daytime sleepiness and, 722–723
Morel, B. A., 28
Mother-infant relationship, and feeding disorders, 545–547
Multi-infarct dementia, sleep disturbances in, 763
Multiple Sleep Latency Test (MSLT), 708, 710–711

N200 waveforms, 141–142
Narcissistic personality disorder, 264
Narcolepsy, 631–632, 641–642, 710, 719
National Alliance for the Mentally Ill (NAMI), 111–112
National Committee for Mental Hygiene, 10
National health care reform, 23–24, 411
National Institutes of Health, research in women's health, 85
National Institute of Mental Health (NIMH)
  discrimination against women, 87
  establishment of, 96–97
National Mental Health Act (1946), 10
Nazis, medical research, 323, 325
Neumann, H., 28
Neurasthenia, 36–37
Neurobiology, of sleep disorders and depression, 669
Neurochemistry
  biological markers
    for affective/impulsive personality disorder, 269
    for alcoholism, 213–215
    for anxiety-related personality disorders, 277–278
    for personality disorders, 260–262
    for schizophrenia, 146–154
    for Tourette's syndrome, 302
  history of psychiatric research, 42–43
Neuroendocrinology, biological markers
  for affective/impulsive personality disorder, 269
  for anxiety-related personality disorders, 277
  for mood disorders, 176–180
  for schizophrenia, 143–146
Neuroimaging, biological markers
  for affective/impulsive personality disorder, 269
  for eating disorders, 245
  for personality disorders, 258–259, 279
  for schizophrenia, 154–161

Neuroimmunology, biological markers for schizophrenia, 142–143
Neuroleptics, gender differences in response to, 79
Neuropeptides
  biological markers for eating disorders, 241–245
  biological markers for schizophrenia, 153
Neuropsychological testing
  affective/impulsive personality disorder, 265
  schizophrenia-related personality disorders, 259
Neurosyphilis, 13
Neurotensin, 153
Neurotransmitters
  biological markers
    for affective/impulsive personality disorder, 270–274, 524
    for attention-deficit hyperactivity disorder, 303, 304
    for eating disorders, 236–241
    for mood disorders, 172–176
    for obsessive-compulsive disorder, 193–194
    for panic disorder, 190
    for personality disorders, **255**
    for posttraumatic stress disorder, 195–196
    for social phobia, 192
    for Tourette's syndrome, 302
  history of psychiatric research, 43
  sleep abnormalities and psychopharmacology, 688–693
  sleep disorders and depression, 670
New York High Risk Project, 574
New York State Psychiatric Institute, 37, 39
Nightmares, 636, 677
Night shifts, 736–748
Night terrors, 634, 635, 642
Night watchers system, 773
Nocturnal penile tumescence (NPT), 659–660

Nontherapeutic research, ethical
issues in, 332–333
Noradrenergic system, biological
markers
for affective/impulsive
personality disorder, 270
for attention-deficit hyperactivity
disorder, 303–304
for obsessive-compulsive disorder,
193–194
for posttraumatic stress disorder,
195
Norepinephrine
biological markers
for eating disorders, 239–241
for mood disorders, 172–173
for schizophrenia, 147–148
insomnia in schizophrenic
patients, 690
Nortriptyline, 658, 661
Nosology
classification of personality
disorders, 280
current classifications for
childhood psychiatric
disorders, 305
history of psychiatric research,
35–38
Nuremberg Trials, 325

Observational studies, research
ethics, 328–331
Obsessive-compulsive disorder
biological markers for, 192–194,
200
clinical characteristics of,
521–523
collaboration with schools in
treatment of, 532
comorbidity with anxiety-related
personality disorders,
275–276
multimodal approaches to
treatment of, 532–536
as neuropsychiatric disorder, 519
psychotherapeutic considerations
in, 524–527
symptoms associated with
Tourette's syndrome, 521

technical and development issues
in psychotherapy for,
527–531
Obsessive Compulsive Foundation,
532
Obstructive sleep apnea syndrome,
630–631, 642, 714, 717–719
Oedipus complex, 494–495
Olds, J., 44
Oligomenorrhea, 234
Operant conditioning paradigm, 468
Opiate system
and eating disorders, 241–243
and posttraumatic stress disorder,
195
Osmond, H., 41
Osteoporosis, 245–246
Outpatient treatment, history of
development, 94
Oxytocin, 244–245

P3 waveforms, 215–216, 221–222
P50 waveforms, 141
P300 waveforms, 139–141, 258
Panic disorder
biological markers for, 188–191,
200
comorbidity with anxiety-related
personality disorder, 276
Paradoxical therapy, 57
Paranoid personality disorder, 256
Paraphilias, 440–441
Parasomnia, 634
Parent movements, for reform of
psychiatric care of chronically
mentally ill, 111–112
Parents. *See also* Family
and psychotherapy of
attention-deficit
hyperactivity disorder,
obsessive-compulsive
disorder, and Tourette's
syndrome, 531
child psychotherapy and, 500
four-phase program of parental
guidance, 501–502
Parkinson's disease, sleep
disturbances in, 764–768,
771–772

Paroxetine, 523
Parran, Thomas, 11
Pathology, history of psychiatric research, 38–46
Patient referrals, and boundary violations, 428
Pauling, Linus, 43
Pavlov, Ivan, 28
Pellagra, 13
Pemoline, 524, 716
Pennsylvania Hospital (Philadelphia), 93
Pergolide, 766, 772
Personality, alcoholism and characteristics of, 217
Personality disorders
  biological markers for
    affective/impulsive personality disorder, 263–275
    anxiety-related personality disorder, 275–278
    schizophrenia-related personality disorder, 255–262
  in children and adolescents, 496–497
  gender and epidemiology of, 280
  psychobiological study of, 281
Phasic-event intrusion hypothesis, 679–680
Phencyclidine/N-methyl-D-aspartate (NMDA), hypothesis of schizophrenia, 152
Phenylketonuria (PKU), 291–292
Phosphatidylinositol, 154
Phosphoinositide system, 181
Phospholipids, 153–154
Physical abuse. See also Child abuse; Sexual abuse
  biological sequelae in borderline personality disorder, 264
  research on children's self-concepts in cases of, 481–482
  sexual abuse compared with, 589–590
Piaget, Jean, 468
Pimozide, 521
Pineal function, biological markers for mood disorders, 182

Pinel, Philippe, 27, 35
Plasma amine oxidase, 260
Play therapy, 500, 512, 579
Pollock, Horatio M., 47
Postpartum women, sleep disturbances in, 621–624, 645
Posttraumatic eating disorder, 552–554
Posttraumatic feeding disorder, 554–556
Posttraumatic stress disorder
  biological markers for, 194–196, **200**
  and biology of personality disorders, 254
  as gender-related disorder, 83
Power seeking, as boundary violation, 427
Preferred provider organizations (PPOs), 390–391
Pregnancy, sleep disturbances in, 621–624, 644–645
Present State Examination, 49
Prevention, history of services for chronically mentally ill, 102–103
Pritchard, J. C., 36
Privacy, definition of, 344
Privilege, legal concept of, 346
Profile of Mood States, 710
Progressive supranuclear palsy, 770
Prolactin
  as biological marker
    for personality disorders, 273
    for mood disorders, 175
    for schizophrenia, 145
  sleep abnormalities in schizophrenic patients, 694
Propranolol, 771
Psychiatrists. See also Education
  contractual obligations and boundary violations, 422
  managed care and changing roles of, 391–394
  roles of in future, 21–24
  sexual discrimination against women, 86–87
Psychodynamics, history of psychiatric research, 44
Psychology, history of psychiatric research, 43–44

Psychoneurosis, concept of in
children and adolescents,
494–496
Psychopathy, affective/impulsive
personality disorder, 264
Psychopharmacology
combined treatment for
attention-deficit
hyperactivity disorder,
obsessive-compulsive
disorder, and Tourette's
syndrome, 533–536
combined treatment of sleep
disorders in depressed
patients, **664, 665**
and deinstitutionalization
movement, 98–99
eating disorders in adolescents,
561, 564–565
future roles of psychiatrist, 22
gender differences in response to,
79–80
of sleep disorders and dementia,
771–773
of sleep disorders and depression,
661–662, 670–671
Psychopharmacology Service
Center, 35
Psychophysiology, biological
markers
for affective/impulsive
personality disorder, 265,
267–269
for schizophrenia, 133, 138–142
Psychosocial function, impact of
sleepiness on, 709
Psychostimulants, biological
markers for schizophrenia,
149–151
Psychosurgery, 32, 323
Psychotherapy. *See also* Treatment
depression and sleep disorders,
662–663, **664, 665**
future of, 67–69
gender differences in response to,
79–80
history of
background information, 56
brief therapy, 58–60
changes in 1950s, 56–58

changes in 1960s and 1970s,
60–62
consolidation and methods of,
62–64
present status of, 64–67
Psychotic disorders, in therapist and
sexual misconduct, 440–443
Psychotropics, history of psychiatric
research and introduction of,
33–35
Public health, role of psychiatrist as
consultant, 23
Publick Hospital (Williamsburg,
Virginia), 93

Quasi-public authorities, 115

Rapport, M. M., 43
Rational emotive therapy, 57–58
Reality-oriented therapy, 577
Recruitment, trends in psychiatric
education, 16–21
Rehabilitation, social and vocational,
111
Reil, J. C., 27
Representational mismatch, 502
Requirements, special for
psychiatric education programs,
14–15
Research
on biological markers
for alcoholism, 208–212
for anxiety disorders,
187–188
in childhood psychiatric
disorders, 305
for mood disorders, 171
for schizophrenia, 161–162
child psychotherapy
methodological flaws in, **474**
on psychodynamics of, 493
reviews of, 475–490
schizophrenia and affective
disorders, 585–586
clinical trial model, 473–474
on confidentiality, 347–352
on effectiveness of psychotherapy,
63–64, 65–67
ethical issues in, 323–337

Seeman, P., 43
Seizures, sleep and, 637–638
Selegiline, 772
Self-defeating personality disorder, 84–85
Self-determination, patient's right to, 326–328
Self-disclosure, as boundary violation, 427
Self-esteem
  child abuse and, 598–599
  gender-related disorders, 81–82
Sensory gating, 141
Serotonin
  aggression and impulsivity, 696
  as biological marker
    for affective/impulsive personality disorder, 272
    for alcoholism, 215
    for autism, 299–300
    for eating disorders, 236–239
    for mood disorders, 174–176
    for obsessive-compulsive disorder, 193
    for schizophrenia, 148–149
  role of in sleep regulation, 688–690
Serotonin reuptake inhibitors, 523
Sertraline, 523
Sertürner, F. A. F., 30
Sexual harassment, 87
Sexism, in psychiatric professions, 86–87
Sexual abuse. *See also* Child abuse
  biological sequelae in borderline personality disorder, 264
  physical abuse compared with, 589–590
Sexuality, sleep disorders and depression, 659–660
Sexual misconduct
  assessment and rehabilitation of accused therapists, 449–451
  ethical guidelines for, 433
  posttermination relationships, 445–446
  prevalence of, 434–437
  prevention of, 451–453
  profile and psychodynamics of therapists in, 438–443

profile of vulnerable patients, 437–438
sanctions against accused therapists, 443–445
treatment of sexually exploited patients, 446–449
Shaw, E., 41–42
Shift work, and sleep disturbance, 736–748, **749**
Simple phobia, biological markers for, 199, **200**
Sinemet, 772
Skin conductance studies, 268
Skinner, B. F., 29, 44, 468
Sleep and sleep disorders
  borderline personality disorder and REM latency, 270
  circadian rhythm system and, 735–736
  in dementia
    Alzheimer's disease, 759–762
    clinical picture of, 757–759
    Creutzfeldt-Jakob disease, 770–771
    Huntington's disease, 768–770
    Parkinson's disease, 764–768
    progressive supranuclear palsy, 770
    treatment of, 771–773
    vascular dementia, 763–768
  depression and
    EEG studies of, 654–656, 661–668
    longitudinal, within-subject studies of, 656–660, 668–672
    population and clinical-sample surveys of, 652–654
  deprivation
    in adolescents, 629–630
    daytime sleepiness and, 712
    in schizophrenia, 679, 682–683
  EEG studies in affective/impulsive personality disorder, 268
  EEG studies in generalized anxiety disorder, 198
  and endocrine activity in depressed patients, 180
  excessive daytime sleepiness (EDS) determinants of, 711–716

differential diagnosis and,
716–724
epidemiology and morbidity
of, 707–708
measurement of, 709–711
genetic influences on, 640–644,
645–646
jet lag and, 748–754
normal development and, 626–627
physiology of, 624–626
in pregnant and postpartum
women, 621–624, 644–645
schizophrenia and
biological mechanisms and
correlates of, 687–695
clinical applications of studies
of, 695–697
differential diagnosis and
abnormalities, 683–687
prolactin responsiveness as
biological marker for, 145
theoretical issues and
directions for future
research, 698–701
shift work and, 736–748
Sleep paralysis, 642, 719
Sleep terrors, 634, 635, 642
Sleep-Wake Activity Inventory, 710
Sleepwalking, 634, 635, 642
Smith, Samuel Mitchel, 9
Smooth pursuit eye movement
(SPEM), 133
Snoring, sleep disorders and, 642, 718
Snyder, S. H., 43
Social bonding, 501
Social phobias
biological markers for, 191–192,
200
comorbidity with anxiety-related
personality disorders,
275–276
Sodium lactate, 189, 197
Sokoloff, L., 41
Somatization disorder, 591
Somatostatin, 153
Southern swing shift schedules, 741
Squires, R. F., 43
Stanford Sleepiness Scale, 710
State markers, definition of, 293
Stimulus-response paradigm, 468

Structural brain imaging, 154–157
Subspecialization, in field of
psychiatry, 15–16
Substituted judgment, 336
Suicide
basal metabolism in personality
disorders, 272–273
insomnia and risk of, 654
serotonin concentrations and risk
of in depressed patients, 174
sexual misconduct and threats or
risk of, 437–438, 446
Sullivan, H. Stack, 44
Sundowning, sleep disturbance in
dementia, 757–759, 773
Suppressive therapy, 577
Suprachiasmatic nucleus (SCN), 730
Surrogates, consent for research,
336–337
Sydenham's chorea, 523
Syphilitic general paresis, 39, **40**

Tarasoff case, 356, 357, 358
Teachers, and treatment of
attention-deficit hyperactivity
disorder, obsessive-compulsive
disorder, and Tourette's
syndrome, 532
Telephone reviews, 395–396
Temperature, circadian rhythm and,
731, 732, 733
Termination, of psychotherapy with
neurotic and conduct disorder
children, 513–515
Therapeutic research, ethical issues
in, 331–332
Therapist-patient sex syndrome,
446, 447
Thioridazine, 579, 771
Thought disorders, 574, 580
Thyroid-stimulating hormone
(TSH), as biological marker
for eating disorders, 231
for mood disorders, 179–180
for schizophrenia, 144
Thyrotropin-releasing hormone
(TRH), as biological marker
for eating disorders, 231
for mood disorders, 179–180

Tourette Syndrome Association, 532
Tourette's syndrome
  biological markers for, 300–303
  clinical characteristics of, 520–521
  collaboration with schools in treatment of, 532
  multimodal approaches to treatment of, 532–536
  as neuropsychiatric disorder, 519
  psychotherapeutic considerations, 524–527
  sleep disturbances in, 640
  technical and development issues in psychotherapy for, 527–531
Trails B Test, 259
Trainee-patient relationship, ethical issues, 337–338
Trainee-supervisor relationship, ethical issues, 338–340
Trait markers, definition of, 293
Transactional analysis, 61–62, 65
Transference, psychotherapy of neurotic children, 506–508
Transinstitutionalization, 107
Transitional experience, 511–512
Treatment. *See also* Child psychotherapy; Psychopharmacology; Psychotherapy
  biology of personality disorders, 280–281
  dementia and sleep disorders, 771–773
  patient's right to refuse, 327
Treponema pallidum, 39
Tricyclic antidepressants, 173, 524
Triiodothyronine, 231
Tuskegee syphilis studies, 325, 330, 334
Twitchell v. McKay (1980), 368

Unipolar depression, sleep abnormalities in, 643–644

Valproic acid, 771
Value systems
  forensic psychiatry and conflicts between medicine and law, 375–377
  and health care reform, 393
Van Gieson, Ira, 39
Van Winkel, E., 41
Vascular dementia, sleep disturbances in, 763–768
Vasopressin, 244–245
Ventriculomegaly, 154–155
Verbal abuse, 427
Veterans Administration, 97
Vietnam War, 61
Visual reaction time, 258
Voluntary choice, 327–328

Walker, Francis A., 47
Watson, J. B., 29, 43–44, 468
Wernicke, G., 28
Willowbrook hepatitis research, 325, 329, 335
Wisconsin Card Sorting Test, 159, 259
Women
  biological and psychosocial factors in eating disorders among, 237
  changing perceptions of gender roles, 85–87
  DSM-IV categories, 84–85
  gender differences in mental disorders, 74–80
  gender-related disorders, 80–84
  shift work and sleep disorders, 745, 748
  sleep disturbance and depression in, 653
  sleep in pregnant and postpartum, 621–624, 644–645
Woolley, D. W., 41–42
World Health Organization, 10
World War I, 12
World War II, 96

Zeitgebers, 735
Zubin, Joseph, 37